Physical Rehabilitation's Role in Disability Management

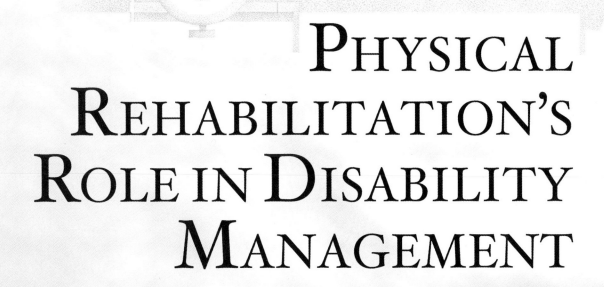

PHYSICAL
REHABILITATION'S
ROLE IN DISABILITY
MANAGEMENT

Unique Perspectives for Success

DAVID W. CLIFTON, Jr., PT

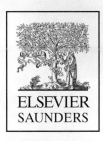

ELSEVIER
SAUNDERS

ELSEVIER
SAUNDERS

11830 Westline Industrial Drive
St. Louis, Missouri 63146

NOTICE

Physical therapy is an ever-changing field. Standard safety precautions must be followed, but as new research and clinical experience broaden our knowledge, changes in treatment and drug therapy may become necessary or appropriate. Readers are advised to check the most current product information provided by the manufacturer of each drug to be administered to verify the recommended dose, the method and duration of administration, and contraindications. It is the responsibility of the licensed prescriber, relying on experience and knowledge of the patient, to determine dosages and the best treatment for each individual patient. Neither the publisher nor the author assumes any liability for any injury and/or damage to persons or property arising from this publication.

International Standard Book Number 0-7216-8474-2

Acquisitions Editor: Marion Waldman
Developmental Editor: Marjory I. Fraser
Publishing Services Manager: Pat Joiner
Project Manager: Sarah E. West
Design Coordinator: Teresa McBryan

Printed in United States of America

Last digit is the print number: 9   8   7   6   5   4   3   2   1

I dedicate this text to my loving family
for their unconditional support and patience
during some very trying times.

For it is my wife, Leslie;
daughters, Brooke and Jena;
and
sons, Taylor and Troy,
who give me purpose for being.

And, in memory of my beloved parents,
David Sr. and Florence,
and
brother Ray
who are in a better place than we.
They did not live to see the text completed,
but their spirits are embodied in my passion and work ethic.

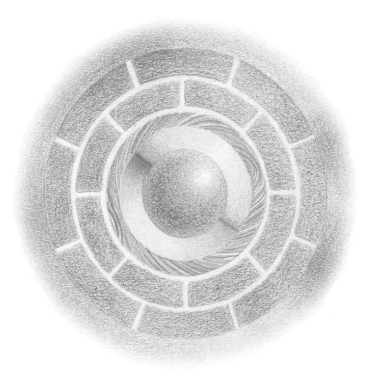

Reviewers

CHRISTINE M. CARPENTER, BA, MA, PhD, DipPT

School of Rehabilitation Services
University of British Columbia
Vancouver, British Columbia

THOMAS MOHR, PT, PhD

Professor and Chairman
Department of Physical Therapy
University of North Dakota
Grand Forks, North Dakota

ARTHUR DELL ORTO, PhD, CRC

Chairman, Department of Rehabilitation Counseling
Boston University
Boston, Massachusetts

SHARI A. RONE-ADAMS, DBA, PT, MS, GCS

Nova Southeastern University
Fort Lauderdale, Florida

JEFFREY ROTHMAN, EdD, PT

Director, Physical Therapy Program
College of Staten Island of the City University of
    New York
Staten Island, New York

DENISE WISE, PT, PhD

Assistant Professor
The College of St. Scholastica
Duluth, Minnesota

vii

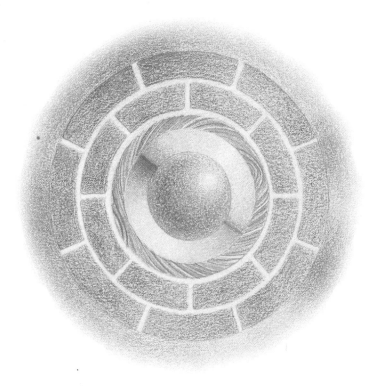

Contributors

Michael R. Burcham, PT, MBA, DHA

Executive Vice President
Paradigm Health;
Adjunct Professor, Vanderbilt University
Brentwood, Tennessee

Ruth Ann Burnett, BSN, CRRN, CCM, CDMS

Disability Consultant
Laurel Springs, New Jersey

David W. Clifton, Jr., PT

Adjunct Professor, Widener University
Institute for Physical Therapy Education,
   Chester, Pennsylvania;
Vice President, Business & Program
   Development
CMA Consultants, Inc.
Reading, Pennsylvania

Elizabeth Genovese, MD, MBA

IMX Medical Management Services
Bala Cynwyd, Pennsylvania

Corrine Propas Parver, JD, PT

Project Director, Health Law Project, LLM Program in
   Law and Government;
Adjunct Professor of Law,
American University Washington College of Law,
Washington, DC
Bachelor and Diploma of Physical Therapy,
   McGill University

Ron Scott, LLM, EdD

Private-Practice Attorney-Mediator;
Adjunct Faculty Member, Physical Therapy Departments,
Husson College, Northern Arizona University,
   Shenandoah University, Rocky Mountain University,
   and the University of Indianapolis

Mark C. Taylor, MS, CDMS, CCM

Director, Claims/Consulting, Disability Reinsurance
ING Re
Minneapolis, Minnesota

Jan Stephen Tecklin, MS, PT

Professor, Department of Physical Therapy
Arcadia University
Glenside, Pennsylvania

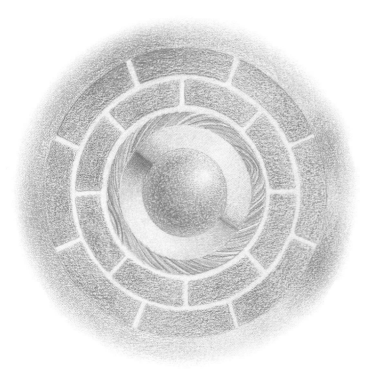

Foreword

Managed care has irrevocably altered the landscape of physical rehabilitation service provision. The dramatic changes in service delivery systems brought about by managed care bring to us both significant challenges as well as unprecedented opportunities to expand our practice roles. To successfully meet our challenges and seize our opportunities, providers of physical rehabilitation services must be capable of functioning within the dynamics of today's health care environment—an environment in which drastic changes have occurred in the funding and delivery of health care. To succeed in this environment, we must continue to evolve our clinical value as we have done in the past. However, now we also must become valued for our economic usefulness. To be valued in this manner, service providers must be able to objectively answer the central question posed by all stakeholders—those who consume our services, those who employ us to provide the services, and by those who pay for our services: *"What is the value, the worth, of what we produce?"*

In the past, quality of care was the watchword. Today, however, the goal of service provision is not merely quality alone but also value. Quality of care is assumed, and value is expected. In the past we were challenged to answer the question, *"Does what we do produce results?"* The question that is asked of us today is quite different. Today, we are asked *"Do the results we produce make a difference—do our outcomes justify the cost of our services?"* That is, are our services of value? In this regard the title and content of this book, *Physical Rehabilitation's Role in Disability Management: Unique Perspectives for Success,* is most applicable because the author presents a wealth of unique and thoroughly referenced ways to respond in the affirmative to this question. The author powerfully challenges prevailing assumptions and conventional wisdom regarding the focus and scope of physical rehabilitation services. The author recognizes

that although many apparently separate and distinct problems may exist, service providers must be focused on the issue that is common to all—namely, service providers must move from an impairment reduction mindset to a disability prevention, disability reduction, and disability management view of their clinical responsibilities. In very practical terms, the author lays out the destination for this paradigm shift and an explicit road map that guides you to that destination. The core of this paradigm shift, and the theme that flows through every chapter of this book, is that a successful outcome is not merely the reduction of impairments. On the contrary, the reduction of impairments without the reduction of disability is an unsuccessful outcome. The author underscores this position in his statements, "Rehabilitation providers are advised to look beyond simply managing impairments as our profession is prone to do. Gains in range of motion, muscle performance, balance along with reductions in pain and swelling should not be the ultimate goals but a means to maximize true function while minimizing disability and maximizing social functioning for those with handicaps." The author makes a strong case for the fact that the attainment of a successful outcome such as this cannot be achieved in isolation of others. The author holds that we must work in a collaborative manner with all stakeholders. In some cases we may function as peer team members, in others as consultants, and in still other situations as educators and/or mentors.

For the provider of physical rehabilitation services, this book will serve as a guide that will enable you to critically evaluate the degree to which you are providing services that are of value to all stakeholders. In this regard, it will provide you with the conceptual framework within which to understand health care's concept of value. It will also provide you with the practical tools required to effectively communicate and objectively define, measure, and demonstrate the value of your services. This book will be extremely valuable for those stakeholders who establish health care payment policy as well as for those who evaluate the appropriateness and effectiveness of our services from a payment perspective. For the medical directors of health care plans, primary care physicians, case managers, risk managers, and claims managers, this book makes a very persuasive argument that it makes economic sense to move the historical focus of payment for impairment reduction to a focus on disability prevention, reduction, and management.

In my experience, David Clifton has always had a clear and practical vision of the direction in which the provision of physical rehabilitation service needed to move in order to remain viable and relevant in the health care system in which we practice. In this book, he has brought that vision into sharp focus.

Mary Foto, OT, FAOTA, CCM

David Clifton's text opens the doors to knowledge and creative thinking that will expand the mind and practice of professionals. It provides an excellent opportunity for clinicians who think outside their own professional walls, who want to understand the complexity of health care and disability management, to change their paradigms. David and the invited authors share vision and new perspectives of insurers, employers, government agencies, case management experts, and specialists in health and disability technology.

The information explored in this text is both extremely interesting and absolutely necessary for the clinician who wishes to make the most of his or her profession, skills, and potential contribution to disability management. David challenges us to learn new concepts; enlarge our capacity; and become consultants, educators, and agents of change.

The text serves professionals who wish to understand how they work best in the context of larger disability and health management issues. The reader will be struck by the diversity of information. The first reading will be of interest, but this text also will become a resource for practice in the entire continuum of disability management.

We can become more proficient, efficient, and effective. But we also can use the text to find a deeper meaning and enjoyment of the complex milieu in which health care today is delivered.

The collaborative care model is of growing importance as we face many challenges in providing good care. By understanding the perspective of others in disability management, disability assessment, health information management, documentation, reimbursement, risk management, ethics, and fraud, we position ourselves to do a better job for the consumers with whom we work, the professionals with whom we interact, and for ourselves in improving our own practices.

Each member of the system has his or her own responsibilities. Each professional wants colleagues in related professions to understand what he or she does, how he or she does it, and how to be best utilized in disability management. In order for us to be understood by others, we must understand them. David Clifton bridges the gap between many professions in his exploration of ideas and new horizons.

This text has three benefactors. The first group is composed of professions such as physical therapy, occupational therapy, medicine, vocational counseling, psychology, and case management. We will find our professions enhanced by myriad points of view. Temporary disability concepts will expand current knowledge, and having all of this information available in one text will allow each professional group to have its own greater reference points.

The second beneficiary is each individual professional. Changes in worker's compensation, long-term care, disability management reimbursement, and legal issues often force a practitioner to change practice patterns. Now, however, one will be able to understand the bases of those actions and participate rather than follow. This text is full of opportunities for new collaborations waiting to be accepted and understood by the individual clinician.

Last, the collaboration of stakeholders in prevention and management of disability will provide benefit to the ultimate stakeholder, the patient in the disability system. If knowledge gives power, each professional's work will become more satisfying, more effective, and able to reduce disability and its effects for those who are served.

Susan J. Isernhagen, PT
President, Susan Isernhagen Consulting

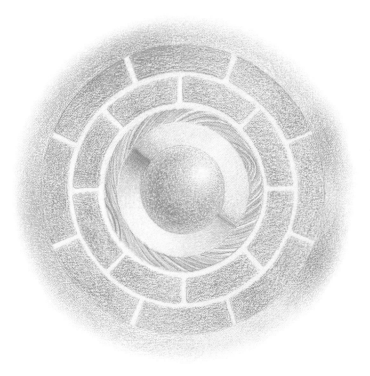

Preface

Physical Rehabilitation's Role in Disability Management: Unique Perspectives for Success was conceived and written as both a textbook and reference, addressing disability management principles, practices, and concepts that transcend "treatment." Disability management involves a constellation of stakeholders, each of whom apply unique experience and skill sets to the prevention, treatment, and management of disability.

If rehabilitation is the unfinished business of medicine, then disability management is the unfinished business of rehabilitation. This text examines the multifactorial nature of disability, including the psychosocioeconomic issues that often determine the success of rehabilitation. The entire disability continuum from preinjury to treatment to post-treatment is explored. Most physical rehabilitation providers reside in the "treatment" portion of this continuum.

In today's era of collaborative care models, it is vital to understand the diverse paradigms coveted by a broad universe of stakeholders. This text is grounded in the premise that physical rehabilitation does not operate in splendid isolation but must become more integrated. Additionally, rehabilitation professionals must learn to effectively transition to change imposed by external elements beyond their direct control. The health care sector's complexity is created by diverse stakeholders who operate from diverse paradigms. This demands inquisitive, agile participants who are willing to understand and actively participate in new paradigms, even when they challenge conventional ways of thinking, alter health care finance and delivery systems, or disrupt business enterprises. Rehabilitation professionals traditionally have been educated and trained under a discipline-specific model. However, this model has limited relevance in today's environment. Today's rehabilitation professional must be equal parts

clinician and business person to effectively compete in an ever-changing market. Providers also must serve as educators, mentors, and consultants to others. This text places an emphasis on being a disability manager and not merely a rehabilitation provider. The text fills a void in the body of knowledge essential to physical therapists, occupational therapists, physicians, nurses, claims managers, employee benefit specialists, case managers, risk managers, and health policy experts.

The text is divided into the following seven sections:

Section I, Understanding Disability, provides an overview of disablement models, costs, and demographics. It emphasizes the importance of distinguishing pathology from impairment, impairment from disability, and disability from handicap status.

Section II, Understanding Disability Management Fundamentals, covers basic disability management principles and practices and applies them to two insurance sectors: worker's compensation and long-term care. Physical rehabilitation services play a significant role in both systems, particularly from a cost perspective. Mark C. Taylor, MS, CDMS, CCM, provides readers with a unique view of disability management from the payer perspective.

Section III, Disability Assessment, describes the art of independent assessment of disability through the use of diversified tools, including independent medical examinations, functional capacity evaluations, and utilization review and management. Elizabeth Genovese, MD, MBA, clearly explains disability determinations and independent medical examination methodologies. David W. Clifton Jr., PT, and Ruth Ann Burnett, BSN, CRRN, CCM, CDMS, jointly cover many elements of functional capacity evaluations from both the payer and provider perspectives. A separate chapter compares and contrasts utilization review and management as well. Section III also includes Jan Stephen

Tecklin's, MS, PT, description of a physical therapy worker's compensation case management program.

Section IV, Health Information Management, was crafted with the following dictum in mind: *"In God we trust, all others bring data."* This section explores the essential topics of information technology, outcomes measures, and quality assurance. Chapter 15, How to Locate Sources of Disability-Related Data, equips readers with tools to independently explore beyond the confines of this text and, in some cases, their own clinical practice.

Section V, Ethical-Legal Regulatory Compliance Issues, features the expertise of two physical therapists who also are practicing attorneys, Corrine Propas Parver, JD, PT, and Ron Scott, LLM, EdD. This section explores issues that have a profound impact on how rehabilitation services are both financed and delivered. Topics include risk management, ethics, reimbursement, and fraud and abuse.

Section VI, Trends and Issues in Health Care Finance and Delivery, includes an exploration of how to transition to change in a complex health care system. New delivery paradigm shifts are described, and complementary and alternative health is examined. Michael R. Burcham, PT, MBA, DHA, a well-known physical therapist and MBA, examines the evolution of managed care, while Clifton

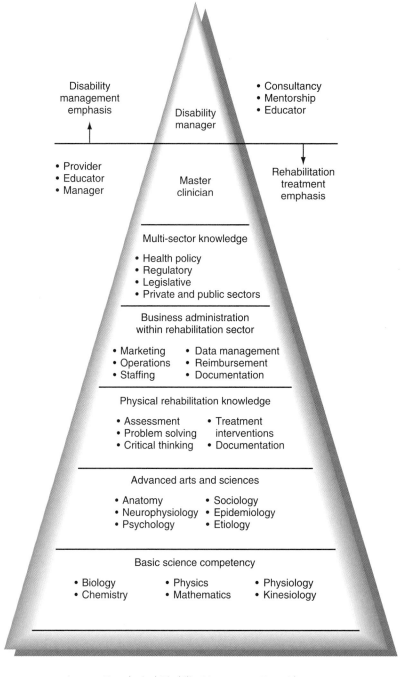

Hypothetical Disability Management Pyramid.

provides a glimpse of the future beyond managed care by offering a compelling case for why chronic injury and illness may be rehabilitation's next horizon.

Section VII, From Clinicians to Consultants, encourages rehabilitation providers to transfer their skills, knowledge, and aptitudes into various consulting capacities. Chapter 26 provides a show-and-tell of persons and organizations that have served as change agents by offering different disability management innovations along the disability continuum. Chapter 27 provides a comprehensive analysis of consulting opportunities and the entire sales/marketing cycle from research to lead prospecting to implementation of consulting services.

SPECIAL FEATURES

The text incorporates a number of unique features that enhance its user friendliness. Most chapters supply *Operational Definitions* and *Suggested Readings* for those who wish to further explore disability management. *Key Points* also provide readers with concise statements that summarize chapter content. Last, the text's *Appendices* provide a plethora of disability-related data for reader reference. Furthermore, the text is lavishly supported by figures, tables, and other visual aids.

Disability Management Pyramid

The disability management pyramid (see figure) is a hypothetical model that portrays various levels of knowledge that must be achieved before one becomes a disability manager. Basic sciences constitute the base of the pyramid. Advanced sciences sit atop basic sciences. Specialized knowledge that is discipline-specific evolves next. A command of business administration skills sets within the rehabilitation sector represents the first foray beyond the clinical realm. Multi-sector knowledge and understanding demonstrate that different paradigms are understood by the individual. One could argue that a master clinician is on par with a disability manager; however, in this model "master clinician" has been placed at the pinnacle of clinical competency but below the first level of business expertise. Of course, there are many individuals who are capable of occupying multiple hierarchal levels. The higher one ascends in the pyramid, the more out-of-the box thinking is required. Also, higher levels generally cannote less treatment and more management and/or consultation. Again, readers are reminded that this is a hypothetical model only.

David W. Clifton, Jr., PT

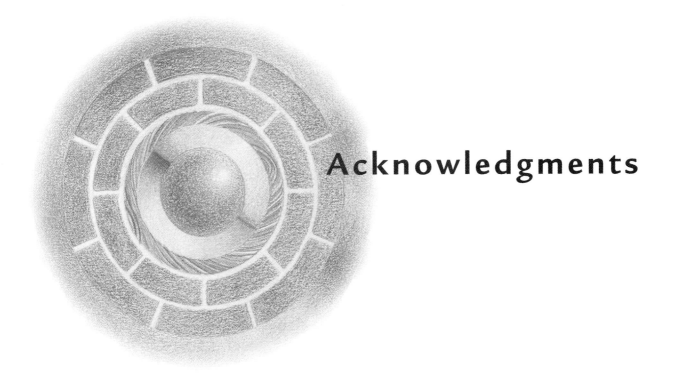

Acknowledgments

There are many others to whom I am indebted for my growth as a clinician, educator, mentor, colleague, writer, student, change agent, and dreamer. These persons hail from diverse backgrounds. This text would not be possible without the belief and support of its earliest champion, Andrew Allen, Elsevier Publishing Director. A special thank you to a diligent taskmaster and mentor, Marjory I. Fraser, Elsevier Senior Developmental Editor. A thank you for the early efforts of Marie Pelcin, Suzanne Hontscharik, and Rachael Zipperlen. Thank you to Marion Waldman, Elsevier Executive Editor, for her "big picture" vision. Out of the bullpen came the consummate closer in Donna Ciccotelli, freelance Developmental Editor. Thank you Donna for your kind spirit and tough love. Your timing of both was exquisite. Thank you also to Sarah West, Elsevier Project Manager, who made this text a reality.

I most heartily thank my contributing authors (Michael R. Burcham, Ruth Ann Burnett, Elizabeth Genovese, Corrine Propas Parver, Ron Scott, Jan Stephen Tecklin, and Mark C. Taylor) for their knowledge; wisdom; and, most important, generosity.

This text at times was like a cork bobbing amidst the waves... the waves of change brought on by mergers, acquisitions, medical emergencies, and other external influences. Like a cork, it never completely sank, but at times it sure felt like it.

I wish to extend a thank you to my classmate, clinical partner, and friend, Steve Buxton, who allowed me the freedom to explore beyond the clinical box. Thank you to Sue Micholovitz, who helped me blaze the utilization/peer review trail that at the time was unknown territory. I also thank my co-instructor Sandy Campbell of Widener University and our physical therapy students for their contributions toward this work, principally through being my sounding board and laboratory.

I also would like to thank Rich Worthington, Edward Palsho, Edward Daley, and John Hart of New Jersey Manufacturers Insurance Group for teaching me about the insurance universe and for allowing us to collaborate for the purpose of ensuring quality care, fair cost, and optimal outcomes. Chapter 11 is their legacy.

A very special thanks to two dear friends and colleagues of the highest order—Mary Foto, OT, FAOTA, CCM, and Susan J. Isernhagen, PT, President, Susan Isernhagen Consulting. The occupational and physical therapy professions, respectively, have been immeasurably enriched through the vision and contributions of these exemplary change agents. Their contribution of the Foreword represents the capstone of this worthy project.

Last, I offer my profound thanks and respect to those who have made physical rehabilitation the great field that it is today. This work stands on the shoulders of giants who dared to lead, risked much, and failed often but who never allowed obstacles to extinguish their flame of passion of service to others. May this text emulate these pioneers by serving others.

David W. Clifton, Jr., PT

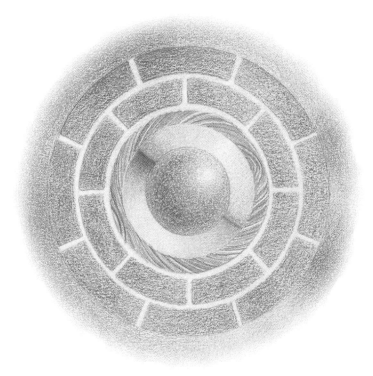

Contents

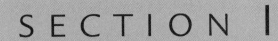

Understanding Disability

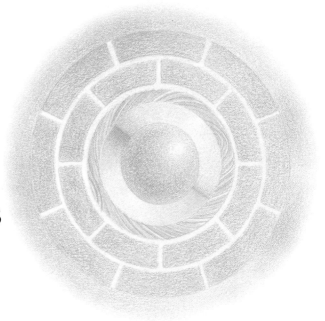

CHAPTER 1

Disablement Models

David W. Clifton, Jr., PT

"Disability description is confounded by divergent use of terminology by governments, professionals, legislators, by people with disabilities themselves and their representative groups."

- Meijers, 1997

KEY POINTS

- Rehabilitation providers must design assessment and management strategies that are geared to the patient at any point along the disablement process from disease to handicap.
- Providers need to ascertain the most authoritative definition of disability for each unique case, whether it is a medical, legal, social, or economic definition.
- Rehabilitation providers must strive to align disability prevention and management goals with those of other health care stakeholders as well as their patients.
- Clinical documentation must address the idiosyncrasies of each case and provide meaningful assessments that can assist others who are involved in disability determinations.
- Rehabilitation providers should strive to make an impact in other non-physical functioning domains (e.g., psychological and social).
- Because of their expertise, skill sets, and focus on function, rehabilitation providers must educate other stakeholders regarding their value and role as disability managers not just treatment providers.

Operational Definitions

Medical Model	The dominant approach to health care in the United States, in which a biomedical cause is the emphasis, with all interventions centering around disease and pathology via passive treatment.
Disability	A relative term describing the actual (objective) or perceived (subjective) dysfunctional status of select individuals or discrete groups.
Impairment	Any loss of psychological, physiological, or anatomical structure or function that may or may not be associated with disability.
Disablement Model	The relationship, or lack thereof, of disease to impairment, impairment to disability, and disability to handicap status.

Different Stakeholders—Different Disability Perspective

Rehabilitation providers vigorously strive to identify, prevent, treat, and manage disability. However, disability remains an enigmatic concept that, depending on the health care stakeholder, is defined in medical, legal, or social terms (Nagi, 1991). The United States begs a universal definition of disability as it struggles with numerous statutes that define this term in various ways. Domzal (1995) has identified at least 50 statutory definitions of disability across federal government acts and programs. This is in addition to 50 separate workers' compensation acts/laws and thousands of disability insurance benefit plans. Table 1-1 provides a sample of disability definitions contained in the clinical literature.

Disability literature contains a bedlam of vocabulary that addresses one common goal shared by diverse interests: discriminating one individual or group from another. Figure 1-1 depicts a diversity of stakeholders who occupy the disability management universe. Disability definitions and interventional strategies can differ greatly among employers, governmental agencies, insurance companies, managed care plans, and health care providers.

Table 1–1 Selective Definitions of Disability

Disability:

Akabas et al, 1992	"Any condition which results in functional limitations that interfere with an individual's ability to perform his or her customary work"
Americans with Disabilities Act (ADA), 1990	"Disability means (A) A physical or mental impairment that substantially limits one or more of the major life activities of such individual; (B) A record of such an impairment; or (C) Being regarded as having such an impairment"
American Medical Association (AMA), 1977	"A patient is "permanently disabled" or "under a permanent disability" when his actual or presumed ability to engage in gainful activity is reduced or absent because of "impairment" which, in turn, may or may not be combined with other factors" (p iii)
American Society of Hand Therapists (ASHT), 1992	"Inability or limitation in performing tasks, activities and roles to levels expected within physical and social contexts"
Brandsma et al, 1995	"A loss or deviation, in both a qualitative and quantitative way, of expected or desired activity performance or behavior of a person, taking into consideration age, gender, physical, and social, and cultural environment"
Finklestein, 1991	"Disadvantage or restriction of activity caused by a social organization, which takes no or little account of people who have physical impairments and thus excludes them from mainstream of social activities"
Greenwood, 1985	"The composite result of individual functional limitations and faults in physical, cultural, social, economic and political environments"
Guralnik, 1994	"Decline in several aspects of functioning" "May be due to different or multiple diseases"
Key, 1995	"An alteration, expressed in non-medical terms, of an individual's capability to meet personal, social, or occupational demands, or to meet statutory or regulatory requirements. The gap between what the individual is required to do and what they are able to do"
Max, Rice, Trupin, 1996	"A child under age 5 with a disability is one who is unable to participate in play activities or is limited in any way" "A child or adolescent aged 5 to 17 with a disability is one who attends or needs to attend special school, is limited in or unable to attend school, or is limited in activities other than school" "An adult with a disability is one who cannot walk or do housework or is limited in the amount or kind of work or housework due to health"
Reith, Ahrens, Cummings, 1995	"Any functional limitation resulting from a physical or mental impairment, however caused, that affects the kind and/or amount of work an individual is capable of performing"
Reusch, Brodsky, 1968	"It is a result of a way of functioning that does not meet the demand of the situation"
Shah, Gerber, 1997	"Disability is an incapacity or perceived inability to perform needed and desirable physical, intellectual, psychosocial, economic, and vocational activities"
Slater et al, 1974	"Disability is an existing limitation in one or more activities which in accordance with the subject's age, sex, and normative social role are generally accepted as essential basic components of daily living"
Social Security Administration (SSA), 1979	"Inability to engage in any substantial gainful activity by reason of a medically determined physical or mental impairment which can be expected to result in death or has lasted or can be expected to last for a continuous period of not less than 12 months"
The Rehabilitation Act of 1973	"A physical or mental impairment that substantially limits one or more major life activities"
World Health Organization, 1980	"Any restriction or lack (resulting from an impairment) of ability to perform an activity in the manner or within the range considered normal for a human being
Wood, 1980	"Represents objectification of an impairment, and as such it represents disturbances at the level of the person"

Handicap:

Guccione, 1993	"The social disadvantage attached to having disease, impairment, functional limitation, or disability" "A reaction to disablement by the society in which an individual lives"
World Health Organization, 1980	"A disadvantage for a given individual, resulting from an impairment or a disability that limits or prevents the fulfillment of a role that is normal (depending on age, sex, social, and cultural factors) for that individual"

From Akabas SH, Gates LB, Galvin DE: Disability Management. New York, American Management Association, 1992, p 282.

Disability may describe the actual or perceived functional or dysfunctional status of select individuals or discrete groups. These persons have distinctive traits when compared with so-called normal or normative populations. Disability definitions discriminate between normal and abnormal populations, healthy and unhealthy groups, functional and dysfunctional groups, and working and non-working groups.

The literature contains a number of dichotomies that describe disability. Koch (2001) provides a contrast between two views of disability. One view portrays disability as a physical fact that affects quality of life (QOL), whereas

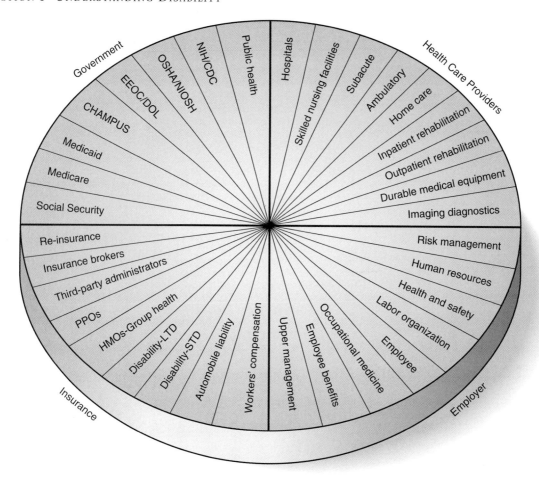

Figure 1–1. Disability management stakeholders' universe. *CDC,* Centers for Disease Control and Prevention; *CHAMPUS,* Civilian Health and Medical Program of the Uniformed Services; *DOL,* U.S. Department of Labor; *EEOC,* Equal Employment Opportunity Commission; *HMOs,* health maintenance organizations; *LTD,* long-term disability; *NIH,* National Institutes of Health; *NIOSH,* National Institute for Occupational Safety and Health; *OSHA,* Occupational Safety and Health Administration; *PPOs,* preferred provider organizations; *STD,* short-term disability.

the other purports that disability is defined by social prejudice. Stated another way, the first view is a patient-centric one, whereas the second is an environmentally driven viewpoint. This could also be construed as actual disability versus perceived disability.

Figure 1–2 illustrates disability defined through two prisms: (1) actual objectively measured disability and (2) subjectively perceived disability. An individual under this model can be labeled disabled through three mechanisms. Quadrant *A* depicts a situation wherein disability has been established through both objective testing and subjective observation. In quadrant *B,* objective clinical testing defines disability, whereas quadrant *C* defines disability subjectively through perception. Non-existence of disability occurs only in quadrant *D* when there is neither objective nor subjective, actual nor perceived disability present. Patients or persons who fall into quadrant *C* present perplexing questions: (1) If a person perceives himself or herself as disabled, either through self-analysis or secondary to labeling by others, is he or she really disabled? (2) Is a perceived disability on par with an actual or measured disability? (3) Are rehabilitation

providers equipped to manage perceived disability in the absence of other disciplines, such as psychology, sociology, or psychiatry? For instance, conditions such as obesity, scar formation, deformity, or psychological problems can rightly or wrongly lead to the conclusion that a person is physically disabled. Subjective perception of disability includes patient self-perception, physician or health care

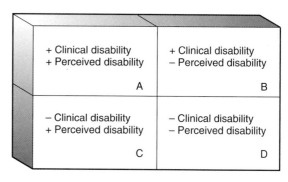

Figure 1–2. Disability rubric.

provider assessment, the absence of functional assessment, health benefit plan definitions, and legal rulings. Any or all of these assessment mechanisms potentially can be devoid of actual disability measures.

Opinions abound concerning what constitutes disability. Cooper (1980) refers to "social disability" and provides a taxonomic hierarchy to describe degrees of disability.

Greenwood (1985) examines disability through a bifurcated approach that contrasts "clinical disability" with "perceived disability." She concludes that handicaps result from a combination of clinical and perceived disability, but asserts that "medicalization of disability" limits its determination to clinical disability. Confusion often results between disability determination by clinical methods and subjective perception of a problem (Jiwa-Boerrigter et al, 1990).

The severity of a disability and the patient's subjective perception of the related problem can be congruent in some cases. In other circumstances, there are significant differences between measured disability and perception. Rehabilitation programs that are designed in consideration of this duality are more likely to address the individual needs of the patient (Jiwa-Boerrigter et al, 1990).

Rehabilitation differs from other medical disciplines because it focuses on the consequences of a disease or injury rather than on the insult itself (Van Bennekom et al, 1995). Table 1–2 depicts the evolution of rehabilitation through five decades (1944 to 1992).

Although rehabilitation has a place of prominence in the management of disability, it remains imperfect. Van Bennekom et al (1995) cite three putative reasons for failure of assessment in rehabilitation medicine:

1. Failure to balance assessment methodology of comprehensiveness and conciseness. Physical rehabilitation assessment should be extensive enough to cover all bases, including the entire disablement model or continuum from disease to handicap. Rehabilitation assessment also must transcend functional domains, including physical, psychological/mental, and social domains.

2. Difficulty with selecting levels for assessment (e.g., impairment versus disability, pathological abnormality versus impairment, disability versus handicap)

3. Failure of standardized assessment methods to consider the patient's perception and to recognize that the patient's perception is likely to have a strong influence on the direction and outcome of rehabilitation

These authors conclude that the patient's perception of his or her condition may be more essential to the design of rehabilitation programs than the disability or handicap itself (Van Bennekom et al, 1995).

There is difficulty associated with applying the disability label to a person or group (Greenwood, 1985). Although disability has gradually become part of the social justice concept in western nations since the seventeenth century and is currently a worldwide concern, it is less clearly definable than other attributes such as race, gender, age, or even poverty (Greenwood, 1985).

The term *disability* has a broad meaning, beyond the strictly physical factors associated with functional impairments in which rehabilitation providers specialize (Miller, 1987; Sandler, 2002). Some people argue against the use of the term *disability*, because it conveys total incapacitation, which is rare (Wolfensberger, 1979).

Disability is a relative term compared with *impairments*, which can be objectively measured and described through various physical or psychological tools (Reusch & Brodsky, 1968). Examination of environmental factors that influence the patient's thoughts and behaviors can be more productive than searching for occult pathological conditions (Waddell, 1991).

Clogston (1990) describes four models of disability:

1. Medical model
2. Social pathology model
3. Minority or civil rights model
4. Cultural pluralism model

These four models can be collapsed into two basic paradigms: the traditional and progressive models. The medical and social models constitute the traditional

 Table 1–2   Definitions of Rehabilitation

Source	Definition
National Council on Rehabilitation (1944)	Restoration of the handicapped to the fullest physical, mental, social, vocational, and economic usefulness of which they are capable
Rusk (1965)	Ultimate restoration of a disabled person to his or her maximal capacity—physical, emotional, and vocational
Krusen, Kottke, Eilwood, (1971)	The process of decreasing dependence of the handicapped or disabled person by developing, to the greatest extent possible, the abilities needed for adequate functioning in the individual situation
Stryker (1977)	A creative process that begins with immediate preventive care in the first stage of an accident or illness, continues throughout the restorative phase of care, and involves adaptation of the whole being to a new life.
Emener, Patrick, Hollingsworth (1984)	A process of helping handicapped individuals move from positions of dependency in their community toward positions of independency in a community of their choice
DeLisa, Martin, Currie (1988)	The development of a person to the fullest physical, psychological, social, vocational, avocational, and educational potential consistent with his or her physiological or anatomical impairment and environmental limitations
Dittmar (1989)	The process by which an individual's movement toward health is facilitated
Hickey (1992)	A dynamic process through which a person achieves optimal physical, emotional, psychological, social, and vocational potential and maintains dignity and self-respect in a life that is as independent and self-fulfilling as possible

From Larsen P: Rehabilitation. In Lubkin IM (ed): Chronic Illness: Impact and Intervention, 3rd ed. Boston, Jones and Barlett, 1995, p 254.

approach to disability definition, because they both focus on the patient or individual. The progressive paradigm includes the minority or civil rights and cultural pluralism models, because both focus on the impact of disability on society. Several watershed pieces of legislation have addressed the importance of a sociopolitical role in disability management in addition to a patient-focused approach. The Rehabilitation Act of 1973, the Education of All Handicapped Children Act of 1975, and the Americans with Disabilities Act of 1990 are examples of legislation that attempts to introduce a shared societal responsibility to address the issue of disability. These and other legislative initiatives strive to enhance the QOL of all persons with disabilities or handicaps (Americans with Disabilities Act [ADA], Public Law No. 101-336, 1990; Education for All Handicapped Children Act, Public Law No. 94-142, 1975; Rehabilitation Act of 1973, Public Law No. 93-112, 1973). Quinn (1995) raises a profound question concerning the role of government in disability: "Does the labeling [disabled or handicapped], which is necessary for qualification as a minority, result in perpetuation of problems rather than their solution?" (p 73).

A non-pejorative paradigm of disability management takes a global view of a person's life rather than a narrow focus on the disability or handicap, which is often the case in rehabilitation (Hahn, 1991).

QOL dimensions identified by patients and their families tend to focus on social issues; however, providers tend to focus on the problem itself, especially the physical elements of impairment, disability, or handicap (Pain et al, 1998). Rehabilitation providers would be better served to focus clinical interventions and select outcome measures based on how their patients view QOL issues rather than focusing on the provider's priorities.

Medical Model of Disability

The traditional medical model of dealing with disability is seriously flawed in several ways. Traditionally, a medical model of disability has dominated conceptions of disability in medical and social sciences through attempts to cure or treat a condition (Imrie, 1997). This construct reduces disability to an individual person's or patient's level without consideration of societal or environmental implications.

Hetherington and Earlam (1994) differentiate disability from handicap. Under their scheme, disability is a measure of the individual's response to illness or injury. Handicap is a concept determined by society's reaction to the person's disability. This view appears to be consistent with Clogston's model (1990). The medical model exists in physical rehabilitation if the therapist focuses on maximizing a patient's function and fails to consider the environment in which the patient must function. Ambulation improvement to 20 feet with the use of a walker does little to obviate a patient's disability if the patient's kitchen or bathroom is 40 feet away or if the patient must navigate stairs. In this example, the patient remains disabled; however, if the person is placed into an environment in which the greatest distance between rooms is 15 feet without stairs as an obstacle, he or she is no longer disabled. Even though this patient is no longer

disabled relative to this new environment, the patient's physical functioning has not improved beyond 20 feet of ambulation. Differences in disability definitions in these examples are not principally caused by the medical condition or the patient; rather they are attributed to environmental elements, stairs, and spatial elements.

Corcoran and Klett (1997) describe the medical model as a dependence model that rests on the assumption that disabled persons are passive recipients of treatment per se. Patients in a passive role are denied access to information and have little contribution to the clinical decision-making process. The sick role or illness model may be an inappropriate paradigm for persons with disabilities (Quinn, 1995). The sick role implies patient passivity, which is the antithesis of physical rehabilitation's focus on function and the inherent premium placed on active participation. The sick role is reinforced by a medical model that traditionally deals with patients who are in the acute stage of injury or illness, when rest and inactivity are commonly prescribed by physicians. This treatment model has limited value in the management of persons with chronic disabilities. Some people contend that a disabled person is not sick and will not get well, because disability is not a temporary condition as is an illness (Quinn, 1995). Quinn (1995) asserts that the medical model is based on the individual but that disability requires a focus on society that deprives the person of an opportunity for success.

Health professionals often recast disability into issues that they can identify and manage (Larson, 1998). This limits the scope of disability to a narrow set of problems instead of viewing the patient from a whole-person perspective.

To the contrary, progressive models empower the individual to be more active, independent, and participatory in the decision-making process. An individual's legal and social rights reinforce the foundation of his or her active involvement in provider choice or refusal of care, goal setting, program design, treatment/management modification, and identification of meaningful outcome measures.

Despite their traditionally narrow focus, physicians often serve as the gatekeepers for many social welfare programs. Physicians are typically the practitioners selected by legislators, policy makers, payers, and employers to make disability decisions. This phenomenon is problematic, because physicians routinely do not possess the skill sets necessary for disability determinations, especially those of a non-organic basis (Loeser & Sullivan, 1997). Physicians generally emphasize pathology, whereas physical rehabilitation professionals address impairments and disability issues. Despite command of medical-related issues, physicians generally do not understand the hazards of disability determination. This shortcoming is acknowledged by the American Medical Association (AMA) in *Guides to the Evaluation of Permanent Impairment.*

"Evaluation (Rating) of Permanent Disability—In the last analysis, this is an administrative and not solely a medical responsibility and function. Evaluation of permanent disability is an appraisal of the patient's present and future ability to engage in gainful activity as it is affected by such diverse factors as age, sex, education,

economic and social environment, in addition to the definite medical factor—permanent impairment. The first group of factors has proved extremely difficult to measure."

- AMA, 1977, p iii

Social Model of Disability

The number and complexity of disability drivers result in a vast number of patients who are deemed disabled even when symptoms do not reflect any discernible abnormality or pathophysiology (Loeser & Sullivan, 1997).

Loeser and Sullivan describe two drivers of disability as pseudodiagnosis or a diagnosis without pathology or true organic cause and pseudoscience.

A plethora of variables directly or indirectly influences disability determinations. These variables transcend medical, legal, social, and health care benefit domains. Figure 1–3 provides a partial listing of factors that influence disability determinations.

Several authors address the social context of disability, specifically social barriers to disability (Finklestein, 1991; Guccione, 1993; Meijers, 1997; Slater & Vukmanovic, 1974). Persons with disabilities under this model face obstacles of a social or environmental nature. Rehabilitation providers often possess a patient-centric approach when they attempt to adapt the individual to the environment.

The social barriers model represents the opposite approach—alteration or elimination of environmental obstacles, policies, and institutions. A new paradigm of disability management dictates a dual focus on both the individual and their environment, addressing both for compatibility.

Greenwood (1985) describes a central semantic problem concerning the terms *disability* and *handicap*. She contends that disability and handicap are intricately woven together, albeit mistakenly so (Greenwood, 1985). These terms may be used interchangeably by both lay persons and health care professionals. Disability is more of an individualistic term, whereas handicap has an environmental connotation. *Disability* can imply that care is directed at accommodating the person to the environment.

Meijers (1997) defines impairment as "a biomedical concept that represents dysfunctions and significant structural abnormalities in an individual's medical status." Meijers also shifts the focus from the individual to the environment when describing the concept of disability as "a discrepancy between individual factors and socio-environmental demands."

Handicap implies that the environment will be adapted to meet the needs of the individual. Both approaches (individual and environment) have value, and rehabilitation providers must design interventions that achieve the

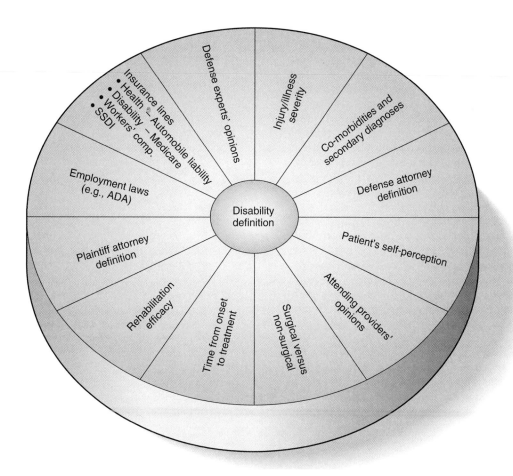

Figure 1–3. Factors that influence disability determinations. *ADA,* Americans with Disabilities Act; *SSDI,* Social Security Disability Insurance.

desired goals of multiple stakeholders. In all likelihood, rehabilitation providers merge both approaches as they attempt to ameliorate disability and its effects on each individual patient. This has been demonstrated in selected sectors wherein the human-environment interface is considered an integral component of disability management. Inpatient rehabilitation of patients with catastrophic cases such as spinal cord injury, traumatic brain injury, and stroke management often involve both approaches. Patients in these treatment settings routinely receive assistive technologies in addition to environmental adaptations. The use of functional capacity evaluations (FCEs), functional job analyses (FJAs), reasonable accommodations, and ergonomics is commonplace in workers' compensation cases.

Greenwood (1985) emphasizes the need to differentiate disability from handicap when establishing goals for rehabilitation programs:

> *"Rehabilitation for handicapping conditions then implies not necessarily the restoration of maximum functional activity or independence, but the restoration of maximum social function, including work and family roles."*

- Greenwood, 1985, p 1241

Legal Model of Disability

The confluence of medical and legal disability determinations creates conflict. It is this conflict that severely challenges disability management, especially under workers' compensation systems, Social Security Disability Insurance (SSDI), and short-term and long-term disability insurance policies, as well as in cases involving the ADA. Health benefit levels in these systems is directly tied to legal definitions of disability. These legal definitions are promulgated through legislation, statutory law, and case law. Medical definitions can drive legal definitions of disability, and inversely, legal definitions can drive medical definitions. The legal definition of disability can, in turn, evolve into the social definition that distinguishes entire populations as disabled or handicapped (Asseo, 1999; Olson, 1999; Savage, 1999).

When these definitions are too vague (as they often are), abuse of special opportunities and services may result (Anonymous, 1999). When disability definitions are too rigid, people who may benefit may be excluded.

Disability semantics can have a profound effect on a patient's life and can mean the difference between a successful clinical outcome and an unsuccessful one, gainful employment and unemployment, and poverty and enrichment.

The legal and insurance sectors depend on the provider as the expert for disability determinations. Rehabilitation providers are uniquely positioned to take a more active role in not supplanting the physician's opinion, but in augmenting it with functionally based data that rehabilitation providers alone are equipped to collect and interpret. Functional capacity evaluations, functional job analyses, implementation of reasonable accommodations under ADA, and return-to-work program design all fall within the unique expertise of rehabilitation professionals.

OVERVIEW OF DISABLEMENT MODELS

The terms *disease, pathology, impairment, disability,* and *handicap,* although potentially connected, are distinct concepts (Greenwood, 1985). Physical rehabilitation providers focus a great deal of their attention, resources, and effort toward discerning the relationship between disease, health, and function (Guccione, 1993).

Guccione (1993) contends that the primary goal of a physical therapy evaluation is to determine the relationship between a patient's impairment and his or her functional limitations. This is significantly different from a medical evaluation that determines the relationship between a disease or pathological abnormality and impairment (Loeser & Sullivan, 1997). Physical rehabilitation practitioners tend to dwell on impairments while attempting to associate them with or disassociate them from function or dysfunction. In doing so, providers typically refer to a disablement model such as the World Health Organization's *International Classification of Impairments, Disabilities, and Handicaps* (ICIDH), Nagi's model, or some variation of the two (Nagi, 1991; World Health Organization [WHO], 1993).

World Health Organization's ICIDH Disablement Model

The International Classification of Impairment, Disability & Handicap (ICIDH) was adopted by WHO in 1976 and amended in 1993.(WHO, 1993). Operational definitions of WHO's disablement model are listed in Table 1-3. The ICIDH was first published in English as a supplement to the *International Classification of Disease* or ICD, Ninth Revision. The original scheme is currently undergoing revision secondary to many constructive criticisms of its design and implementation (Brandsma et al, 1995). A sampling of these criticisms can be found subsequently.

Despite its imperfections, the WHO nomenclature is one of the most widely embraced disablement models within the physical rehabilitation community (Brandsma et al, 1995). As such, review of its basic components is worthwhile. The original schematic viewed health as a

 Table 1-3 World Health Organization Definitions

The World Health Organization, through its *International Classification of Impairments, Disabilities, and Handicaps,* has promulgated the following definitions:

Disease:	"any pathological process associated with a characteristic identifiable set of symptoms"
Disorder:	"any morbid process or functional abnormality"
Impairment:	"any loss or abnormality of psychological, physiological, or anatomical structure or function"
Disability:	"any restriction or lack (resulting from impairment) of ability to perform an activity in the manner or within the range considered normal for a human being"
Handicap:	"is a disadvantage for a given individual, resulting from an impairment or disability, that limits or prevents fulfillment of a role that is normal (depending on age, sex, and social and cultural factors) for that individual"

From Duckworth D: Measuring disability: The role of the ICIDH. Disabil Rehabil 7:338–343, 1995.

linear or sequential phenomenon, with disease leading to impairments, impairments leading to disabilities, and disabilities leading to handicaps. However, one of the most commonly articulated criticisms centers around the notion that disability is not a linear process and that not all diseases necessarily lead to impairments, not all impairments lead to disabilities, and not all disabilities lead to handicaps. In fact, in its *Guides to Evaluation of Permanent Impairment,* the AMA acknowledges that health is not always a linear process: "It is unrealistic to presume that all of these impairments especially those of a minor nature, will necessarily at some time result in disability" (AMA, 1977). As previously mentioned, there is almost universal recognition that non-medical issues (e.g., psychosocial issues) contribute to the disability equation. Impairment as a medical factor does not operate in isolation from other variables. The AMA considers the evaluation or rating of permanent disability to be an administrative, and not solely a medical, responsibility. Disability, unlike impairment, cannot be measured with a reasonable degree of precision and standardization. The ICIDH cautions that "the situation [disability assessment] is in fact more complex" (WHO, 1993, p 30).

The WHO definitions have spawned a number of derivative definitions of disability that focus on a host of variables, including age, time, orientation (duration of illness), irritability stage (acute-subacute-chronic), legal statutes, insurance policy language, psychological function, physical function, and social function.

Wood (1980), a principal contributor to the ICIDH classification scheme, affirms disablement language confusion. He describes disablement as "a collective descriptor referring to any experience identified variously by the terms impairment, disability and handicap" (Wood, 1980).

ICIDH Criticisms

Although the ICIDH enjoys worldwide acceptance, it is not without its critics. Table 1-4 lists a sampling of criticisms cited in the literature.

Several experts have outlined problems encountered in the use of ICIDH, especially problems related to differentiating between disability and handicap (Chamie, 1990; Chapireau & Colvez, 1998; Nagi, 1991).

Chamie (1990) describes three broad categories associated with ICIDH caveats:

1. Isolating and differentiating the impairment, disability, and handicap concepts through descriptors of behavior
2. Training persons who come from disparate backgrounds and experience in the use of the concepts, particularly coding classifications, in a standardized manner
3. Applying the classification scheme across various theories and models of disablement

Isolating and differentiating impairment, disability, and handicap can be problematic when two different classifications have functional overlapping. For example, Chamie (1990) points out that dressing disabilities can be classified under disability codes 35 and 36 or under physical independence handicaps using handicap code 2. This example represents a disparity regarding how specific behavior is viewed and how this could mistakenly lead to a misclassification, especially when disciplines use different classification schemes.

Chapireau and Colvez (1998) note that the ICIDH describes handicap as a social phenomenon with classification directed at circumstances and not at the individual's attributes. However, the ICIDH does not describe circumstances but instead describes individuals' attributes.

Table 1-4 Criticisms of the ICIDH Scheme by Authors

Author	Criticism
Brandsma et al, 1995	(1) change "impairments of structure" to "impairments of function" because some functions are difficult to differentiate (e.g., loss of appetite, resulting from physiological versus psychological reason)
Chapireau, Colvez, 1998	(1) overlap between disability and handicap (2) recommends the use of "social disability" in place of "handicap"
Chamie, 1980	(1) classify disabilities into two broad categories, "functional limitations" and "activity restrictions" (2) there are no well-established recommendations for classifying physical independence, mobility, social integration, and communication roles
Duckworth, 1995	(1) cites that "the obvious, direct way of using the ICIDH classification within rehabilitation medicine is as a checklist for recording patient's impairments, disabilities, and handicaps at the start of the rehabilitation process" (p 339); however, this is very time-consuming (2) including a "dependency" measure raises the question of the relationship between disability severity and degree of dependency
Nagi, 1991	(1) identifies overlap between disability and handicap attributes (2) "the ICIDH fails to meet norms of coherence necessary for any conceptual scheme" (p 326)
Wood, 1980	(1) difficulty of translating ICIDH into other languages (e.g., limited vocabulary, especially adjectives) (2) use of the same terms in the context of impairment, disability, and handicap should be avoided (3) "the same word may have both a loose colloquial meaning and be used in a highly specific technical sense" (e.g., degenerative) (p 87)
Thuriax, 1995	(1) suggest improving the presentation of the way in which external or environmental factors affect the ICIDH (2) impairment classifications need to consider non-health professionals (3) need to grade severity of conditions

Note: This listing is not intended to be exhaustive, nor is it intended to portray only a negative view of ICIDH. The author affirms the valuable contribution of the ICIDH schematic.
From Thuriax Mc: The ICIDH: Evolution, status and prospects. Disabil Rehabil 17(3-4): 112-118, 1995.

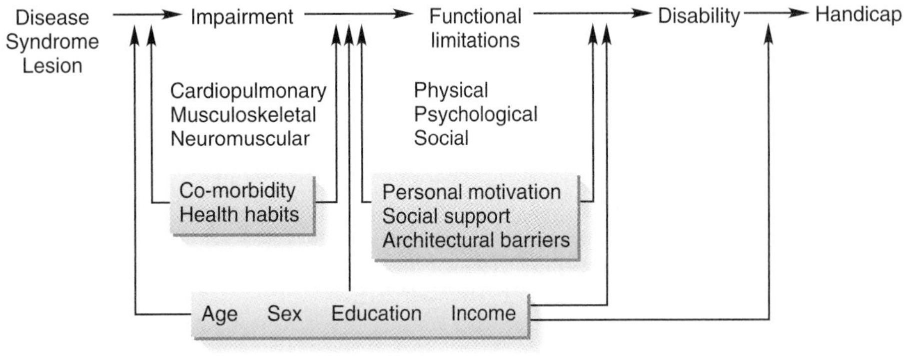

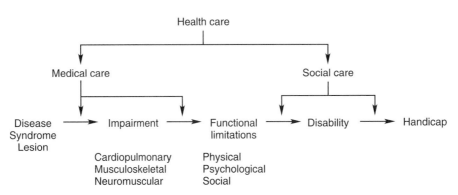

Disease → Impairment → Functional → Disability → Handicap
Syndrome   limitations
Lesion

Cardiopulmonary   Physical
Musculoskeletal   Psychological
Neuromuscular   Social

Co-morbidity   Personal motivation
Health habits   Social support
                       Architectural barriers

Age   Sex   Education   Income

Figure 1–4. Personal factors that affect the trajectory of disability. (From Guccione AA [ed]: Geriatric Physical Therapy. St Louis, Mosby, 1993.)

These authors prefer the term *social disability* to *handicap* as a means of clarifying disability and handicap.

Nagi's Disablement Model

Nagi's model (1991) involves four separate yet related concepts: disease, impairment, functional limitation, and disability. Nagi is a sociologist by training, and his theory of disease stems from the principle of homeostasis, which is threatened by infection, trauma, degenerative processes, or other causes. Impairments represent the second level of his disablement model (Nagi, 1991). Impairments can result from pathological conditions but are not necessarily the consequence of them. Functional limitations represent the next stage of Nagi's model. Functional limitations may flow from impairments or be altogether unrelated. Again, there is no absolute linear relationship between stages. Functional limitations are delineated as physical function, psychological function, and social function. Physical function is the principal target of rehabilitation professionals, although providers must be mindful of other domains.

Guccione's Adaptation of the Nagi Model

Figures 1–4, 1–5, and 1–6 portray Guccione's expansion of Nagi's basic disablement model. Function (or a lack thereof) is commonly used as an important criterion for determining disability (Guccione, 1993). In Figure 1–4, functional limitations transcend three domains of function: physical, psychological, and social. Physical function is the intended focus of most physical rehabilitation assessments and interventions. Although physical rehabilitation professionals focus primarily on physical functioning, Guccione (1993) appropriately points out that rehabilitation impacts on all three domains. Nagi (1991) does not include the concept of handicap in his disablement model, because he considers it to be a social disadvantage based on societal reaction versus the result of any of the earlier stages of his model: disease, impairment, and disability. Stated another way, Nagi prefers the patient-centric approach rather than the environmentally driven paradigm. This is most interesting given that he is a sociologist and not a medical practitioner per se.

> *Disability depends on both the capacities of the individual and the expectations that are imposed on the individual by those in the immediate social environment, most often the patient's family and caregivers.*
>
> - Guccione, 1993

Attention to impairments is assumed to address physical functioning, either directly or indirectly, although there is a paucity of empirical data to unequivocally demonstrate it.

Health care

Medical care   Social care

Disease → Impairment → Functional → Disability → Handicap
Syndrome   limitations
Lesion

Cardiopulmonary   Physical
Musculoskeletal   Psychological
Neuromuscular   Social

Figure 1–5. The health care continuum from disease to handicap. (From Guccione AA [ed]: Geriatric Physical Therapy. St Louis, Mosby, 1993.)

Figure 1–6. Expansion of the Nagi disablement model. (From Guccione AA: Physical therapy diagnosis and the relationship between impairments and function. Phys Ther 71:499-504, 1991.)

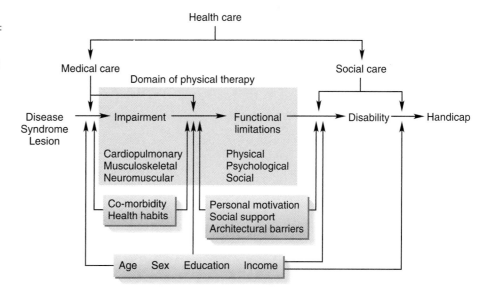

Disability represents the end stage of Nagi's model. It is generally understood that disability occurs over time if impairments are not appropriately addressed or are neglected altogether.

Figure 1-7 illustrates the relative frequency or occurrence of disability and handicap within the Nagi Disablement Model. Persons with handicaps are the fewest in number relative to the general population. Persons with disability are the next largest group but are fewer in number than those with functional limitations. More individuals have a pathological abnormality than a functional limitation, disability, or handicap. Persons with impairments represent a larger group than those with diagnosed pathological conditions. This recognizes the high prevalence of impairments in the absence of known pathological findings (e.g., mental, emotional).

Economic Disablement Model

There is no true economic disablement model, but rehabilitation providers must appreciate that disablement is often tied to an individual's ability to participate in gainful employment (Alston, 1997; Kennedy & Minkler, 1998).

Disability is defined with an economic bias in certain benefit structures such as workers' compensation, SSDI,

Figure 1–7. Relative prevalence of disability, functional limitations, pathology, and impairment. (Data from Nagi SZ: Some conceptual issues in disability and rehabilitation. In Sussman MB [ed]: Sociology and Rehabilitation. Washington, DC, American Sociological Association, 1965.)

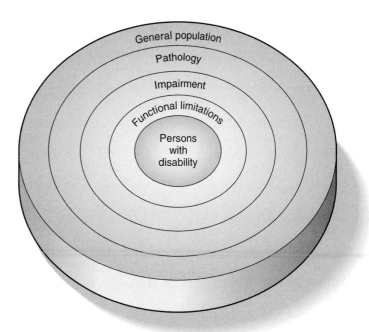

and short-term and long-term disability policies. Successful disability management warrants that providers ascertain operational definitions for impairment, disability, and handicap, because these concepts often vary from policy to policy, state to state (workers' compensation or automobile liability cases), benefit structure to benefit structure, or case to case.

Advice for Rehabilitation Providers

The ADA of 1990 describes disability as a natural part of the human experience and in no way diminishes the right of individuals to do the following:

- Live independently
- Enjoy self-determination
- Make choices
- Contribute to society
- Pursue meaningful careers
- Enjoy full inclusion and integration in the economic, political, social, cultural, and educational mainstream of U.S. society

These goals have relevance for rehabilitation providers who wish to engage in disability management of the whole person by looking beyond their clinical treatment and the patient's diagnosis/condition.

Rehabilitation providers cannot assume that their own disability definition has utility when dealing with various insurance companies, government entities, the legal community, patients, or other health professionals; nor can a health care organization assume that all clinicians embrace the same concept of disability.

Rehabilitation providers are advised to look beyond simply managing impairments, as our profession is prone to doing. Gains in range of motion, muscle performance, and balance, along with reductions in pain and swelling, should not be ultimate goals of rehabilitation but rather a means to maximize true function while minimizing disability and maximizing social functioning for those with handicaps. Providers should learn to appreciate the views of other health care stakeholders and factor these views into assessment, treatment, and management interventions. Last, physical rehabilitation providers must make every attempt to influence, either directly or indirectly, dysfunction that falls outside of physical function and that is housed in the psychological and social functioning domains.

References

Alston RJ: Disability and health care reform: Principles, practices and politics. J Rehabil 63(3):15-19, 1997.

American Medical Association: Guides to the Evaluation of Permanent Impairment, Chicago, 1977, American Medical Association.

Americans with Disabilities Act of 1990. Public Law 101-336, U.S.C. 104, Statute 329; July 26, 1990.

Anonymous: The spectrum of disability. Lancet 354(9180):693, 1999 (editorial).

Asseo L: High court query: Who is disabled? Philadelphia Inquirer, p A28, April 29, 1999.

Brandsma JW, Lakerveld-Heyl K, Van Ravensberg CD et al: Reflection of the definition of impairment and disability as defined by the World Health Organization. Disabil Rehabil 17(3-4):119-127, 1995.

Chamie M: The status and use of the *International Classification of Impairments, Disabilities, and Handicaps* (ICIDH). World Health Stat Q 43(4):273-280, 1990.

Chapireau F, Colvez A: Social disadvantage in the *International Classification of Impairments, Disabilities and Handicaps.* Soc Sci Med 47(1):59-66, 1998.

Clogston JS: A content analysis of disability coverage in 16 newspapers. Louisville, KY, Avocado Press, 1990.

Cooper JE: The description and classification of social disability by means of a taxonomic hierarchy. Acta Psychiatr 27:140-146, 1980.

Corcoran TR, Klett TE: Managed disability—Past, present and future. Benefits Q 13(4):8-13, 1997.

Domzal C: Federal Statutory Definition of Disability. Washington, DC, National Institute on Disability and Rehabilitation (NIDRR), United States Department of Education, 1995.

Education for All Handicapped Children Act of 1975. Public Law 94-142 (Section 6); November 29, 1975.

Finklestein V: Disability: An administrative challenge? In Oliver M (ed): Social Work, Disabled People, and Disabling Environments. London, Kingsley, 1991, pp 19-39.

Greenwood JG: Disability dilemmas and rehabilitation tensions: A twentieth century inheritance. Soc Sci Med 20(12):1241-1252, 1985.

Guccione AA: Health status: A conceptual framework and terminology for assessment in geriatric physical therapy. In Guccione AA (ed): Geriatric Physical Therapy. St Louis, Mosby, 1993, pp 101-111.

Hahn H: Alternative views of empowerment: Social services and civil rights. J Rehabil 57(4):17-19, 1991.

Hetherington H, Earlam RJ: Rehabilitation after injury and the need for coordination. Injury J 25(8):527-531, 1994.

Imrie R: Rethinking the relationships between disability, rehabilitation and society. Disabil Rehabil 19(7):263-271, 1997.

Jiwa-Boerrigter H, van Engelen HG, Lankhorst GJ: Application of the ICIDH in rehabilitation medicine. Int Disabil Stud 12(1):17-19, 1990.

Kennedy J, Minkler M: Disability theory and public policy: Implications for critical gerontology. Int J Health Law 28(4):757-776, 1998.

Koch T: Disability and difference: Balancing social and physical constructions. J Med Ethics 27(6):370-376, 2001.

Larson E: Reframing the meaning of disability to families: The embrace of paradox. Soc Sci Med 7:865-875, 1998.

Loeser JD, Sullivan M: Doctors, diagnosis and disability: A disastrous diversion. Clin Orthop 336:61-66, 1997.

Meijers JM: Work-related disability assessment: A study on credibility and applicability. Amsterdam, July 1997, Maastricht University, Faculty of Health Sciences, www.gladnet.org/index. cfm?fuseaction=research.SearchResultsDisplay&FileToReturn =444.htm, accessed August 12, 2000.

Miller TR: Evaluating Orthopedic Disability: A Commonsense Approach, 2nd ed. Radell, NJ, Medical Economics Books, 1987.

Nagi SZ: Disability concepts revisited. In Pope AM, Tarlov AR (eds): Disability in America: Toward a national agenda. Washington, DC, National Academy Press, 1991, pp 309-327.

Olson W: Under the ADA, we may all be disabled. Wall Street Journal, p A27, May 17, 1999.

Pain K, Dunn M, Anderson G: Quality of life: What does it mean in rehabilitation? J Rehabil 64(2):5-11, 1998.

Quinn P: Social work and disability management policy: Yesterday, today and tomorrow. Soc Work Health Care 20(3):67-82, 1995.

Rehabilitation Act of 1973. Section 202(i)(1); 29 U.S.C. 761a(I)(i); 1973.

Reusch J, Brodsky CM: The social concept of disability. Arch Gen Psychiatry 19:394-403, 1968.

Sandler A: Disability defined. Psychology Today 35(4):34, 2002.

Savage DG: Disability question to be weighed by high court in employment case. Philadelphia Inquirer, April 20, 1999.

Slater SB, Vukmanovic C, Macukanovic P et al: The definition and measurement of disability. Soc Sci Med 8(5):305-308, 1974.

Van Bennekom CAM, Jelles F, Lankhorst GJ: Rehabilitation activities profiles: The ICIDH framework for a problem-oriented assessment method in rehabilitation medicine. Disabil Rehabil J 17(3-4):169-175, 1995.

Waddell G: Occupational low back pain, illness behavior and disability. Spine J 16:683-685, 1991.

Wolfensberger W: The case against the use of the term "disability." Rehabil Lit 40(10):309, 1979.

Wood PHN: The language of disablement: A glossary relating to disease and its consequences. Int Rehabil Med 2:86-92, 1980.

World Health Organization: International Classification of Impairments, Disabilities, and Handicaps: A Manual Relating to the Consequences of Disease, vol 41, Geneva, WHO, 1993 (originally published in 1980).

SUGGESTED READINGS

Domzal C: Federal Statutory Definitions of Disability. Prepared for the National Institute on Disability and Rehabilitation Research, Office of Special Education and Rehabilitative Services, from Conwal Inc., 510 N. Washington Street, Suite 200, Falls Church, VA 22046, 1995.

Guccione AA: Physical therapy diagnosis and the relationship between impairment and function. Phys Ther 71:499-504, 1991.

National Council on Disability (NCD): NCD Bulletins, www.ncd.gov/newsroom/bulletins/04bulletins.html, accessed August 8, 2002.

Shah JP, Gerber LH: Evaluation of musculoskeletal disability: Current concepts and practice. Am J Phys Med Rehabil 76(4): 344-347, 1997.

## CHAPTER 2

Disability Costs and Demographics

David W. Clifton, Jr., PT

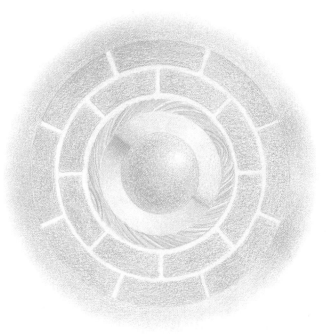

"Americans with disabilities spend more than four times as much on medical care, services and equipment, on average, as their non-disabled counterparts."

- Max et al, 1996

KEY POINTS

- Rehabilitation providers can collect, analyze, and apply disability-related data for both clinical and business purposes.
- Disability data are invaluable in identifying emerging trends and targeting underserved populations with new services.
- Physical rehabilitation is a leading cost driver and can directly or indirectly impact other costs including direct medical costs, indemnity or wage replacement, and administrative and legal costs.
- Rehabilitation providers can demonstrate their cost-effectiveness and efficiency by comparing/contrasting financial data with other databases composed of similar demographic groups.

Operational Definitions

Costs	Any and all costs associated with a diagnosed condition or disability. These include direct and indirect medical costs and non-medical costs such as administrative, indemnity, and legal costs.
Disability	The actual (objective) or perceived (subjective) dysfunctional status of select individuals or discrete groups.
Demographics	The study of human population and statistics including population size and characteristics (e.g., age, gender, diagnoses, condition).
Payer or Payor	Party or entity responsible for payment of medical bills. May include employers, insurance companies, managed care organizations, government sources, or patients themselves.

Why Should Rehabilitation Providers Examine Disability Data?

The purpose of this chapter is to familiarize readers with some of the costs associated with disability. These costs are enormous and portend a bright future for rehabilitation professionals and disability managers who offer cost-effective, efficacious, and efficient services.

Disability-related data can be studied from a variety of perspectives depending on the purpose of the data analysis, collection, and application. Rehabilitation providers can use data in a number of applications that enhance both the clinical and business aspects of their practices. Disability data can be used for strategic planning and marketing (business) or for facility and provider profiling purposes (clinical).

Disability-related costs and demographics can be examined across age, gender, medical conditions, occupations, provider types, treatment settings, and insurance lines. Providers are cautioned to carefully review sources of data and to find corroborative evidence before using data for business or clinical decision making. Poor sources and/or corrupt data can lead to poor clinical and business decisions. Accurate and timely data can be invaluable to rehabilitation providers for the following reasons:

1. To identify emerging population trends
2. To provide baseline cost data against which the rehabilitation provider's clinical data can be compared.
3. To identify and target demographic groups for current and new services
4. To assist in strategic planning, particularly regarding resource allocation

Rehabilitation providers who directly engage in strategic planning with specific emphasis on program development can benefit from identifying potential markets or patient populations. Market size and potential target populations can be predicted through data collection and analysis. The following examples provide insight into the types of data that are available to providers.

For example, a rehabilitation provider specializing in orthopedics might examine data samples from the National Ambulatory Medical Care Survey conducted by the National Center for Health Statistics in order to identify patient trends and unfulfilled needs (NCHS, 1998a).

Example 1: Office Visits to Orthopedic Surgeons: 1995-1996

- 76.5 million office visits over two year period or 38.3 million visits per year
- Prevalence rate: 14.5 visits per 100 persons
- 6 of 10 visits were injury related
- Visit rate increased with age
- 6 of 10 visits resulted from musculoskeletal system symptoms
- Most common complaint: knee symptoms
- Between 1975 and 1996, the visit rate to orthopedists did not significantly change for persons younger than 45 years but increased for persons between 45 and 64 years, between 65 and 74 years, and older than 74 years.

These data support a growing need for rehabilitation services of persons with knee conditions and treatment of age-related conditions (persons older than 45 years).

Example 2 suggests several unmet needs. One, alternatives to emergency room facilities are needed, especially for black populations (NCHS, 1998a). These data also may suggest a triage role for physical rehabilitation providers to alleviate the visit burden from other settings, especially those for elder populations (persons older than 75 years). Rehabilitation professionals are equipped to screen for various conditions that may be more amenable to their services than to traditional medical care. This does not equate to expanded scope of practice, rather to an additional portal into the medical system. For instance, referrals to the appropriate specialist are incumbent on physical therapists who practice under direct access.

Example 2: Summary from the National Ambulatory Medical Care Survey 1998

- In 1997, 787 million visits were made to physicians
- Women are more likely to visit a doctor than are men, especially younger men
- 50% of visits were covered by private insurance, 30% by health maintenance organizations
- 15% of visits were referred by another physician
- Approximately 50% of visits were made to primary care physicians
- 25% of visits were made to family practice physicians, 15% to internists, 12% to pediatricians, and 9% to obstetricians/gynecologists
- 75% of visits were made to physician group practices
- 10% of visits were to hospital-employed physicians
- There were 36 visits per 100 persons
- Patients older than 75 years had the highest rate of doctor visits

- Emergency room visits for black persons were 80% higher than for white persons
- There were 77 million visits to hospital outpatient services or 18.9 per 100 persons

Fiscal Therapy

Disability management through a myriad of interventions attempts to control costs, enhance quality, and optimize functional outcomes. Outcomes are multidimensional and include both clinical and economic measures. Health care today is big business, which requires providers to be both effective clinicians and sound business persons. To remain competitive in a dynamic market, providers must be cognizant of the financial consequences of their health care services and clinical decision making (Gleckman, 2002; Jackson 2002; Lauer 2002). Ideally, they must achieve a delicate balance between humanitarian concern and economic accountability. Prudent providers strive to select and implement cost-effective, value-driven services. This cannot be accomplished in the absence of data.

Clinicians with a desire to demonstrate value (cost/benefit ratio) can do so only by comparing their utilization and cost data with industry standards or benchmarks. These benchmarks are available through a wide spectrum of sources in both the private and public sectors. Readers are encouraged to refer to Chapter 15.

General Disability Demographic and Cost Data

More than $1 trillion was spent on health care in the United States during 1997 (Levit et al, 1998). This is significant because it represents the first time in history that more than $1 trillion was spent on health care. Private sources of funding (non-governmental) were responsible for 53.6%, or $585.3 billion, of this spending. Public funding (governmental) was responsible for 46.4%, or approximately $507.1 billion. Consumer out-of-pocket spending, which included co-payments and deductibles, amounted to $187.6 billion.

The number of persons with disabilities differs by source and by how one defines disability. Disability is a health care challenge, especially for physical rehabilitation providers who directly treat and manage key demographic groups.

Disability Prevalence

The Economic and Social Research Institute, using data from the 1994 National Health Survey, estimates that 20.7% of all non-institutionalized Americans have at least one disability (Economic and Social Research Institute, 1999). This amounts to 53.9 million persons. Specific, chronic disability challenges 37.1 million, or 14.3% of all Americans. Major life-limiting disability is experienced by 6.6% of the population, or 17 million individuals (Figure 2–1). McNeal (1993) estimates the total U.S. population with disabilities to be approximately 50 million.

The World Health Organization (WHO) has long recognized the prevalence of persons with disabilities

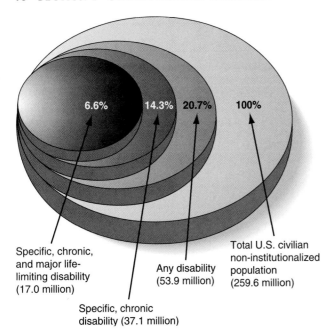

Specific, chronic,
and major life-
limiting disability
(17.0 million)

Any disability
(53.9 million)

Total U.S. civilian
non-institutionalized
population
(259.6 million)

Specific, chronic
disability (37.1 million)

Figure 2–1. Alternative definitions of disability and their impact on population estimates. (Based on data from the 1994 National Health Survey Disability Supplement. Economic and Social Research Institute, Phase 1, Washington, DC, April 1999.)

(WHO, 1980). An estimated 450 to 500 million persons worldwide are disabled according to WHO's definition. This represents an astonishing global prevalence rate of 1 in every 10 persons.

Who Pays and How Much?

The nation's health care dollar is divided among numerous sources of funding. Private insurance or an employer-based system remains the largest single source of funding at approximately 32% of the total (Health Care Financing Administration [HCFA], 1998). Medicare is next by underwriting roughly 20% of total costs. Medicaid, the federal-state joint health care financing program, subsidizes 15% of all health care costs. Private pay or out-of-pocket costs account for roughly 17% of the total. Other public sources cover close to 12% of expenditures and other private sources cover nearly 5% of all costs (Figure 2–2).

Payment sources shift along with patient populations. For instance, although employers shoulder the largest burden across all age groups for health care, the Federal government through its Medicare and Medicaid programs is the largest purchaser of long-term care (Congressional Budget Office, 1999).

A Minority of Cases Drives Costs

It is well established that a minority of conditions or cases consumes a disproportionate share of costs. One sixth of the population with disabilities consumes more than half of total health care costs (Figure 2–3) (Max et al, 1996). In workers' compensation, 20% of reported claims consume 60% of total system costs (National Council on Compensation Insurance [NCCI], 1994). Hashemi et al (1998)

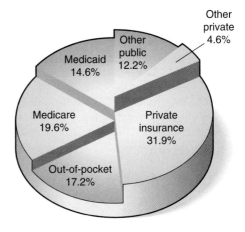

Figure 2–2. Health care cost allocation. (Health Care Financing Administration: National Health Expenditures 1977, Washington, DC, HCFA. Available at www.hcfa.gov, accessed April 14, 1999.)

found a correlation between length of disability (LOD) and workers' compensation costs. Reese (1998) reported that 68% of claims with an LOD of more than 1 year accounted for 89.9% of total costs and 75% of total disability days. The lesson here is that chronic conditions consume immense sums of money. This fact alone supports the need for more physical rehabilitation expertise.

Low back pain with less than 1 month duration accounted for 85.5% of all claims. However, this group accounted for only 10.9% of all costs. To the contrary, the 4.6% of claims with LOD of more than 1 year consumed more than 64.9% of costs. This reinforces the idea that chronic cases are more expensive; however, they are not routinely subject to managed care interventions. Managed

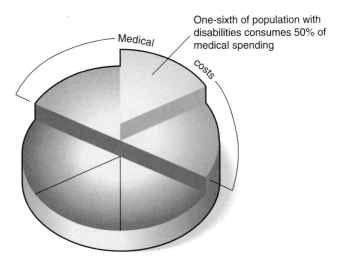

Total medical costs for population with disability

Figure 2–3. One sixth of the population with disabilities consumes half of total medical costs. (Based on data from Max W, Rice DP, Trupin L: Medical expenditures for people with disabilities. Disability Statistics Abstract, No. 12. Washington, DC, US Department of Education, National Institute on Disability and Rehabilitation Research, 1996.)

care has done a reasonably good job with acute conditions but has achieved modest success in dealing with chronic conditions.

Disability Trends: Who Becomes Disabled?

The proportion of the U.S. population with disabilities has dramatically risen during the past 25 years. Two distinct trends have contributed to this increase: an aging population and more reporting of children and young adults with disabilities (Kaye et al, 1996). The National Health Interview Survey (NHIS) is a household survey of the non-institutionalized U.S. population taken annually since 1970 (Trupin & Rice, 1993). Data from this survey are valuable in forecasting health care service needs and

in identifying expanding populations of persons with disabilities. Disability under the NHIS is defined as limitation in activity resulting from chronic health conditions and impairments. According to the NHIS, 15% of the non-institutionalized U.S. population has disabilities. This amounts to approximately 37.7 million persons.

There is an increasing trend of activity limitation (11.7% of the population in 1970 versus 15% in 1990). Men have consistently reported lower disability rates than women during the past 25 years, but the difference is attributed primarily to the greater average longevity of women to men. Figure 2–4 illustrates age-adjusted disability prevalence over the past 25 years. Adults 65 years or older experience disability at approximately twice the rate of younger working-age adults (45 to 64 years) and

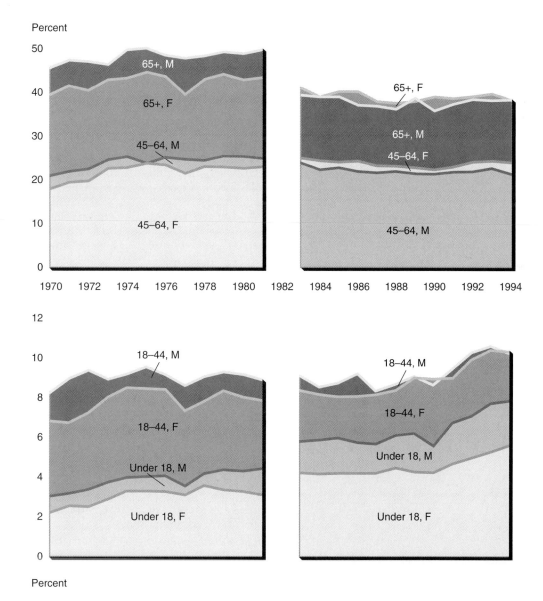

Figure 2–4. Proportion of U.S. population with activity limitation by age and gender (1970-1994). National Health Interview Survey. National Center for Health Statistics. (Tabulations compiled by the Disability Statistics Rehabilitation Research and Training Center, University of California, San Francisco, 1997.)

four times the prevalence of young adults (18 to 44 years). However, significant increases in disability prevalence occurred during the 1990s among persons younger than 45 years of age. These increases are principally attributed to the identification of learning disabilities and to the prevalence of asthma and mental conditions. During this same time span, the prevalence of orthopedic, neurological, and mental disorders, especially cumulative trauma disorders (CTDs), rose for young adults. Last, the Americans with Disabilities Act (ADA) impacted prevalence through an expanded definition of *disability* (ADA, 1990). Figure 2–4 illustrates the proportion of the U.S. population with activity limitations. These data are depicted by age and gender.

Americans spend more than $1.4 trillion, or 14% of the gross domestic product, on health care (Gleckman, 2002). These costs are expected to spiral to $3 trillion within the next decade, creating exceptional opportunities for those engaged in new services and treatments, biotechnology, and prevention (Gleckman, 2002; Mandel, 2002). Rehabilitation professionals are uniquely positioned to participate in this growth, especially in treatment, management, prevention, and consultation directed at chronic illnesses and injuries. Consulting opportunities are explored in Chapter 27.

However, not all of the anticipated spending will present opportunity. For some providers, a bloated health care budget may represent a threat, specifically via claims denials. Rising health care costs are often associated with intensified scrutiny of provider credentials, treatment selection, costs, and clinical outcomes. Gleckman (2002) notes that perhaps one third of all expenditures, approximately $600 billion, may be for "unnecessary, out-of-date, or even dangerous treatments."

Is There a Correlation between Health Care Cost and Patient Satisfaction?

Figure 2–5 represents a theoretical model that portrays relationships between health care costs and patient satisfaction. In this model, Group 1 patients incur relatively high costs but have relatively high patient-satisfaction rates. Inversely, Group 4 patients incur low cost with resultant low patient satisfaction. Group 2 patients,

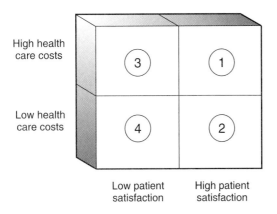

Figure 2–5. Relationship between health care costs and patient satisfaction.

despite having lower health care costs, report high satisfaction levels. Group 3 patients, despite high cost, report low satisfaction. It is possible that persons with chronic conditions often fall into this last category. The point of this exercise is to illustrate that greater health care expenditures may or may not equate with the perception of better care or clinical outcomes. There may be a general tendency for Americans to equate higher cost with higher quality. This inclination may or may not manifest itself in the purchase of health care services. Rehabilitation providers are encouraged to track patient satisfaction relative to treatment expenditure in order to gain a better understanding of the relationship between cost and perceived quality.

According to Mandel (2002), there have been relatively few attempts to both demonstrate and measure the health benefits of health care spending, especially increased spending. Rehabilitation providers must be aware of the fiscal impact of their clinical decision making while being prepared to demonstrate value to various stakeholders, including patients and their families, insurers, employers, and society. This can be accomplished only through careful data collection, analysis, and implementation.

Rehabilitation Cost and Utilization

Physical rehabilitation's greatest prominence is found in the following two insurance sectors as a result of the relative stability of these funding sources: long-term–care (LTC) and workers' compensation. Rehabilitation services under the LTC sector are substantially funded by Medicare and Medicaid, whereas workers' compensation systems are funded by employers. Workers' compensation systems are set up with the basic tenets of first dollar coverage and hypothetically unlimited care. First dollar coverage means the absence of co-payments or deductibles by the patient. Other insurance lines are less friendly and impose obstacles to physical rehabilitation's fullest participation, namely group or general health plans with their gatekeeper model (Beard 1998, Hurley et al, 1991; Bodenheimer et al, 1999). Primary care physicians (PCPs), or gatekeepers, serve to restrict access to specialty services as one means of cost containment. Physical rehabilitation services under managed care are routinely considered a specialty or discretionary service. Restricting or delaying beneficiaries' choice can potentially drive costs higher, especially when a chronic condition arises as a result of neglect. Some would contend that gatekeepers prevent and/or delay referral for rehabilitation. However, this appears to be changing as the managed care backlash continues. The "graying of America" also should open more gates in terms of increased number of and expedited referrals for rehabilitation.

Tracking physical rehabilitation costs and utilization rates is problematic for several reasons. Rehabilitation costs are routinely embedded in other categories of costs, such as "physician services," "ancillary," or the vague "other" category. Rehabilitation costs also are consolidated under treatment settings such as outpatient costs; hospital costs; inpatient, home care, or skilled nursing facilities; or other suppliers (Mehn, 1997).

Absence of Provider Identifiers in Billing

There is also a relative absence of provider identifiers or codes, especially within the private insurance sector, including workers' compensation, and automobile liability). For instance, all providers who use the Current Procedural Terminology (CPT) 97000 series may be aggregated under one identifier code by an insurance company. This makes it difficult to ascertain which discipline is responsible for which costs. Although the American Medical Association owns the copyright to the CPTs, no one discipline commands exclusive use of these codes; it is common for codes to be shared among disciplines. For instance, the 97000 series is commonly used for billing purposes by chiropractors, physicians (MD, DO), kinesiotherapists, athletic trainers, and massage therapists, as well as physical therapists. In turn, insurance companies may assign an identical provider code to anyone using a specific code, such as an electrical stimulation code (CPT 97014.4). Discipline-specific identifiers would allow for more accurate cost accounting. This also would serve to discern physical therapist services from physical therapy services. The former requires a licensed physical therapist, whereas the latter is a generic term inappropriately used by a variety of disciplines to describe interventions typically, but not exclusively, falling under the 97000 series codes. Databases that lump "physical therapy" services with care provided by a "physical therapist" may be at best misleading and at worst corrupted.

Referral for Profit Potential

Mitchell and Scott (1992) exposed the comparatively higher cost of physical therapy services rendered through physician-owned centers when compared to non-physician joint ventures. The authors reviewed data from 118 outpatient physical therapy centers and 63 outpatient comprehensive rehabilitation facilities in Florida (Mitchell & Scott, 1992). They studied the following variables: visits per patient, average revenue per patient, percent operating income, percent markup, profits per patient, licensed therapist to patient time per visit, and licensed and unlicensed medical worker time per visit. Their findings indicate that visits per patient were significantly higher in physician joint ventures when compared with non-physician joint ventures. Utilization rates were 39% to 45% higher, whereas gross and net revenue per patient was 30% to 40% greater in physician-owned centers (Mitchell & Scott, 1992). Referring physicians' investments in health care–related businesses to which they refer remain a focus of much attention and national legislative efforts (Crane, 1992; HCFA, 2002; Iglehart, 1990; U.S. Department of Health and Human Services, 1989; Stark II 2002). The American Physical Therapy Association's (APTA's) *Guide to Physical Therapists Practice*, Parts I and II provide some general cost estimates based on general conditions (Figure 2–6) (APTA, 1999). Estimated Physical Therapy Costs by Diagnosis enables a provider to compare or contrast his or her clinical costs on an episodic basis. The APTA Guide uses a per visit estimate of $100 as a baseline for calculation. The Guide also provides a range of number of visits or length of stay by diagnosis. These are guides only, but they provide useful reference points.

DISABILITY DATA BY PAYER SOURCE

Medicare

Long-term–care in the United States consumed more than $76 billion in 1993 but rose dramatically to $351 billion by 1996 (Moerschel & Saltzman, 1995; Waid, 1998). These are staggering figures when considering that Medicare pays only 6% to 8% of all nursing home costs (Government Accounting Office, 1995). Medicare Part A pays for only 100 days per illness episode and imposes co-payments after the twenty-first day. Financing of LTC in the future will be a daunting task because the Congressional Budget Office (CBO) expects national expenditures for long-term–care services for the older adult population to escalate each year through 2040 (CBO, 1999).

Table 2–1 provides CBO projections of long-term–care through 2040 broken down by payer source. These include Medicare, Medicaid, private long-term–care insurance, private insurance, self-pay or out-of-pocket, and others. These costs are segregated in the table by treatment setting (e.g., institutional care, skilled nursing facilities [SNFs], home care). Medicare and Medicaid finances three quarters of all public spending (Waid, 1998).

A disproportionate concentration of Medicare's beneficiaries, costs, and utilization rates are in just six states. These include California, Florida, Illinois, New York, Pennsylvania, and Texas. Two Northeastern states, New York and Pennsylvania, have the highest average total short-term hospital days at 6.7 and 6.6 days, respectively (Table 2–2).

It is estimated that one in seven persons are disabled by the age of 65 (Beger, 1998). Beger defines disability as chronic pain, fatigue, or an emotional disorder. Seventy-eight million baby boomers, or almost one in four Americans, meet these criteria for disability. These data may be conservative, because a comprehensive estimate of the number of persons with disabilities requires consideration of institutionalized as well as non-institutionalized individuals (Figure 2–7, p. 22).

Rehabilitation services are popular in SNFs. According to the Government Accounting Office (GAO), 60% of nursing home residents receive some form of therapy (GAO, 1995). SNFs provide therapies either through their own staff or by outsourcing to contract vendors. In 1995, 75% of SNFs relied on specialized rehabilitation agencies, also termed *outpatient therapy agencies* (OPT). However, this number has dropped precipitously as many SNF owners moved rehabilitation in-house. All SNFs bill Medicare by either the facility or the contract service company (OPT).

Figure 2–8 (p. 23) depicts the expanding role played by rehabilitation services in SNFs. Rehabilitation in 1990 consumed 18% of SNF services compared with 30.1% in 1996 (HCFA, 1998). The exponential rise in utilization rates of three major ancillary services—physical, occupational, and speech therapies—between 1989 and 1993 contributed to aggressive cost-containment interventions, which continues today (Figure 2–9, p. 23) (GAO, 1995).

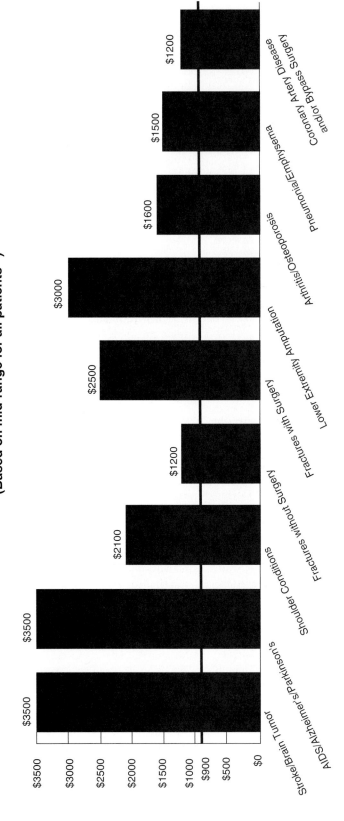

Figure 2–6. Estimated physical therapy costs by diagnosis. (Data based on information from PT Bulletin, 1999.)

Table 2-1 Projections of National Long-Term-Care Expenditures for the Elderly (in billions of dollars)

Payer	2000	2010	2020	2030*	2040*
Services Provided in an Institutional Setting					
Medicare	12.3	16.0	19.5		
Medicaid	36.2	52.0	57.7		
Private long-term care insurance	†	11.2	25.9		
Out-of-pocket	34.3	29.3	35.6		
Other payer	†	†	†		
Total	85.8	108.5	138.7	191.7	217.9
Services Provided in the Home					
Medicare	17.1	23.8	31.0		
Medicaid	7.1	14.9	17.7		
Private long-term care insurance	†	5.5	10.2		
Out-of-pocket	8.5	6.3	7.3		
Other payer	†	†	†		
Total	37.2	52.2	68.6	103.3	128.2
Total Long-Term Care Services					
Medicare	29.4	39.8	50.6		
Medicaid	43.3	66.9	75.4		
Private long-term care insurance	5.0	16.7	36.2		
Out-of-pocket	42.8	35.5	42.9		
Other payer	†	†	†		
Total	123.1	160.7	207.3	295.0	346.1

Data from Congressional Budget Office. Available at www.cbo.gov.

*Estimates of each payer's expenditures cannot be determined.

†Less than $5 billion.

Occupational therapy costs rose most dramatically at 870%, from $8 million in 1989 to $856 million in 1993. Despite these gargantuan increases, Medicare remains an insignificant payer of SNF services, accounting for only 6% to 8% of the total expenditure, or $6 billion, annually (GAO, 1995).

However, perceived and real abuses within the Medicare program contributed to the implementation of the agency's largest and most aggressive antifraud initiative, "Operation Restore Trust" (U.S. Department of Health and Human Services, 1995). This initiative coupled with the 1997 Balanced Budget Act has substantially curtailed Medicare expenditures across a number of treatment settings including home care and SNFs (Balanced Budget Act, 1997).

Rehabilitation's impact on Medicare SNF charges leaped dramatically between 1990 and 1996 (Figure 2-10, p. 24).

In 1990, rehabilitation (18.5%) was second only to "accommodations" (58.5%) as a percentage of total cost drivers. By 1996, rehabilitation's share of the SNF pie expanded to 30.1%, significantly closing the gap with accommodations (44.7%).

Figure 2-11 (p. 25) contrasts the use of physical therapy services in home care between 1988 and 1996 (HCFA, 1998). Note that although the physical therapy utilization (visits) and charges decreased by percentage between 1988 and 1996, both aggregate visits and charges increased.

Medicare Part B

Buchanan et al (1996) describe Medicare Part B rehabilitation costs across six treatment settings: hospital outpatient, rehabilitation hospitals, SNFs, independent rehabilitation agencies, comprehensive outpatient rehabilitation facilities, and home health agencies. Rehabilitation costs between 1987 and 1990 spiraled upward by 86% across these settings. Hospital outpatient costs were consistently found to be the lowest, whereas independent rehabilitation agencies were found to be the highest-cost alternative. The authors claim that increases cannot be explained by Medicare eligibility changes, population shifts, aging, or economic inflation (Buchanan et al, 1996). The highest growth differentials were found among new provider types and proprietary organizations. These data strongly suggest a profit margin incentive versus medical necessity for services.

Workers' Compensation

The prevalence and cost impact of rehabilitation in workers' compensation systems is significant. Workers' compensation is a patchwork of 50 different state laws, and as such, operates more like a legal than a medical system. Workers' compensation is a casualty insurance system, which is employer-funded, but is overseen by state agencies. The reader is advised to refer to Chapter 5 for a more detailed exploration.

LaPlante (1997c) reports that 9% of, or 14.2 million, working-age people in the United States have a work disability based on results of the U.S. Current Population Survey. The proportion of persons with a work disability escalates with age. For instance, although only 1.8% of persons 16 to 24 years of age are limited in work performance, 7.9% of those between 55 and 64 years are disabled.

Table 2-2 Medicare Inpatient Short Stay by Top Six States

Top Six States	Total Medicare Charges (billion)	Covered Charges (billion)	Medicare Reimbursement (billion)	Total Hospital Days	Average Total Days (per patient)
California	$18.1	$17.9	$6.7	5,020,430	5.6
Florida	$12.2	$12.1	$4.9	4,477,273	6.0
Illinois	$8.0	$7.9	$3.8	3,323,942	6.2
New York	$11.6	$11.5	$5.1	4,864,657	6.7
Pennsylvania	$11.8	$11.5	$7.3	7,394,307	6.6
Texas	$10.7	$10.5	$5.0	4,440,432	6.2

Data from Health Care Financing Administration, 1998 Statistical Supplement.

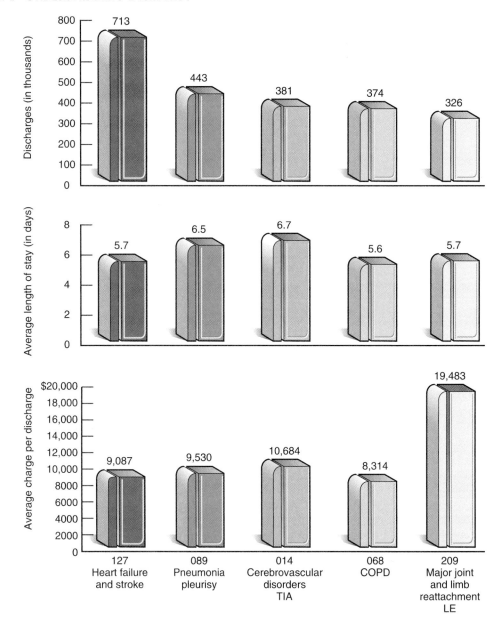

Figure 2–7. The five most prevalent Medicare diagnosis-related groups (1996). *COPD,* Chronic obstructive pulmonary disease; *LE,* lower extremity; *TIA,* transient ischemic attack. (Data from Health Care Financing Administration, Statistical Supplement 1998. Office of Information Services. Medicare Decision Support System. Office of Strategic Planning. Washington, DC, US Department of Health and Human Services, Health Care Financing Review, 1998.)

Cumulative trauma disorders

CTD, or repetitive strain injury, is a highly controversial category of workplace injury or illness. Debate rages on many fronts concerning medicolegal liability, disability definitions, prevalence, cost, and the work relation to CTDs (Anderson, 1998; Hays, 1998; Lankford, 1997; Wojcik, 1997).

The U.S. Department of Labor Bureau of Labor Statistics reported 332,000 CTDs in 1994—a rate four times that of 1991 (U.S. Department of Labor, Bureau of Labor Statistics, 1995). Total costs to employers in 1994 exceeded $10.8 billion.

Physical therapy utilization

The NCCI, one of the two primary workers' compensation research trade associations, estimates that physical therapy is responsible for 8% to 16% of all workers' compensation medical costs (NCCI, 1994). Physical therapy is involved in 35% of all workers' compensation cases, most notably for musculoskeletal injury. However, what is not revealed by these data is the percentage of costs attributed to physical therapists.

The Workers' Compensation Research Institute (WCRI), a professional trade group, conducts workers' compensation research, including state-by-state profiles.

Figure 2–8. Percent distribution of Medicare skilled nursing facility charges by type of service. (Data from Health Care Financing Administration, Office of Information Services: Data from the Medicare Decision Support System. Data developed by the Office of Strategic Planning. 1998 Statistical Supplement.)

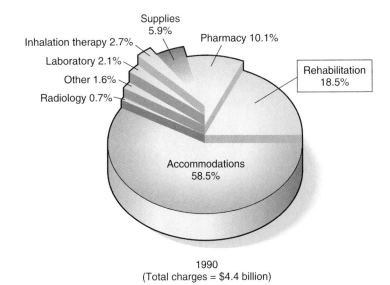

1990
(Total charges = $4.4 billion)

1996
(Total charges = $20.4 billion)

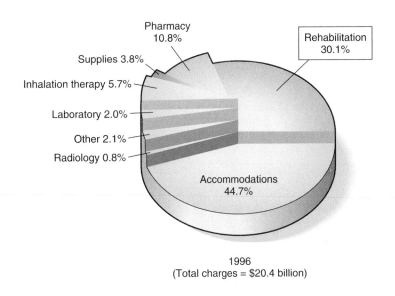

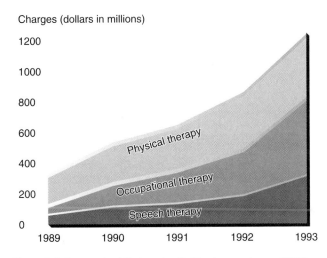

Figure 2–9. Increase in skilled nursing facility therapy charges (1989-1993). (Data from US General Accounting Office, Health Education and Human Services Division. [GAO/HEHS] Publication 98-23. Washington, DC, GAO/HEHS, 1998.)

In profiling New Jersey's workers' compensation system, WCRI noted that growth in medical costs was largely fueled by two significant cost drivers: chiropractic services and physical therapy (WCRI, 1994). Again, it is unclear what percentage of physical therapy services was billed by physical therapists versus others using similar CPT codes.

Swanson (1995) reports the involvement of physical therapy in 16% of all low back cases.

Physical rehabilitation utilization rates are substantially higher in workers' compensation versus group or general health insurance. The average visit number is 12.3 visits under workers' compensation compared with 5.4 visits under group health (Swanson, 1995). Physical rehabilitation is often the primary reason a case remains open under workers' compensation; thus it also drives other costs including administrative, legal, medical (especially orthopedic and neurological), and indemnity or wage replacement. When a therapy case remains open, the injured worker continues follow-up visits to primary care physicians and specialists, including orthopedists, neurologists,

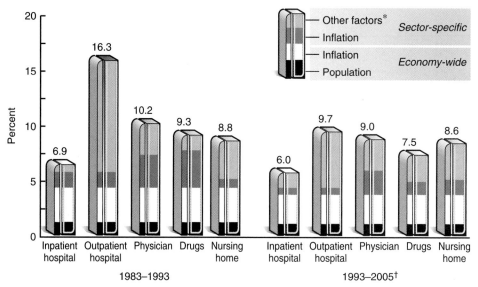

*Other factors include joint effects of the factors shown.
†Some years' data are projected.

Figure 2-10. Factors accounting for average annual growth, selected types of national health expenditures (1983-2005). (Data from Health Care Financing Administration. 1998 Statistical Supplement.)

and neurosurgeons. Therefore, other medical costs grow along with therapy expenditures. According to NCCI, treatment durations for workers' compensation are four times greater than in group health (206.6 versus 51.9 days, respectively).

Jette et al (1994) discovered that physical therapy charges were 36% higher for workers' compensation cases than for similar cases funded by other insurance sources.

Deyo and Tsui-Wu (1987), reporting on the second annual National Health and Nutrition Examination Survey, noted that 16% of those who sought care from a health provider received care from physical therapists.

Williams et al (1998) reported that physical therapy combined with diagnostic procedures and surgery consumed 66% of expenditures related to workers' compensation cases associated with low back pain (Figure 2-12, p. 26).

Chronic Conditions

There are 9.5 million persons described with conditions serious enough to limit their major activity (LaPlante, 1997b). These conditions overwhelmingly tend to be chronic in nature. The true prevalence and costs of chronic conditions has rarely been determined because the U.S. health care system traditionally has been geared (e.g., hospital-driven) toward acute-condition management. Only in the past few decades have hospital stays sharply declined in favor of outpatient visits. See Chapter 22 for a more expanded discussion of chronic illness and injury.

Hoffman et al (1996) opine that, "Our health care system remains firmly rooted in episodic and acute care, but is unlikely to continue this way in the next century." Regrettably, managed care plans often avoid chronic conditions because they encumber increased utilization

and specialist services (e.g., rheumatology, neurology, cardiology). Further compounding this situation is the fact that 44% of persons with chronic conditions have more than one chronic condition that requires management (Hoffman et al, 1996).

Figure 2-13 (p. 26) depicts chronic conditions across a broad spectrum of disabilities. Figure 2-14 (p. 26) describes the five most disabling chronic conditions.

Of all individuals with chronic conditions, 46% accounted for 76% of all direct medical costs in 1987 and incurred annual costs that averaged $3074 compared with $817 dollars for persons with only acute conditions (Hoffman et al, 1996).

Hoffman et al (1996) report that persons with multiple conditions generate significantly greater medical costs: $4672 in annual average costs versus $1829 per single condition. The site of care also greatly influences the costs of care. Nearly 40% of the total direct costs for chronic conditions in 1990 were expended for hospital-based care, whereas almost 25% were spent on physician services (Hoffman et al, 1996).

Acute Care Services

Hospitals remain the single greatest cost driver despite managed care's impact on marked reduction in hospital length of stay. Hospitals were responsible for $128 billion, or 45%, of the total cost of disabilities (Max et al, 1996).

The NCHS reported 71.9 million procedures performed on 39.9 million discharges from hospitals and freestanding centers in 1996 (NCHS, 1998b). More than 40.4 million procedures were inpatient based compared with 31.5 million ambulatory cases. Of all procedures, 65% were categorized as surgical, whereas 35% were non-surgical.

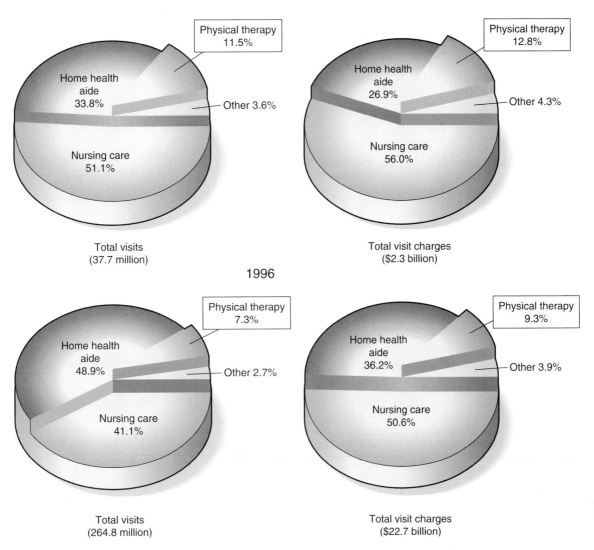

Figure 2–11. Percent distribution of Medicare home health visits and charges by type of visit. (Source: Health Care Financing Administration, Office of Information Services. Data from the Medicare Decision Support System. Data developed by the Office of Strategic Planning. 1998 Statistical Supplement.)

Physician services are second, with total expenditures of $70 billion. Results of the National Ambulatory Medical Care Survey indicate that 787 million visits were made to physicians in 1997 (NCHS, 1998a). Private insurance was responsible for 50% of these visits and managed care for 30% of all payments. LaPlante et al (1997) reports that people who visited physicians more frequently or had longer hospital stays were more likely to be functionally limited. Research has shown that adults who are unable to perform their major activity (e.g., gainful employment) contact their physicians nearly 20 times a year compared with 3.9 visits for those without disability. A comparable association was found with regard to hospital use. Approximately 18% of people who did not use the hospital were considered functionally limited. Not surprisingly, 73% of persons who had hospital stays of 3 weeks or longer reported functional impairments (LaPlante, 1997c).

So-called "other professional services" generated $22 billion in costs (Max et al, 1996). It is presumed that physical rehabilitation falls within this last category of expenditure.

Disability Prevalence and Cost by Diagnosis/Condition

There are data available that segregate disability costs by diagnosis, condition, body region, or system (Table 2–3). These are helpful to rehabilitation providers for the identification of potential markets by matching the provider's services to demographic populations. Data serve to predict service demand, use, and cost (Forer, 1997). Sound, strategic planning incorporates comparisons of at-risk populations with health plan enrollees or beneficiaries, especially if a provider engages in a risk-based contract such as capitation wherein utilization drives profits or lack

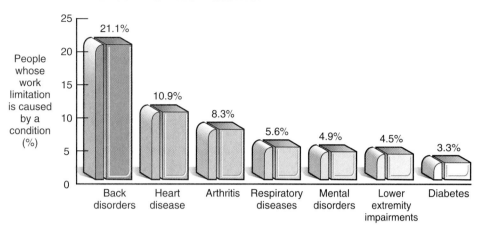

Figure 2-12. The top seven chronic conditions causing work limitation. (Data from LaPlante MP, Carlson D: Disability in the United States: Prevalence and Causes. 1993 Disability Statistics Report 7, Washington, DC, US Department of Education, National Institute on Disability and Rehabilitation Research, 1996.)

Main causes of work limitation

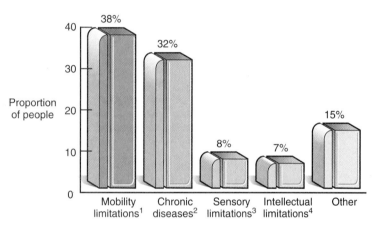

Figure 2-13. Chronic conditions include a broad spectrum of disabilities. (Data from Pope A, Tarlov A [eds]: Disability in America: Toward a National Agenda for Prevention. Washington, DC, Institute of Medicine, National Academy Press, 1991.)

Categories of disabling
chronic conditions

Examples:
1. Arthritis, paralysis
2. Asthma, heart disease, cancer, diabetes
3. Blindness, hearing impairment
4. Mental retardation, senility

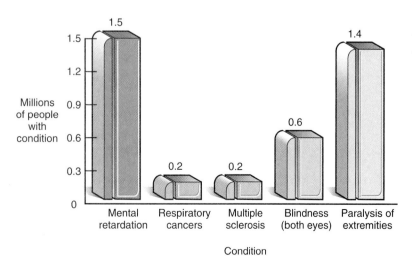

Figure 2-14. The five most disabling chronic conditions. (Data from Collins JG: Prevalence of selected chronic conditions: United States, 1986-88. Vital Health Stat 10[182]: 1-87, 1993.)

Condition

Table 2-3 Incidence Rates

Impairment Group	Incidence Rate/1000
Stroke	1.6490
Orthopedic	2.0000
Amputee	0.1002
Spinal cord injury	0.1619
Brain injury	1.3666
Neurological conditions	0.0350
Arthritis	0.1259
Pain	0.3996
Cardiac	0.1341
Pulmonary conditions	1.0460
Burns	0.0300
Congenital deformities	0.0036
Major multiple trauma	0.0025
Development disabilities	0.0025
Other debility	0.0250
Postsurgical	0.3600
Complex medical	1.6690
Metabolic disorders	1.2130
Injured workers	4.1087

Data from Forer S: The Meaning of Change—Yesterday and Tommorow: Today No Longer Exists. Lecture Presented at the Ninth Annual Medical Rehabilitation: Managing Managed Care Through Research Conference, Buffalo, NY, 1997.

thereof. Table 2-4 presents survivorship data segregated by treatment setting. These data can assist providers in predicting patient volumes, resource allocation needs, and potential marketing targets. Of course, these data are highly malleable and subject to the following marketing influences: health benefit plan design, reimbursement schemes, facility accreditation, staff allocation, patient preferences, self-pay, and regulatory demands.

Uninsured/Underinsured Population

A discussion of health care costs and demographics would be incomplete without addressing the uninsured and underinsured populations. These groups represent a large, untapped market for physical rehabilitation providers once funding mechanisms are secured. In the meantime, providers must select whether to render pro bono services, assuming of course that these persons are even referred for treatment. The Institute of Medicine (IOM) reports that uninsured adults are less than half as likely to receive needed care for serious medical conditions as those with insurance (IOM, 2001). IOM data indicate that the number of uninsured or underinsured is approximately 40 million, or greater than the combined populations of Texas, Florida, and Connecticut.

Rehabilitation providers should be aware of several myths and realities centering around the uninsured or underinsured population. (IOM, 2001).

Myth 1: People without health insurance get the health care services they need ("They just go to the hospital emergency room").

Reality: These persons are far less likely to visit a doctor or receive preventive services for chronic conditions.

Myth 2: People without health insurance are young, healthy adults who actually decline employer-sponsored benefit coverage.

Reality: Young adults between 19 and 34 years are uninsured more often than any other demographic group, largely because they are ineligible for workplace health insurance. Only 4% actually decline insurance (IOM, 2001).

Myth 3: The number of uninsured Americans is not that large and is actually declining.

Table 2-4 Sample Condition Prevalence by Setting Type

Condition	Acute Rehab Setting	Subacute Setting	Outpatient Rehab Setting	Home Health Setting
Stroke	40%	61%	63%	35%
Orthopedic	33%	61%	62%	25%
Amputee	79%	10%	75%	30%
Spinal cord injury	92%	5%	75%	25%
Brain injury	9%	1%	9%	3%
Neurological conditions	50%	20%	50%	25%
Arthritis	5%	5%	50%	25%
Pain	1%	0%	10%	0%
Cardiac (medical)	2%	20%	10%	20%
Pulmonary (medical)	1%	10%	1%	10%
Burns (medical)	5%	20%	20%	25%
Congenital deformities	23%	10%	30%	25%
Major multiple trauma	50%	40%	80%	20%
Developmental disabilities	25%	10%	50%	15%
Other disabilities	10%	30%	20%	25%
Postsurgical (medical)	0%	20%	0%	20%
Complex medical	0%	10%	0%	25%
Metabolic disorders	0%	15%	0%	20%
Injured worker	0%	0%	15%	0%

Data from Forer S: The Meaning of Change-Yesterday and Tomorrow: Today No Longer Exists. Lecture Presented at the Ninth Annual Medical Rehabilitation: Managing Managed Care Through Research Conference, Buffalo, NY, 1997.

Reality: Although the uninsured population slightly declined in 1999, future projections indicate continued growth unless there is substantial restructuring of the opportunities for coverage.

Myth 4: Most uninsured persons do not work or have a family member working.

Reality: Of all uninsured persons, more than 80% younger than 65 years of age live in working families (IOM, 2001).

Myth 5: Immigration is the chief reason for the growing uninsured population.

Reality: More than 80% of all uninsured persons are U.S. citizens

The focus of rehabilitation will likely need to be on disability management of chronic conditions when uninsured persons finally receive necessary health care funding.

SUMMARY

Physical rehabilitation providers are encouraged to identify and utilize data in their design and execution of disability management programs. The dictum "if you don't measure it, you can't manage it" resonates in today's highly competitive managed care market. However, readers are cautioned concerning a second dictum: "Figures lie, and liars figure." Selective use of data is critical if one is to arrive at accurate conclusions, especially when comparing databases. For the foreseeable future, segregated data remains enigmatic for physical rehabilitation providers, but this should not dampen the quest for data.

References

American Physical Therapy Association: Guide to Physical Therapist Practice. Physical Therapy 81(1):S3-S738, Alexandria, VA, American Physical Therapy Association, 2001.

Americans with Disabilities Act of 1990. Public Law 101-336, U.S.C. 1201, Statute 329; July 26, 1990.

Anderson D: RSI can strain the bottom line. Business & Health 16(1): 44-45, 1998.

Balanced Budget Act (BBA) of 1997: Public Law No. 105-133; August, 1997.

Beard PL: Specialty empowerment: A new trend in managed care. Healthcare Financial Manage 52(3):62-64, 1998.

Beger CS: Disability trends and management. Broker World 18(3):16-20, 1998.

Bodenheimer T, Lo B, Casalino L: Primary care physicians should be coordinators, not gatekeepers. JAMA 281(21):2045-2049, 1999.

Buchanan JL, Rumpel JP, Hoenig H: Charges for outpatient rehabilitation: Growth and differences in provider types. Arch Phys Med Rehabil 77(4):320-328, 1996.

Congressional Budget Office: Projections of expenditures for long-term care services for the elderly. March 1999, www.cbo.gov, accessed August 17, 1999.

Crane TS: The problem of physician self-referral under the Medicare and Medicaid antikickback statute: The Hanlester Network case and the safe harbor regulations. JAMA 268:85-91, 1992.

Deyo R, Tsui-Wu YJ: Descriptive epidemiology of low back pain and its related medical care in the United States. Spine 12:264-268, 1987.

Economic and Social Research Institute (ESRI): 1994 National Health Interview Survey, Disability Supplement, phase 1 Washington, DC, ESRI, April, 1999.

Forer S: The meaning of change—Yesterday and tomorrow: Today no longer exists. Ninth Annual Medical Rehabilitation: Managing Managed Care Through Research Conference, Buffalo, NY, 1997.

Gleckman H: Welcome to the health-care economy. Business Week 3796:144, 2002.

Government Accounting Office (GAO): Medicare: Tighter Rules Needed to Curtail Overcharges for Therapy in Nursing Homes. Office of Health, Education and Human Services (GAO/HEHS) Publication 95-23. Washington, DC, GAO/HEHS, 1995.

Hashemi L, Webster BS, Clancy EA: Trends in disability duration and cost of workers' compensation low back pain claims (1988-1996). J Occup Environ Med 40(12):1110-1119, 1998.

Hays D: Doubts raised about drop in workplace injuries. National Underwriter 102(1):6, 1998.

Health Care Financing Administration (HCFA): Statistical Supplement 1998. Office of Information Services. Medicare Decision Support System. Office of Strategic Planning. Washington, DC, US Department of Health and Human Services, Health Care Financing Review, 1998.

Hoffman C, Rice D, Sung HY: Persons with chronic conditions: Their prevalence and costs. JAMA 276(18):1473-1479, 1996.

Hurley RE, Gage BJ, Freund DA: Rollover effects in gatekeeper programs: Cushioning the impact of restricted choice. Inquiry 28(4):375-384, 1991.

Iglehart JK: Congress moves to regulate self referral and physician ownership of clinical laboratories. New Engl J Med 322(23): 1682-1687, 1990.

Institute of Medicine, Committee on the Consequences of Uninsurance. Board on Health Care Services: Coverage Matters: Insurance and Health Care. Washington, DC, National Academy Press, 2001, pp 1-8.

Jackson RL: The business of surgery. Health Manage Technol 23(7): 20-22, 2002.

Jette AM, Smith K, Haley SM et al: Physical therapy episodes of care for patients with low back pain. Phys Ther 74:101-105, 1994.

Kaye HS, LaPlante MP, Carlson D et al: Trends in disability rates in the United States, 1970-1994: Disability Statistics Abstracts, No 17. Washington, DC, US Department of Education, National Institute on Disability and Rehabilitation Research, 1996.

Lankford K: Enormous employer disability costs. Life Assoc News 92(1): 36, 1997.

LaPlante MP: People with functional limitations in the United States. Disability Statistics Abstract, No 1. Washington, DC, US Department of Education, National Institute on Disability and Rehabilitation Research, 1997a.

LaPlante MP: People with disabilities in basic life activities in the U.S. Disability Statistics Abstract, No 3; 1997b, www.dsc.ucsf.edu, accessed June 29, 1999.

LaPlante MP: People with work disability in the U.S. Disability Statistics Abstract, No 4; 1997c, www.dsc.ucsf.edu, accessed June 29, 1999.

LaPlante MP, Cyril J: Disability in the States. Disability Statistics Abstract, No 6. Washington, DC, US Department of Education, National Institute on Disability and Rehabilitation Research, 1993.

LaPlante MP, Rice DP, Wenger BL: Medical care use, health insurance, and disability in the United States–#8, Disability Statistics Abstract, Disability Statistics Research and Training Center, Institute for Health & Aging, School of Nursing, University of California, San Francisco, 1997.

Lauer CS: A wake-up call for the industry. Modern Healthcare 32(28):23, 2002.

Levit K, Cowan C, Braden B et al: National Health Expenditures in 1997: More slow growth. Health Affairs 17(6):99-110, 1998.

Mandel MJ: Health care's economic payoff. Business Week 3780: 28, 2002.

Max W, Rice D, Trupin L: Medical expenditures for people with disabilities. Disability Statistics Abstracts, No 12. Washington, DC, US Department of Education, National Institute on Disability and Rehabilitation Research, 1996.

McNeal JM: Americans with Disabilities, 1991–92: Data from the Survey of Income and Program Participation. Bureau of the Census, Current Population Reports, P 70-33. Washington, DC, US Department of Commerce, 1993, p 9.

Mehn JH: Understanding and interpreting the changing health care environment, McKinsey and Co. Inc. Presentation sponsored by the Foundation for Physical Therapy Research, Ft Lauderdale, FL, February 18, 1997.

Mitchell JM, Scott E: Physician ownership of physical therapy services: Effects on charges, utilization, profits and service characteristics. JAMA 268(15):2055-2059, 1992.

Moerschel GA, Saltzman S: The long-term care industry: Beneficiaries of change. Chicago, The Chicago Corporation: The Chicago Dearborn Company, 1995, pp 1-52.

National Center for Health Statistics: Office Visits to Orthopedic Surgeons, (1995-1996), Advance Number 302. Based on the National Ambulatory Medical Care Survey, 98-1250, 1998a, www.cdc.gov/nchswww/releases/98facts/98sheets/ortho.htm, accessed August 12, 1999.

National Center for Health Statistics: Vital and Health Statistics, Ambulatory and Inpatient Procedures in the United States, 1996, Series 13. National Health Care Survey No. 139. Washington, DC, US Department of Health and Human Services, Centers for Disease Control and Prevention, National Center for Health Statistics, DHHS Pub. No. 99-170, 1998b.

National Council on Compensation Insurance (NCCI): Medical expenditures in workers' compensation: Utilization of service drives cost. Boca Raton, FL, NCCI, 1994.

Reese S: Integration: The case for blended benefits. Business Health 16(4):62-65, 68-69, 1998.

Stark: II, 42 USC sec 1395nn, Jan. 4, 2002.

Swanson GH: Use of outcome reports: Justifying the need for physical therapy services. Orthop Phys Ther Clin North Am 4(2):253-268, 1995.

Trupin L, Rice DP: Health Status, Medical Care Use, and Number of Disabling Conditions in the United States, Disability Statistics Abstract, No 9. Washington, DC, US Department of Education, National Institute on Disability and Rehabilitation Research, 1993.

US Department of Health and Human Services: Financial arrangements between physicians and health care businesses. Washington, DC, Office of the Inspector General, 1989.

US Department of Health and Human Services: Secretary Shalala launches new "Operation Restore Trust," press release, Washington, DC, May 3, 1995, www.os.hhs.gov/news/press/1997/pres/970520.html, accessed July 20, 2000.

US Bureau of Labor Statistics, US Department of Labor: Occupational injuries and illnesses: Costs, rates, and characteristics, Bulletin 2455.Washington, DC, US Bureau of Labor Statistics, 1996.

Waid MO: Overview of the Medicare and Medicaid programs. Health Care Financing Review, Statistical Supplement. Baltimore, US Department of Health and Human Services, Health Care Financing Administration, Office of Strategic Planning, 1998.

Williams DA, Feuerstein M, Durbin D et al: Health care indemnity costs across the natural history of disability in occupational low back pain. Spine J 23(21):2329-2336, 1998.

Wojcik J: Experts dispute 'epidemic' of strain disorders. Business Insurance 31(27):59, 1997.

Workers' Compensation Research Institute (WCRI): Cost drivers in New Jersey. WCRI Research Brief, 10(7):1994, Cambridge, MA, 1994.

World Health Organization (WHO): International classification of impairments, disabilities, and handicaps: A manual of classification relating to the consequence of disease. Geneva, Switzerland, World Health Organization, 1980.

SUGGESTED READINGS

Cardenas DD, Haselkom JK, McElligott JM, Gnatz SM: A bibliography of cost-effectiveness practices in physical medicine and rehabilitation: AAPM&R white paper. Arch Phys Med Rehabil 82(5):711-719, 2001.

Disability Statistics Abstracts series. Available at www.dsc.ucsf.edu.

National Center for Health Statistics: Ambulatory and Inpatient Procedures. Available at www.cdc.gov/nchs.

Stoddard S, Jans L, Ripple J, Kraus L: Chartbook on Work and Disability in the United States. Washington, DC, US Department of Education, National Institute on Disability and Rehabilitation Research, 1998.

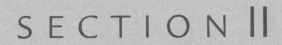

Understanding Disability Management Fundamentals

CHAPTER 3

Disability Management: Principles and Practices

David W. Clifton, Jr., PT

"Integrated disability management coordinates occupational and non-occupational disability programs and other related health programs—such as group health plans, health promotion programs and employee assistance programs (EAPs)—to bring down costs, improve overall workforce health and make administration easier. Such integration encompasses illness and injury, prevention efforts, rehabilitation, medical case management, and return-to-work (RTW) programs for all causes of disability."

- Watson Wyatt Worldwide, 1998/1999

 KEY POINTS

- Rehabilitation providers must understand and apply fundamental disability management (DM) principles and practices if their treatment is to be successful.
- DM in today's health care system(s) is a multivariate challenge that requires a multidisciplinary approach.
- DM connotes different meanings depending on the health care stakeholder involved.
- DM spans the entire injury continuum from prevention/ wellness to treatment and beyond.

 Operational Definitions

Case Management (CM)	A service embedded in DM that on a case-by-case basis attempts to control health care costs while preserving quality care through coordination of medical, vocational, and rehabilitation services.
Disability Management (DM)	Skillful handling of people and details in a systematic, cohesive, functionally oriented application of services and resources to minimize the effect of disease, injury, impairment, and disability. DM spans the entire health care continuum from prevention to treatment to post-treatment consultation.
Disability Treatment	Direct provision of health care to a patient or client.

Integrated Disability Management (IDM)	A blending of DM interventions into one cohesive program that crosses insurance lines and/or health benefit plans.

A DISABILITY MANAGEMENT LEXICON

There is no universal definition of DM, because it crosses many literature sources, including vocational, medical, human resources, ergonomic, safety and health, and legal. However, the quotation at the opening of this chapter captures the multidimensional nature of DM.

The clinical literature represents a lexicon of DM concepts, practices, and principles (Akabas et al, 1992; Huffman & Johnson, 1994; Lukes & Wachs, 1996; Schwartz et al, 1989; Shrey & LaCerte, 1995; Smith, 1997; Tate, 1992; Walker, 1998). The term *disability management* is used to describe a plethora of interventions, each of which is geared toward some aspect of disability prevention, treatment, and management.

Today's disability managers, including physical therapists (PTs), occupational therapists (OTs), and case managers, must have a command of a complex array of issues. These issues fall within diverse domains of knowledge shown in Table 3-1. It is incumbent that clinicians who wish to expand their role into DM possess working knowledge that typically resides in non-medical domains. These domains include legal, human resources, technology, risk management, ethics, utilization review/management, insurance, reimbursement, labor relations, business, and accreditation.

Table 3–1 Domains of Knowledge Required of Disability Management Professionals

Medical	Legal	Human Resources
Pathology	Workers' compensation	Employee-assistance programs
Impairment	Americans with Disabilities Act (ADA)	Benefit structures
Diagnostics	Family Medical Leave Act (FMLA)	"Modified duty"
"Maximum Medical Improvement (MMI)"	"Medical necessity"	"Reasonable accommodation"
Irritability stages	Any Willing Provider Laws (AWPs)	Vocational training
Treatment protocols	"Community standards of care"	Health policy
Ethics	**Utilization Review/Management**	**Insurance**
Patient confidentiality	Preauthorization	STD/LTD
Ombudsman role	Medical records review	SSDI/SSI
Patient abandonment	Telephonic review	Medicare
"Do no harm"	Criteria review	Medicaid
Informed consent	Independent medical examinations	MCOs
Professional versus business duty	Bill audits	Integrated benefits
Technology	**Risk Management**	**Accreditation**
Diagnostic	Business and professional risks	Joint Commission for the Accreditation of Health Care Organizations (JCAHO)
Treatment	Professional liability	Commission for the Accreditation of Rehabilitation Facilities (CARF)
Documentation	Medicare fraud and abuse	National Committee for Quality Assurance (NCQA)
Health Evaluation Data Information Sets (HEDIS)		
Electronic commerce	Risk indicators	Medicare
Outcomes management	Fault tree analysis	State insurance/Health departments
Labor Relations	**Business**	**Reimbursement**
Management-labor Contracts/agreements	Finance	Fee for service
U.S. Department of Labor	Staffing	Prospective payment
Occupational Safety and Health Administration (OSHA)	Operations	Resource-based utilization groups (RUGs)
National Institute of Occupational Safety and Health (NIOSH)		
Equal Employment Opportunity Commission (EEOC)	Marketing	Capitation
Americans with Disabilities Act	Strategic planning	Cost reports
Collective bargaining	Productivity	Diagnosis-related groups (DRGs); ambulatory payment groups (APGs)

LTD, Long-term disability; *MCOs*, managed care organizations; *SSDI*, Social Security Disability Insurance; *SSI*, Social Security Insurance; *STD*, short-term disability.

Chapter 1 provides an overview of disablement models and definitions of *disability*. By extension, this chapter addresses DM principles and practices that can be applied within most disablement models and rehabilitation programs.

What Is Disability Management?

DM is an intervention or interventions designed to address *discrepancies between an individual's functional level and socioenvironmental demands*. This definition implies that DM considers the individual's functional status, as well as his or her social and environmental needs.

DM programs view the individual in the context of his or her environment and focus on the following:

- The patient's condition and his or her worksite demands
- Impairment and disability
- Disability and handicap
- Treatment and management

- Medical and non-medical challenges
- Health care and business

Disability Management: A Multivariate Challenge Requiring a Multidisciplinary Approach

Rehabilitation providers can be more effective when dealing with disability across different health insurance or benefit plans. To become more effective in DM, providers must understand the system within which they ply their trade. This means looking beyond the confines of the clinic, the patient's condition, and the therapy intervention itself. An injured employee's insurance benefits may substantially dictate how a therapy program is designed in terms of preauthorization requirements, frequency and duration of services, cost of services, and coverage/noncoverage itself. In addition, payer goals may differ. For instance, a group or general health claim may emphasize the need to achieve "maximum medical improvement" or "maximum medical benefit," whereas a workers' compensation case demands a greater emphasis on function, specifically return-to-work (RTW). An impairment-based rehabilitation program may be acceptable under a group health plan but unacceptable under workers' compensation.

DM demands a multidisciplinary approach commensurate with the multivariate nature of disability. Theoretically, no two cases are identical because of the variables, introduced by payers, patients, and others. DM is not defined by a single profession because of its broad context (Akabas et al, 1992; Rosenthal & Olsheski, 1999). This means that education and communication are cornerstones of every DM program.

Disability's Perception as a Medical Problem

Some employers and providers view disability as a medical problem that is best addressed through medical personnel, when in reality, disability is both a medical and a non-medical phenomenon that requires multiple and diverse disciplines in its prevention, treatment, and management. In one survey, 52 employers were asked which profession was best suited to provide comprehensive DM services (Rosenthal & Olsheski, 1999). Survey respondents viewed disability as a medical issue when asked a question concerning which type of professional is best suited to provide DM services (Rosenthal & Olsheski, 1999):

Which profession is best suited to manage disability?

- 22% or 42% of employers indicated an occupational health nurse
- 14% or 27% of employers indicated human resources staff
- 8% or 15% of employers indicated PTs
- 6% or 12% of employers indicated rehabilitation/vocational counselor

These data suggest that DM is fragmented and is in need of a multidisciplinary approach. This presents opportunities for therapists to take a lead role in DM interventions. Eight to fifteen percent of employer respondents cited PTs as the professionals best suited to manage disability. Again, this does not imply that PTs can manage disability alone.

Disability Treatment Versus Management

Shrey and LaCerte (1995) provide a description of DM that reinforces the desirability of a proactive approach based on management, not treatment per se:

"Disability management is the proactive process of minimizing the impact of injury, disability or disease on the worker's capacity to perform work. Disability management is an interdisciplinary concept that includes physical, emotional, vocational, medical, and organizational factors that impact on employment."

- Shrey & LaCerte, 1995

This definition of DM acknowledges the multivariate nature of disability and the interface between a person's individual condition and his or her work environment. Shrey and LaCerte (1995) developed a "workability box" to display the relationship between what an injured person would do, wants to do, can do, and could do. These constructs describe a patient's motivation, intent, capability, and capacity, which can be assessed through four DM tools: medical disability assessment, work capacity evaluation, vocational rehabilitation, and ergonomic job analysis (Figure 3–1).

Patient needs, goals, and expectations extend well beyond the confines of disease, impairment, and clinical treatment, and in many cases, transcend physical functioning altogether. Master clinicians may well be those therapists who have a command of both clinically based knowledge and skill sets associated with non-medical or psychosocioeconomic issues commonly associated with disability.

This paradigm shift is closely related to others: the transfer of rehabilitation services from a clinical focus to a worksite focus. Early intervention programs use the worksite as a therapeutic environment via work conditioning, work hardening, and transitional or modified duty. There is a shift from principally focusing on the individual to considering his or her environment as well. The growth in the use of functional job analysis, ergonomics, reasonable accommodations, and functional capacity evaluations is evidence of this shift. Rehabilitation providers who wish to excel in solving employer-based disability challenges must embrace a new mindset that

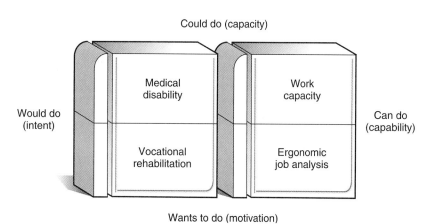

Could do (capacity)

Would do (intent)

Medical disability

Vocational rehabilitation

Work capacity

Ergonomic job analysis

Can do (capability)

Wants to do (motivation)

Figure 3–1. Return-to-work environment: The workability box. (From Lacerte M, Desjardins L: Evaluation of work disability from a worker-work environment perspective. In Shrey DE, LaCerte M [eds]: Principles and Practices of Disability Management in Industry. Winter Park, FL, GR Press, Inc, 1995, p 211.)

extends beyond that of clinician. Clinicians are traditionally educated and trained with a focus on "treatment." Today's reality is that disability *management* has supplanted injury *treatment.* A treatment paradigm involves direct hands-on care, whereas a management paradigm suggests augmentation of treatment through case management, coordination, education, and communication. A management approach is especially crucial when patients or clients are in the chronic stage of a disability when the signs and symptoms of the initial injury can be inconsequential, but psychosocial issues can be very important.

Psychosocial and economic issues have been known to demand and respond better to management skills than to treatment skills per se (Clifton, 1992; Fritz & George, 2002; Lemstra & Olszynski, 2003; Polatin et al, 1989). These factors are considered by some to be the best predictors of chronicity (Kendall, 1999). Clinical management that ignores psychosocial issues can result in more patients entering the chronic phase of injury or illness. Psychosocial issues are more thoroughly explored in Chapter 7.

Optimal success in rehabilitation may be predicated on a blending of treatment and management skills. Successful DM professionals may be those who possess knowledge, experience, and understanding outside of the "clinical box" or beyond the medical model (Lerner, 1998). Relatively few practicing therapists have a substantial opportunity to explore other domains of knowledge, and most physical or occupational therapy programs typically have only one or two issues classes that incorporate this knowledge.

Clinical treatment is embedded in an extensive matrix that includes external drivers that constantly shape and reshape actual treatment. This is especially true when considering the effect of shifting reimbursement schemes on rehabilitation service delivery. Shrinking reimbursement resulting from diagnosis-related groups, Medicare caps on outpatient physical therapy (since repealed), managed care capitation, and prospective payment can potentially have a direct effect on resource allocation, which imminently leads to changes in health care delivery.

Domains of knowledge listed in Table 3–1 represent a linkage between the medical aspects of treatment and the business aspects of DM. Domains include medical, legal, risk management, human resources, ethics, utilization review and management, accreditation, technology, labor relations, and reimbursement. It is difficult to covet knowledge in all of these areas; therefore a partnership approach provides enormous advantages to those who possess a global view of disability (Hintzman & Farrell, 1997).

Need for Disability Management

A brief discussion of disability-related costs is warranted to document the considerable opportunity for participation of physical rehabilitation providers in both the design and the implementation of DM programs (Table 3–2). Providers who wish to justify their involvement in DM can use these data in marketing efforts directed at employers and insurers.

 Table 3–2 Roster of Disability Management Definitions

The following list of DM definitions has highlighted concepts that distinguish critical issues.

Smith (1997)
"A systematic, cohesive, and goal-oriented approach that seeks to (a) minimize the impact that reduced functioning may have on an individual's social and vocational roles and (b) maximize the health of employees in order to prevent disability or further deterioration when a disability is present."

Schwartz et al (1989)
"Disability management involves the use of services, people and materials to minimize the impact and cost of disability to employers and employees and encourages return to work for employees with disability."

Huffman & Johnson (1994)
"Disability management—managing the costs of disability through aggressive coordination of medical care, focusing on appropriate return to work and productivity."

Tate (1992)
"A strategy that can be used to maximize the health of an employee population and their dependents."

Shrey & LaCerte (1995)
"Disability management is the proactive process of minimizing the impact of injury, disability or disease on the workers' capacity to perform work. Disability management is an interdisciplinary concept that includes physical, emotional, vocational, medical, and organizational factors that impact on employment."

Akabas et al (1992)
"Disability management is a well coordinated, cost-effective prevention and early intervention effort, the purpose of which is to eliminate as many situations that cause disability as possible and to assist a newly disabled worker in successful job maintenance or return to work."

Lukes & Wachs (1996)
"In an effective disability management program, efforts are made to keep employees healthy and safe in all aspects of their lives, not just at work." "Disability management begins before any injury or illness occurs, before anyone is disabled." "It is a proactive, anticipatory strategy."

Several non-medical cost indicators illustrate the enormity of disability and the growing need for disability managers. These indicators include disability costs as a percentage of payroll, lost productivity costs, long-term disability (LTD) rate, worker replacement costs, fraud costs, and lost work days (Nelson, 1991; Wolfe & Haveman, 1990).

Disability is increasingly expensive for employers, who fund the majority of health care in the United States. According to a Dupont Corporation study, the estimated average cost to a corporation for one missed work day per employee is $13,000 (Matthes, 1992). The Bureau of Labor Statistics (BLS) reports that 6.7 of every 100 workers suffer a work-related disability (BLS, 1999). Almost half of all work-related disabilities reported result in lost-time incidents. This partly explains why health benefits as a percentage of payroll ranged from 1.7% to 12% through most of the 1990s, depending on the industry, its population, and insurance lines (Nelson, 1991; Strosahl & Johnson, 1998; Watson Wyatt, 1998/1999; Winslow, 1999). LTD rates are commonly measured per 1000 employees. The average LTD rate has risen from 6.7 incidents in 1981 to 8.7 in 1994 per 1000 employees (Accum & Bellman, 1996).

Fraud is another cost of special concern to employers. Fraudulent claims can run as high as 25% of total health care costs, although this figure may be inflated. A more accurate estimate of fraud costs is in the 1% to 3% range (Lerner, 1998).

A Disability Management Triad

Figure 3–2 depicts a conceptual triad that integrates three DM components: treatment/management, education, and consultation. As the triangle is traversed from the outer to the inner levels, the specificity of action increases. For example, "treatment-education-consultation" resides on the outermost plane, because these encompass a broader array of possibilities than elements on the inner levels. Treatment that addresses an individual's disability is rehabilitation focused, depicted in the second level. Rehabilitation that focuses on the injured worker's capabilities and limitations represents the next level. The greatest specificity involves the focus-on-function approach to DM, depicted in the innermost level.

PARADIGM SHIFTS

Rehabilitation provider understanding of new paradigms may facilitate participation in a broader context (beyond treatment) with other DM team members. This is essential, because today's clinician faces an increasingly complex health care system that engages a diverse range of stakeholders. Each of these stakeholders, including physical rehabilitation providers, views and shapes disability through his or her own unique prism. It should be noted, however, that not all experts believe a multidisciplinary team yields superior outcomes (Stucki, 2003).

Disability: From an Individual Focus to a Socioenvironmental Focus

"Traditional rehabilitation service models developed from a medically-based conceptualization of disability and treatment. Within this framework, the individual was viewed as having an impairment that needed to be evaluated (diagnosed) in order for services to be provided to the individual (treatment) by trained professionals."

- Hursch, 1995

The individual-based approach to rehabilitation represents the traditional model of care. Raman and Levi (2002) note that PT guiding documents routinely articulate disability in the context of an individual's limitations versus disability as a societal phenomenon. The patient-centric view of disability is consistent with the medical model of disability, which reinforces passive receipt of services

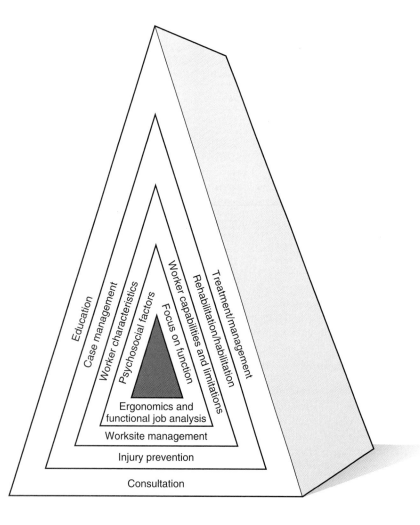

Figure 3–2. The disability management triad.

delivered by the provider, principally during the acute stage of injury or illness (Corcoran & Klett, 1997; Quinn 1995). However, this treatment-oriented view is in conflict with an evolving paradigm of disability as a societal or environmental phenomenon (Hahn, 1991; Pain et al, 1998; Hursch, 1995).

> *"It is believed that a concept of disability that is more inclusive of broad, as well as specific, contexts of disability may lead to improved physical therapy management for individuals with a wide range of performance capacities."*
>
> - Raman & Levi, 2002

The Raman and Levi (2002) study suggests a trend toward individualization of disability, but readers are cautioned that only selected core documents from the physical therapy profession were examined. This study did not constitute a comprehensive analysis of the literature. For example, literature pertaining to industrial, physical, or occupational therapy routinely addresses both the individual and his or her environment within a disability model (Leone, 1995; McKenney, 2000; Shrey & LaCerte, 1995).

From Clinic to Worksite

Opportunities exist to participate in DM, especially for those providers who embrace a paradigm shift away from clinically based services and toward worksite-based or employee-specific interventions (Hursch, 1995; Lemstra & Olszynski, 2003; Shrey, 2000). Hursch coined the phrase "ecological paradigm" to describe the individual-worksite interface. An ecological paradigm shift demands that providers look to the employer as their "other customer." Employers finance the majority of health care in the United States. Therefore it is incumbent on rehabilitation providers to learn more about employer needs and expectations in the context of managing their employees at risk of disability and its consequences. One means of acquiring this knowledge and understanding is to step out of the clinic and into their world. Onsite (employer location) therapists tend to be more familiar with employee work demands, company injury reporting and management systems, labor-management relations, and injury trends than are offsite practitioners. Basic elements of an effective onsite DM program include the following (Vance & Brown, 1995):

- Team approach
- Functional outcome–based
- Early intervention
- Active versus passive treatment
- Communication
- Education

Rehabilitation providers can integrate with employers for both occupationally based and non-occupational injuries, even if rehabilitation itself is clinically based. DM programs can be devised that satisfy the needs of multiple insurance lines and benefit plans, including workers' compensation, long-term care, disability insurance (short-term disability [STD] and LTD), and group or general health.

A host of interventions can prevent and/or minimize the effects of disability. Workers' compensation carriers may indicate a preference for functional capacity evaluation (FCE), work hardening, and functional job analysis (FJA) for the management of disability. When combined, these strategies address both the individual (FCE, work hardening) and his or her environment (job analysis). Therapists who develop and use FJAs are better positioned to link their patient's disability with worksite demands. The FJA becomes the blueprint for a clinically based RTW program that can consist of work conditioning or work hardening. The FJA can also serve as a template for the design and performance of FCEs. Employee and management education and training can be provided at the employer location. Programs for cumulative trauma prevention, good posture, ergonomics, and employee health and wellness can be provided proactively, or before injury occurs.

Providers cannot assume that employers have well-established or fundamentally sound DM programs in place. Therapists may initially need to serve as educators assisting employers in the development of DM programs.

Early intervention is a distinguishing feature of DM and third-party–paid rehabilitation services that are typically initiated well after the onset of disability (Rosenthal & Olsheski, 1999). Habeck (1996) contends that DM is not the equivalent of individually oriented rehabilitation services in terms of the goals, outcome measures, and strategies used. This represents a major departure from traditional rehabilitation services, especially outpatient services.

From Individual Silos to Teams

A partnership approach to DM removes providers from their silos or individual departments or settings (e.g., physical therapy and occupational therapy departments) and engages them in a collaborative strategy. Integrated disability management (IDM) conveys several meanings depending on the stakeholder and his or her domain of influence. Integration can describe benefit structures, DM strategies, medical and non-medical staff collaborations, and occupational (workers' compensation) and non-occupational insurance benefits (disability insurance, group or general health insurance). Figure 3–3 depicts integration of insurance benefits across four benefit schemes. Employers who integrate health benefits attempt to use similar claims management practices but rarely truly integrate health care delivery. For example, an employer may choose to use different provider networks for group health (i.e., managed care) and workers' compensation (i.e., non-managed care). Although claims management can be somewhat standardized or integrated, care management may or may not be integrated.

Disability and its management are clearly in the eye of the beholder. As an example, Figure 3–4 depicts a person with a low back injury, a herniated nucleus pulposus. DM views in this case may dramatically vary, because each health care stakeholder has a different approach to treatment and/or management based on his or her experience, goals, knowledge, and skill sets. For instance, the primary care or family physician may focus on the diagnostic

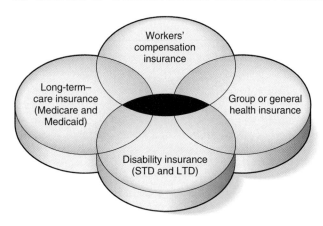

Figure 3–3. Integrated disability across insurance benefit plans. *LTD,* Long-term disability; *STD,* short-term disability.

workup in search of an organic cause of the problem. An orthopedist or neurosurgeon may be consulted during or after the initial diagnostic workup to determine the patient's surgical candidacy.

PTs involved in the case formulate a *functional diagnosis* and encourage early movement and restorative activities to avoid medical procedures and/or surgery.

From Case Management to Disability Management

Case management (CM) is a vital component or subset of DM (Lukes & Wachs, 1996).

Case managers use a number of professional designations after their names to signify certification. These include the following:

- Certified Case Manager (CCM)
- Certified Rehabilitation Counselor (CRC)

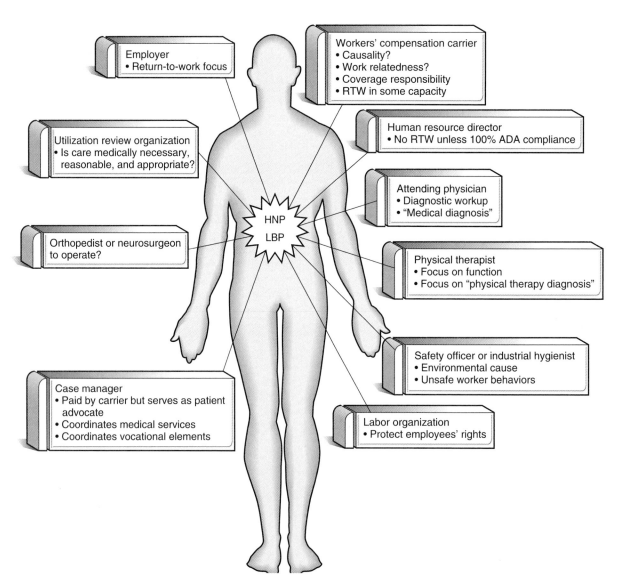

Figure 3–4. Low back pain: Different stakeholder paradigms. *ADA,* Americans with Disabilities Act of 1990; *HNP,* herniated nucleus pulposus; *LBP,* low back pain; *RTW,* return-to-work.

Table 3-3 Case Management Versus Disability Management

Case Management	Disability Management
Individual case focus	Population focus
Less emphasis on prevention	More emphasis on prevention
Paid to manage cases	Paid to avoid management of cases
Focus on high-cost or catastrophic cases	Focus on all employees
Principal emphasis on cost-reduction	Principal focus on health
Traditionally applied to acute conditions	Traditionally applied to chronic conditions

NOTE: Case management is a component of disability management and, as such, may share attributes listed in the disability management column.

- Certified Insurance Rehabilitation Specialist (CIRS)
- Certified Disability Manager (CDM)

DM necessitates a broader vision from injury and illness prevention to treatment to post-treatment management, whereas case managers are typically engaged after the injury or illness has occurred. Not all disability cases receive CM. Traditionally, the need for case management was triggered by high medical costs, protracted treatment, or "red flag" conditions.

Today, case managers tend to be involved earlier on a case-by-case basis. Case managers are used in every insurance line and for a variety of conditions. Case managers are typically paid by insurance companies or employers while serving as patient advocates. This dual master relationship is most challenging for case managers when balancing the needs of various parties who reside in different domains (see Table 3-1).

CM is not a profession unto itself but a certification for those who possess a primary degree or degrees in other fields. CM is no longer defined by registered nurses, because a diversity of disciplines is now represented. In fact, physical rehabilitation providers may be uniquely qualified to sit for certification examinations that enable them to serve as case managers.

Case managers occupy several different employment domains. Case managers can be independently employed, contracting their services directly to employers or insurers. In some circumstances, case managers are employees of the employer or insurance entity. However, this relationship can be perceived as a potential conflict of interest when compared with independent case managers. Case managers also work for provider organizations in a variety of roles, including quality assurance, peer review, provider credentialing, or marketing (Table 3-3).

INTEGRATED DISABILITY MANAGEMENT

IDM commonly describes health benefit packages that combine one or more insurance lines, typically to capture claims administration efficiencies under one umbrella. Another name for benefits consolidation is 24-hour coverage (Kunnes & Hellwig, 1995; Smith, 1997). When benefits are integrated, a centralized claims administration process may manage workers' compensation, group health, disability insurance, and long-term–care claims through one body of claims adjusters. When this occurs,

occupational benefits administration and non-occupational benefits administration are integrated. Although simplistic on the surface, these integrated models can be overwhelmingly complex because of different benefit structures. The same diagnosis or condition may be handled differently because of varying insurance benefits.

For example, workers' compensation, when coupled with group health or general insurance, has not been an overwhelming success for a variety of reasons. Namely, workers' compensation involves a patchwork of 50 state laws regulated by government agencies. Benefit structures are statutorily promulgated and cannot be altered as readily by insurers as in group or general health policies (Vash, 1991). Workers' compensation has a high degree of litigation associated with it relative to group health. Beneficiaries under workers' compensation do not share financial risk and thus may not have the incentive for an early RTW or disability resolution. In fact, it is common to find injured workers receiving more take-home pay while getting workers' compensation indemnity payments because of its non-taxation status.

Clinicians are advised to learn as much as possible about each health benefit structure, because the design of the system may have as much impact on recovery cycles, clinical outcomes, and cost as the treatment itself (Table 3-4).

Labor-Management Synergy

Development of an employee-employer synergy may be the most difficult aspect of an IDM program. Companies that encourage this collaboration may view individual performance and corporate performance as mutually exclusive concepts (Tortarolo & Polakoff, 1995).

Despite the obvious barriers to IDM, support for IDM has been overwhelming (Bousquet, 1992; Burns, 1997;

 Table 3-4 Selected Components of DM

- CM
- Vocational rehabilitation and counseling
- Pain clinics
- RTW programs and early interventions
- EAPs
- Psychological evaluations
- Functional capacity evaluations
- ADLs assessments
- Restorative rehabilitation
- Functional job analyses
- Identification of architectural barriers
- Ergonomics
- Reasonable accommodations
- Safety and health programs
- Work hardening
- Utilization review and management
- Patient and family education
- Management (employer) education
- Pre-employment or post-offer (ADA) examinations
- "Light," "modified," or "transitional" duty design and identification

ADA, Americans with Disabilities Act of 1990; ADLs, activities of daily living; EAPs, employee assistance programs; RTW, return-to-work.
Data modified from Lipow VA: Aging workers: Disability management strategies. Rehabil Manage 10(1):32-36, 1997; Smith D: Implementing disability management: A review of basic concepts and essential components. Employee Assist Q 12(4):37-50, 1997.

Cohen, 1998; Flectcher, 1997; Fruen, 1992; Hergenrader, 1997; Matthes, 1992; McShulkis, 1997; Owens, 1998; Watson & Huban, 1997).

Disability Continuum

IDM can have various meanings depending on the stakeholder. IDM to a provider may mean a continuum of disability: prevention/treatment/management services spanning pre-injury to post-injury.

For the sake of this discussion, IDM is viewed as a blending of disability interventions into one cohesive program within one or more insurance lines. For instance, an IDM program in workers' compensation insurance may involve pre-injury or prevention strategies, treatment-based interventions, and post-treatment controls.

EMPLOYER AND INSURER INTEGRATED DISABILITY MANAGEMENT EFFORTS

Who Manages Disability?

Employers potentially face several competing challenges when attempting to manage disability. The employer's medical director may establish appropriate "work restrictions" to encourage expeditious RTW. However, the human resources director may forbid RTW without 100% recovery. The human resources director may also be responsible for "reasonable accommodations" under the Americans with Disabilities Act of 1990 (ADA) without adequate knowledge of the employee's limitations or critical job demands. Similarly, externally based health care providers may possess adequate medical knowledge but remain ignorant of the critical job demands required of employees. Relatively few external health care providers take the time to visit the worksite. Those professionals who take the time to visit the worksite are often ill-trained and/or poorly educated regarding human factors and ergonomics, two essential foundations for reasonable accommodations. In turn, safety officers, industrial hygienists, or ergonomists may be recruited to engineer reasonable accommodations such as job redesign or equipment adaptations.

Clearly, the complexity of a given case is commensurate with the number of persons involved and the diversity of issues confronted during DM. Both medical and non-medical challenges are confronted in this hypothetical case. Shared DM practices and principles among stakeholders are vital; otherwise, fragmentation of services and interventions results. DM requires aggressive coordination between medical, vocational, and organizational aspects. DM requires a delicate balance between preserving and/or restoring the health of the worker while preserving the financial interests of the employer (Schwartz et al, 1989; Shrey & LaCerte, 1995).

Which Cases Are Managed?

Some employers and insurers engage in targeted IDM, wherein high-risk, high-cost, or high-prevalence conditions are initially integrated. These cases constitute roughly 80% of health care dollars but only 5% of all employees (Luke & Wachs, 1996). Companies target these cost-driver groups because of the savings potential associated with a relatively small percentage of the working population. Cumulative trauma cases are one example of an employer cost driver that is ideally suited for rehabilitation providers' participation in DM.

In its survey of large employers with more than 1000 employees, Watson Wyatt Worldwide (1998/1999), a well-known employer consulting firm, found that 42% of these employers used IDM programs. This figure is up from 20% of employers responding to the 1996/1997 survey (Watson Wyatt Worldwide, 1998/1999). In the 1998/1999 survey, IDM was defined as a coordination of occupational and non-occupational disability programs and other related programs such as group health plans, health promotion programs, and employee assistance programs (EAPs). Companies that reported IDM blended their STD, LTD, sick pay, and workers' compensation programs. Readers are advised to secure a copy of Watson Wyatt Worldwide's report, "Staying @ Work" (1998/1999), because it contains insightful information about employer DM initiatives.

Although many midsize to large American employers use some component of DM (e.g., case management), few have truly integrated STD, LTD, workers' compensation, and group health beyond a purely claims administration function. Few employers have integration across the continuum from prevention to treatment and post-treatment. Smaller employers are extremely disadvantaged, because they lack the necessary resources to blend benefits and services. Instead, they use managed care organizations (MCOs) and traditional indemnity carriers to manage their risk.

Ten Commandments of Disability Management

Through the mid-1990s, employers typically depended on the efforts of third-party insurers or MCOs to protect their assets. Many employers adopted the attitude that medical costs, although rising, are simply "a cost of doing business." They initially responded to the rising costs of the 1980s through a curtailment in benefit structures or with frozen wages. Some employers converted to "cafeteria plans," wherein each individual employee selected only the coverage he or she or his or her dependents were likely to need. This allowed employers to avoid financing insurance benefits (paying insurance premiums) that only a minority of employees required. Relatively few employers aggressively managed their health care costs, and when they did, they typically managed a small minority of high-cost or catastrophic cases. These efforts focused on the roughly 5% of workers who consume 80% of the health care dollars (Lukes & Wachs, 1996). It was this group of workers that was targeted through an insurance or medical model.

Table 3–5 presents "10 Commandments of Employer-Based Disability Management" (Lerner, 1998). These DM principles offer a humane approach to DM that balances business interests with interests of injured employees. Integrated DM begins with agreement among stakeholders regarding goals and expectations of DM (e.g., RTW, incentives and penalties, rules and guidelines, communication needs). These and other DM components are supported

Table 3–5 10 Commandments of Employer-Based Disability Management

One	Make return-to-work a clear focus.
Two	Provide strong incentives and no penalties for attempting some type of work.
Three	Use the rules as guidelines, but be creative in making the most of the benefits available.
Four	Put understanding, compassionate people in positions involving contact with claimants.
Five	Establish clear and ongoing communication between claimants and the workplace.
Six	Set clear expectations of who will be involved and what, when, where, why, and how things will happen.
Seven	Pay attention to actual details of the plan in any denials and provide proper support and documentation, taking pains to comply with ERISA (Employee Retirement Insurance Security Act).
Eight	Do not operate from the point of view that claimants are abusers and malingerers until proven otherwise.
Nine	Avoid the abuses, excuses, delays, and deceit tactics for which some disability carriers are known.
Ten	Understand that disability is a human problem.

Data from Lerner JR: The new direction in disability management. Business & Health 16(10):36-45, 1998.

by a foundation of trust among stakeholders, especially between the employee and the employer (Lewin & Schecter, 1995).

Under new DM models, employers and providers do not operate from the point of view that claimants are abusers and/or malingerers. Visionary employers provide strong incentives for a RTW without penalty for failed attempts. These employers understand that disability is a human problem and therefore avoid deceitful tactics in their DM programs.

Human Resources Integrated Disability Management Model

Employers seem to be moving toward a human resources model of DM that looks beyond "treatment" or insurance underwriting to prevention and management of all employees and their health care needs, not just a selected few. A human resources model of DM embraces a wellness and general health philosophy. Injury and illness prevention programs are an integral component of this model. Employee screenings, vaccinations, health club memberships, and educational programs are designed to prevent disability while enhancing employee productivity. Physical rehabilitation providers have played a relatively minor role in these initiatives and are advised to diversify their offerings beyond treatment. Evidence suggests that support for IDM continues to grow among employers nationwide. However, this new paradigm has been problematic for several reasons (Ceniceros, 1998). Namely, few employers commit funds to prevention strategies. Instead, they often rely on insurance policies to fund losses.

Labor-Management Synergy

Successful DM programs are able to balance labor-management needs and overcome inherent differences

in expectations. This balance is forged through mutual trust and understanding (Mills, 1995). Employer-based health care benefits were created because of unions and labor organizations.

However, employers have abdicated a great deal of control over health care finance and delivery to third-party payers, especially MCOs. Only recently have employers begun to reassert their leverage over third-party payers, with some electing self-insurance or self-funding as an alternative. A self-funded employer does not pre-pay insurance premiums; instead it sets aside "company reserves" to cover losses as they occur. Company reserves are a calculation of the amount of money needed to cover an injured or ill employee throughout his or her disability period. This money comes out of a company's budget and is set aside in an escrow account earmarked for the employee only. Employers assume great financial risk under self-insurance if they experience an injury run or prevalence and/or if they realize an increase in injury or illness severity. Self-funded employers have greater incentives to invest in prevention and early intervention services when compared with those that are third-party insured.

For example, a worker develops job-related carpal tunnel syndrome (CTS), and his or her employer is self-insured for workers' compensation. Under this scenario, injury or disease (the Occupational Safety and Health Administration [OSHA] considers CTS an occupational disease) costs are not paid for through insurance premiums. The employer must put aside company reserves that involve calculations of anticipated direct medical costs and indemnity or wage replacement losses. If the insured worker is a well-paid young person, his or her lifetime earnings and medical bills can be substantial.

An employee-employer or labor-management synergy may be the most difficult to achieve within an IDM model. Mills (1995) suggests that the key to successful integration hinges on "demystifying disability management and making it a workable business strategy." Companies that encourage this collaboration view individual health and performance and corporate performance as mutually inclusive concepts (Tortarolo & Polakoff, 1995).

Employers routinely experience interdepartmental tension or rifts, which inhibit the acceptance of IDM strategies. This is not unlike the problems associated with a fragmented health care system that attempts to provide integrated services along the continuum of care. In both situations, corporate and personal attitudinal adjustments are necessary for successful implementation.

Providers indoctrinated with a "treatment" mindset are encouraged in this DM model to embrace a prevention mode as well. Proactive strategies are vital in DM, and they displace or, at a minimum, augment reactionary strategies (e.g., "treat it"). This new paradigm requires employers to engage in programs such as ergonomics *before* an injury is incurred, or the employer receives an OSHA citation. An enormous opportunity exists for PTs or OTs to participate earlier in the disability continuum or before injury occurs. In addition, providers accustomed to giving care are positioned to mentor other caregivers (e.g., worker's family, corporate nurse, safety officer, industrial hygienist, human resources staff) and the workers themselves.

MCOs, through primary care physicians (PCPs) or "gatekeepers," are principally responsible for relegating rehabilitation to discretionary or elective service status. When a health care service is labeled as "elective," it tends to receive low priority. In the case of physical rehabilitation, low priority means reduced or delayed referrals from PCPs. The demand for ancillary services, which include physical rehabilitation, has essentially resulted from an employer desire to stem costs (Gallagher & Granahan, 1995). Providers must assume a stronger role in educating PCPs regarding the benefits of early intervention and the consequences of delayed referral.

Enlightened employers will become one of rehabilitation's potential partners as they continue to take responsibility to not only finance but also to manage health care. The incentive to use physical rehabilitation expertise should grow along with an aging American workforce and with dissipation of managed care cost savings (Clifton, 1996). Physical rehabilitation providers add value to an employer's DM program, because their non-clinical treatment and services are appropriate at virtually any point along the injury or illness continuum—from prevention to treatment to management. Capturing new business is only one challenge that rehabilitation providers must accept; production of favorable clinical and economic outcomes is another.

Disability Management Opportunities in Workers' Compensation

Workers' compensation systems may present the greatest opportunity for rehabilitation providers to participate in DM along its entire spectrum. MCOs are now responding to employer needs in a variety of ways. Of 135 HMOs surveyed by Milliman and Robertson (Gallagher & Granahan, 1995), 72% had established workers' compensation provider networks. This trend combined with high visibility of rehabilitation in workers' compensation (35% to 40% of all cases) creates a fertile arena for DM and rehabilitation. Those MCOs accustomed to managing disability under group or general health claims are met with a number of confounding obstacles unique to the workers' compensation environment. Effective managed workers' compensation is built on three cornerstones: pre-accident management, DM, and rehabilitation. Rehabilitation providers are routinely involved in all three of these activities (Ryan, 1992).

Injury causality disputes are common in workers' compensation and may invite the professional opinion of a PT or an OT. Work restrictions or limitations associated with RTW determinations also present opportunity. For instance, FCEs play an integral role in facilitating safe worker-worksite matches or in identifying elements of disability.

The high degree of litigation in workers' compensation relative to group health creates an environment for those with medicolegal expertise. MCOs that ignore these ingredients run the risk of losing more employers in the exodus toward self-insurance.

Goals of Disability Management

Early DM efforts were spearheaded by a desire to reduce costs. Today's DM targets newly disabled persons to prevent chronicity, maximize function, enhance worker productivity, reduce cost, and facilitate an earlier RTW.

DM as a coordination of prevention, early intervention, and RTW programs enjoys broad-based support as compared with first-generation "shotgun" approaches or those that focused only on one point along the injury continuum (Beger, 1998; Corcoran & Klett, 1997; Fenelle, 1997; Hintzman & Farrell, 1997).

Why Do Workers Remain Disabled?

Ultimately, all IDM programs strive to maintain or return persons to gainful employment whether they become disabled under STD, LTD, workers' compensation, sick pay, or group health. Therefore it is essential that providers understand why there are low employment rates for persons with disabilities. Only then can a market-driven approach be developed. Table 3–6 contains a partial listing of reasons for these low employment rates. Note that this list does not address the typical medical or treatment issues with which providers often concern themselves: severity, patient age and gender, co-morbidities, secondary diagnoses, and pain level. To the contrary, this list is highly skewed toward psychosocial issues such as access to services, delayed referral, and employer ignorance.

Systems Approach to Disability Management

DM as a "systems approach" implicates not only the worker but also the supervisor, management, and co-workers, who are encumbered with heightened responsibilities and productivity demands when others have disabilities (Smith, 1997). One disabled worker can impose organization-wide morale problems, stress, and absenteeism by proxy. Therefore it behooves the employer to involve a systems approach to disability prevention and management. Disability should not be viewed as an isolated event in the life of the affected person.

 Table 3–6 Reasons for Low Employment Rates Among Persons with Disabilities

- Lack of access to health insurance through the private sector
- Lack of access to personal assistance services
- Stereotypes and discrimination
- Lack of motivation
- Inadequate rehabilitation
- Lack of access to housing
- Lack of access to transportation
- Lack of access to assistive technology
- Employer ignorance
- Non-referral to specialists under managed care
- Failure to accommodate the workplace
- Delayed referral to rehabilitation
- "Treatment" versus "management" approach
- Medical paradigm predominates instead of an independent-living paradigm

The traditional method that employers used in dealing with disability was to remove the involved person from the work environment and to isolate him or her within a highly fragmented health care system. New DM practices recognize the catabolic effect that isolation has on an injured or ill employee. Today's programs strive to keep workers in the workforce or to reintegrate them as quickly as possible, before they become entrenched in the "sick role" through disassociation from their "worker" context. Clinicians recognize that increased activity does not positively correlate with an increase in symptoms (e.g., increased pain) (Vowles & Gross, 2003). Back pain management exemplifies this paradigm shift. For years, conventional wisdom dictated upward of 2 weeks of bed rest. The catabolic effects of bed rest (e.g., reduced cardiac function, decreased muscle performance, reduction in bone density) coupled with the permeation of psychosocial problems often eclipsed the magnitude of the original insult. Prolonged bed rest is virtually unheard of today, because *reactivation* is the operative word. Often, rehabilitation providers do not see these persons until they are fully entrenched in the chronic stage of irritability. Providers find themselves addressing non-physical or organic problems associated with or, in some cases, caused by delayed referral to rehabilitation. This problem is aggravated under managed care as rehabilitation is pushed further down the referral chain. In this system, PCPs are rewarded for cost savings attributed to non-referrals for specialist services. Rehabilitation under this scenario is considered a specialty and, as such, a "discretionary" or "elective" service.

At times, rehabilitation providers under this model become equated with chronic care or specialization, when in fact many of their skills, as well as their knowledge and aptitudes, are appropriate for early intervention during the acute or subacute stages of irritability. Regrettably, DM has traditionally been reserved for chronic or permanent disability cases, some the result of the system itself (Galvin, 1986; Tate et al, 1986).

PCPs, most of whom have little or no theoretical or didactic training in physical rehabilitation, are assigned the task of dealing with one of the largest and most expensive categories of conditions: musculoskeletal. If physical rehabilitation providers are to be included in DM programs, they must educate PCPs about treatment interventions. Specific information that may enlighten PCPs about rehabilitation's role in DM includes the following:

- Rehabilitation admission criteria, which are condition driven
- Clinical evaluation, testing, and assessment methods
- Objective functional measures
- Development of functional diagnoses
- Deciphering of billing and reimbursement codes
- Demonstration of clinical outcome measures with supportive literature
- Condition-driven discharge criteria

What Does the Future Hold?

There are few professionals who are as uniquely trained and competent as PTs and OTs for working with the

 Table 3–7 Projected Disability Population Versus Population Capacity of Rehabilitation Resources

Year	Projected	Possible
2000	2,673,000	1,791,000
2005	2,965,000	1,957,000
2010	3,297,000	2,143,000
2015	3,483,000	2,229,000
2020	3,545,000	2,233,000

Data from Hester EJ, Decelles P, Faimon GR: Return to work: Policy implications. In Fuhrer MJ (ed): Rehabilitation Outcomes Analysis and Measurement. Baltimore, Brooke, 1987, pp 243-254.

musculoskeletal population. These professionals are highly recognized as critical components of many DMs programs, yet Hester et al (1987) prophetically predicted labor shortages through the first two decades of this millennium (Table 3–7).

The second column of Table 3–7 illustrates the projected number of workers within the disability support system through 2020. The third column indicates the manageable population based on available rehabilitation resources, including personnel. The future looks positive under this projection for therapists who covet DM knowledge, experience, and skill sets.

REHABILITATION'S ROLE IN PREVENTION

Employers, especially small to midsize ones, generally do not possess adequate resident knowledge or resources concerning workplace safety and health. This heightens the need for outsourced solutions. Figure 3–5 depicts the percentage of employers that use various interventions for specific conditions. Musculoskeletal conditions are the most prevalent reason for lost work days (Watson Wyatt Worldwide, 1998/1999).

Rehabilitation providers can play a pivotal role in disability prevention through various employer-based health, wellness, and safety programs (Baum, 1995; Kornblau & Ellexson, 1995; Leone 1995; Mistral, 1995). Several experts support ergonomics focused on low back and upper extremity cumulative trauma as particularly fertile areas for prevention services (Anderson, 1995; Melink, 1996; Mital, 1995).

DM programs are not truly integrated without proactive or prevention-based programs (Burns, 1997; Fruen, 1992; Walker et al, 1995). Many of these programs are natural extensions of rehabilitation professionals' fundamental education and training in human anatomy, kinesiology, human physiology, biomechanics, neurophysiology, and orthopedics. Involvement in onsite injury-prevention services not only ensures fewer injuries but also improves RTW decision making through an appropriate worker-worksite match. This matching process can occur following either treatment or the conducting of an FCE.

Rehabilitation's participation in disability prevention programs can be facilitated through a variety of mechanisms, including workers' compensation insurers, self-funded or self-insured employers, various safety counsels,

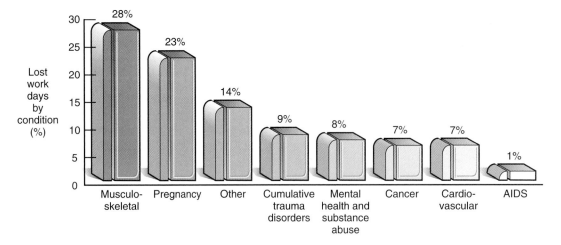

Figure 3–5. Percentage of lost work days by condition. *AIDS,* Acquired immunodeficiency syndrome.

EAPs, ADA, and OSHA. Readers are referred to Chapter 27 for an expanded view of opportunities.

WHAT CONSTITUTES SUCCESSFUL DISABILITY MANAGEMENT?

Cost Data

Ample data are available to support the cost benefits of DM (Beger, 1998; Laabs, 1993; Lewis, 1993; Shamie, 1994; Smith, 1997; Wyatt Watson Worldwide, 1998/1999). Of those large employers (more than 1000 employees) surveyed by Wyatt Watson Worldwide, 42% realized costs savings of 19% of their total disability bill.

The U.S. Department of Labor, Bureau of Labor Statistics reports that for every dollar spent in EAPs, there is a return-on-investment of $16. The seminal studies by Northwestern Life Insurance Company (now ING Financial Services) illustrated that for every dollar spent on rehabilitation, the return-on-investment is approximately $31 (Northwestern Life Insurance Company, 1988). Integrated health care routinely yields savings of approximately 15% from total disability costs (Reith et al, 1995).

One of the best and most-often cited examples of DM savings is reported by Steelcase (Laabs, 1993). This company's underlying principle of DM is that all employees must be treated as management would like to be treated. This approach saved the company more than $24 million between 1986 and 1993. This company essentially cut its average cost per claim by 50%. All of these gains were made without deterioration in quality of care or labor-management relations. This example speaks to the importance of a corporate attitude or culture that fully supports the principles and practices inherent in DM. Positive and negative incentive approaches are often referred to as *carrots and sticks.* A combination of carrots and sticks that maximizes the advantages and minimizes the disadvantages of each provides the most effective long-term solution for disability-related costs. This approach is referred to by some as the *sticks that look like carrots* method (Axene & Lucas, 1996).

Worker-Worksite Matching

The rights of people with disabilities mandates an approach to DM that balances both the economic and the humanistic needs of two important stakeholders in disability: employees and employers (Giordano & D'Alonzo, 1995; Habeck & Hunt, 1999; Owens, 1998).

Evidence suggests that employment, staying on the job, or RTW is the single biggest key to DM (Crook et al, 1998; McKenney, 2000). Simply stated, work is therapeutic!

What Determines Return-to-Work ?

RTW or gainful employment represents an optimal functional outcome measure. Disability prognosticators are important to consider when assessing persons with disabilities. Krause et al (2001) identified 100 different determinants of RTW outcomes through a literature search. Some variables facilitate RTW, whereas others have an inhibitory effect. Because the direct effects of an injury rarely determine RTW status, it is essential for therapists to identify disability prognosticators. Psychosocial or non-medical factors are more prognostic than are medical factors, according to experts (Akabas et al, 1992; Fritz & George, 2002; Galizzi, 1996; Krause et al, 2001; Mitchell, 1998; Suter, 2002).

Worker characteristics and workplace accommodations such as modified or transitional duty have been positively associated with RTW (Roessler & Rumrill, 1993). Efficacy has been established when physical conditioning is combined with a cognitive behavioral approach to DM (Schonstein et al, 2003). Shrey and LaCerte (1995) purport that once the injured worker has moved beyond the acute stage of rehabilitation, the workplace should be considered the therapeutic environment of choice.

The worker-worksite match forms the foundation of a successful DM program. This pairing requires assessment and management of both worker and worksite (Toeppen-Sprigg, 2000). Examination of the worksite is not restricted to the physical plant itself, but incorporates policies and procedures, personnel relationships, corporate culture, and a host of other variables. Availability of workplace accommodations plays a critical role in RTW decisions (Shaw et al, 2001).

Disability prognosticators include the following:

- Low workplace support
- Lack of modified or transitional duty
- Delayed reporting of injury
- Short job tenure
- Prior episodes
- Seniority issues
- Job dissatisfaction
- Injured worker's dislike of the first-line supervisor
- Compensation benefit levels

There is substantial evidence to suggest that, whenever possible, workplaces that do not match a worker's functional capabilities must be modified if long-term or permanent disability is to be avoided (Crook et al, 1998; McKenney, 2000; Shaw et al, 2001; Vierling, 2000; Ward, 2001; Williams & Westmoreland, 2002).

Employers' changes in the work environment serve an important role in work reintegration and account for approximately 80% of workers who resume employment and exit the Social Security disability rolls (Wheeler et al, 2001-2002). Employers who offer prompt and appropriate accommodations can reduce lost time per episode and recidivism or reinjury rates by 50% (Crook et al, 1998; Frank et al, 1998). They also have reduced their safety-related incidents substantially. All of these gains were made without deterioration in quality of care or labor-management relations.

Poor labor-management relations can sabotage a sound DM or rehabilitation program. There is an invaluable lesson here for rehabilitation providers. A patient can make remarkable progress during rehabilitation, which is then undermined by management attitudes and behaviors. Again, rehabilitation providers must be aware of labor-management relations if they are to fully understand the dynamics of recovery, including threats and opportunities. Mills (1995) cites an old adage, "employers get the union they deserve." This quote cuts both ways: An employer that respects its employees in turn has respectful employees. Conversely, employers with cynical or condescending attitudes toward employees spawn disrespectful employees. Unions may also get the kind of employers they deserve. Overly aggressive or greedy unions can contribute to similar behaviors in management.

Clinical skill alone or well-designed jobs may not be enough to overcome barriers to employment erected through poor labor-management relations. Cooperation between workers and management is essential in facilitating RTW (Williams & Westmoreland, 2002).

Rehabilitation interventions that incorporate work conditioning and work hardening have been shown to facilitate restoration of function (Feuerstein et al, 1999; Lemstra & Olszynski, 2003).

There is significant evidence to suggest that disability compensation levels have a negative effect on RTW status and other clinical outcomes (Hee et al, 2002; Lopez et al, 2000; Drew et al, 2001; Atlas et al, 2000). Suter (2002) found that presence of litigation can hamper disability recovery and RTW (Suter 2002).

An expanded discussion of these and other variables associated with disability outcomes can be found in Chapter 7.

Ten Rehabilitation Principles for Disability Management

Education is the bedrock on which DM programs are erected. TEACH CORP is an acronym presented here for the first time as a means of reminding rehabilitation providers of a core skill set—teaching. Rehabilitation providers perhaps spend more time both qualitatively and quantitatively with their patients than do professionals of any other medical profession. Often, a therapist explains a patient's medical condition, a side effect of treatment, or a surgical procedure. This by no means implies that therapists are practicing medicine or usurping the attending physician's power. Instead, therapists practice the art of teaching, because their patients are in acute need of both timely and accurate information. However, teaching is not limited to patients. Therapists routinely teach family members, claims adjusters, corporate nurses and physicians, risk managers, case managers, and others about the varied aspects of physical rehabilitation and DM. Teaching opportunities abound during the pre-injury phase, treatment phase, and post-treatment period or consultation phase of injury or illness.

T	imeliness	*C*	ontinuum
E	ducation	*O*	utcomes
A	ssessment	*R*	esearch
C	ollaboration	*P*	revention
H	abilitation		

Timeliness

Galvin (1985) was among the first rehabilitation professionals to observe that *to delay rehabilitation is to compromise rehabilitation.* Data have shown that early referral to rehabilitation yields better outcomes. Rehabilitation providers can educate employers in using rehabilitation providers in a triage capacity, particularly under workers' compensation directive states. In these states, employers and/or insurers can direct an injured worker to preferred providers. Although a common trait of managed care and general health, this practice is less prevalent in workers' compensation. Those therapists who practice in direct-access states are well positioned to serve in a triage capacity. Perhaps outcomes data from these states will support early intervention as a universal practice!

Education

To truly be successful in DM, rehabilitation providers must educate others regarding their value. This is especially critical in times when rehabilitation interventions are being challenged regarding their efficacy and cost-effectiveness.

This may require a greater understanding of one's audience and their beliefs, values, and perceptions of rehabilitation's role. Therapists who find the time and means to step out of the clinic and into the world of employers, insurers, third-party administrators, case managers, disability managers, attorneys, and health care policy makers enhance their individual and their profession's potential for participation at *every* point along the disability continuum.

Assessment

Disability assessment must precede any treatment or management, because *if you don't measure it, you can't manage it.* Assessment in a DM program transcends impairment and disability determination. Therapists who acquire information about non-medical issues or psychosocial barriers to recovery command a greater understanding of the worker's disability status. In summary, assessment must include the patient's workplace issues, family support structures, psychological response to illness/injury, and compensability of a claim. Non-RTW has been associated with higher psychosocial morbidity (Mason et al, 2002).

Continuum

The disability continuum offers an opportunity for PTs and OTs to offer their expertise in the health-wellness-prevention; treatment; and post-treatment, or consultation, stages (Isernhagen, 1992). Table 3-8 demonstrates the diversity of skills, knowledge, and aptitude that a therapist competent in upper extremity musculoskeletal management possesses.

Habilitation

Physical rehabilitation has operated predominantly under the notion of restoration or rehabilitation of health (Remenyi, 1995). Although both a desirable and a noble goal, full restoration of function may not be feasible. DM strives to maximize function, although function may be well short of a person's pre-morbid functional status. Shifting the focus to workplace accommodation may be the most realistic approach to DM.

Collaboration

Successful rehabilitation within a DM paradigm requires collaboration both within and beyond provider ranks. Employers, insurers, case managers, attorneys, and employees operate from different paradigms and belief structures, which must be understood and taken into account. Partnering with other medical professionals, including psychologists, psychiatrists, sociologists, and vocational specialists, may require acquisition of new knowledge and skill sets.

Outcomes

DM outcomes are multidimensional and include both clinical and financial measures. These outcomes may be influenced only partly by the patient's condition and provider's interventions. Again, worker-workplace interactions must be considered for successful outcomes (Brines et al, 1999). However, providers are cautioned about the use of RTW as a stable outcome measure because of the high recurrence of injury. RTW may not be a stable outcome measure of a DM program (Butler et al, 1995). Enriched disability compensation programs can discourage full participation and compromise outcomes of vocational rehabilitation programs (Drew et al, 2001).

Research

Providers are encouraged to conduct periodic literature reviews, to convene practice consensus panels, and to conduct clinical trials pertaining to their interventions. Delineation of what works from what does not work is critical to ensuring the integrity of one's practice and profession. Research fuels innovations in treatment and DM.

Prevention

There is a growing role for rehabilitation providers in the realm of injury and illness prevention. This may not involve the acquisition of new knowledge and skills sets as much as an attitudinal adjustment. Therapists covet inherent knowledge and skill sets that simply have to be unleashed in a preventive mode.

 Table 3-8 An Example of the Diversity of Skills Needed by an OT and PT in the Treatment of an Upper Extremity Musculoskeletal Disorder

Prevention	Treatment	Consultation
Ergonomic analysis	Acute-stage antiinflammatory modalities	Functional capacity evaluation
Post-offer functional screening	Therapeutic exercise	Functional job analysis
Cumulative trauma education and training for employees	Work conditioning and work hardening	Job accommodation or reasonable accommodations
Employer/insurer educational modules	Assistive technology and adaptive equipment	ADA and OSHA compliance

ADA, Americans with Disabilities Act of 1990; *OSHA*, Occupational Safety and Health Administration.

CONCLUSION

DM requires a paradigm shift on the part of providers, as well as on the part of employers and employees. It is especially critical that providers embrace a collaborative approach to DM. Providers who wish to be successful within IDM systems must accept that they are not simply rehabilitation professionals who occupy a niche within the treatment model. In doing so, these providers may lose their relevancy as DM continues to evolve. Instead, rehabilitation providers can serve as disability managers engaged in a collaborative, versus an isolationist, approach.

Patients are not the only customers. A "management" mindset displaces a "treatment" mindset when describing the provider's future role in DM. When this occurs, disability prevention and consultation occupy their rightful place alongside treatment and DM.

Last, physical rehabilitation has an amazing opportunity to flourish within DM programs; however, this may require abandonment of some traditional ways of viewing one's profession. When asked, "What do you do for a living?" therapists may wish to choose alternative responses to "I'm a PT" or "I'm an OT," because these labels merely describe one's professional training and licensure but fail to fully articulate the potential for a more expanded role in disability prevention and DM. The new paradigm may sound something like this, "What do you do for a living?" "I prevent, manage, and provide consultation regarding disability. Oh, and I happen to be a physical therapist!"

REFERENCES

Accum C, Bellman M: Relieving the pain of disability costs. Group Insurance Solutions Jan:19-23, 1996.

Akabas S, Gates L, Galvin D: Disability Management: A Complete System to Reduce Costs, Increase Productivity, Meet Employee Needs and Ensure Legal Compliance. New York, American Management Association, 1992.

Anderson MA: Ergonomics: Analyzing Work from a Physiological Perspective. In Isernhagen SJ (ed): The Comprehensive Guide to Work Injury Management. Gaithersburg, MD, Aspen, 1995, pp 3-39.

Atlas SJ, Chang Y, Kammann E: Long-term disability and return to work among patients who have herniated lumbar disc: The effect of disability compensation. J Bone Joint Surg Am 82(1):4-15, 2000.

Axene DV, Lucas OM: Research Report: Provider Incentives in the Optimally Managed Delivery System. Seattle, WA, Milliman & Robertson, Inc., 1996, pp 1-13.

Baum B: Working with the workers: The "buy in" to maintenance of wellness. In Isernhagen SJ (ed): The Comprehensive Guide to Work Injury Management. Gaithersburg, MD, Aspen, 1995, pp 254-263.

Beger SS: Disability trends and management. Broker World 18(3): 16-20, 1998.

Bousquet C: Integrated disability benefits plans on the rise. National Underwriter 96(38):20-21, 1992.

Brines J, Salazaar MK, Graham KY: Return to work experience of injured workers in a case management program. Am Assn Occup Health Nurses 47(8):365-372, 1999.

Bureau of Labor Statistics (BLS): Survey of occupational injuries and illnesses: 1998. Washington, DC, US Department of Labor, BLS, 1999.

Burns J: This coalition has some big shoes to fill. Managed Healthcare 7(10):56, 1997.

Butler RJ, Johnson WG, Baldwin ML: Managing work disability: Why first return to work is not a measure of success. Ind Labor Relations Rev 48:452-469, 1995.

Ceniceros R: Disability integration makes slow gains study shows. Business Insurance 32(16):1, 1998.

Clifton DW: Critical issues for determining work hardening outcomes. PT Pract 1(3):52-60, 1992.

Clifton DW: Payor-provider alliances. Rehabil Manage: The Interdisciplinary J Rehabil 9(5):100-102, 1996.

Cohen T: STD/LTD integration points the way to future. National Underwriter 102(2):9-10, 1998.

Corcoran TR, Klett TE: Managed disability: Past, present and future. Benefits Q 13(4):8-13, 1997.

Crook J, Moldofsky H, Shannon H: Determinants of disability after work-related musculoskeletal injury. J Rheumatol 25(8):454-1456, 1998.

Drew D, Drebing CE, Van Orner A, et al: Effects of disability compensation on participation in and outcomes of vocational rehabilitation. Psychiatr Serv 52(11):1421, 2001.

Fenelle C: New trends and approaches: Keeping track of disability management. Risk Management 44(6):76, 1997.

Feuerstein M, Burrell LM, Miller VI et al: Clinical management of carpal tunnel syndrome: A 12-year review of outcomes. Am J Ind Med 35(3):232-245, 1999.

Fletcher M: Disability management integration growing. Business Insurance 10(12):92, 1997.

Frank J, Sinclair S, Hogg-Johnson S et al: Preventing disability from work-related low-back pain. New evidence gives new hope—if we can just get all the players onside. Can Med Assn J 166(158):1625-1631, 1998.

Fritz JM, George SZ: Identifying psychosocial variables in patients with acute work-related low back pain: The importance of fear-avoidance beliefs. Phys Ther 82(10):973-983, 2002.

Fruen M: Disability management focuses on prevention. Business & Health 10(12):24-29, 1992.

Galizzi M, Boden LI: What are the most important factors shaping return to work? Evidence from Wisconsin Workers' Compensation Research Institute. Cambridge, MA, 1996, Wisconsin Workers' Compensation Research Institute.

Gallagher PA, Granahan WL: HMO Managed Workers' Compensation Strategies and Products. Report on the Second Annual Milliman & Robertson Survey. Seattle, WA, Milliman & Robertson, Inc, 1995.

Galvin DE: Employer-based disability management and rehabilitation programs. In Pan EL et al (eds): Annual Review of Rehabilitation, vol. New York, Springer, 1985.

Galvin DE: Health promotion, disability management, and rehabilitation in the workplace. Rehabil Lit 47:218-223, 1986.

Giordano G, D'Alonzo BJ: Challenge and progress in rehabilitation: A review of the past 25 years and a preview of the future. Am Rehabil 21(3):14-21, 1995.

Habeck R: Differentiating disability management and rehabilitation: A distinction worth making. NARPPS J 11(2):8-20, 1996.

Habeck RV, Hunt HA: Disability management perspectives: Developing accommodating work environments through disability management. Am Rehabil 25(2):18-25, 1999.

Hahn H: Alternative views of empowerment: Social services and civil rights. J Rehabil 57(4):17-19, 1991.

Hee HT, Whitecloud TS III, Myers L et al: Do worker's compensation patients with neck pain have lower SF-36 scores? Eur Spine J 11(4):375-381, 2002.

Hergenrader R: Hands-on disability management on the rise. National Underwriter 101(7):8-10, 1997.

Hester EJ, Decelles P, Faimon GR: Return to work: Policy implications. In Fuhrer MJ (ed): Rehabilitation Outcomes Analysis and Measurement. Baltimore, Brooke, 1987, pp 243-254.

Hintzman D, Farrell C: The benefits of a partnership approach to disability management. Benefits Q 13(4):14-18, 1997.

Huffman D, Johnson C: Developing work injury disability provider networks. Risk Manage 41(11):49-56, 1994.

Hursch NC: Essential competencies in industrial rehabilitation and disability management practice: A skills-based training model. In Shrey DE, LaCerte M (eds): Principles and Practices of Disability Management in Industry. Winter Park, FL, GR Press, 1995, pp 303-352.

Isernhagen D: The continuum of care in industrial physical therapy. Orthopaedic Phys Therapy Clin North Am 1(1):7-14, 1992.

Kendall NA: Psychosocial approaches to the prevention of chronic pain: The low back paradigm. Bailleres Best Pract Res Clin Rheumatol 13(3):545-554, 1999.

Kenney D, Powell NJ, Reynolds-Lynch K: Trends in industrial rehabilitation, ergonomics and cumulative trauma disorders. WORK 5(2): 133-142, 1995.

Kornblau BL, Ellexson MT: Reasonable accommodation and the Americans with Disabilities Act. In Isernhagen SJ (ed): The Comprehensive Guide to Work Injury Management. Gaithersburg, MD, Aspen, 1995, pp 781-795.

Krause N, Dasinger LK, Deegan LJ et al: Psychosocial job factors and return-to-work after compensated low back injury: a disability phase-specific analysis. Am J Ind Med 40(4):374-392, 2001.

Kunnes R, Hellwig VM: Reaching the final frontier: Managing disability gives employers newfound opportunity to control costs. Business Insurance, Aug 21, 1995, p 13.

Laabs J: Steelcase slashes workers' comp costs. Personnel J 72(2):72-73, 1993.

Lechner DE: Work hardening and work conditioning interventions: do they affect disability? Phys Ther 74(5):471-493, 1994.

Lemstra M, Olszynski WP: The effectiveness of standard care, early intervention, and occupational management in workers' compensation claims. Spine J 28(3):299-304, 2003.

Leone FH: Developing an occupational medicine programs and systems. In Isernhagen SJ (ed): The Comprehensive Guide to Work Injury Management. Gaithersburg, MD, Aspen, 1995, pp 613-633.

Lerner JR: The new direction in disability management. Business & Health 16(10):36-45, 1998.

Lewin D, Schecter S: Four factors lower disability rates. Personnel J November:14, 1995.

Lewis L: Employers place more emphasis on managing employee stress. Business & Health 11(2):46-50, 1993.

Lipow VA: Aging workers: Disability management strategies. Rehabil Manage 10(1):3234,36, 1997.

Lopez JG, Ernst MD, Wright TW: Acromioplasty: comparison of outcome in patients with and without workers' compensation. J Southern Orthop Assn 9(4):262-266, 2000.

Lukes E, Wachs JE: Keys to disability management. AAOHN J 44(3):141-147, 1996.

Mason S, Wardrope J, Turpin G et al: Outcomes after injury: A comparison of workplace and nonworkplace injury. J Trauma 53(1):98-103, 2002.

Matthes K: Companies have the ability to manage disability. Human Resource Focus 69(4):3, 1992.

McKenney S: Working with industry: Matching the work and worker. WORK 15(2):121-124, 2000.

McShulkis E: Integrated health care services slash costs. Human Resource (HR) Magazine 42(8):27, 1997.

Melnik MS: Upper extremity injury prevention. In Key GL (ed): Industrial Therapy. St Louis, Mosby, 1996, pp 148-180.

Mills D: Building joint labor-management initiatives for worksite disability management. In Shrey DE, LaCerte M (eds): Principles and Practices of Disability Management in Industry. Winter Park, FL, GR Press, 1995, pp 225-247.

Mistal M: Establishing an industrial prevention program. In Isernhagen SJ (ed): The Comprehensive Guide to Work Injury Management. Gaithersburg, MD, Aspen, 1995, pp 118-126.

Mital A: Ergonomics, injury prevention, and disability management. In Shrey DE, LaCerte M (eds): Principles and Practices of Disability Management in Industry. Winter Park, FL, GR Press, 1995, pp 157-171.

Mitchell K: Working with the employer organization as client. Presented at Second Disability Managers Conference, 1998.

Nelson W: Workers' compensation: 1984-1991 benchmark revision. Soc Secur Bull 55:365-390, 1991.

Northwestern Life Insurance Company: Second chance: Rehabilitating the American worker. Minneapolis, Northwestern Life Insurance Company, March 1988.

Owens P: Integrated health and disability management in the workplace. Compensation and Benefits 13(3):31-36, 1998.

Pain K, Dunn M, Anderson G: Quality of life: What does it mean in rehabilitation? J Rehabil 64(2):5-11, 1998.

Polatin P et al: A psychosociomedical prediction model of response to treatment by chronically disabled workers with low-back pain. Spine 14(9):956-961, 1989.

Quinn P: Social work and disability management policy: Yesterday, today and tomorrow. Social Work in Healthcare 20(3):67-82, 1995.

Raman S, Levi SJ: Concepts of disablement in documents guiding physical therapy practice. Disabil Rehabil 24(15):790-797, 2002.

Reith L, Ahrens A, Cummings D: Integrated disability management: Taking a coordinated approach to managing employee disabilities. AAOHN J 43(5):270-275, 1995.

Remenyi AG: An international view of older workers and work disability: Trends and implications for occupational rehabilitation. In Shrey DE & Lacerte M (eds), Principles and Practices of Disability Management in Industry. Winter Park, FL, 1995, GR Press, pp 555-602.

Roessler RT, Rumrill PD Jr: Enhancing productivity of your job! The "win-win" approach to reasonable accommodations. Fayetteville, AR, 1993, Arkansas Research and Training Center in Vocational Rehabilitation.

Rosenthal DA, Olsheski JA: Disability management and rehabilitation counseling: Present and future opportunities. J Rehabil 65(1):31-38, 1999.

Rhomberg S, Wolf L, Evanoff B: An integrated program for the prevention and management of musculoskeletal work injuries. WORK 5(2):115-122, 1995.

Ryan J: A broad brush approach to managed care. Risk Manage 39(6):46-52, 1992.

Saunders RL, Anderson MA: Early treatment intervention in industrial physical therapy. Orthop Phys Ther Clin North Am 1(1):67-74, 1992.

Schonstein E et al: Work conditioning, work hardening and functional restoration for workers with back and neck pain. In: The Cochrane Library: The Cochrane Database of Systematic Reviews (Complete Reviews), (1): CD001822, www.ncbi.n/m.nih. gov, accessed March 27, 2003.

Shaw WS, Feuerstein M, Lincoln AE: Case management services for work related upper extremity disorders. Integrating workplace accommodation and problem solving. Am Assn Occup Health Nurses J 49(8):378-389, 2001.

Schwartz G et al: The disability management sourcebook. Washington, DC, Washington Business Group on Health, 1989.

Shamie L: EAPs and disability management. Employee Assistance Programs. EAP Digest, September:1994.

Shaw WS, Fuerstein M, Lincoln AE et al: Case management services for work related upper extremity disorders. Integrating workplace accommodation and problem solving. Am Assn Occup Health Nurses J 49(8):378-389, 2001.

Shrey DE: Worksite disability management model for effective return-to-work planning. Occup Med 15(4):789-801, 2000.

Shrey DE, LaCerte M (eds): Principles and Practices of Disability Management in Industry. Winter Park, FL, GR Press, 1995.

Smith D: Implementing disability management: A review of basic concepts and essential components. Employee Assistance Q 12(4):37-50, 1997.

Strosahl K, Johnson P: Tactical teamwork: The new direction of disability management. Business and Health 16(12):21-24, 1998.

Stucki G: Understanding disability. Ann Rheum Dis 62:289-290, 2003.

Suter PB: Employment and litigation: Improved by work, assisted by verdict. Pain J 100(3):249-257, 2002.

Tate DG: Workers' disability and return to work. Am J Phys Med Rehabil 71:92-96, 1992.

Tate DG, Habeck RV, Schwartz G: Disability management: A comprehensive framework for prevention and rehabilitation in the workplace. Rehabil Lit 47:230-235, 1986.

Toeppen-Sprigg B: Importance of job analysis with functional capacity matching in medical case management: A physician's perspective. WORK 15(2):133-137, 2000.

Tortarolo JS, Polakoff PL: The future of disability management is ... integration. Benefits Q 11(3):49-55, 1995.

Vance SR, Brown AM: On-site medical care and physical therapy impact. In Isernhagen SJ (ed): The Comprehensive Guide to Work Injury Management. Gaithersburg, MD, Aspen, 1995, pp 269-279.

Vash CL: Improving disability management in the workplace. Insurance implications. J Insur Med 23(2):112-115, 1991.

Vierling L: The Americans with Disability Act: implications of Supreme Court decisions for case managers. Case Manager J 11(1):47-49, 2000.

Vowles KE, Gross RT: Work-related beliefs about injury and physical capability for work in individuals with chronic pain. Pain 101(3):291-298, 2003.

Walker JM: Understanding disability: A lexicon. Risk Manage 45(11):14-22, 1998.

Walker JM, Heile G, Heffner F: 10 Tips for disability management programs. Risk Manage 42(6):57-61, 1995.

Ward MD: Unum Provident's WorkRX program manages lost time. Case Manager J 12(5):32, 2001.

Watson RM, Huban SP: Managing disabilities in an integrated health environment: The experience of Aetna. Benefits Q 13(4):65-71, 1997.

Watson Wyatt Worldwide Third Annual Report: "Staying @ Work" 1998/99, Bethesda, MD, Watson Wyatt Worldwide, 1998/1999, p 2, www.watsonwyatt.com.

Wheeler PM, Kearney JR, Harrison CA: The U.S. study of work incapacity and reintegration. Soc Security Bull 64(1):32-44, 2001-2002.

Williams RM, Westmoreland M: Perspectives on workplace disability management: A review of the literature. WORK 19(1):87-93, 2002.

Winslow R: Aetna program aims to get workers on disability back on job more quickly. Wall Street J, September 9, 1999.

Wolfe BL, Haveman R: Trends in the prevalence of work disability from 1962-1984, and their correlates. Milbank Q 68(1):53-80, 1990.

SUGGESTED READINGS

Falvo D: Medical and psychosocial aspects of chronic illness and disability, ed. 2, Gaithersburg, MD, Aspen, 1999.

National Institute of Disability Management and Research: Occupational standards in disability management, Port Alberni, British Columbia, 1999, http://www.nidmar.ca, accessed 1999.

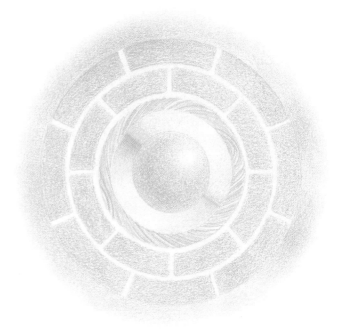

CHAPTER 4

Disability Management in Long-Term Care

David W. Clifton, Jr., PT

"Skills to meet those requirements [older Americans] are often as much 'high touch' as 'high tech', based as much in common sense and emotional intelligence as in the reductionistic simplistic approach to problem-solving that dominates scientific medicine, and require deep commitment to the humanistic, holistic, and ethical dimensions of patient care, including acceptance of and expertise in care of the very old, frail and often dying."

- Hazzard et al, 1997

Health care benefits are generally poorly understood by current and potential beneficiaries, as well as by providers. It is incumbent that rehabilitation providers better understand the benefit structures that either directly or indirectly affect their services. This chapter strives to demystify elements of Medicare, Medicaid, and Social Security Disability Insurance (SSDI) programs. However, it is likely that by the time this book is published, rules, procedures, and benefits structures once again will have evolved. Change and uncertainty appear to be the norm, especially in publicly sponsored health care benefits. Providers who have a command of insurance benefit language, policy inclusions and exclusions, and appeal processes are better positioned to serve their patients both as a caregiver and as ombudsman.

KEY POINTS

- Disability prevention programs will play an increasingly important role in disability management. These programs will use physical rehabilitation providers in the following roles: educational, consultative, and mentoring, and as ombudsman.
- Rehabilitation professionals should recognize the contribution of non-physical-function (e.g., psychosocial function) domains on disability status and disposition.

- Management of multiple chronic disorders has emerged as a central paradigm in geriatrics. This is a departure from health care's traditional focus on single disease interventions.
- A "Disability Management Triad" that addresses the interface of an individual's function, assistive devices, and environment offers a more holistic approach to disability.
- Payers, especially government-based funding sources, continue to encourage the use of function-based outcome measures.
- Funding sources will provide opportunities for rehabilitation providers to participate more fully in disability determinations. Rehabilitation providers will augment the role of physicians in benefits (e.g., Social Security Disability Insurance), eligibility determinations, medical necessity decisions, and treatment setting recommendations.
- Emerging demographics combined with the knowledge, experience, and skill sets of physical rehabilitation providers will fuel the renewal of rehabilitation, especially when directed at chronic conditions. These groups have been largely ignored, underserved, or poorly served by managed care organizations (MCOs) that have tended to focus on acute hospital-based care.

Operational Definitions

Long-Term Care	Medical care, health care, personal care, social care, and supportive services rendered to individuals with chronic conditions or those in the postacute phase of irritability who have lost the ability for self-care and who typically receive services in nursing facilities, assisted-living centers, subacute care centers, and home care.
Subacute Care	Care that falls between acute care and chronic care; comprehensive inpatient care rendered as an alternative to acute hospitalization for acute illness or injury or for exacerbation of a disease process.
Independent-Living Model	A treatment model that deemphasizes a focus on an individual's anatomical or physiological impairment and that instead focuses on social functioning and the human-environment interface.
Patient-Centered Practice	A model of care delivery that considers the holistic needs and responsibilities of the patient versus the traditional regionalization approach to medicine and rehabilitation. Patient-centered practice examines and addresses non-medical domains beyond just physical function (e.g., psychosocial issues).
Mandated Assessment	State or federal government-mandated assessments that focus principally on physical function, which is used to establish patient eligibility for institutionalization, typically in nursing facilities or long-term-care facilities.

FOCUS ON FUNCTION

Society has elected to support disabled individuals partly through government-sponsored health care funding and delivery mechanisms. Regrettably, as well-intentioned as these initiatives are, there are always individuals who are underserved or poorly served. This problem is not going to vanish easily, because of a phenomenon known as *demographic shock* (Table 4–1).

Aging citizens in today's U.S. health care systems face a conundrum of logistical challenges. Fragmentation of services, including trips to numerous providers, durable medical equipment suppliers, and laboratories, frustrates many individuals who are trapped between acute care and long-term care.

Function-Function-Function

"Location, location, location" may ensure success in real estate, but "function, function, function" is a requirement

 Table 4–1 Demographic Shock

- Early retirement
- Baby boomers followed by fewer tax-paying workers
- Increased life expectancy
- Growth in chronic illnesses and conditions
- Decline in employer contributions to private insurance

Data from Burman L, Penner R, Steuerle G et al: Policy changes posed by the Aging of America Urban Institute, 1998, www.urban.org, accessed September 14, 2000.

for success in disability management. Without question, the most distinguishing feature of physical rehabilitation is its focus on function. Few medical disciplines possess the skills, knowledge, or aptitude that rehabilitation professionals possess in terms of functional assessment and the design of functionally based programs.

The assessment of physical functioning is one of the most critical aspects of long-term care (Schmid, 1998). Securing a physical rehabilitation assessment is especially challenging in persons with chronic conditions, particularly when mental conditions are involved. Long-term care relies heavily on these assessments for the determination of eligibility and payment for services. These assessments often form the basis for care planning, yet many beneficiaries are not expeditiously referred to qualified providers. Some attribute this problem to a stark, historical underrepresentation of geriatrics in medical education and training in the United States (Hazzard et al, 1997).

Ideally, a long-term–care assessment is multidisciplinary and considers a person's physical functioning, affect, social function, cognition, pain, discomfort, and satisfaction. This cluster is referred to as *quality-of-life* (QOL) indicators (Kane & Kane, 2000). A QOL approach may require a paradigm shift for some therapists accustomed to uni-disciplinary practice with a focus on impairments, not on holistic assessment.

EDUCATED PATIENTS AND CONSUMERS

Long-Term–Care Benefits

"If consumers do not understand their choices and do not have the information to successfully navigate their health care delivery systems, their potential for receiving high quality care is diminished from the outset."

- Hibberd et al, 1998

Research has shown that few beneficiaries are well-informed about their choices, and most of them derive their information from health maintenance organization (HMO) advertisements or through word-of-mouth (Hibberd et al, 1998). Some Medicare enrollees falsely view HMOs and fee-for-service (FFS) as offering essentially the same benefit structures and choices despite their obvious differences. The choice between Medicare supplemental plans, also known as Medicare +, has been described as "mind numbing" (Hibberd et al, 1998). This poises a critical question that each rehabilitation provider must ask himself or herself:

Are health care providers professionally obligated to educate beneficiaries about their benefit plans so that they can become more informed consumers of health care services?

or

Does this responsibility belong to the patient, his or her family and friends, or advocacy groups, such as the AARP (American Association of Retired Persons)?

Every clinician must answer these questions from his or her unique perspective. However, uninformed patients may suffer the consequences when providers fail to enlighten them. Rehabilitation providers may at a minimum be responsible for educating Medicare beneficiaries about what constitutes medical necessity, skilled services, and maintenance care.

When insurance plans require co-payments or deductibles, providers are obligated to inform patients of their financial responsibility before commencement of care. This responsibility falls under one's business contract or fiduciary duty, not under one's professional or clinical ethics.

Table 4–2 provides a sample of free Medicare publications that can assist consumers and providers in better understanding long-term–care benefits and help providers convey the benefits to their patients. These materials are general in nature. Of course, current benefits data must be analyzed on a case-by-case or patient-by-patient basis.

MEDICARE OVERVIEW

Congress created Medicare in 1965 as a national health care program for seniors and disabled persons. Medicare rules and regulations are established by the Centers for Medicare & Medicaid Services (CMS), formerly known as the Health Care Financing Administration (HCFA). Daily claims administration operations are handled by fiscal intermediaries (FIs), such as Blue Cross Plans, Aetna, or other health care insurers. The CMS is organized around the following three centers with distinct roles:

- The Center for Beneficiary Choices, which focuses on Medicare + Choice programs
- The Center for Medicare Management, which focuses on the traditional Medicare program
- The Center for Medicaid and State Operations, which focuses on state-administered programs

Beneficiary Financial Responsibility

Medicare is an insurance program like managed care that involves beneficiaries in at-risk contracts. For instance, in 1998 Medicare beneficiaries paid, on average, $2600 in out-of-pocket expenses for co-insurance, deductibles, and premiums. This is an enormous sum of money, considering that more than half (54%) of all beneficiaries are on fixed incomes, earning less than $15,000 a year

 Table 4–2 Free Medicare Publications

- Does Your Doctor or Supplier Accept Assignment?
- Guide to Choosing a Nursing Home
- Guide to Health Insurance for People with Medicare
- Health Plan Comparison Information
- Learning about Medicare Health Plans
- Medicare Coverage of Kidney Dialysis
- Medicare Health Plan Quality and Satisfaction Information
- Medicare Home Health Care Services
- Medicare Hospice Services
- Medicare Supplemental Insurance (Medigap) Policies and Protections
- Medicare & You (available in English, in Spanish, on audiotape, and in Braille)
- Worksheet for Comparing Medicare Health Plans
- Your Guide to Medicare Medical Savings Accounts
- Your Guide to Private Fee-for-Service Plans

Contact information: Telephone (800)633-4227; Website, www.medicare.gov.

(Medicare: New Choices, New Worries, 1998). Rehabilitation providers must be prudent in the delivery of care, ensuring that it is medically necessary, reasonable in cost, and requires skilled services, especially in light of the financial strain imposed on senior citizens and those with disabilities.

Medicare Parts A and B

Medicare has two principal parts. Part A is financed through a payroll tax, whereas Part B is funded through general government revenues in addition to beneficiary premium payments. Part A, also known as *Hospital Insurance (HI),* covers hospital stays in semiprivate rooms, nursing (except private-duty nursing), and medical expenses. Skilled nursing facility (SNF) care, including rehabilitation services, is also funded. Rehabilitation consumes an increasing portion of the Medicare dollar (Figure 4–1).

SNF stays must follow a hospitalization of at least 3 days to be covered. Home health services are available, including ancillary care in the form of physical therapy and speech-language therapy. Medicare-approved hospice services are covered under Part A.

Figure 4–2 depicts the steady decline over a 24–year period (1972 to 1996) of Medicare funding for short-stay hospital payments. This reduction in overall funding is in direct conflict with an increasing life expectancy and aging of Americans.

Part B is referred to as *Medical Insurance (MI)* and funds physician visits, outpatient rehabilitation (physical, occupational, and speech and language therapy), ambulatory surgery, and durable medical equipment. The Balanced Budget Act (BBA) of 1997 changed Medicare reimbursement for outpatient rehabilitation by imposing an arbitrary limit of $1500. This provision established caps of $1500 on occupational therapy and $1500 on physical therapy and speech-language pathology combined. For example, a patient falls and breaks her hip, requiring physical therapy. Once the $1500 cap is reached, no additional therapy would be reimbursed in that calendar year, even in the event that she suffers a stroke. Fortunately, this cap has been repealed.

Home health care is also covered under Part B, provided certain conditions are met. Part B also finances a host of preventive services, including bone mass measurements, colorectal cancer screening, diabetes monitoring, mammogram screening, Pap smear and pelvic examinations, prostate cancer screening, and vaccinations. An assortment of other services is covered under Part B, including chiropractic, orthotics and prosthetics, emergency care, clinical psychology, and diagnostic testing. Twenty-percent deductibles are routine expenses for beneficiaries in addition to their premium payments (Table 4–3, p. 55).

Most Medicare beneficiaries do not pay monthly premiums for Part A, but in 1999, beneficiaries paid a total of $768 for a hospital stay of 1 to 60 days, $192 per day for days 61 to 90, and $384 per day for days 91 to 150 (HCFA, 1999). Scheduled benefits are always subject to policy changes; however, in 1999, Medicare fully covered 20 days in SNFs and paid $95.50 per day from 21 to 100 days. Medicare paid nothing after 100 SNF days.

Part A can be viewed as analogous to Blue Cross, whereas Part B is analogous to Blue Shield plans. In 1999,

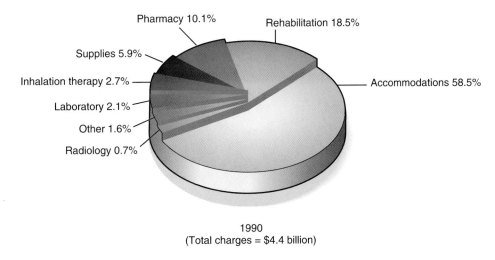

1990
(Total charges = $4.4 billion)

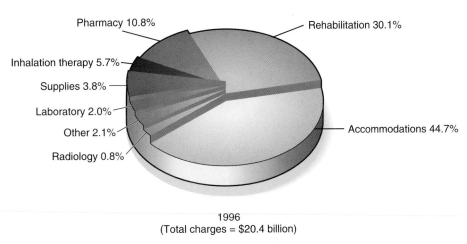

1996
(Total charges = $20.4 billion)

NOTE: Medicare program payment data are not available by type of service.

Figure 4–1. Percent distribution of Medicare skilled nursing facility charges by type of service: Calendar years 1990 and 1996. (Data from Healthcare Financing Administration [HCFA], Office of Information Services. Data developed by the Office of Strategic Planning, HCFA Financing Review, 1998 Statistical Supplement.)

Part B involved a $45.50 per-month premium along with deductibles, co-insurance, or co-payments. Under Part B, Medicare pays 80% or the "allowable charge," and the beneficiary pays 20%.

Medigap plans are supplemental Medicare plans regulated at the state level that help beneficiaries finance the deductibles in Parts A and B. Most states adopt the regulations of the National Association of Insurance Commissioners (NAIC).

Medicare Part C: Medicare + Choice

The BBA of 1997 established a new Medicare Part C, commonly known as *Medicare + Choice*. This supplemental coverage offers an option to Medicaid, Medigap, and other retiree plans. According to the Physician Payment Review Commission (PPRC), only 10% of all seniors are without supplemental plans that augment the coverage of Parts A and B (PPRC, 1997).

Nugent (1996) provides a comprehensive description of four types of "Medicare + Choice" plans offered by MCOs:

1. Risk-based models involve HMOs and capitation reimbursement. This is the most prevalent Medicare + Choice model. Nugent provides an example from the reimbursement structure for this model. The HMO receives payment based on utilization rates. These plans reimburse providers on a per-capita basis using a formula called the *adjusted average per-capita cost* (AAPCC). The AAPCC is based on a 5-year weighted average of fee-for-service (FFS) costs in a given county. A Medicare HMO is then reimbursed at a flat 95% of the calculated AAPCC. This calculation assumes that the HMO is 5% more efficient than an FFS plan. In reality, this simply has not been the case, and subsequently, there has been a mass exodus of HMOs from the Medicare market (Benko, 2000; Medicare HMO

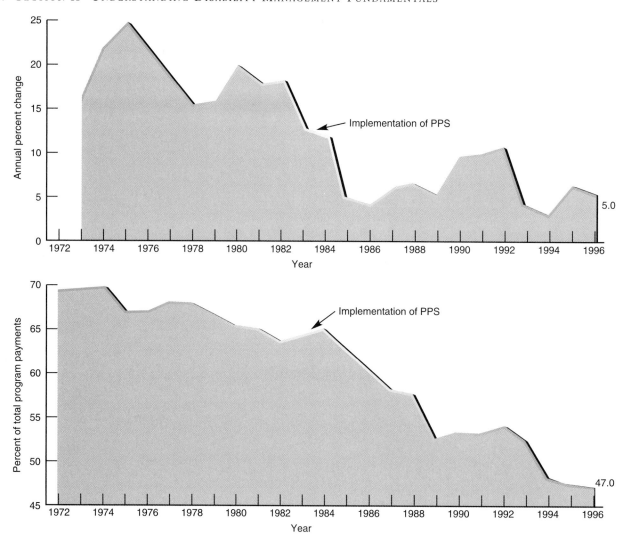

Figure 4–2. Changes in Medicare short-stay hospital program payments: Calendar years 1972 to 1996. (Data from Healthcare Financing Administration [HCFA], Office of Information Services. Data developed by the Office of Strategic Planning, HCFA Financing Review, 1998 Statistical Supplement.) *PPS*, Prospective payment system.

Data Report, 2000). Sixty-five Medicare + Choice HMOs elected to withdrawal contracts, and 53% reduced their service areas, affecting nearly 1 million beneficiaries (Medicare HMO Data Report, 2000). All Medicare beneficiaries who are dropped from Medicare HMOs may return to traditional FFS models. Several insurers (Aetna, Cigna, Foundation Health Plan, Humana, Oxford Health Plan, Pacificare, United Healthcare, and Anthem Blue Cross) have either abandoned markets altogether or dramatically curtailed offerings.

2. Cost-based HMOs pay on a cost-related basis, provided that care is rendered by an affiliated provider.
3. Selected preferred provider organizations (PPOs) are also paid on a cost basis, but they provide limited coverage for non-affiliated provider services.
4. Residual categories describe those plans that are typically operated by businesses, MCOs, or labor organizations.

These health care prepayment plans are also known as *social HMOs.* Membership is more exclusive than in other models.

The aforementioned models may use the same preferred provider networks for both group or general health and long-term care. This practice is generally fraught with problems, because long-term care involves chronic conditions, whereas group health focuses on acute conditions. Long-term care also involves older persons who may have secondary diagnoses or co-morbidities. Group health is principally managed by primary care physicians (PCPs) who are generalists. Long-term care demands specialized providers.

In general, HMOs have had a modicum of success in restraining acute care costs but have failed miserably at controlling costs associated with postacute and chronic conditions. These cases are principally treated in SNFs,

Table 4–3 Stakeholder Responsibilities Associated with Medicare

Fiscal Intermediary
- Determine allowable cost and reimbursement amounts
- Maintain records
- Establish quality controls
- Assist in fraud and abuse initiatives
- Conduct focused and random medical record reviews and audits

Providers/Suppliers
- Establish medical necessity of care
- Demonstrate reasonable care
- Maintain sound functionally based clinical documentation
- Avoid and report potential fraud and abuse

Beneficiaries
- Pay appropriate premiums and deductibles
- Avoid and report potential fraud and abuse
- Actively participate in the health care plan

Data modified from Waid MO: Overview of the Medicare and Medicaid Programs, Health Care Financing Review, 1998 Statistical Supplement.

 Table 4–4 Controlling Utilization: How Does Medicare Evaluate a Coverage Issue?

Step 1	An internal evaluation of the issue is conducted: • Medical literature review • Review of other HCFA/Medicare documentation • Consultation with other federal agencies • Consultation with HCFA contractors
Step 2	A recommendation is made secondary to staff review and research
	or
Step 3	The issue is referred to the Advisory Committee process (Federal Advisory Committee Act)
Step 4	The issue is referred to an independent or unbiased technology-assessment organization: • Medical literature review • Consultation with other federal agencies or health programs • Consultation with HCFA contractors • Consultation with interested fiscal intermediaries • Consultation with professional medical societies/trade groups • Consultation with technology manufacturers • Consultation with beneficiaries or consumer groups
Step 5	Policy development decision memorandum is submitted to HCFA's Director of the Office of Clinical Standards and Quality (OCSQ)
Step 6	The policy decision is approved or modified by the OCSQ
Step 7	Policy is issued, with Medicare manual instructions given

Data from Kurlander SS: HCFA opens up: Understanding the Medicare coverage process for medical technology and services. Rehab Manag 11(6):66-67, 1998. *HCFA,* Health Care Financing Administration.

rehabilitation hospitals, long-term–care hospitals, and home care. MCOs have had the greatest impact in the hospital and outpatient sectors.

Nearly all inpatient rehabilitation and most SNF services are postacute. Postacute care also involves 75% of all long-term–care hospital services, approximately one third of home health care cases, and one fifth of outpatient rehabilitation services. A disproportionate percentage of postacute costs is driven by a limited number of diagnosis-related groups (DRGs) as part of a prospective payment system (PPS). Acute hospital inpatient admissions are classified into one of 494 DRGs. HCFA uses an algorithm that ties a patient's International Classification of Diseases diagnosis code to a DRG. Rasmussen (1996) points out that PPS is intended to pay for "necessary" costs for an "average" patient with a specific DRG. Welch (1998b) reports that 14 DRGs account for half of the costs, whereas 30 DRGs account for two thirds of all expenditures.

The effect of PPS on rehabilitation is profound, with some hospitals reducing the role of rehabilitation because they are reimbursed on a fixed-payment per-case basis. Although rehabilitation produces lower profits for hospitals today, it can assist hospitals in controlling costs. Rehabilitation, when used in the context of overall disease state or condition management, can reduce the expenditures associated with traditionally more expensive interventions (e.g., surgical or medical interventions).

How Does Medicare Evaluate a Coverage Issue?

Medicare periodically conducts an extensive study of a coverage issue. This process involves several stages and can take years before a final determination is made. Rehabilitation providers may be aware of the lengthy deliberations surrounding coverage of electrical stimulation in wound healing. Table 4–4 illustrates Medicare's process.

Ultimately, to be considered reasonable and necessary, therapy interventions must meet Medicare criteria as outlined in the Medicare Manual. Table 4–5 describes conditions that must be met for a provider's services to be covered.

Managed Savings Accounts

Some Medicare + Choice plans allow for participation in medical savings accounts (Benko, 2000; Waid, 1998). These tend to be high-deductible health plans to which the federal government pays a portion of the capitation rate. Managed savings accounts are plans with finite spending limits that require discretionary purchases of health care services. Consumers retain the authority to determine how their money is allocated.

Prospective Payment System

A significant shift in long-term–care reimbursement occurred on July 1, 1998, when the BBA was enacted. PPS was proposed for SNFs. The reimbursement system known as *RUG-III,* or resource-based utilization groups version III, serves as the cornerstone. RUG-III uses federally mandated standardized clinical assessment to classify SNF residents into one of 44 payment categories. This classification system is known as *MDS* (minimum data set). Each MDS category describes patient needs and the anticipated intensity of service, including treatment time. The greater the skilled needs of the SNF resident or

Table 4–5 Medicare's Criteria for Reasonable and Necessary Physical, Occupational, and Speech Therapy Services

To be considered reasonable and necessary therapy, the following conditions must be met:
- Services must be considered, under accepted standards of medical practice, to be specific and effective treatment for the patient's condition.
- Services must be of such a level of complexity and sophistication or the condition of the patient must be such that the services required can be performed safely and effectively only by a qualified physical therapist or under his or her supervision.
- There must be an expectation that the condition will improve significantly in a reasonable (and generally predictable) period of time, based on the physician's assessment of the patient's restoration potential after any needed consultation with the qualified physical therapist, or the services must be necessary to the establishment of a safe and effective maintenance program required in connection with a specific disease state.
- The amount, frequency, and duration of the services must be reasonable.

Data from Health Care Financing Administration (HCFA), Publication 12, Medicare Manual; §230.3: Physical, Speech, and Occupational Therapy. Furnished by the Skilled Nursing Facility or Others under Arrangements with the Facility under its Supervision, copyright 1998, Commerce Clearing House Incorporated.

category, the greater the reimbursement. The following seven resident/patient categories compose the 44 groups in RUG-III (Table 4-6):

- Rehabilitation
- Extensive services
- Special care
- Clinically complex
- Impaired cognition
- Behavioral problems
- Reduced physical function

The complexity of RUG-III classification necessitates computer software programs that group residents into a RUG category, taking into consideration the aforementioned seven categories. HCFA provides its "Raven" software program free of charge to provider organizations that participate in Medicare.

Diagnosis-Related Groups

In 1983, a patient classification system was ushered in when inpatient hospital services were converted to a PPS. Case mix adjustment is the method that assigns patients, according to different attributes, to a DRG. Attributes include diagnosis, surgery, age, gender, and treatment setting during discharge. A total of 511 DRGs has led to earlier hospital discharges under PPS (Menke et al, 1998). Table 4-7 presents a list of the top 20 most common DRGs.

The demand for both physical and occupational therapy skyrocketed with early discharge from inpatient hospital services (Sandstrom et al, 2003). Services that were once delivered through inpatient care are now transferred to alternative, typically less expensive, settings

 Table 4–6 Seven Major Resident or Patient Types Under the RUG-III System

1. Rehabilitation
   - Physical, occupational, or speech therapy
   - Therapy required minimum three times per week
   - 45 minutes of direct patient care per session
   - Represents 12 of 44 payment groups based on ADLs score, therapy minutes, therapy days, need for rehabilitation nursing
2. Extensive Services
   - Suctioning, tracheostomy care, ventilator/respirator, parenteral feedings
   - Represents 3 of 44 payment groups
   - Considers ADLs score plus treatment sessions per day
3. Special Care
   - Burns, quadriplegia, stage 3 to 4 pressure ulcers, feeding tube, multiple sclerosis, intravenous medications
   - Represents 3 of 44 payment groups according to ADLs score
4. Clinically Complex
   - Dehydration, respiratory therapy, stasis ulcers, oxygen therapy, pneumonia, terminal diagnoses
   - Represents 8 of 44 payment groups
   - Considers ADLs score plus need for rehabilitation nursing
5. Impaired Cognition
   - Short-term memory, orientation recall, decision-making impairments
   - Represents 4 of 44 groups
   - Considers ADLs score plus need for rehabilitation nursing
6. Behavioral Problems
   - Wandering, verbal abuse, physical abuse, inappropriate behavior, delusions, hallucinations
   - Represents 4 of 44 groups
   - Considers ADLs score plus need for rehabilitation nursing
7. Reduced Physical Functions
   - Represents 10 of 44 groups
   - Considers ADLs score plus need for rehabilitation nursing

ADLs, Activities of daily living.
Data modified from American Health Information Management Association, 1999, www.ahima.org/members/quiz/articles/dougherty.html, accessed October 31, 2002.

 Table 4–7 20 Most Common Diagnosis-Related Groups (DRGs)

Condition	DRG
1. Heart failure	127
2. Simple pneumonia and pleurisy	89
3. Chronic obstructive pulmonary disease	88
4. Specific cerebrovascular disorders	14
5. Major joint and limb reattachment—lower extremities	209
6. Gastrointestinal hemorrhage	174
7. Esophagitis	182
8. Nutritional disorders	296
9. Respiratory infections/inflammations	79
10. Cardiac arrhythmia	136
11. Angina pectoris	140
12. Percutaneous cardiovascular procedures	112
13. Septicemia	416
14. Kidney and urinary tract infection	320
15. Circulatory disorders/anterior myocardial infarction	121
16. Major small/large bowel procedures	148
17. Hip and femur procedures except major joint	210
18. Circulatory disorders except anterior myocardial infarction	124
19. Transient ischemic attack/precerebral occlusions	15
20. Chest pain	143

Data modified from Welch WP: Bundled Medicare payment for acute and postacute care. Health Affairs 17(6):69-81, 1998b.

(home care, SNFs, outpatient centers, assisted-living centers).

Ambulatory Payment Classification

The BBA also contains a provision for PPS under hospital outpatient Medicare services. Part B, or supplemental medical insurance (SMI), is furnished to hospital inpatients without Part A (health insurance), and outpatient services are covered. Outpatient hospital services are classified into an ambulatory payment classification (APC) much like RUG-III. Like RUG, each APC receives its own unique reimbursement value. This system replaced the previous cost-based payment policy.

Does a Prospective Payment System Erode the Quality of Care?

A research collaboration between Rand Corporation and the University of California at Los Angeles (UCLA) studied the question of how the PPS reform affected the quality of care afforded Medicare beneficiaries (Rand Corporation, 1998). Researchers concluded that PPS did not have an adverse effect on patient outcomes despite shorter hospital lengths of stay. However, Medicare patients were discharged in more unstable conditions when compared with groups of FFS patients. This study involved 16,758 Medicare patients hospitalized throughout 300 hospitals located in five states (California, Florida, Indiana, Pennsylvania, and Texas). Of the patients studied, 50% were covered under FFS between 1981 and 1982. The remaining 50% of the patients were covered under inpatient PPS between 1985 and 1986. Patients involved in this study fell into five condition categories: congestive heart failure (CHF), acute myocardial infarction, pneumonia, hip fracture, and cerebrovascular accident (CVA).

Principal outcome measures consisted of short-term mortality, medium-term mortality, length of stay, living status at discharge (home or care facility), SNF stays, and readmissions. Researchers found that measures of quality of care improved for the PPS-covered subjects. Although short-term mortality increased in association with unstable condition at discharge (within 90 days of discharge), overall mortality dropped.

MEDICAID

Medicaid is a means-tested entitlement program and the single largest insurance program in the United States in terms of persons covered, with more than 41 million eligible beneficiaries (Iglehart, 1999). Medicaid is *not* a program that exclusively addresses the health care needs of the impoverished. Almost 7 million eligible beneficiaries had qualifying disabilities under Medicaid according to Urban Institute estimates (Meyer & Zeller, 1999).

Who does Medicaid cover?

- 21.3 million children
- 9.2 million adults with families
- 4.1 million older adults
- 6.7 million blind or disabled persons

- Iglehart, 1999

Medicaid represents a joint federal-state government program that serves the most vulnerable population, the poor. However, states administer their own programs and determine eligibility requirements, covered benefits, and fee schedules. Iglehart (1999) reports that Medicaid represents 40% of all federal dollars invested in state programs.

In general, inner-city hospitals and facilities attend to this large poor population. Some facilities go so far as to refer Medicaid cases to competing facilities, a practice known as *patient dumping*. Some states take advantage of a Medicaid loophole that enables them to inflate medical charges paid by the federal government. Most states operate under a 50:50 ratio, with the federal government and state government each financing 50% of Medicaid costs.

Medicaid Quality Review

Medicaid managed care plans are subject to quality review. The Medicaid Health Plan Employer Data and Information Set (HEDIS) was developed in collaboration with the National Committee for Quality Assurance (NCQA). This version of HEDIS has been adapted and modified to reflect the unique needs and expectations of Medicaid programs. This data set provides individual states, MCOs, health care providers, and consumers with quality-related data and resources. Several other quality assessment initiatives are directed at Medicaid (UCLA, 1999). These include the following:

- Foundation for Accountability (FACCT): A collaboration among various stakeholders including private and public payers, consumers, and HCFA. FACCT has been instrumental in the development of several condition- or disease-specific outcome measures (e.g., for diabetes, mental depression, breast cancer).
- Quality Assurance Reform Initiative (QARI): Similar stakeholders have collaborated to produce means of monitoring and improving quality of managed Medicaid services. QARI has published "A Health Care Quality Improvement System for Managed Care." These guides were tested by the Kaiser Family Foundation and released through the National Academy for State Health Policy's *Quality Improvement Primer for Medicaid Managed Care.*

Providers would be well advised to secure summaries of these guidelines to better understand the needs and expectations of other stakeholders in the long-term–care sector.

Managed Medicaid

States were granted authority to enter into managed Medicaid arrangements under the BBA of 1997. By 1998, every state except Alaska offered some form of managed Medicaid in which PCPs serve as gatekeepers. As with managed Medicare programs, many of these PCPs are unaccustomed to dealing with aging or chronically ill populations. PCPs under managed care plans are accustomed to dealing with single acute disease or injury. However, Medicaid populations often suffer from multiple

Table 4–8 Comparison Between Medicare and Medicaid

	Medicare	Medicaid
Establishment	Social Security Act, Title XVIII	Social Security Act, Title XIV
Funding	Public-federal	Public-federal and state
Governance	Federal under U.S. Department of Health and Human Services	Federal-state
Demographics	Largest source of funding for the older-than-65-years age bracket	Largest source of funding for poor
Policymaking	Federal and fiscal intermediaries (FIs)	States establish eligibility policy
Eligibility	Inconsistent among FIs	Inconsistent across states
Reimbursement	Generally lower than private insurance	Generally the lowest level
Children	Not covered	Covered
Managed care	Yes	Yes
Cost sharing	Yes, annual premiums (Part C), co-payments and deductibles (Parts A and B)	Yes, deductibles, co-payments for some services
Prescription coverage	Yes	No

chronic conditions and a constellation of psycho-social-economic issues.

There are three basic types of managed Medicaid (Holahan et al, 1998):

1. Primary care case management
2. Full-risk HMOs
3. Prepaid health plans

The primary care case management model matches beneficiaries with providers who are responsible for coordination of care; utilization; and referral monitoring, especially to specialists for emergency services. Full-risk model HMOs (as in group health) offer a full range of services across a continuum that includes preventive services and acute primary care. Prepaid plans typically use the services of clinics or large group practices that do not assume the degree of financial risk (under capitation) of a provider in a full-risk HMO arrangement. In fact, ambulatory services are often the only at-risk service for providers.

One can easily become confused concerning the similarities and differences between Medicare and Medicaid financing systems. Table 4–8 provides a comparison between Medicare and Medicaid.

Obstacles to Managed Medicaid

Medicaid is difficult to manage from an MCO perspective. Typically, MCOs seek to identify a homogeneous population that will respond well to preventive or acute care services. Medicaid covers an extremely heterogeneous population spanning all ages and a multitude of conditions. Managed care attempts to structure benefit programs through a variety of incentives and disincentives. Medicaid has little or no ability to financially reward providers for risk sharing. Managed Medicaid represents a real paradox. Managed care preferences for selective enrollment coupled with the gatekeeper model of restricted access to care (e.g., specialist care) represents the antithesis of Medicaid. Medicaid seeks to be more all-inclusive and to essentially accept enrollees that other plans do not desire.

Managed care plans make use of risk adjustments to manage certain conditions more efficiently. Medicaid currently has inadequate risk adjustment methodologies (Holahan et al, 1998). Last, Medicaid has a poor image that does little to entice managed care participation or provider recruitment (Table 4–9).

WHAT IS REHABILITATION'S BITE OUT OF THE MEDICARE PIE?

Disaggregated or rehabilitation-specific data are difficult to accurately ascertain because of the plethora of rehabilitation settings, disciplines, FI preferences, ambiguity of provider identifier codes, diversity among FIs, and divergent billing and collections software. Rehabilitation services consume approximately 10% of the Part B pie (Welch, 1998a). In 1996, rehabilitation revenues, when broken down, included 6% for SNFs ($1.052 billion), 3% for outpatient therapy provider ($528 million), and 1% for comprehensive outpatient rehabilitation facilities ($103 million). Medicare payments to hospital outpatient departments have been described as an $11 billion "black box," but it is estimated that 3% of all Medicare billings ($358 million) involve rehabilitation (Welch, 1998a).

Physical rehabilitation plays a major role in Medicare and promises to play an even greater role as Americans age. Sixty percent of all nursing home patients receive some form of therapy (General Accounting Office [GAO], 1998). The GAO (1998) described rehabilitation's high profile as having "problems involving billings

 Table 4–9 Obstacles to Managed Medicaid

- Medically needy beneficiaries are a complex heterogeneous group.
- High-cost cases are involved.
- Medicaid has minimum financial leverage over providers.
- Public and private providers may potentially absorb costs associated with specialty or emergency department visits (full-risk model).
- Managed care potentially limits access to services.
- Risk adjustment methods are rudimentary.
- Medicaid suffers from a poor image.

Data modified from Holahan J et al: Medicaid managed care in thirteen states. Health Affairs 17(3):43-63, 1998.

for overpriced, inappropriate, or undelivered therapy services."

Outpatient physical therapy charges submitted by rehabilitation agencies rose from $1 billion in 1990 to $3 billion in 1993. Occupational therapy billings rose an astronomical 879% between 1989 and 1993 (from $88 million to $856 million). Certainly, some of these increases result from greater awareness of the value that therapies offer to the aging population, in addition to overuse, misuse, and abuse of services.

Consequently, rehabilitation providers now face both threat and opportunity. Opportunity is driven by demographics (e.g., aging baby boomers), but it is threatened because of increasing scrutiny (through fraud and abuse initiatives). Selected rehabilitation providers can expect continued retrospective scrutiny of their Medicare billings, and those providers with documented poor profiles may be subjected to 100% prepayment review or retrospective medical records review.

However, a discussion of responsibility or lack thereof would be incomplete without equal apportionment of culpability for escalating costs. The GAO, the fiscal watchdog of the federal government, allocates some blame for escalating costs to CMS (formerly HCFA) and Medicare fiscal intermediaries.

Increased auditing of Medicare cases has resulted in medical record review of 3% to 5% of therapy cases and 100% prepayment review for selected providers or suppliers.

SOCIAL SECURITY DISABILITY INSURANCE

The Social Security Act was passed in 1965 and was amended in 1983 with the introduction of PPS. Both Medicare and Medicaid were provisions of the Social Security Act.

In addition to Medicare and Medicaid, two disability programs are housed within the Social Security Administration (SSA): Social Security Disability Insurance (SSDI) and Supplemental Security Income (SSI).

The SSDI program is funded through employee and employer contributions and covers injured workers and their widows or widowers, dependents, and adult disabled children. Eligibility requirements are calculated based on the amount of benefit tied to an individual's work history and earnings. SSI is a needs-based program for disabled or blind adults and children. A fixed monthly payment is provided, with some states supplementing this amount. By the end of 1998, the SSI paid benefits to more than 5.2 million needy, blind, and disabled beneficiaries. This group accounted for total expenditures of $129 billion. Predicted costs over the ensuing years are expected to amount to $122,000 per recipient (GAO, 1999).

The following five major categories of benefits are covered through Social Security taxes: retirement, disability, family benefits, survivors, and Medicare (SSA, 1998).

Social Security Administration's Disability Determination Process

The SSA defines *disability* in its disability benefit brochure as follows:

"If you cannot do work you did before and we decide that you cannot adjust to other work because of your medical condition(s). Your disability also must last or be expected to last for at least a year or to result in death."

- SSA, 1998

How is disability determined under SSDI?

The Social Security Office forwards a case to a statewide Disability Determination Services (DDS) office once the basic requirements for benefits have been met. The DDS examines the medical evidence from physicians, hospitals, therapists, and others. The beneficiary's ability to perform critical job demands (e.g., walking, sitting, lifting, carrying) is then ascertained through an interview process. DDS may require traditional medical information or refer a claimant for a "consultative examination." This examination may be conducted by an independent physician or facility or by an attending doctor. In each case, the SSA pays for the examination, including travel expenses incurred by the beneficiary. The disability determination process involves five steps:

Step 1: Determination of whether a claimant is gainfully employed. The following formula is applied: Earnings of more than $500 per month for sighted persons and more than $930 per month for blind individuals. If "yes," the disability is denied; if "no," the case proceeds to Step 2.

Step 2: Determination of the presence or absence of a severe impairment. Severe impairments are those that significantly limit an individual's ability to physically or mentally perform basic work activities. If "yes," the case proceeds to Step 3; if "no," disability is denied.

Step 3: "Medical listings" are used to determine if an impairment is consistent with a diagnosis or condition. If "yes," disability benefits are allowed; if "no," the case proceeds to Step 4.

Step 4: Determination of impairment severity is then made relative to the beneficiary's ability to work. During this stage, the residual functional ability of the claimant is assessed and compared with the critical job demands. If "yes," case proceeds to Step 5; if "no," the disability is denied.

Step 5: Determination of whether the impairment prevents the claimant from performing any other form of work. If "yes," disability is allowed; if "no," the disability is denied.

Figure 4-3 depicts the five steps in the SSA disability determination process.

A letter of determination then follows and describes benefits entitlement or the rationale for a denial of the claim.

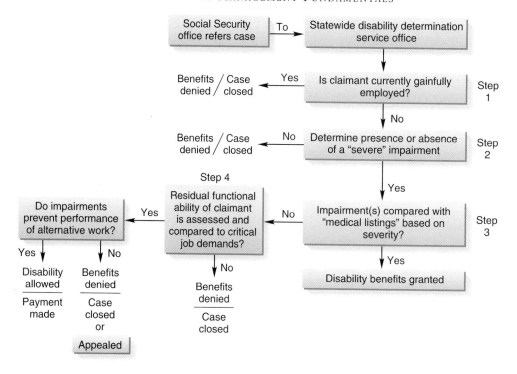

Figure 4–3. 5-Step Social Security Administration disability determination process.

If the claim is denied, the claimant has 60 days in which to file an appeal. There are three levels of appeal:

Social Security Appeal Levels

Level One:	Hearing by an administrative law judge
Level Two:	Review by the Appeals Council
Level Three:	Federal court review

The SSA allows beneficiaries to secure an attorney for appeals, or an SSA representative is assigned. This representative cannot charge a fee to the beneficiary. Beneficiaries also are entitled to a free fact sheet called "Social Security and Your Right to Representation" (Publication No. 05-10075).

The SSA's disability program provides incentives to transition back to work, including continuation of benefits and health coverage, while a person attempts to return to gainful employment.

Despite these incentives, it is virtually an axiom that, "once on the disability rolls, always on the disability rolls." Some assert that changes in the Social Security law and interpretations throughout the 1980s have led to a system that encourages disability and discourages a return to gainful employment—the very antithesis of physical rehabilitation (Quadagno, 1997). This presents enormous challenges, particularly to vocational and rehabilitation providers who have more to offer than traditional medical assessments of pathological conditions and impairments. Vocational specialists, occupational therapists, and physical therapists can be invaluable assets to the disability assessment process. However, to date, these disciplines are under-represented in the SSDI process, which tends to be physician-centric in nature. Although the SSA's system for disability determination is seriously flawed, efforts have been made to improve the process, including the

development of a taxonomy of functional assessment constructs (Halpern, 2001).

The final disposition of SSDI cases varies. Individuals can remain on the disability roll until death. Persons may be converted to SSI from SSDI when they turn 65 years old or have experienced a medical recovery. SSDI beneficiaries who return-to-work can be dropped from disabilities rolls, albeit this rarely happens (Quadagno, 1997).

SSA is obligated by law to every three years conduct reviews of disability cases. However, there is an incredible backlog of cases reported, and even when reviews are performed, most maintain their disability status.

SUBACUTE CARE

During the 1990s subacute care was one of the fastest growing health care sectors (Parakh, 1994).

What Is Subacute Care?

Subacute care occupies the middle ground between acute illness and injuries and chronic conditions. Subacute care has been defined across a number of dimensions, including time from injury or illness onset, severity of condition, provider type, reimbursement scheme, and treatment settings (Levenson, 2000; Chen et al, 2002). The term *subacute* elicits a strange dichotomy. On one hand, it is used to describe a narrow patient population (e.g., ventilator dependent), but paradoxically, it also serves as a safety net for those cases that do not fit neatly into the acute or chronic categories. Thus, *subacute care* as a term remains enigmatic. However, most subacute programs share the attributes listed in Table 4–10.

In an attempt to demystify the term *subacute care,* the American Health Care Association (AHCA), the Joint

Table 4–10 *Subacute Care Attributes*

- Conditions that require skilled monitoring
- Conditions that require high-level or expensive technology
- Extended treatment periods
- Specialist-driven care
- Conditions that require services historically delivered via inpatient hospitalization
- Complex or numerous diagnoses
- Interdisciplinary coordinated services
- More intensive than skilled nursing facility services
- Less intensive than acute care hospitalization services
- Effect of a cure is not a primary goal
- Stabilization of a condition may be the principal goal
- Generally less expensive than acute hospital-based services

Commission on Accreditation of Healthcare Organizations, and the Association of Hospital-Based Skilled Nursing Facilities promulgated the following definition:

> *"Subacute care is comprehensive inpatient care designed for someone who has an acute illness, injury, or exacerbation of a disease process. It is goal oriented treatment rendered immediately after, or instead of, acute hospitalization to treat one or more specific active complex medical conditions or to administer one or more technically complex treatments, in the context of a person's underlying long-term conditions and overall situation."*

- AHCA, 2000

The discussion of subacute care is included in this long-term–care chapter because many individuals go on to develop chronic conditions that require postacute care along the treatment continuum after the acute phases of service. Many of these persons owe their lives to modern technology because in earlier days of medicine, they would not have survived the acute incident, nevertheless make it into the chronic phase of recovery. However, appropriate rehabilitation services rendered during the subacute stage of irritability can potentially reduce the number and severity of cases that evolve into chronic conditions.

Which Conditions Fall Under the Subacute Label?

The acute phase of injury or illness is generally agreed to be that time in which clinical signs and symptoms are greatest (e.g., pain and swelling). This phase lasts approximately 1 to 2 weeks for musculoskeletal soft tissue injury. However, for neurological conditions, the acute phase of the recovery trajectory can be longer. Specific timeframes defining acute, subacute, and chronic phases of conditions are unnecessary for the sake of this discussion. Again, subacute or intermediate care falls between the acute and chronic phases. However, the following timeframes are offered as guidelines for each irritability stage. These timeframes may be collapsed or expanded, depending on secondary diagnoses, psychosocial issues, co-morbidities, and other extenuating or mitigating circumstances.

- Acute phase   1 to 2 weeks
- Subacute phase   2 to 6 weeks
- Chronic phase   6 to 8 weeks or more

In general, by the time an individual reaches the chronic phase of treatment, his or her anatomical and physiological tissue healing may have been achieved. Of course, there are always those who heal more quickly or slowly, depending on circulatory, endocrine, or other factors. These cases may expand or contract irritability timeframes.

Where are Subacute Cases Treated and Managed?

Subacute facilities exist within traditional hospitals, in SNFs, or in stand-alone centers. Parker et al (2000) examined 25 databases to assess the evaluative research literature on the costs, quality, and effectiveness of different locations of care for elderly populations. A total of 84 papers from 45 clinical trials were examined. Parker et al (2000) found that although new delivery models have been developed recently, evidence concerning effectiveness and costs is weak.

According to the AHCA, most subacute patients are older adults, with only one third younger than 65 years of age. Of discharged subacute patients, 22% return home for self-care, whereas 34% require home health care services.

Patients treated at subacute centers include those with orthopedic, neurological, and cardiopulmonary conditions and those who have specialized needs but do not require the intensity of an acute care stay. The line between acute care and subacute care can be fuzzy; thus two similar cases can be treated in two different treatment settings.

Critics may argue that subacute care replaces acute care simply to preserve reimbursement, which may be reduced by managed care if care is rendered in an acute care setting or is monitored by a PCP. Subacute care remains a controversial area with concerns raised about profiteering, value, and clinical effectiveness (Burns, 1995; Haffey & Welsh, 1995; Hill-Lamb, 1995; Infante, 1994). Most notably, cost differentials between hospital-based services and free-standing facilities have been studied (Liu & Black, 2003; Chen et al, 2002).

Rehabilitation providers may offer interventions in the subacute setting that are similar to interventions offered in other settings. However, considering the explosive growth in subacute care and the surrounding controversy, treatment goals and functionally based outcomes must be even more clearly established. At least one study has shown no significant difference in functional outcomes between nursing facilities that provide traditional rehabilitation and nursing facilities with specialized rehabilitation capabilities such as subacute care (Kane et al, 1996). Other researchers have demonstrated weak evidence about effectiveness and cost of subacute services (Parker et al, 2000; Evans & Hendricks, 2001).

Only 6.4% of patients who receive therapy in SNFs receive an amount or intensity of services that would qualify them for an acute rehabilitation unit (Kane et al, 1996). More than 50% of all patients newly admitted to SNFs receive "substantial" amounts of rehabilitation on admission (Murray et al, 1999). These and other data may partly explain why payers focus on cost when selecting a treatment setting:

> *"Because there are few controlled studies of rehabilitation outcome at any level of care, insurers may focus only on the issue of cost and increasingly use nursing homes as a major site for rehabilitation care."*
>
> - Murray et al, 1999

Furthermore, Medicare's current payment system for inpatient rehabilitation encourages earlier discharges to nursing homes regardless of individual patient characteristics (Chan & Ciol, 2000). Scrutiny of nursing facility rehabilitation services is certain to escalate in light of the following variables: growth in an aging population, expansion of SNF service offerings, paucity of outcomes data, and provider alteration of services in response to new financial incentives (White, 2003; Shatto, 2002).

DISABILITY MANAGEMENT: ROLE IN LONG-TERM CARE

Physical rehabilitation is routinely involved in the treatment and management of chronic conditions at a time when managed care principally addresses acute-stage injury and illness. The length of this chapter is indicative of the vital role physical rehabilitation will play as Americans continue to age and as alternative funding sources for long-term care are explored by both the private and public sectors.

The role of PCPs has dampened the effect of rehabilitation in group health or general health situations. However, the gatekeeper model is severely challenged by an aging America coupled with the growth in chronicity.

New Paradigm Shifts are Required

Long-term care represents an opportunity for physical rehabilitation's renewal efforts. Few can disagree that rehabilitation took its lumps during the 1990s, partly because of managed care; restrictive Medicare reimbursement policies; and the sector's collective failure to shift paradigms and to recognize that other health care stakeholders held different beliefs, needs, and expectations. However, demographic shifts are undeniably in rehabilitation's favor, with aging baby boomers and the rise in the number of persons with chronic conditions. Ironically, it was Medicare that first spurred the demand for physical rehabilitation by offering a nationwide financing mechanism, and it may be Medicare that stimulates a second growth curve. Despite its intensified antifraud and antiabuse efforts targeting rehabilitation ("Operation Restore Trust," U.S. Department of Health and Human Services, 1995), Medicare may, in the future, embrace rehabilitation as one of its solutions to the aging population dilemma.

Population-based disease modeling, patient screening, and patient monitoring may minimize the prevalence and severity of chronic conditions (Tompkins et al, 1999). Physical rehabilitation needs to find a way to participate in these treatments or, better yet, in new management paradigms.

In the 1970s, a dramatic paradigm shift began, and it continues today. This involves a shift away from the paternalistic medical model of care and toward an independent-living model. This shift uniquely positions rehabilitation specialists for the future (DeJong, 1979).

Rehabilitation will play a vital role in reducing the effects of chronic conditions such as diabetes, chronic obstructive pulmonary disease (COPD), stroke, and other conditions that previously were principally managed through medical interventions. Traditionally, rehabilitation has rendered its services after the patient has been stabilized. Then for a finite period, either inpatient or outpatient services are rendered. However, there is much that rehabilitation can accomplish in persons who are at initial risk or at risk of secondary incidents. This preventive rehabilitation approach is relatively untested. Tompkins et al (1999) recognize the value in this approach:

> *"Medicare reflects the long-term public perspective, and thus should further this new direction by supporting education, reimbursing for prevention efforts and allied health services, encouraging efficiency, and monitoring cost and quality outcomes."*

Disability management in the aging population is a question of balance—balance between economic and professional pressures, medical and functional diagnoses, physical and psychosocial elements, clinically based care and self-care, and treatment and management.

The aging population presents unique challenges to the rehabilitation specialist, that transcend the medical condition or dysfunction being treated. In many cases, "management" completely supplants "treatment," because conditions may be terminal, highly progressive, or static, with little or no prospect for a cure or remission. Many of these persons require some form of adaptive or mobility equipment (Table 4–11).

Williams (1997) describes several common physiological phenomena that challenge rehabilitation providers and complicate case management of elder persons:

- Normal decrease in bone density
- Decrease in dermal thickness and reduced subdermal fat
- Decrease in balance
- Increased risk of falls
- Contractures
- Decreased aerobic capacity
- Decreased connective tissue elasticity
- Pain

Factors that interplay in long-term care demand a collaboration of medical specialists and generalists, community resources, assistive technologies, and environmental experts.

Disability Management Triad

Many components of disability management can be condensed into three categories of intervention. All three of these categories apply to disability prevention, treatment, and management (Figure 4–4):

1. Functionality
2. Assistive technology
3. Environmental

Table 4–11 Frequency of Equipment Needs in Older Persons with Long-Term Physical Disability

Equipment	Percent of Older Population
Manual wheelchair	32%
Power wheelchair	13%
Scooter	27%
Cane: indoor use only	22%
Cane: outdoor use only	37%
Walker	8%
Orthosis	48%

Data from Williams A: More than surviving: Aging persons with long-term physical disability. Proceedings of the 12th International Congress of the World Confederation for Physical Therapy, PL-RR-0631-TH, 631. American Physical Therapy Association, Alexandria, VA, 1995.

Disability management principally involves enhancing a patient's functional ability, securing the necessary personal assistive technology, and screening and modifying his or her environment to maximize both function and implementation of assistive technology.

As medical technology continues to rapidly expand, therapists need to familiarize themselves with emerging technologies that can be coupled with their function-based rehabilitation programs. This necessitates studying and understanding developments from bioengineers, computer-based companies, architects, ergonomists, industrial hygienists, safety engineers, and the information technology sector. The U.S. government is also an invaluable source of information that is both free and useful in this regard. A good example is the Department of Veteran Affairs (VA) *Rehabilitation R&D Progress Reports* (published annually).

In an ideal model, these three elements (functionality, assistive technology, environmental) of disability management may be in balance; however, in reality, this is seldom the case. Patients require varying degrees of emphasis on function, assistive technology, and environmental factors. One overwhelming attribute is that all three elements require a high degree of education and emphasis placed on self-care, consistent with an independent-living model.

Interventions may be of a preventive, restorative, or maintenance nature in any of the triad components. For example, for some patients, a power wheelchair may prevent a disability (e.g., fractures resulting from falls and osteoporosis), whereas for others, it may improve mobility. It is conceivable that prevention, restoration, and maintenance of function are all concurrently achieved.

Many exciting developments in assistive technology are augmenting the efforts of rehabilitation professionals. Computer applications offer some of the most promising technologies. The use of virtual-reality techniques for fall prevention is one example (Jaffe, 1998). Researchers use images from a videocamera with a computer simulation program that is superimposed with a videomixer. This allows subjects to walk on a motorized treadmill while wearing a high-resolution head-mounted display. For safety purposes, an overhead harness is attached while the subject navigates a course consisting of various computer-generated obstacles. This computer simulation enhances the effects of gait training (functionality) along with environmental screening (home-safety checkout).

A patient's performance in activities of daily living (ADLs) and instrumental activities of daily living (IADLs) directly describe QOL or lack thereof. IADLs are those tasks that generally command a higher cognitive functional level in addition to greater physical functioning. IADLs are more complex and describe independent living beyond personal hygiene, including meal preparation, shopping, laundering, driving, and financial management.

There is an inverse relationship between decreased function in ADLs and IADLs and any number of QOL indicators (Figure 4–5).

Exercise decreases both pain and disability (Mangione, 2001). However, experts have pointed out the need for greater understanding of activity patterns beyond conventional therapeutic exercises and ADLs (Nagi, 1979). Physical rehabilitation is in the throes of a paradigm shift toward a more global view of a patient's functional ability (Berg & Cassells, 1990; Bond et al, 1995). A new independent-living model has been supported by disability management and rehabilitation experts (DeJong, 1979).

Figure 4–4. Disability management triad. *ADLs,* Activities of daily living; *IADLs,* instrumental activities of daily living.

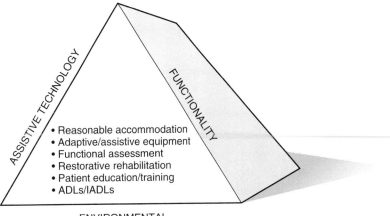

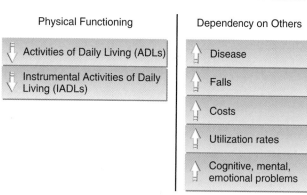

Figure 4–5. Inverse relationship between decreased function and other issues.

The traditional paternalistic biomedical model of care yields to a model that deemphasizes focus on an individual's anatomical and physiological problems and instead favors social functioning and the human-environment interface. New disability assessment and management tools focus on lifestyle activities in the context of social functioning. Bond et al (1995) review the six survival roles necessary to avoid a handicap label. These are defined by the World Health Organization's *International Classification of Impairments, Disabilities, and Handicaps* (ICIDH) (World Health Organization [WHO], 1993).

1. *Orientation:* An individual's ability to orient himself or herself to his or her surroundings
2. *Physical independence:* Ability of individuals to remain effectively independent regardless of their immediate bodily needs
3. *Mobility:* Ability of individuals to move within their environments
4. *Occupation:* Ability of individuals to engage in employment, play, or recreation
5. *Social integration:* Ability of individuals to actively participate in social relationships
6. *Economic self-sufficiency:* Ability of individuals to successfully engage in socioeconomic activities

Therapists as Case Managers

New treatment and management paradigms may require that a physical or occupational therapist operate in more of a case management role than in a caregiver role. Therapists in collaboration with others may become the architects of a treatment program implemented by another person or other persons. If this occurs, management will supplant treatment. This may be a difficult concept for some rehabilitation professionals to embrace, because rehabilitation goals often center around hands-on restoration or rehabilitation. In older adult populations or in those with chronic conditions, restoration or rehabilitation may not be the principle clinical goal. Many conditions are not amenable to rehabilitation in a traditional sense. Adaptation and accommodation to one's environment may be more appropriate and achievable goals. Ultimately, rehabilitation must integrate cognitive, affective, and social issues to be maximally effective (Lusardi, 1997).

If You Don't Measure It, You Can't Manage It

Functional assessment of a geriatric population requires knowledge that is unique. For instance, a straightforward musculoskeletal evaluation of a younger person is significantly different from that of an older patient, who may be on 10 to 14 medications and suffer from COPD, CHF, osteoporosis, IDDM, hearing and vision loss, and cognitive impairment. Providers must learn to piece together tattered medical histories that, under the best of circumstances, are eroded by time, multiple admissions, innumerable treatment interventions, and countless providers. Clinicians and researchers have described a plethora of assessment tools that are applied to the older adult population (Applegate et al, 1990; Fleming et al, 1995; Guccione & Jette, 1990; Rubenstein, 1983). All of these assessment tools probably have a place in long-term care, but many obstacles remain.

Drug-related illness is a significant problem in this population, accounting for 5% to 23% of all hospitalizations (Tamblyn, 1996). Cardiovascular, psychotrophic, and nonsteroidal anti-inflammatory drugs, or NSAIDs, are the most-commonly implicated drugs. Tamblyn describes the following three mechanisms that may have either an associative or causative influence on drug-related illness:

1. Increased sensitivity of diseased tissues to drug toxicity
2. Potential drug interactions
3. Patient compliance difficulties as the number of drugs increases

Physical rehabilitation providers must assess polypharmacy of their patients as a component of a comprehensive assessment approach. Various behaviors commonly found among the elderly (e.g., lethargy, confusion, aggressiveness, balance disruptions, pain, and sensory disturbances) may have their genesis in drug responses versus the illness itself.

Huijbregts and Gruber (1997) describe the principal steps in a measurement process that can be applied to older populations:

Step 1: *Clarify the variable to be measured.* Assessment methods used in physical rehabilitation generally fall into the impairment and disability domains described by WHO's disablement model (WHO, 1993).

Step 2: *Determine the reason or purpose for measurement.* Purposes of measurement include a disability assessment to discriminate between a disabled person and a non-disabled person. Patient clinical improvement as measured between two points in time (e.g., admission and discharge) represents a second measurement function. Effectiveness of treatment demands an outcome measure that demonstrates the value of a given intervention.

Step 3: *Use a patient-centered practice model based on the holistic needs and responsibilities of the patient.* A patient-centered approach may necessitate assessment of physical domain factors, as well as non-medical or psychosocial issues, especially as they relate to the operational definition of disability.

Table 4–12 Partial Listing of Geriatric Functional Assessment Tools

Arthritis Impact Measurement Scale (AIMS)	Minor et al, 1989
Berg Balance Scale	Berg et al, 1995
Continuing Care Disability Measure (CCDM)	Huijbregts & Kay, 1995
Disability Inventory (DI) of the Chedoke-McMaster Stroke Assessment	Gowland et al, 1995
Elderly Mobility Scale (EMS)	Smith, 1994
Frail Elderly Functional Assessment (FEFA)	Gloth et al, 1995
Functional Inventory Measures (FIM)	Granger et al, 1990
Functional Reach (Goal Attainment Scaling [GAS])	Duncan et al, 1990
Katz Index	Katz, 1963
Multilevel Assessment Instrument (MAI)	Lawton et al, 1989
Older American Resources and Services (OARS)	Fillenbaum & Smyer, 1981
Osteoarthritis Screening Index (OASI)	Schilke et al, 1996
Resident Assessment Instrument (RAI)	American Health Care Association, 1989
Two-Minute Walking Test	Stewart et al, 1990
Western Ontario and McMaster Universities Osteoarthritis Index (WOMAC)	Deyle et al, 2000

Mandated assessments that include physical function are often used as a basis for SNF eligibility and payment for services (Kane & Kane, 2000). Mandated functional assessments are now required for home health services and rehabilitation (Kane & Kane, 2000).

Table 4–12 provides a partial list of geriatric functional assessment tools.

Certificate of Need: Obstacle or Opportunity?

Under the current Medicare system, physicians complete a "Certificate of Medical Necessity" (CMN) for durable medical equipment and must certify the need for rehabilitation services. Physicians determine the need for and use of rehabilitation services or length of stay in rehabilitation cases. CMNs do not authorize physical or occupational therapists to determine medical necessity or reasonableness of care, despite their unparalleled expertise in the care and management of long-term–care conditions. Physicians alone are not equipped to manage disability. Research has shown that a multidisciplinary approach to disability is more beneficial than evaluation by physicians alone, even when they are physiatrists (Haig et al, 1995).

DISABILITY PREVENTION

If You Don't Use It, You Lose It: Disuse and the Elderly

There is compelling evidence that indicates physical disability associated with aging is principally caused by disuse and secondary conditions (Ashworth et al, 1994; Fiatarone et al, 1990; Kohrt et al, 1991; Rogers et al, 1990a; Rogers et al, 1990b; Skelton et al, 1994).

Disuse is clearly avoidable through various preventive activities. Physical rehabilitation providers can play a significant role in prevention of dysfunction for both healthy and frail persons (Lusardi, 1997). The best disability management tool is prevention, and the best preventive approach is physical activity. Disability management in an elderly population may be synonymous with prevention.

The U.S. Surgeon General's Office has published a report touting the benefits of physical activity (Table 4–13). Physical activity in older adults may not prevent the onset of primary conditions, but it has potential value in the prevention of secondary conditions and co-morbidities.

Rimmer (1999) describes a paradigm shift from disability prevention to prevention of secondary conditions, which may be a more appropriate strategy in long-term care. It is rare to treat an older-adult patient who is devoid of secondary diagnoses or morbidities. It is not unusual for secondary problems to have more predictive value in terms of functional outcome (Williams, 1997). These secondary problems often interfere with aggressive therapies. Generalized weakness is a classic example under Medicare. This condition, particularly following a prolonged hospitalization, is underappreciated and subsequently devalued by FIs. A general fixation on new or acute problems is associated with both MCOs and Medicare.

Therapists as Educators

Rehabilitation providers must serve in at least two educator capacities. One, they must educate others concerning

 Table 4–13 Benefits of Physical Activity

- Maintains the capability for independent living while reducing the prevalence and severity of falls and fractures
- Reduces the risk of dying from coronary heart disease and of developing hypertension (HTN), colon cancer, or diabetes
- Reduces HTN is some persons
- Helps persons with chronic, disabling conditions improve their stamina and muscle performance
- Reduces symptoms associated with anxiety and depression while fostering improvements in mood and sense of well-being
- Helps maintain and delay deterioration of healthy bones, muscles, and joints
- Helps control joint pain and swelling associated with arthritis

Data modified from National Center for Chronic Disease, Prevention and Health Promotion: Physical Activity and Health: Older Adults. A report of the United States Surgeon General, Centers for Disease Control and Prevention, www.cdc.gov/nccdphp/sgr/olderad.htm, accessed October 14, 2000.

Table 4–14 Model of the Comparative Importance of Benefits from Participation in Resistance Exercise Programs for Each Age Group from Children to Older Adults

	Children	Adolescents	Young Adults	Middle-Aged Adults	Older Adults
Muscle hypertrophy	NA	+	+++	++	++
Neural adaptation	++	+	+	+	++
Improved skill	+++	++	++	+	+
Muscular endurance	+	++	++	++	+++
Injury prevention	+	++	++	+++	++
Recreation	++	+++	++	++	++

Data from Vandervoort AA: Resistance exercise throughout life. Orthop Phys Ther Clin North Am 10(2):229, 2001.

+, Important; ++, moderately important; +++, very important; *NA*, not applicable.

NOTE: Subjective rankings are suggested by the author for healthy children and adults who are active but not training elite athletes. The basis of the relative rankings arises from the physiological potential for adaptation in each age group and the presumed needs of the normal patterns of work, leisure, and activities of daily living. Males and females may have different priorities in some age groups.

the efficacy and effectiveness of their interventions, whether they be preventive, treatment, or management in nature. Secondly, providers need to educate elders about the anatomical, physiological, psychological, and sociological changes that occur with aging.

Guccione (2000) challenges physical rehabilitation providers to demonstrate the value of their interventions. He asserts that the perception of rehabilitation specialists regarding their service effectiveness may not be commensurate with the true picture:

"Rehabilitation specialists are quick to assume that merely offering their services to elders living in the community will delay functional decline and reduce the threat of institutionalization. Unfortunately, little evidence exists to support this assumption."

- Guccione, 2000, p 13

It is imperative that therapists educate other health care stakeholders regarding the cost-benefit ratio of preventive and early intervention programs. Mangione (2001) notes that medical and physical rehabilitation providers have traditionally directed their interventions at the amelioration of pain, rather than focusing on providing interventions to mitigate decreased activity and physical deconditioning. When rehabilitation programs address restoration and maximization of function, they have been shown to be effective in staving off problems associated with aging (Grounds, 1998; Thompson et al, 1999; Tracy et al, 1999). For example, resistance exercise throughout all phases of life (children, adolescents, young adults, middle-aged adults, and older adults) has proven efficacious (Vandervoort, 2001) (Table 4–14).

"An Ounce of Prevention Is Worth a Pound of Treatment"

Physical rehabilitation providers have been relatively slow to embrace opportunities in geriatric disability prevention, despite a relative abundance of literature supportive of these programs for elderly populations (McCloy, 2001; Lexell, 2000; Sharkey & Williams, 2000).

For example, Chandler (2000) advocates a comprehensive assessment designed for older persons who may be prone to falling. This requires a methodological, or systems, approach. "Systems" in this case does not imply anatomical

systems, although these, too, must be considered. First, a multidisciplinary team is assembled that includes a physician, social worker, nurse, psychologist, physical therapist, and occupational therapist.

The addition of an optometrist or ophthalmologist is recommended because of the link between visual acuity and falls. Second, a medication review is conducted to identify potential or experienced side effects and interactions that may precipitate a fall. Medications include hypnotics, tranquilizers, sedatives, tricyclic antidepressants, antihypertensives, muscle relaxants, and pain medications. The social worker and/or psychologist can conduct interviews with the person, his or her family, and medical staff. Occupational and physical therapists accumulate impairment-specific and disability-specific data that may be associated with falls. Therapists also can perform an environmental screening to minimize fall risk. Adaptive and assistive device analysis should be a component of the program. These data can be assembled and reviewed by the team, who in turn can customize a prevention program that takes into consideration the most salient variables.

Rehabilitation providers can offer a variety of prevention programs designed to address the needs of an aging population. The most prevalent causes of morbidity and mortality involve congestive heart disease (CHD), cancer, and stroke. CHD accounts for 31% of all deaths, whereas cancer claims 21% of all older adults (Bush et al, 1994). Rehabilitation plays a major role in these and other conditions across every treatment setting. There is potential benefit from rehabilitation before the first incident of stroke or myocardial infarction. Yet, under the medical model, medications and surgery are the principal means of controlling symptoms and preventing incidents. There has been significant concern about the amount of medication given to geriatric populations (Beers et al, 1992; Gerety et al, 1993; Stein, 1994).

Despite the availability of preventive technologies, rehabilitation typically is prescribed after the fact or during the step-down phase following a serious incident. Rehabilitation providers are viewed more as treaters and less as health and wellness experts. Our health care system has the available medical technology to identify persons at risk of developing various conditions, including CHD and CVA. These persons could be referred to a preventive

Table 4–15 Disability Management in Long-Term Care: A 12-Step Administrative Plan

1. Understand the health care plan benefits and be sure that your patients understand them as well.
2. Articulate a clear medical necessity statement to support the scope of care. Include literature citations, treatment algorithms, guidelines, standards, clinical research, physical rehabilitation curriculum, and expert consensus documents.
3. Document in functional terms that are consistent with the plan's requirements (e.g., activities of daily living, instrumental activities of daily living, quality-of-life measures).
4. Understand and execute insurance denial appeals processes. Demand a true peer review for treatment-based denials (versus technical or administratively based denials).
5. Engage the patient in every phase of treatment and management from goal setting to discharge planning, as well as in the appeal processes.
6. Use an outcome measures system that is appropriate to your patient population.
7. Emphasize education and mentoring versus a hands-on treatment approach alone.
8. Encourage prevention programs targeting specific populations and/or conditions that are largely preventable. These may include osteoporosis and fall prevention.
9. Stress self-care, responsibility, and accountability with patients.
10. Coordinate rehabilitation services with other elements of the disability management plan. Use every patient encounter as an opportunity to teach another medical discipline about the value of rehabilitation.
11. Identify and encourage participation of the patient's family and other support structures.
12. Design a repeatable model that minimizes treatment variations while harmonizing treatment and management practices and principles

cardiovascular program that is monitored by rehabilitation personnel.

Rehabilitation professionals can participate in the union between technology and rehabilitative interventions that will facilitate improved clinical outcomes while opening renewed opportunities for participation in exciting long-term–care initiatives (Christenson, 1987; Frain & Carr, 1996; Mann, 1994) (Table 4–15).

Fall Prevention

There are many injury prevention strategies that can address the needs of a geriatric population. Fall prevention commands its own spotlight because of the profound effect that falls have on this population. Fall prevention is a major goal of rehabilitation for both providers and patients in addition to increased functionality and independence (Chandler, 2000; El-Faizy & Reinsch, 1994; Englander et al, 1996; Lach et al, 1991).

Most falls occur in persons older than 70 years old, with a mode of 86 years (Charron et al, 1995). Females incur 76.4% of all non-fatal accidents and a majority of falls (Charron et al, 1995). This is believed to be associated with the longevity demographics associated with females versus males.

Falls occur in persons with or without ambulatory assistive devices, including walkers. According to the U.S. Bureau of the Census (1993), there were an estimated 1,693,512 walker users in 1990. Falls were overwhelmingly the principal cause of non-fatal injury, accounting for 95.8% of such injuries (Charron et al, 1995). Fractured hip is the most common serious injury, and nearly one third of all fall victims are hospitalized. Falls also are a major cause of death from injury in the elderly. Falls are the cause in two thirds of injury-related deaths in persons 85 years or older (Baker & Harvey, 1985).

Fall prevention requires a multifactorial approach because falls are a heterogeneous phenomenon (Chandler, 2000; Lusardi, 1997; Tinetti et al, 1994; Tinetti et al, 1996). Fall prevention also requires a multivariate analysis of risk factors (Oliver et al, 2004). Providers are cautioned against focusing solely on one impairment measure or physiological factor associated with falls. Many factors, including confidence-building strategies, also should be incorporated into any fall prevention program (Petrella et al, 2000). Strength or lack thereof is a major factor in balance, gait, and the occurrence of falls (Wolfson et al, 1995). Musculoskeletal and postural deficits have been linked to falls (Kaufmann, 1990; Chandler et al, 1990) as well as various physiological factors (Lord et al, 1994). Falls also can be attributed to sensorimotor deficiencies (Stelmach & Worringham, 1985) and poor vision (Lord et al, 1991). Cognition deficits also contribute to fall risk (Rappaport et al, 1998).

In a fall prevention model, purposeful movement results from the interaction of environmental conditions; one's past experience; and one's present cognitive, sensory, motivational, motor, and musculoskeletal systems. The integration of functional systems within a given environment requires that therapists engage in a bifurcated process: assessment of the individual and environment. Robbins et al (1989) categorize fall risk factors as intrinsic (person) or extrinsic (environmental). Although fall prevention is a straightforward goal, it requires an understanding of complicated anatomical, physiological, and biomechanical factors that either individually or collectively place a person at risk. Chandler (2000) cautions against working from a laundry list of fall risk factors (intrinsic and extrinsic). Each case demands its own comprehensive analysis of risk factors in order to craft an effective prevention approach.

Age-related changes in a person's sensory and effector systems are critical indicators of gait quality (Lusardi, 1997; Palta, 1995). Sensory system changes affect visual acuity, depth perception, and sensitivity to visual flow. Effector system changes impact muscle performance, posture, joint range of motion, flexibility, and aerobic conditioning (Frontera et al, 1991; Hollenberg et al, 1998; Horak et al, 1989; Hu & Woollacott, 1994; Judge et al, 1995; Vandervoort, 1999).

Although functional kinematic measures of gait are found to decrease with age, it is difficult to associate

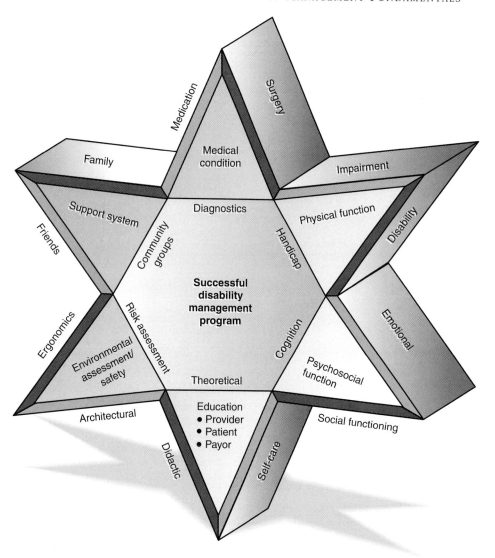

Figure 4–6. Successful disability management.

specific impairments with gait difficulties (Bohannon et al, 1996; Frank et al, 1996; Kaneko et al, 1991).

Osteoporosis is a prime example of a largely preventable condition (McCloy, 1998). Prevention activities can reduce pain and suffering, cost, morbidity, and mortality associated with osteoporosis-related fractures (McCloy, 1998). Osteoporosis accounts for 300,000 hospitalizations for hip fractures along with 1.5 million total fractures each year (Chrischilles et al, 1994; Looker et al, 1995). Looker et al (1995) report annual health costs exceeding $8 million for hip fractures associated with osteoporosis. Hip fractures account for 25% of all mortalities in older-adult populations (Guccione, 2000). Public health initiatives welcome the input of physical rehabilitation and exercise experts through consumer education, exercise, and healthy lifestyle encouragement (McCloy, 1998; Tompkins et al, 1999; U.S. Department of Health and Human Services, 1990).

McCloy (1998) provides a comprehensive collection of resources directed at osteoporosis prevention, including professional trade associations, advocacy groups, public health services, government agencies, information services, and Internet sites.

A number of researchers have demonstrated the effect of exercise on bone mineral density (Inman, 1998; Carter et al, 2002). Successful programs share three basic components: early diagnosis, comprehensive treatment (diet, pharmacology, strength training, and weight-bearing activities), and consumer education. Carter et al (2002) report improvements in dynamic balance and strength after exercise programs designed for elder populations (65- to 75-year-old women). These among other variables are critical determinants of fall risk, particularly in women with osteoporosis.

The effectiveness and efficacy of fall prevention programs are subjects of debate. Some contend that effectiveness of fall prevention programs is non-definitive (Vassallo et al, 2004). A systematic review and meta-analysis of clinical literature concluded that interventions to prevent falls in elderly populations are effective in both reducing the risk of falling and monthly rates of falling, especially when a multifactorial program is implemented (Chang et al, 2004). Kerse et al (2004) in a randomized controlled trial describe a fall prevention program that did not reduce falls or subsequent injuries from falls.

Elements of an Effective Disability Management Program

The disability management star illustrated in Figure 4–6 depicts the elements of an effective disability prevention and management program. Each point of the star represents key components of a disability management program:

- Medical condition
- Physical function
- Psychosocial function
- Education
- Environmental assessment/safety
- Support system

Successful disability management hinges on the education of all stakeholders, especially patients, providers, and payers. These parties must understand the perspective, concerns, and needs of other participants. Psychosocial variables, including patient social functioning, cognition, and emotional state, are addressed in addition to customary medical and physical functioning elements. The patient's support system and primary environment (work, school, sports, institution) require analysis. Risk assessment is crucial in the identification of architectural barriers and the development of ergonomic solutions for the facilitation of safe patient-environment interfacement. To be effective, rehabilitation providers must assess the relative strength or weakness of a patient's support system. The active involvement of family, friends, and community groups can have a direct impact on a number of things, namely, treatment setting, use of adaptive or assistive technology, and educational and training requirements.

REFERENCES

American Health Care Association (AHCA): 1989, www.ahca.org, accessed July, 27, 2004.

American Health Care Association (AHCA): Nursing facility subacute care: The quality and cost-effective alternative to hospital care, 1996, www.ahca.org, accessed July 27, 2004.

American Health Care Association et al: 2000, www.ahca.org, accessed July 27, 2004.

American Hospital Association website, www.ahca.org/brief/bg-sa.htm, accessed October 9, 2000.

Applegate WB, Blass JP, Williams TF: Instruments for the functional assessment of older patients. New Engl J Med 322:1207-1214, 1990.

Ashworth JB, Reuben DB, Benton LA: Functional profiles of healthy persons. Age Aging 23:34–39, 1994.

Baker SP, Harvey AH: Fall injuries in the elderly. Clin Geriatr Med 1(3):501-512, 1985.

Beers MH et al: Inappropriate medication prescribing in skilled-nursing facilities. Ann Intern Med 117:684–689, 1992.

Benko LB: The exodus escalates. Modern Healthcare 30(27):14, 2000.

Berg K, Wood-Dauphinee S, Williams J: The balance scale: Reliability assessment with elderly residents and patients with acute stroke. Scand J Rehabil Med 27:27-36, 1995.

Berg RL, Cassells JS: The Second Fifty Years: Promoting Health and Preventing Disability. Washington, DC, National Academy Press, 1990.

Bohannon RW, Andrews AW, Thomas MW: Walking speed: Reference values and correlates for older adults. J Orthop Sports Phys Ther 24:86-90, 1996.

Bond MJ et al: Lifestyle activities of the elderly: Composition and determinants. Disabil Rehabil 17(2):63-69, 1995.

Boyle J: An overview of today's Medicare managed care market. In Reichard J, Rosenthal B: (eds): 1996 Health Network and Alliance Sourcebook. New York, Faulkner & Gray, 1996, pp E16-E24.

Burman L et al: Policy Challenges Posed by the Aging of America, Urban Institute, 1998, www.urban.org/health/oldpol.html, accessed September 14, 2000.

Burns J: HHS plans further study of subacute-care sector (News). Modern Healthcare 25(13):22, 1995.

Bush TL et al: Risk factors for morbidity and mortality in older populations: An epidemiologic approach. In Hazzard WR et al (eds): Principles of Geriatric Medicine and Gerontology, 3rd ed. New York, McGraw-Hill, 1994.

Carter ND, Khan KM, McKay HA et al: Community-based exercise program reduces risk factors for falls in 65 to 75 year-old women with osteoporosis: Randomized controlled trial. Can Med Assoc J 167(9):997-1004, 2002.

Chan L, Ciol M: Medicare's payment system: Its effect on discharges to skilled nursing facilities from rehabilitation hospitals. Arch Phys Med Rehabil 81(6):715-719, 2000.

Chandler JM, Duncan PW, Studenski SA: Comparison of postural responses in young adults, healthy elderly and fallers using postural stress test. Phys Ther 70:410-415, 1990.

Chandler JM: Balance and falls in the elderly: Issues in evaluation and treatment. In Guccione AA (ed): Geriatric Physical Therapy. St. Louis, Mosby, 2000, pp 280-292.

Chang JT, Morton SC, Rubenstein LZ et al: Interventions for the prevention of falls in older adults: Systematic review and meta-analysis of randomized clinical trials. BMJ 328(7441):653-654, 2004.

Charron PM, Kirby RL, MacLeod DA: Epidemiology of walker-related injuries and deaths in the United States. Am J Phys Med Rehabil 74(3):237-239, 1995.

Chen CC, Heinemann AW, Granger CV et al: Functional gains and therapy intensity during subacute rehabilitation: A study of 20 facilities. Arch Phys Med Rehabil 83(11):1514-1523, 2002.

Chrischilles E, Shireman T, Wallace R: Costs and health effects of osteoporosis fractures. Bone 15:377-396, 1994.

Christenson MA: The therapist as geriatric environmental consultant. Topics Geriatr Rehabil 3:79-83, 1987.

DeJong G: Independent living: From social movement to analytic paradigm. Arch Phys Med Rehabil 60:435-446, 1979.

Department of Veteran Affairs: Rehabilitation R&D Progress Reports. Veterans Administration, Rehabilitation Research and Development Service, Scientific and Technical Publications Section (122), 103 South Gay Street, Baltimore, MD 21202-4051.

Deyle GD et al: Effectiveness of manual physical therapy and exercise in osteoarthritis of the knee: A randomized controlled trial. Ann Intern Med 132:173, 2000.

Duncan P et al: Functional reach: A new clinical measure of balance. J Gerontol 45(6):M192-7, 1990.

El-Faizy M, Reinsch S: Home safety intervention for the prevention of falls. Phys Occup Ther Geriatr 12(3):33-49, 1994.

Englander F, Hodson TJ, Terregrossa RA: Economic dimensions of slip and fall injuries. J Forensic Sci 41(5):733-746, 1996.

Evans RL, Hendricks RD: Comparison of subacute rehabilitative care with outpatient primary medical care. Disabil Rehabil 23(12):531-538, 2001.

Fiatarone MA et al: High intensity strength training in nonagenarians: Effects on skeletal muscle. JAMA 263:3029-3034, 1990.

Fleming KC et al: Practical functional assessment of elderly persons: A primary care approach. Mayo Clin Proc 70:890-910, 1995.

Frain JP, Carr PH: Is the typical modern house designed for future adaptations for disabled older people? Age Ageing 25:398-401, 1996.

Frank JS, Winter DA, Craik RL: Gait disorders and falls in the elderly. In Bronstein AF, Brandt T, Woollacott M (eds): Clinical Disorders of Balance, Posture, and Gait. London, Arnold, 1996, p 287-300.

Frontera W et al: A cross-sectional study of muscle strength and mass in 45 to 78 year old men and women. J Appl Physiol 71:644–650, 1991.

General Accounting Office (GAO): Tighter Rules are Needed to Curtail Overcharges for Therapy in Nursing Homes. Report to the Ranking Minority Member, Committee on Commerce, US House of Representatives, March 1998.

General Accounting Office (GAO): Supplementary Security Income Additional Actions Needed to Reduce Program Vulnerability to Fraud and Abuse. Report to the Honorable Henry A. Waxman, Ranking Minority Member, Committee on Government Reform, US House of Representatives, (GAO/HEHS-99-151), September 1999.

Gerety MB et al: Adverse events related to drugs and drug withdrawal in nursing home residents. J Am Geriatr Soc 41:1326-1332, 1993.

Gloth PM III, Scheve AA, Shah S: The frail elderly functional assessment questionnaire: Its responsiveness and validity in alternative settings. Arch Phys Med Rehabil 80(12):1572-1576, 1999.

Gowland C et al: Chedoke-McMaster Stroke Assessment: Development, Validation and Administration Manual. Hamilton, Ontario, Canada, Chedoke-McMaster Hospitals and McMaster University, 1995.

Grounds MD: Age-associated changes in the response of skeletal muscle cells to exercise and regeneration. Ann Acad Sci 854: 78-91, 1998.

Guccione AA: Implications of an aging population for rehabilitation: Demography, mortality, and morbidity in the elderly. In Guccione AA (ed): Geriatric Physical Therapy, 2nd ed. St Louis, Mosby, 2000.

Guccione AA, Jette AM: Multidimensional assessment of functional limitations in patients with arthritis. Arthritis Care Res 3:44–52, 1990.

Haig AJ et al: Outpatient planning for persons with physical disabilities: A randomized prospective trial of physiatrist alone versus a multidisciplinary team. Arch Phys Med Rehabil 76(4):341-348, 1995.

Haffey WJ, Welsh JH: Subacute care evolution in search of value. Arch Phys Med Rehabil 76(12 suppl):SC2-4, 1995.

Halpern M: Functional assessment taxonomy relevant to low-back impairments. J Occup Rehabil 11(3):201-215, 2001.

Hazzard WR, Woolard N, Regenstreif DI: Integrating geriatrics into the subspecialties of internal medicine: The Hartford Foundation/ American Geriatrics Society/Wake Forrest University Bowman Gray School of Medicine Initiative. J Am Geriatr Soc 45(5):638-640, 1997.

Health Care Financing Administration (HCFA): Medicare and You 2000. HCFA Publication No. 10050, revised 1999.

Hibberd JH et al: Can Medicare beneficiaries make informed choices? Health Affairs 17(6):181-193, 1998.

Hill-Lamb ML: More alphabet soup—LTAC. How does long-term acute care fit into the health care continuum? Surg Serv Manage 1(3):37-40, 1995.

Holahan J et al: Medicaid managed care in thirteen states. Health Affairs 17(3):43-63, 1998.

Hollenberg M et al: Treadmill exercise testing in an epidemiologic study of elderly subjects. J Gerontol Biol Sci Med Sci 53A:B259-B267, 1998.

Horak FB, Shupert CL, Morka A: Components of postural dyscontrol in the elderly. Neurobiol Aging 10:727-738, 1989.

Hu MH, Woollacott M: Multisensory training for standing balance in older adults: I. Postural stability and one-leg standing balance. J Gerontol 49:M52-61, 1994.

Huijbregts MPJ, Gruber RA: Functional outcome measurement in the elderly. Orthop Phys Ther Clin North Am 6(3):383-401, 1997.

Huijbregts MPJ, Kay T: The Continuing Care Disability Measure (CCDM): A Gross Motor Function And Mobility Outcome Measure For Continuing Care Clients. Proceedings of Congress of the World Confederation for Physical Therapy, Washington, DC, June 3-5, 1995.

Iglehart JK: The American health care system: Medicaid. New Engl J Med 340(5):403-408, 1999.

Infante M: Subacute units need to be aware of standards. Contemporary Long Term Care 17(4):64, 1994.

Inman CL, Warren GL, Hogan HA et al: Mechanical loading attenuates bone loss due to immobilization and calcium deficiency. J Appl Physiol 87(1):189-195, 1999.

Jaffe DL: Use of Virtual Reality Techniques to Train Elderly People to Step Over Obstacles (abstract), 1998, www.dinf.org/csun_98/csun98_001.htm, accessed October 15, 2000.

Judge JO et al: Dynamic balance in older persons: Effects of reduced visual and proprioceptive input. J Gerontol 50A:M263-M270, 1995.

Kane RL et al: Do rehabilitative nursing homes improve outcomes of care? J Am Geriatr Soc 44:545-554, 1996.

Kane RL, Kane RA: Assessment in long-term care. Annu Rev Public Health 21:659-686, 2000.

Kaneko M et al: A kinematic analysis of walking and physical fitness testing in elderly women. Can J Sport Sci 16:233-238, 1991.

Kauffman T: Impact of aging-related musculoskeletal and postural changes on falls. Top Geriatr Rehabil 5(2):34-43, 1990.

Katz S et al: Studies of illness in the aged. The index of ADL: A standardized measure of biological and psychosocial function. JAMA 185:914-919, 1963.

Kerse N, Butler M, Robinson E et al: Fall prevention in residential care: A cluster, randomized, controlled trial. J Am Geriatr Soc 52(4):524-531, 2004.

Kohrt WM et al: Effects of gender, age and fitness level on response of VO_2 max to training in 6-71 yr olds. J Appl Physiol 71:2004-2111, 1991.

Kurlander SS: HCFA opens up: Understanding the Medicare coverage process for medical technology and services. Rehab Manag 11(6):66-67, 1998.

Lach HW et al: Falls in the elderly: Reliability of a classification system. J Am Geriatr Soc 39:197-202, 1991.

Levenson S. The future of subacute care. Clin Geriatr Med 16(4):683-700, 2000.

Lexell J: Strength training and muscle hypertrophy in older men and women. Topics Geriatr Rehabil 15:41-46, 2000.

Liu K, Black KJ: Hospital-based and freestanding skilled nursing facilities: Any cause for differential Medicare payments? Inquiry 40(1):94-104, 2003.

Looker A et al: Prevalence of low femoral bone density in older U.S. women from NHANES III. J Bone Miner Res 10:796-802, 1995.

Lord SR, Ward JA, Williams P et al: Physiological factors associated with falls in older community dwelling women. J Geriatr Soc 42:1110-1117, 1994.

Lord SR, Clark RD, Webster IW: Visual acuity and contrast sensitivity in relation to falls in a population of aged persons. J Gerontol 46:M69-M76, 1991.

Lusardi MM: Mobility and balance in later life. Orthop Phys Ther Clin North Am 6(3):305-328, 1997.

Mangione KK: Exercise prescription for osteoarthritis of the knee. Orthop Phys Ther Clin North Am 10(2):279-289, 2001.

Mann WC: Technology. In Border BR, Wagner MB (eds): Functional Performance in Older Adults. Philadelphia, FA Davis, 1994.

McCloy CM: Prevention and health promotion strategies in osteoporosis management. Orthop Phys Ther Clin North Am 7(2):235-249, 1998.

McCloy CM: Can the physical therapist make the paradigm shift from health to wellness? Orthop Phys Ther Clin North Am 10(2):303-328, 2001.

Medicare HMO Data Report: Medicare + Choice Plan Withdrawals, 2000. Available at www.medicarehmo.com, accessed October 7, 2000.

Medicare: New choices, new worries. Consumers Reports 3(9):27-38, September 1998.

Menke TJ et al: Impact of all-inclusive diagnosis-related group payment system on inpatient utilization. Med Care 36(8):1126-1137, 1998.

Meyer JA, Zeller PJ: Kaiser Commission, Medicaid and the Uninsured: Profiles of Disability, Employment and Health Coverage. Report prepared for The Kaiser Commission on Medicaid and the Uninsured, September 1999.

Minor MA et al: Efficacy of physical conditioning exercise in patients with rheumatoid arthritis and osteoarthritis. Arthritis Rheum 32:1396, 1989.

Murray PK et al: Rapid growth of rehabilitation services in traditional community-based nursing homes. Arch Phys Med Rehabil 80(4):372-378, 1999.

Nagi SZ: The concept and measurement of disability. In Berkowitz ED (ed): Disability Policies and Government Programs. New York, Praeger, 1979, pp 1-15.

Nugent J: PT reimbursement in Medicare managed care. American Physical Therapy Association, Reimbursement News, 3(5):1-4, 1996.

Oliver D, Daly F, Martin FC et al: Risk factors and risk assessment tool for falls in hospital in-patients: A systematic review. Age Aging 33(2):122-130, 2004.

Palta AE: A framework for understanding mobility problems in the elderly. In Craik RL, Oatis CA (eds): Gait Analysis: Theory and Application. St Louis, Mosby, 1995, pp 436-449.

Parakh B: Unleashing the potential of subacute care. Medical Interface 7(10):95-97, 1994.

Parker G, Bhaktra P, Katbamna S et al: Best place of care for older people after acute and during subacute illness: A systematic review. J Health Serv Res Policy 5(3):176-189, 2000.

Petrella RJ et al: Physical function and fear of falling after hip fracture rehabilitation in the elderly. Am J Phys Med Rehabil 79(2):154–160, 2000.

Physician Payment Review Commission (PPRC): Annual Report to Congress. Washington, DC, PPRC, 1997.

Quadagno J: Incentives to disability in federal disability insurance and supplemental security income. Clin Orthop 336:11-17, 1997.

Rand Corporation: Research Highlights: Effects of Medicare's Prospective Payment System on the Quality of Hospital Care, 1998. Available at www.rand.org/publications, accessed October 31, 2002.

Rapport L et al: Executive functioning and predictors of falls in rehabilitation setting. Arch Phys Med Rehabil 79:629-633, 1998.

Rasmussen B: The Rehabilitation Therapist's Guide to Capitation and Per-Case Payment. Alexandria, VA, American Physical Therapy Association, 1996.

Rimmer J: Health promotion for people with disabilities: The emerging paradigm shift from disability prevention to prevention of secondary conditions. Phys Ther 79:495-502, 1999.

Robbins AS et al: Predictors of falls among elderly people: Results of two population-based studies. Arch Intern Med 149:1628-1633, 1989.

Rogers MA et al: Decline in VO$_2$ max with aging in master athletes and sedentary men. J Appl Physiol 68:2195-2199, 1990.

Rogers MA et al: Effect of 10 days of inactivity on glucose tolerance in master athletes. J Appl Physiol 68:1883-1837, 1990.

Rubenstein L: The clinical effectiveness of multidimensional geriatric assessment. J Am Geriatr Soc 31(12):758-763, 1983.

Sandstrom RW, Lohman H, Bramble JD: Health Services: Policy and Systems for Therapists. Upper Saddle River, NJ, Prentice Hall, 2003.

Schilke JM et al: Effects of muscle-strength training on the functional status of patients with osteoarthritis of the knee joint. Nurs Res 45:68, 1996.

Schmid N: Acute care and long term care partner to provide better services for seniors. Ambulatory Outreach Summer:15-17, 1998.

Sharkey NA, Williams NI: The role of exercise in the prevention and treatment of osteoporosis and osteoarthritis. Nurs Clin North Am 35:209-221, 2000.

Shatto A: Comapring Medicare beneficiaries, by type of post-acute care received: 1999. Health Care Financ Rev 24(2):137-142, 2002.

Skelton DA et al: Strength, power and related functional ability of healthy people aged 65-89 years. Age Ageing 23:371-377, 1994.

Smith R: Validation and reliability of the elderly mobility scale. Physiotherapy 80:744, 1994.

Social Security Administration: Social Security: A "Snapshot." SSA Pub. No. 05-10006, March 1998.

Stein BE: Avoiding drug reactions: Seven steps to writing safe prescriptions. Geriatrics 49(9):28-36, 1994.

Stewart DA et al: The two minute walking test: A sensitive index of mobility in the rehabilitation of elderly patients. Clin Rehabil 2:273, 1990.

Stelmach GE, Worringham CJ: Sensorimotor deficits related to postural stability: Implication for falling in elderly, Clin Geriatr Med 1(3):679-694, 1985.

Tamblyn RM, McLeod PJ, Abramhamowicz M et al: Do too many cooks spoil the broth? Multiple physician involvement in medical management of elderly patients and potentially inappropriate drug combinations. CMAJ 158(8):1177-1184, 1996.

Tamblyn RM: Medication use in seniors: Challenges and solutions. Therapie 51(3):269-282, 1996.

Tinetti M, Speechley M, Ginter S: Risk factors for falls among elderly persons living in the community. New Engl J Med 319:1707, 1988.

Tinetti ME et al: A multifactorial intervention to reduce risk of falling among elderly people living in the community. New Engl J Med 331:821-827, 1994.

Tompkins CP et al: Applying disease management strategies to Medicare. Milbank Q 77(4):461-484, 1999.

Thompson E et al: Cardiovascular response to submaximal concentric and eccentric isokinetic exercise in older adults. J Aging Phys Activity 7:20-31, 1999.

Tracy BL et al: Muscle quality: II. Effects of strength training in 65-75 yr-old men and women. J Appl Physiol 86:195-201, 1999.

United States Department of Health and Human Services: Operation restore trust. 1995.

United States Department of Health and Human Services: Healthy People 2000: National Health Promotion and Disease Prevention Objectives. Washington, DC, US Government Printing Office, 1990.

University of California Los Angeles, http://geronet.ph.ucla.edu/managed_care/fact_sheet.htm, accessed March 9, 2002.

Vandervoort AA: Ankle mobility and postural stability. Physiother Theory Pract 15:91-103, 1999.

Vandervoort AA: Resistance exercise throughout life. Orthop Phys Ther Clin North Am 10(2):227-240, 2001.

Vassallo M, Vignaraja R, Sharma JC et al: The effect of changing practice on fall prevention in a rehabilitative hospital: the hospital injury prevention study. J Am Geriatr Soc 52(3):335-339, 2004.

Waid MO: Overview of the Medicare and Medicaid Programs. Health Care Financing Review, 1998 Statistical Supplement. Baltimore, US Department of Health and Human Services, Health Care Financing Administration, Office of Strategic Planning, 1998.

Welch WP: What does Medicare pay for? Disentangling the flow of funds to health care providers. Health Affairs 17(4):184-197, 1998a.

Welch WP: Bundled Medicare payment for acute and postacute care. Health Affairs 17(6):69-81, 1998b.

White C: Rehabilitation therapy in skilled nursing facilities: Effects of Medicare's new prospective payment system. Health Affairs (Millwood) 22(3):214-223, 2003.

Williams AK: Aging persons with long-term physical disabilities. Orthop Phys Ther Clin North Am 6(3):357-367, 1997.

Wolfson L, Judge J, Whipple R et al: Strength is a major factor in balance, gait and the occurrence of falls. J Gerontol 50A:64-67, 1995.

World Health Organization: International Classification of Impairments, Disabilities, and Handicaps: A Manual Relating to the Consequences of Disease, vol 41, Geneva, WHO, 1993 (originally published in 1980).

SUGGESTED READINGS

Congressional Budget Office: Long-Term Budgetary Pressures and Policy Options. Washington, DC, US Government Printing Office, 1997.

Guccione AA: Geriatric Physical Therapy, 2nd ed. St Louis, Mosby, 2000.

Health Care Financing Review: 1998 Statistical Supplement. Baltimore, US Department of Health and Human Services, Health Care Financing Administration, Office of Strategic Planning, 1998.

Health Affairs: January/February 1999, vol 18, no 1, 269 pp. Special issue covering The Future of Medicare.

Slifkin RT et al: Medical managed care programs in rural areas: A fifty-state overview. Health Affairs 17(6):217-227, 1998.

Social Security Administration: Disability benefits. SSA Pub. No. 05-10029, September 1999.

Stuck AE et al: Comprehensive geriatric assessment: A meta-analysis of controlled trial. Lancet 342:1032-1036, 1993.

Ting H: Subacute care: Analysis of the market opportunities and competitors. Center for Healthcare Information, 2000, www.healthcare-info.com/sca.htm, accessed September 22, 2000.

Wharton MA: Environmental design: Accommodating sensory changes in the elderly. In Guccione AA (ed): Geriatric Physical Therapy, 2nd ed. St Louis, Mosby, 2000.

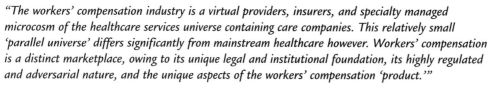

CHAPTER 5

Disability Management in Workers' Compensation

David W. Clifton, Jr., PT

"The workers' compensation industry is a virtual providers, insurers, and specialty managed microcosm of the healthcare services universe containing care companies. This relatively small 'parallel universe' differs significantly from mainstream healthcare however. Workers' compensation is a distinct marketplace, owing to its unique legal and institutional foundation, its highly regulated and adversarial nature, and the unique aspects of the workers' compensation 'product.'"

- Lunbeck et al, 1997

KEY POINTS

- Workers' compensation (WC), unlike other health care systems, is a legal system, not a medical one. Workers' compensation involves statutory law.
- WC structure and processes present unique barriers to successful disability management outcomes. These must be understood; addressed; and in some cases, overcome by rehabilitation professionals.
- Non-medical issues (e.g., psychosocial variables) directly and indirectly affect disability management within workers' compensation systems. These variables can drive cost, utilization, provider type, and clinical outcomes.
- Rehabilitation professionals play a significant role under WC and are well positioned to have positive impact. This impact spans the following three points along the disability continuum: from injury/illness prevention, through treatment, and post-treatment.
- Return-to-work (RTW), not maximum medical improvement, is the outcomes litmus test in WC cases. RTW or gainful employment represents the ultimate goal of work-related disability management and rehabilitation.

Operational Definitions

Incidence	A measure of injury or illness frequency in WC.
Indemnity	WC or disability benefits that are paid in place of lost wages. These replacement wages are determined by each state's workers' compensation act or law. However, this typically is non-taxable income paid at two thirds of the worker's average weekly wage.
Integrated Benefits	The blending of WC with other insurance lines, such as group health or long-term disability insurance. Joint administration of lines achieves greater efficiencies and/or cost controls; also known as *24-hour coverage.*
Loss	Injury or illness that leads to lost time from work.
Loss Prevention	Interventions designed to prevent and/or reduce the frequency/severity of losses.
Permanent Partial Disability (PPD)	A disability (physical or mental) that is expected to last a lifetime but that renders the worker only partially unable to earn a living.
Permanent Total Disability (PTD)	A disability that is so severe that it renders a person unable to engage in any degree of gainful employment. Compensation may have limits in time, or it may run an entire lifetime in the rarest form of disability.

Reasonable Accommodations	Terminology used under the Americans with Disabilities Act of 1990 (ADA) for interventions designed to ensure a safe but expedient worker-workplace match; generally a combination of administrative and/or engineering controls.
Return-To-Work (RTW)	An aggressive job-specific restorative program designed with outcomes based on injured or ill persons' reentry into gainful employment at some level with or without reasonable accommodations.
Temporary Partial Disability (TPD)	A disability wherein all earning capability is lost, but only temporarily. Insurance benefits continue until the person is capable of some form of RTW. TPD is the most common disability category in WC.

WORKERS' COMPENSATION OVERVIEW

Common Benefit Design Features

Worker's compensation (WC) programs were developed in the early 1900s through state acts or laws. The United States currently has a patchwork of 50 state WC laws. These laws each have unique elements, but they also share common attributes. Unlike other insurance lines, WC is a legal, not a medical, benefits system (Durbin, 1993; Palczynski, 1993). WC was designed as a no-fault system that protects both employers and employees. Employers are protected from legal actions arising from workplace accidents, whereas a worker's right to employability is preserved. Hypothetically, in the case of an injury, employers cannot fire injured workers, who in turn cannot sue employers under a liability theory.

More than 80% of workers in the United States are covered by WC (Durbin, 1993). Workers who have transitory jobs or fail to meet the domicile (residence) requirements of a given state are covered under separate federal workers' compensation acts. These include harbor workers (e.g., longshoremen, military personnel, railroad workers). There are also categories of workers who are exempted from WC coverage altogether: employees of non-profit organizations, religious groups, domestic service workers, farm employees, casual laborers, and state and local government workers.

WC acts provide varying degrees of coverage for medical costs, indemnity or lost wage replacement, vocational services, and death benefits (Table 5–1).

Because each state has its own unique WC law, bureau, or commission, these state authorities, not insurance companies, establish program eligibility criteria, coverage parameters, and provider participation rules. This represents a significant departure from other insurance lines wherein benefit structures are established by the insurance company itself.

Unlike group health or managed care, WC provides first-dollar coverage for medical treatment, including physical rehabilitation. This means that WC beneficiaries do not share financial risks, as do their managed care counterparts via co-payments or deductibles. Hypothetically, WC medical coverage is unlimited in terms of duration and cost. However, several issues serve to create an adversarial system. These issues are discussed later in this chapter.

How Is Workers' Compensation Financed?

WC insurance is underwritten by private insurers in most states, although employers ultimately finance WC costs. In other states, WC is provided by the state in direct competition with private insurers. The most common form involves high-risk pools or state-funded programs. These exist for those employers who have difficulty securing private insurance, are too small to constitute their own group, or were dropped from other workers' compensation programs because of excessive risk underwriting or actual losses that exceed industrial sector norms. A small number of WC systems are "monopolistic," meaning the state is the only authorized source of WC coverage. Under this scenario, the state itself serves as the insurance company. State funds fall within the "other" category depicted in Figure 5–1.

Most WC insurance is underwritten through traditional property and casualty insurers such as Liberty Mutual, Wausau, and New Jersey Manufacturers.

Many states allow employers to use "alternative markets" for WC coverage. Alternative markets include deductible policies, retro-rated policies, dividend policies, and self-insurance. Self-insurance is the most pertinent to

Table 5–1 Workers' Compensation Benefits Coverage	
Direct medical coverage	Hospitalization, physician services, medications, rehabilitation, durable medical equipment
Disability coverage	Indemnity or lost wages for temporary or permanent conditions that involve partial or full disability
Vocational services	Job placement, vocational assessment, retraining
Death benefits	Survivors receive death benefit payments if the death is work related

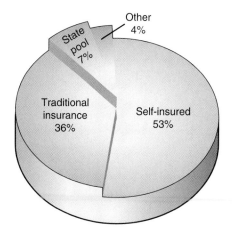

Figure 5–1. Workers' compensation: Market share by insured type. (Data from Lunbeck RA, Johnson JT, Lee R: Workers' Compensation: A Not-So-Parallel Universe. Boston, Hambrecht and Quist Capital Management LLC Company Report, March 20, 1997.)

the rehabilitation provider in terms of consultative opportunities with employers for both disability prevention and management programs. More than 50% of all WC insurance is self-funded or self-insured (see Figure 5–1). Generally, employers may self-insure for WC provided they can demonstrate financial solvency. Self-insurance alleviates the need to pay insurance premiums because costs are paid as losses (e.g., accidents, injuries, illnesses) are incurred. An employer who is self-insured must set aside "company reserves" when a loss occurs. A loss under WC occurs when a reportable injury or illness results in lost time from the job. The company reserve is an amount of money calculated to cover the loss, both medical and indemnity (wage replacement) costs for the lifetime of a disability. The lifetime of a disability is determined by a host of variables including injury or illness severity, establishment of medically necessary care, employment status, and litigation. In catastrophic cases such as spinal cord injury, head trauma, asbestosis, and other chronic conditions, company reserves can run into the millions of dollars. Therefore self-insurance carries greater risk, since an insurance policy does not pay for the loss because there is no prepayment of insurance premiums. Instead, a "pay as you go" mechanism results, in which money comes directly out of the employer's coffers. Company reserves cannot be used for any other purpose but to fund the loss. This can make disability prevention programs appealing to self-insured employers. Company reserves are escrowed in interest-bearing accounts that are exclusively earmarked for the injured or ill employee. This takes money out of a company's cash flow and thus the appeal of loss prevention programs. Should the employee not require the full amount of money reserved, the funds are rolled back into the employer's accounts after the case is closed. A "closed case" is one in which any of the following occurs:

- Injured worker returns to his or her previous job (with or without restriction or limitations)
- Injured worker dies
- Injured work retires
- Injured worker is transferred to a new job
- Injured worker receives a court or workers' compensation judge award (e.g., permanent total disability [PTD])
- Injured worker changes employer

Self-insured employers are a hotbed of opportunity for rehabilitation providers because of the heightened degree of risk taking and the need to aggressively prevent injury and control medical costs. Physical rehabilitation providers have both the education and the clinical experience to effectively offer injury prevention or risk management programs (Table 5–2) (Huhn & Volski, 1985).

THE LANGUAGE OF WORKERS' COMPENSATION

WC, previously known as *workmen's compensation,* has its own unique dialect. Because it is a legal or disability management system, many of its associated terms are unfamiliar to providers. A brief review of the most common terms confronting rehabilitation providers is provided.

Causality

Causality describes the linkage between a work-related incident, event, trauma, or accident that directly leads to an impairment or disability. In WC, only those losses that have a proximate link to the workplace are considered covered expenses. The burden of proof rests with the employer to disprove the work-relatedness of a claim. This is typically accomplished through a combination of engineering studies, independent medical examinations, and medical expert testimony. Considering their knowledge of anatomy, biomechanics, kinesiology, and injury mechanisms, rehabilitation providers are invaluable adjuncts to these determinations. Physical or occupational therapists' professional opinions are occasionally used in concert with the medical opinions of orthopedists, occupational medicine physicians, neurologists, and physiatrists.

Medical Necessity

Medical necessity is a concept that denotes that causality or work-relatedness has been established for an injury or loss and that medical treatment is required for an impairment or disability. Some persons misinterpret medical necessity and use it interchangeably with "reasonable" and "appropriate" care. *Reasonable and appropriate care* does not directly address the issue of causality or question the legitimacy of a condition. These concepts are two steps removed from causality or work-relatedness determinations and one step removed from medical necessity determinations. Once an injury or illness has been declared compensable because work-related causality has been established, the question then becomes, "Is there an organic basis for treatment?" Diagnostic workups generally establish the anatomical, physiological, or neuropsychiatric nature of a problem. After cause has been determined and a diagnosis rendered, determination can be made regarding whether care is reasonable and appropriate. A case can have causality established, but not medical necessity. Similarly, a case may be work related and an employee may have a genuine diagnosis, yet care is deemed unreasonable or inappropriate. Reasonable and appropriate care for a condition is that which is consistent with a community standard of care. A community standard

Table 5–2 Rehabilitation Provider's Role in Workers' Compensation

Intervention	Preinjury	Postinjury
Ergonomic assessment	✓	✓
Functional job analysis	✓	✓
Functional capacity evaluation	✓	✓
Employee education and training (e.g., cumulative trauma, back injury, proper lifting, manual material handling)	✓	✓
Management education and training (e.g., worker-worksite matching, prevention/wellness programs)	✓	✓
Work conditioning and work hardening	✓	✓
Early intervention programs		✓
Medicolegal consultation		✓
Post offer evaluation (Americans with Disabilities Act)	✓	

of care is established through clinical literature (peer-reviewed), peer consensus, curriculum, and prevailing practice standards.

Compensable

A *compensable* case under WC is one in which benefits eligibility, causality, and reasonableness have been established in accordance with statutory requirements. These cases are deserved of medical treatment and indemnity or lost wages if time away from work resulted from the injury or illness. Case law forms the foundation of administrative decisions pertaining to benefits by establishing compensability of injury or illness. Again, providers must remember that they are operating under a legal, not a medical, system. Therefore it is incumbent on providers to become well versed in WC case law, especially if they conduct functional capacity evaluations (FCEs) for the purpose of disability or RTW determinations.

Aggravation of Pre-Existing Condition

In most WC jurisdictions, coverage is provided for cases in which a preexisting injury was aggravated by a workplace variable. These cases are considered as new injuries or illnesses under the law. Employees do not relinquish their right to benefits simply because they have a preexisting injury or illness, as is the case in other forms of insurance (e.g., group health).

Work Relatedness

Under WC, injuries or illnesses must be related to the workplace, typically through a proximate cause, to be covered. This is a highly controversial and litigated issue in WC, and an ever-growing body of case law addresses it on a state-by-state basis. In recent years, the work relatedness, and ultimately compensability, of what constitutes a WC claim has been markedly expanded. Most notably, cumulative trauma disorders (CTDs) or repetitive strain disorders (RSDs) and mental stress claims have expanded the notion of compensability (Anderson, 1998; Hays, 1998; Lankford, 1997).

Experience Modification

WC rating bureaus (e.g., National Council on Compensation Insurance [NCCI]) promulgate *experience modifiers* or *modifications* (known as *mods*) based on the loss experience of an insured business. Experience mods cause insurance premiums to move up or down from year to year, because they compare a company's loss experience with past years and adjust rates accordingly. In addition, a company's loss experience can be compared with a "community standard" or against similar businesses. Rehabilitation providers who wish to consult with employers need to recognize this term to demonstrate the effectiveness of cost-containment or consultative programs.

Combined Ratio

Combined ratio describes the sum of loss and expense ratio. It is also referred to as the *combined loss and expense ratio.*

The loss ratio is the percentage of insurance premiums that are applied against losses. The expense ratio is the percentage of insurance premium that is directed toward an insurance company's operational costs. When the combined ratio is 100%, this means that every premium dollar collected was used to pay down losses and operating expenses. In this example, there is no profit reaped by the insurer. When the ratio is less than 100%, there is profit, or what is called an *underwriting gain*. More than 100% ratios represent business losses and unprofitable insurance lines. Throughout most of the 1980s and into the mid-1990s, WC carriers sustained combined ratios well in excess of 100%, reaching as high as 123% (NCCI, 1999). Essentially, for every dollar collected as insurance premium in 1991, $1.23 was expended to cover both medical and indemnity payments. Managed WC strategies curtailed these losses in the second half of the 1990s, but they have begun to rise again in typical WC cycles.

Disability Ratings

Disability determinations are scaled under WC along at least two planes. Disability awards are driven by a temporal plane (time-based) in which the duration of a disability determines whether a claim is temporary or permanent. Second, the extent of disability or severity index dictates whether a claim involves *partial* or *total* disability. When a claim results in a nil chance of the employee ever returning to gainful employment (in any capacity), a PTD award is granted. As one might expect, PTD awards are relatively rare, but this does not prevent some injured employees (and their attorneys) from filing for this designation.

Of all WC injuries, 76% require medical services only and do not lead to any disability rating (NCCI, 1996). A mere 0.1% of all claims result in a disability rating of PTD or death.

Permanent partial diability (PPD) results when a person in all probability will not work again in his or her former position or preinjury/preloss job. PPD claims account for 8% of all disability ratings (NCCI, 1996).

Temporary total disability (TTD) and temporary partial disability (TPD) depict the individual who is temporarily out of work or is working in a reduced capacity. In this scenario, there is a full expectation of a full RTW in his or her previous position or job after appropriate medical and rehabilitation services have been rendered. TTDs compose 16% of all disability ratings (NCCI, 1996).

Scheduled Versus Non-Scheduled Losses

Scheduled injuries are those that typically involve very specific injury to specific body parts (e.g., amputated limbs, deafened ears, or blinded eyes). These claims are compensated based solely on medical impairment or loss versus lost earning capacity (as in disability insurance claims). Each body part or loss is associated with a payment schedule based on a precalculated number of weeks. For instance, a loss of a thumb may result in a 60-week payout of indemnity that is about 66⅔rds of the worker's average weekly wage (AWW) over the last quarter. The loss of a second finger may result in a 30-week payout of about 66⅔rds of the AWW. Loss of hearing in both ears may result in 175 weeks of payment. Scheduled injuries are also referred to as *specific losses,* because they lend themselves to objective measures of disability. Specific losses, unlike soft tissue sprain or strain, tend to be unequivocal relative to the degree or severity of resultant disability.

To the contrary, *non-scheduled injuries* involve more subjective areas such as the trunk, internal organs, neck, or psychological conditions. These conditions may require an independent medical examination (IME) or an FCE. Indemnity compensation levels are determined by functional impairment measure or as a prediction of loss of earning capacity. Some states require specific impairment/disability measures, whereas others do not. Readers are encouraged to read Chapter 8.

Experience Rating

A state agency may rate an employer by its claims experience as compared with a normative database consisting of comparable companies in comparable industrial sectors. A 1.0 experience rating represents the average for a given industry sector. Companies with experience modifiers greater than 1.0 typically enjoy better WC rates or premiums. When this occurs, it is called a *credit mod.* A *debit mod* results when a company underperforms relative to a sector facing similar exposures and experiences greater than average losses.

Reportable Injury

Reportable injuries are more of an OSHA term than a WC concept per se. However, because employers are required to record (on OSHA 200 logs) any reportable injuries or illness resulting from workplace exposures, it is included for discussion here. Reportable injuries are those that satisfy one of the following criteria:

- Days away from work result
- Days of restricted, "modified," "transitional," or "light" duty
- Medical treatment extends beyond immediate first aid

Lost Time Accident

Lost time injuries or *illnesses,* as the name suggests, involve conditions that result in lost work time. Lost time injuries are OSHA reportable occurrences. If an employer experiences a disproportionate number by percentage (population versus man hours worked) of lost time accidents, a federal inquiry can be triggered. OSHA can use WC injury logs or the OSHA 200 log to investigate jobs with injury rates that are higher than the industrial sector average.

Whole Man/Whole Person

WC disability rating schemes may use the *whole man* or *whole person* method in determination of the degree of disability and payment for the disability. Essentially, impairment and disability are rated based on how much function has been lost as a result of an injury expressed as a percentage of the total body (100%). Obviously, the higher the percentage, the greater the payment.

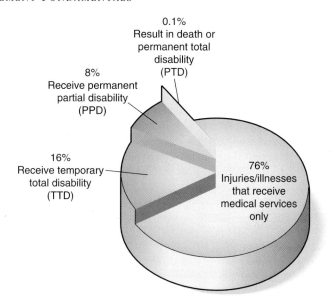

Figure 5–2. Workers' compensation disability categories by prevalence. (Data from National Council on Compensation Insurance [NCCI]: Annual Statistical Bulletin. Boca Raton, FL, NCCI, 1996.)

Permanancy

Permanency addresses the time dimension associated with WC and disability. A person can be described as having a temporary or permanent disability in terms of the disability's duration. A *permanent disability* obviously implies no chances of recovery, whereas a label of *temporary* implies some degree of recovery. Most claims (76%) receive only medical services and are without disability labels (temporary versus permanent and partial versus total) (Figure 5–2).

WORKERS' COMPENSATION DEMOGRAPHIC AND COST DATA

Aggregate Costs

WC has been estimated to be a $54.5 to $96.6 billion market in direct medical and indemnity payments (Miller, 1995; Neumark et al, 1991). Over one decade alone (1981 to 1991), the average medical costs per case more than tripled (Durbin, 1993).

When indirect costs such as administrative expenses, legal fees, employee replacement, and lost productivity are factored in, estimates rise exponentially. An extensive analysis of costs for 1992, a peak year, revealed that direct and indirect workplace costs exceeded $145 billion (Leigh et al, 1997). Indirect costs accounted for 66% of total costs ($96 billion). There were more than 13 million non-fatal WC injuries, with 6 million disabling injuries, in 1992.

Medical costs spiraled out of control between the 1980s and 1990s. In 1981, the average medical cost per case was $2134 compared with $7817 in 1991 (Durbin, 1993).

Who and What Is Injured?

WC is an outpatient phenomenon versus the traditional hospital-based group or general health system. A financial analysis of this sector concluded, "Highly fragmented outpatient physician and therapist providers comprise the front line of the workers' compensation industry" (Lunbeck et al, 1997).

Rehabilitation providers can access several sources for data specific to work-related disability. These include the following:

- OSHA
- National Institute for Occupational Safety and Health
- Bureau of the Census
- State workers' compensation bureaus
- National Safety Council
- NCCI
- Workers' Compensation Research Institute (WCRI)
- National Center for Health Statistics
- U.S. Department of Labor

More than 13 million non-fatal injuries and more than 860,000 illnesses occur annually among American workers (Leigh et al, 1997). When combined for these incidents, direct and non-direct medical costs topped $145 billion. Leigh et al (1997) consider these estimates to be low because of underreporting.

Back disorders are the number one cause of work-related disability (LaPlante & Carlson, 1996). Heart disease is second, at 10% of all incidents. Arthritis (8.3%), respiratory diseases (5.6%), mental disorders (4.9%), lower extremity impairments (4.5%), and diabetes (3.3%) round out the top categories of work-related disability.

Musculoskeletal conditions account for 28% of lost work days, the greatest percentage of any category (Watson Wyatt Worldwide, 1998/1999). "Soft tissue" injuries account for an increasing number/percentage of claims (Butler et al, 1996). Next is pregnancy (23%), "other" (14%), CTDs (9%), mental health and substance abuse (8%), cancer (7%), cardiovascular conditions (7%), and AIDS (1%).

A WC injury profile performed by the NCCI found that 32.7% of all injuries are associated with the back, followed by upper extremities, which incur a 26.5% prevalence rate (Table 5-3).

Sprains and strains are the most prevalent musculoskeletal injuries (52% prevalence). Strains due to overexertion are associated with the highest cause of injury (43.3% of all cases). Slips and falls are the second-leading cause of injury (21.2% of all cases).

Liberty Mutual's "Workplace Safety Index" ranked the 10 top causes of WC-based injuries (Roberts, 2002). Nationwide, overexertion injuries accounted for roughly $10.3 billion in wage and direct medical payments during 1999. This represents 25.5% of all WC, according to Liberty Mutual, the largest underwriter of WC in the United States.

Table 5-3 Workers' Compensation Injury Profile

A. BODY PART

Injury Type	Percentage of Cases	Percentage of Medical Benefits
Head	3.90%	4.20%
Neck	2.60%	3.10%
Back	32.70%	39.90%
Trunk (excluding back)	7.70%	8.50%
Upper extremities	26.50%	17.50%
Lower extremities	18.60%	16.10%
Multiple injuries	7.90%	10.60%
Other	0.01%	0.01%

B. NATURE OF INJURY

Injury Type	Percentage of Cases	Percentage of Medical Benefits
Contusion	8.4%	7.4%
Crushing, fracture	12.9%	13.3%
Hernia	1.7%	0.7%
Rupture	1.6%	2.6%
Sprain, strain	52.0%	55.6%
Amputation	1.3%	1.4%
Vision loss	0.1%	0.1%
Occupational disease/cumulative injury	3.6%	3.6%
Other	18.5%	15.3%

C. CAUSE OF INJURY

Cause	Percentage of Cases	Percentage of Medical Benefits
Burn or extreme cold	2.6%	2.3%
Caught in or between	3.7%	9.5%
Cut, puncture, scrape	3.3%	1.4%
Fall or slip	21.2%	18.9%
Motor vehicle	4.7%	5.6%
Strain or jumping	43.3%	44.1%
Striking against or stepping on	3.6%	2.8%
Struck by object	7.7%	6.8%
Miscellaneous	9.8%	8.7%

Data from National Council on Compensation Insurance: Annual Statistical Bulletin. Boca Raton, FL, NCCI, 1996.

Employers ranked repetitive motion injuries (RMIs) as their most important priority ("Executive Survey of Workplace Safety") despite ranking sixth among costs. Direct costs associated with RMIs involved $2.7 billion nationwide. Liberty Mutual's "Workplace Safety Index" top 10 injuries in 1999 are as follows:

Loss Mechanism	Annual Costs
1. Overexertion	$10.3 billion
2. Falls on the same level	$4.6 billion
3. Bodily reaction (e.g., bending, slipping without falling)	$3.8 billion
4. Falls to lower level	$3.7 billion
5. Being struck by an object	$3.4 billion
6. Repetitive motion	$2.7 billion
7. Highway accidents	$2.4 billion
8. Being struck against an object	$1.7 billion
9. Becoming caught in or compressed by machinery	$1.6 billion
10. Exposure to temperature extremes	$400 million

U.S. Bureau of Census data reveal similar rates of work disability between men and women across all ages (McNeil, 1997). These data refute a commonly held belief that WC is a man's domain. These data may reflect entry of more women into the workplace and might represent a niche market for rehabilitation providers.

Workers' Compensation Versus Non–Workers' Compensation Cost-Duration Data

Data from the NCCI indicate significant differences between WC cases and non-WC cases in the following areas: duration of treatment, visits to providers, and case costs (Durbin et al, 1996).

These data were derived from four geographically diverse states: Florida, Illinois, Pennsylvania, and Oregon. Fifteen WC carriers provided data descriptive of the following: (1) total payment, (2) total service per episode duration, and (3) outpatient dates of service. WC cases, with one exception (hernia), were consistently more costly than non-WC cases (Durbin et al, 1996).

Duration of care, otherwise known as *length of stay,* is significantly longer in WC cases than in non-WC cases (Durbin et al, 1996). WC beneficiaries visit their providers 2.2 times more frequently than do non-WC beneficiaries, partly due to the paucity of cost and utilization controls. Duration of care or length of stay in WC is significantly greater than in similar non-WC cases (207 versus 52 days, respectively). Likewise, WC cases are more expensive at 1.7 times the cost of non-WC cases. These data illustrate an extreme need for disability management in WC.

Rehabilitation as a Workers' Compensation Cost Driver

"Much workers' compensation medical care is delivered through the general healthcare system, which has different imperatives, creating inefficiencies in the workers' compensation sphere and, therefore, a huge opportunity for focused compensation providers."

- Lunbeck et al, 1997

In 1972, the National Commission on State Workmans' Compensation set forth its mission or foundation for modern WC laws (National Commission on State Workmans' Compensation Laws, 1972). The term *workers'* replaced "workmens'" to reflect the importance of women in the workforce. This commission identified and strongly encouraged the adoption of the following five objectives:

1. To provide broad coverage of employees for work-related injuries and disease
2. To provide substantial protection against loss of income
3. *To provide appropriate medical care and rehabilitation services* [emphasis added]
4. To encourage safety
5. To effectively deliver benefits and services

Rehabilitation services command an extremely high profile in WC, as evidenced by objective No. 3. Utilization rates for rehabilitation in WC exceeds rates in other insurance lines. Despite this fertile environment, relatively few providers have chosen to specialize in this area. Lost work days appear to drive the type of service required in WC cases. Surgery, diagnostic, and rehabilitation are the top three interventions in the management of low back disorders (Williams et al, 1998).

Financial Impact of Physical Rehabilitation

Cost data associated with physical and occupational therapy services under WC are rarely segregated from total costs; however, limited data are available that suggest the prominent role played by rehabilitation professionals. Physical therapy and chiropractic services have been shown to be the greatest medical cost drivers in some WC systems, such as New Jersey's (Gardner et al, 1994). Physical therapy accounts for 8% to 16% of all WC costs and was involved in 35% of all cases in Florida (NCCI, 1994). WC utilization rates eclipse those of other insurance lines for similar conditions. The average rate of outpatient physical therapy covered by WC was 12.3 visits compared with 5.4 under group health. The average treatment duration under WC is four times greater than that of non-WC. NCCI reports 206.6 days for WC cases compared with 51.9 for non-WC. Jette et al (1994) noted that physical therapy charges for low back pain management were 36% higher for WC cases than for non-WC.

The WCRI documents that physical and occupational therapy combined accounts for 10% of all medical payments and 37% of all claims, averaging 14.4 visits per claim at an average cost of $1237 (Eccleston, 2000).

According to the NCCI, physical therapy is involved in 35% of all WC cases, compared with less than 4% in non-WC (e.g., group health) (Durbin, 1993). WC cases involving physical therapy costs are nearly three times as costly as similar cases treated under non-WC insurance lines. This ratio exceeds the ratio for pure "medical" services, which are, on average, twice as expensive under WC than under non-WC plans (Pozzebon, 1993). WC low back cases receiving physical therapy incur costs that are 62% higher than non-WC back claims. This additional expense may be partly justified by the unique rehabilitation focus associated with WC. However, this may not account for all of its disproportionality. In WC, the focus is on RTW. This requires a more functional approach and grappling with a host of psychosocioeconomic issues (Meerding et al, 2004; Schultz et al, 2004).

Readers are referred to Chapter 7 for a more detailed description of these variables. The very structure of WC makes it a more challenging environment because of its first-dollar coverage (no financial risk for patient), hypothetically unlimited care, and high degree of litigation, to name a few. Durbin (1993) reports that the average physical therapy case cost under WC is $1777, compared with $597 for non-WC cases.

SPECIFIC BARRIERS TO DISABILITY MANAGEMENT

"The contour of the land is an aid to an army; sizing up the opponents to determine victory, assessing dangers and distances, is the proper course of action for military leaders. Those who do battle knowing these will win, those who do battle without knowing these will lose."

- Tzu, 1991

This war-related quotation by Tsu could very well be mistaken for a disability manager's survival guide. Providers must engage in the analysis of multiple variables associated with disability management and physical rehabilitation. Smail (1995) breaks these into the following three categories:

1. Variables related to the individual
2. Variables related to employment
3. Variables related to society

Krause et al (2001) identified about 100 different determinants of RTW outcomes through an extensive literature review. WC, partly due to a disproportionate number of chronic cases, is a system of "specialists" versus the "generalist" or primary care focus of group health. Persons with disabilities require a comprehensive array of health care services and providers (Beatty et al, 2003). WC systems are constructed and operated in a manner that provides multiple and diverse barriers to successful RTW outcomes (Clifton, 1995). Perhaps this explains why relatively few providers specialize in this area (Table 5-4).

Regardless of WC's barriers, providers must become familiar with the external influences that serve to influence their treatment programs. Providers must learn to control those variables within their domain and to collaborate with others when necessary. Disability management of a typical WC case involves a community context: injured employee, first-line supervisor, primary care physician (PCP), orthopedist, neurologist, physical or occupational therapist, case manager (insurance company's), claims adjuster, human resources department, attorney, third-party administrator (in self-insured employers), and vocational rehabilitation specialist. These persons confront a plethora of issues specific to WC. Time and space constraints preclude a full-blown discussion of each listed obstacle. Key obstacles that are discussed in detail include litigation, delayed rehabilitation, poorly trained physicians,

Table 5–4 Workers' Compensation: Disability Management Obstacles

- Cost shifting from other insurance lines (e.g., employee claims of work relatedness)
- Lack of financial risk for patients (e.g., co-payments, deductibles)
- Absence of standardized disability determination standards
- Patchwork of state laws
- A legal, not medical, system
- Expanded definition of disability (e.g., psychiatric, cumulative trauma disorders)
- Hypothetically unlimited medical care
- Highly litigious
- Dueling doctors
- Focus on RTW, not just "maximum medical benefit"
- High degree of fraud and abuse
- Paucity of providers trained in occupational medicine and WC
- Delayed rehabilitation and ineffective postinjury communications
- Generous indemnity or wage replacement
- High prevalence of unnecessary medical care
- Loosely and poorly designed provider networks
- Driven more by cost-containment versus quality enhancement (e.g., preferred provider organizations' "discount fees")

consumer ignorance, worker profiles, fraud and abuse, expanded disability definition, and disability determinations.

These issues have been selected for an expanded view because they are areas in which rehabilitation providers can have direct impact. In contrast, providers realistically can effect little change in WC system structural or design elements because these require legislative, regulatory, litigation, or electoral initiatives.

Delayed Rehabilitation

It is a long-held belief by some that to delay rehabilitation is to compromise rehabilitation in a WC system (Ehrmann-Feldman et al, 1996; Galvin, 1986; Haig et al, 1990; Lemstra & Olszynski, 2003). Poor communication is one of the disadvantages of WC, and it begins with the employer. Following a work-related incident, employers are legally obligated to complete and file an "Employer's First Report of Injury" form.

This officially opens a case for medical benefits. A critical success indicator is how expeditiously the employer files this form. It has been estimated that how an employer responds within the first 24 hours following injury determines 50% of future claim costs and outcomes (Miller, 1995). The national average between the time an incident occurs and the time the adjuster receives the claim is 21 days. This is a critical timeframe for many rehabilitation cases, sespecially those that involve soft tissue injury with accompanying inflammatory responses, collagen formation, range-of-motion restrictions, and pain. For instance, 21 days can make the difference between a frozen shoulder (adhesive capsulitis) and a shoulder with good ROM. A full 30% of first reports of injury are delayed, according to the Wyatt Company (Miller, 1995). Some occupational medicine companies assist employers in the completion of these forms to expedite referral for treatment. Next, the employee schedules and completes a visit to one of the employer's posted panel physicians. This may further delay a referral for rehabilitation. A PCP may then refer the injured worker to a medical specialist. The medical specialist, who commonly is an orthopedist, neurologist, physiatrist or physical medicine and rehabilitation physician, may then make a referral for physical rehabilitation. Weeks or months may pass before the injured worker is seen by a physical or occupational therapist. At this late juncture, the therapist is often confronted with confounding obstacles that may or may not be related to the original insult. Fortunately, orthopedic surgeon visits covered by WC or managed care are more likely to result in a rehabilitation referral than are noncovered visits (Freburger et al, 2003).

Workers' Compensation Suffers from "Information Asymmetry"

For years, WC has been defined by "information asymmetry," in which the injured worker, supervisor, and attending health practitioners have lacked critical information for safe, expeditious, and cost-effective RTW (Margoshes, 1998). A disconnect between various WC stakeholders is common concerning important issues, including causality, availability of "modified" or "transitional" duty, "reasonable accommodations" (in accordance with the Americans with Disabilities Act), and disability definitions. Therapists speak a functionally based language, whereas referring physicians are entrenched in the medical model of thinking (e.g., biopathology). Rehabilitation providers need to engage in self-education about key WC issues, selected language, and the paradigms from which other stakeholders view rehabilitation. Many local insurance associations or WC bureaus offer educational courses for both claims staff and providers. This provides an ideal environment for provider-payer dialogue and exchange of information, rather than waiting until *after* a claims denial has resulted. Providers can also familiarize themselves with the literature of other disciplines. Providers can further their knowledge and understanding of how insurance works by subscribing to claims newsletters and publications, by ordering materials from insurance trade groups and educational sources (e.g., WCRI, NCCI, International Association of Accident Boards and Commissions [IAABC], Insurance Institute of America), and by attending claims conferences. Readers should note that these and other data sources are contained in Appendix E and Suggested Readings.

Physician Limitations

There is an acknowledged lack of training and knowledge among many physicians regarding recognition and prevention of occupational illness and injury (Castorina & Rosenstock, 1990; Levy, 1985; Newman, 1995; Rosenstock et al, 1991). Physicians routinely lack expertise in WC laws, causality determinations, objective disability rating schemes, and RTW planning. Many WC physicians are PCPs who, under managed care, assume greater control over diagnostic workups, referrals to specialists, utilization controls, treatment protocols, and risk management. Despite these shortcomings, physicians are the ones within WC who initiate and terminate physical rehabilitation services. In addition, they also are the health care providers who are most-often called on to provide professional opinion about the functionality (ability/disability) of the patient, a task more suited to rehabilitation professionals.

Rehabilitation providers can enhance their role in WC by educating physicians, especially PCPs, about rehabilitation issues. Some entrepreneurial therapists have developed referring physician educational kits that describe physical therapy diagnoses, treatment protocols and measures, and service offerings. These "infomercials" straddle both the educational and marketing spheres and can be an effective means of positioning one's practice for increased referrals and/or consultative opportunities.

Consumer Education

In general, consumers are not interested in highly technical or clinically based information or satisfaction measures (Darby & Dervin, 1997). Consumers have an interest in measures that may be incongruent with those preferred by rehabilitation providers. Therefore incorporating patient goals and expectations into the treatment plan is critical when evaluating and establishing a rehabilitation program. Although the importance of incorporating patient goals and expectations is obvious, it is seldom performed in WC cases.

Patient Profiles

A great deal of research has been conducted in an attempt to identify patient profiles that generate high costs, delayed RTW, and poor outcomes. The fact that a minority of cases generates a majority of costs in WC is universally understood (Galizzi & Boden, 1996; Hester & Decelles, 1986; Westmorland & Pennock, 1995). To remain competitive, providers must become more educated about patient or injured employee profiles that predict both good and bad outcomes.

Aging Workers

Aging workers present a unique challenge in WC, because employers have voraciously downsized at a time when baby boomers have pushed into their 50s (Isokowe et al, 1990; Lipow, 1997; Smith, 1996).

Reasonable logic indicates that injured workers on average will be older than those in previous decades. This demographic demands a different approach and heightened awareness about chronic illnesses and injuries, namely disease state management. An aging WC population presents greater potential for aggravation of preexisting injury. Chapter 22 provides interesting insight into these and other issues confronting future rehabilitation professionals.

Fraud and Abuse

Fraud and abuse have been described as "the twin parasites" that "drained away what remained of the line's [workers' compensation's] vitality" (NCCI, 1999). Physical rehabilitation's high profile in WC injuries intensified scrutiny in the form of medical record reviews, service pre-certification, provider credentialing/re-credentialing, independent evaluations or second opinions, fee schedules, and other cost-containment strategies. Fraud and abuse referrels also have escalated (Butler et al, 1996).

Litigation

It is curious how perceptions of attorneys tend to be bipolar. On one hand, some, like Shakespeare in Henry VI, want to "kill all the attorneys." Yet, who is the first person to whom many of us run when in trouble—an attorney? In some cases, attorneys serve a vital role in WC; in others, they serve as an unnecessary expense and obstacle to RTW. Each WC case must be judged on its own merit. One thing is clear, however: rehabilitation providers can expect far more litigation under WC than under any other insurance or health care system.

In WC, a hypothetically no-fault system, 5% to 10% of all patients retain lawyers; this is a significant percentage. There is a positive correlation between attorney involvement and the percentage of "open cases" (Durbin, 1995, 1997). There also is a positive correlation between attorney involvement and higher WC costs. The WCRI reports that lawyers are retained, on average, in 80% of high-cost PPD cases. In some states, this figure is even higher (e.g., Illinois, 92%; Tennessee, 90%) (Durbin, 1995, 1997). Attorney fees accounted for 30% of the costs of fractures and for 50% of the costs for sprains, strains, or soft tissue injury (Durbin, 1995, 1997). Litigation increases average costs for disability ratings, even with a small number of law firms involved:

> "The top five [law] firms in New Jersey represented workers in 40% of 1991 claims versus 30% of 1989 claims, and the top five firms responsible for occupational disease and cumulative injury claims filed 86% of those claims in 1991."
>
> - Gardner et al, 1994

Rehabilitation providers must prepare themselves for practice within a litigious WC system. The best disability management professionals are cognizant of both legal and human considerations that arise in many cases (Lerner, 1998). Specifically, clinical documentation must be clear and defensible. Second, providers must prepare themselves to serve as medical experts. Perhaps most importantly, providers should be capable of linking a patient's functionality to the critical job demands of work.

Dueling Doctors

Disability determinations are one of the most highly controversial elements of a WC system. It is not uncommon for injured workers with similar conditions to receive divergent disability ratings or awards (Durbin & Kish, 1998).

Variation is the norm in WC disability determinations. Some variation results from a lack of disability determination standards, whereas some of it results from the litigation phenomenon previously discussed. In WC, the plaintiff filing for disability (injured employee) may retain a "medical expert" (through his or her attorney). The insurance company or self-funded employer retains a defense medical expert. These experts are usually doctors, but therapists can also be included because of their functional expertise. In fact, it is perplexing that the medical expert (e.g., orthopedist, neurologist) often uses data excerpted from a therapist's clinical records or FCE report, yet the therapist is seldom called as a medical expert in these cases. In addition to expressing his or her own medical judgments, the physician will often convey the therapist's opinion (secondhand), provided it is harmonious with the physician's opinion. This represents a ripe opportunity for rehabilitation providers to participate in the medico-legal realm of WC. Augmenting the physician's role in disability determinations is a reasonable option for physical and occupational therapists that may lead to expert testimony.

Disability determinations are not rendered based on lost earning capacity but on the degree of physical or mental impairment. Disability assessment has been described as "a construct that straddles medicine and society" (Carey, 1999). Disability determination approaches differ between, and generally involve one of, the following:

- Adversary experts: plaintiff or employee versus defense or payer
- Independent examiners who conduct fitness-for-duty examinations, independent medical examinations, or disability assessments
- Standardized evaluation guidelines (e.g., *AMA Guides to the Evaluation of Permanent Impairment*)
- Functional capacity evaluations

The use of adversarial experts is by far the most prevalent disability determination approach, with standardized guidelines the rarest. Not surprisingly, most plaintiff expert opinions favor the injured employee, whereas defense expert opinions favor the payer. Final PPD benefits vary between 16.6% and 39% across states for similar sample cases (Durbin, 1997). Results from New Jersey WC low back cases corroborate the disparity between plaintiff and defense opinions (Boden, 1987). Using a point system for rating disability, the average difference between orthopedic opinions (plaintiff versus defense) was 27. Neuropsychiatric opinions varied by an average of 28 points. Extreme ratings such as these are commonly found in WC (Boden, 1987).

1. Defense experts (orthopedic and neuropsychiatric) gave "zero" disability ratings in 35% and 60% of the cases, respectively.
2. Defense experts gave 15% or higher disability ratings in only 5% of total cases.
3. Plaintiff experts gave 15% or lower disability ratings in only 4% to 6% of all cases.
4. Plaintiff experts gave 30% or higher disability ratings in 67% of the orthopedic cases and in 35% of the neuropsychiatric cases.

These data raise serious questions and doubts about the objectivity of paid experts when examining the same groups of patients and perhaps encourage increased use of FCEs. In reality, final disability judgments generally tend to split the difference between experts (plaintiff/worker and defense/insurer/employer). Boden's (1987) study essentially concluded the following:

1. Plaintiff experts exaggerate disability.
2. Defense experts understate disability.
3. Final judgments generally split the difference mathematically.
4. The use of dueling experts prolongs the claims resolution process.
5. There is no accepted method for transforming functional limitations into numerical ratings.

On the basis of these data, one could argue that functionally based professional opinions are preferred over medically based ones. Physical rehabilitation providers who perform FCEs and FJAs (functional job analyses) may be well positioned to seize an opportunity for objective ability/disability assessments. Readers are referred to Chapter 9.

Expanded Definition of Compensability

Expansion of what constitutes a compensable injury or illness is a strong current trend in WC claims (Anderson, 1998; Bennett & Meyer, 1991; Carter, 1991; Cross, 1998). OSHA's aggressive initiatives throughout the 1980s and 1990s provided much of the impetus regarding CTDs or RSDs. The prevalence and causality of CTDs remain a controversy despite the national attention CTDs have received. Some purport that the claims of CTDs are exaggerated or are actually decreasing (Anonymous, 1997; Brostoff, 1997; LaBarr, 1997; Wojcik, 1997). Others claim that CTDs are underreported by as much as 60% (Nelson et al, 1992). This trend should continue to uniquely position rehabilitation providers within WC, both as providers and in a consultative role.

Mental health claims represent a second trend regarding expanded compensability (Harris, 1999; Ozersky, 1998; Sanders, 2000).

Employer Choice of Physician or Provider

WC systems tend to be cyclical and dependent on bias swings between different stakeholders. During one cycle, a system may have an employer bias, whereas during another phase, the bias may favor the employee. The WC pendulum during the past two decades has swung closer toward an employer bias. Employers impanel providers as part of their WC panel or preferred network. The initial choice, number, and timing of provider changes fall within the purview of employers in many WC programs. The cost savings of this movement remain mixed; some studies illustrate savings, whereas others do not (Boden & Fleischman, 1989; Durbin & Appel, 1991; Pozzebon, 1993; Victor & Fleischman, 1990).

WC provider panels customarily include physicians and occasionally include chiropractors. In general, physical and occupational therapists are not considered PCPs in WC and hence do not enjoy widespread panel listings.

However, this may change as the value of rehabilitation services becomes more fully appreciated and may potentially become a byproduct of direct access legislation sweeping the United States. This can happen only if providers enhance their profiles, especially among employers who finance WC.

There is a general trend toward prolonging the time period during which employers can direct care to preferred providers under WC. When this period expires, employees are free to choose providers rather than relying on employer-selected ones.

Fee Schedules

WC fee schedules use a host of benchmarks, including the following:

- Other states' WC schedules, especially adjacent or similar socioeconomic states
- Third-party payers (e.g., Blue Cross/Blue Shield)
- Medicare

A growing trend correlates WC fee schedules with Medicare levels. However, in doing so, there is a great deal of irrationality (Lunbeck et al, 1997). There does not appear to be any systematic relationship to charges across various states based on provider costs of delivering services. Medicare fee schedules are usually lower than WC rates by 30% in median states. Fee schedules are baffling, because states with more generous fees have providers who can generally render services less expensively. It also is not uncommon for some states to have extremely low reimbursement rates relative to high practice expenses.

STATE WORKERS' COMPENSATION REFORM ACTIVITY

Virtually every state has reexamined its WC system, and several states have emerged as barometers of change. According to Eccleston (1997), states generally have the following four gradations of "managed workers' compensation":

1. Mandatory use of managed care within WC
2. Regulating WC managed care acts
3. Using a "permissive" managed care policy
4. Allowing limited use of managed care

Most states fall into the last category, although at least six have managed WC (Himmelstein, 1996). Nearly half of all states have or are developing treatment guidelines. Adherence to guidelines is mandatory in some states, but voluntary for most. Providers who wish to stay apprised of state-by-state developments should refer to WCRI's analyses.

Integrated Benefits

WC remains a fragmented market dominated by small, local provider organizations. One of the reasons for paucity of managed care in WC (compared with group health) is that few companies are confident enough to accept both medical and indemnity risk. Of 22 managed care organizations surveyed, only four accept medical and indemnity risks (Penshorn & Johnson, 1995). The litigious nature of WC combined with its indemnity basis has resulted in what some have called a "stock leadership vacuum in the managed workers' compensation insurance niche" (Lunbeck et al, 1997).

Integrated benefits is a hybrid of 24-hour coverage, which describes two basic arrangements: (1) blended WC and group health or (2) combined WC and disability programs (STD and LTD).

Although integration has been challenging, there are definite benefits, and seven states (Florida, Georgia, Kentucky, Louisiana, Minnesota, Oklahoma, and Massachusetts) have mandated 24-hour coverage in one form or the other. Integration of claims management eliminates "double dippers" (i.e., persons who receive dual benefits from different insurance lines). Streamlined administration enables insurers to avoid redundancy in claims functions (Fletcher, 1997). Lost time cases are easier to track when benefit plans are merged. Last, disability definitions and assessment schemes can be standardized along with treatment interventions.

Integrated benefits are not without detractors, who claim that costs may outweigh savings or that regulatory variations are too great (Fletcher, 1995).

WC has attracted a variety of cost-containment initiatives that have yielded divergent savings. Fee schedules have been reported to save up to 54% of medical costs (Eccleston et al, 1997). Preferred provider networks have reduced utilization rates (visits) by between 14% and 50%. Utilization review and management have reduced costs 5% to 15% on average. Application of an HMO or capitation model in WC has dropped costs between 10% to 43%. The use of practice guidelines has

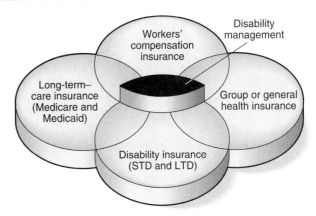

Figure 5–3. Integrated disability management across benefit scheme. *LTD,* Long-term disability; *STD,* short-term disability.

resulted in cost reductions of between 17% and 33% (Granneman, 1994).

PHYSICAL REHABILITATION PROVIDERS' ROLE IN WORKERS' COMPENSATION

A disability management program can be designed to span all insurance lines, including WC, if providers understand the relationship between a worker and his or her worksite within the context of system-specific variables (Figure 5–3).

Figure 5–4 depicts a disability management program that addresses the needs of various benefits programs. Providers who manage a variety of patients from diverse

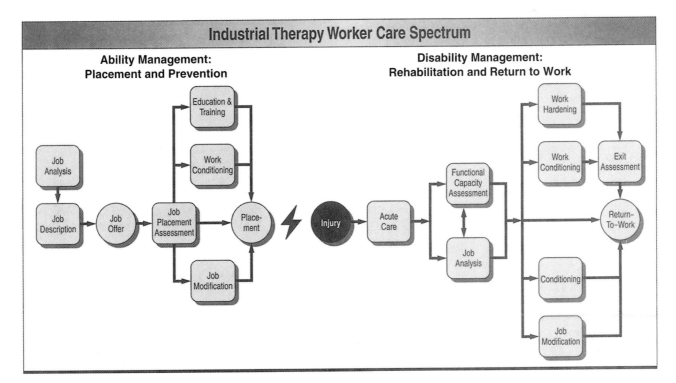

Figure 5–4. Industrial therapy worker care spectrum. (From Key GL [ed]: Industrial Therapy. St Louis, Mosby, 1995.)

industries and insurance lines need to establish standardized procedures that enable a focus-on-function through worker-worksite matching. Providers who accomplish this should do well, particularly under 24-hour or integrated benefit plans. Some of these plans roll claims and medical management together regardless of which insurance line is involved. For example, group or general health may be administered along with WC or disability insurance (STD or LTD). These plans may or may not jointly manage medical and indemnity issues.

Open Cases

Rehabilitation providers must realize that when protracted rehabilitation is involved, a case remains "open." Open cases incur a multitude of costs beyond those of rehabilitation. Rehabilitation drives other medical costs, because it is generally rendered based on a referral from a physician. As long as the patient is engaged in physical therapy, he or she may also periodically visit the orthopedist, neurologist, or occupational medicine specialist. Thus therapists are in a powerful position (fiscally speaking) of driving both indirect and direct WC costs.

This high profile can result in an expanded role or in intensified claims scrutiny. Open cases accumulate administrative, legal, lost productivity, indemnity, worker replacement, hiring and training, supervisory, and overtime costs. The cost to the employer greatly exceeds the billing rate of the therapist. Certainly, some of these costs accrue with or without the presence of rehabilitation, but providers should be mindful of the economic impact their clinical decisions have on aggregate system costs (Table 5-5).

Disability management in WC requires a comprehensive approach through integrated programs (Margoshes, 1998). Physical rehabilitation providers can serve a variety of worker and employer needs through a host of interventions that span the entire disability continuum, from injury and illness prevention to treatment to post-treatment consultation (Huhn & Volski, 1985; Isernhagen, 1995; Smith, 1997). Services can be designed and implemented within three general domains, each of which includes service subsets:

1. Loss prevention domain
   - Ergonomics
   - Employee education/training
   - Management education/training
   - CTD screenings
   - Employment evaluations (e.g., post-offer evaluations)
   - FJA
   - ADA compliance

2. Treatment domain
   - Work conditioning
   - Work hardening
   - Vocational retraining
   - Pain management
   - Restorative therapy
   - Employee education/training
   - Management education/training
   - Ergonomics
   - ADA compliance

3. Post-treatment or consultative domain
   - Medico-legal testimony
   - OSHA consultation
   - ADA consultation
   - Employee education/training
   - Management education/training
   - Ergonomics
   - ADA compliance

Physical rehabilitation providers are historically most active in the disability treatment domain; however, they covet skills, knowledge, experience, and aptitudes that would allow a relatively easy transition into the other two domains: loss prevention and post-treatment consultation.

Key's *Industrial Therapy* (1995) provides a comprehensive depiction of the need for preventive services focusing on "ability management" and rehabilitation or "disability management" (see Figure 5-4).

Prevention services in this model include job analysis, job description education and training, work conditioning, job modification, and placement. A proper worker-worksite match should serve to reduce the incidence and severity of work-related injuries. However, injuries inevitably occur, and Key's model provides a functionally based treatment or disability management protocol. The right side of Figure 5-5 shows the rehabilitation and RTW process.

Following acute care, injured workers are assessed with functional capacity assessments, which are compared with their job analyses. Restorative therapies follow in the form of work hardening, work conditioning, and job modification (e.g., transitional duty). An exit assessment then determines RTW disposition and identifies relevant work restriction and limitations.

WC is undoubtedly one of the most fertile venues for disability management because of its demographics, the

 Table 5-5 WC Costs that Are Driven by "Open" Rehabilitation Cases

Direct Medical Costs

- Rehabilitation costs
- Visits to referring physician (e.g., primary care physicians, occupational medicine)
- Visits to specialty physicians (e.g., orthopedists, neurologists)

Direct Administrative Costs

- Case management
- Indemnity payments or lost wage replacement
- Claims management
- Vocational counseling or vocational rehabilitation

Indirect Medical Costs

- Independent medical examinations
- Medical records review or utilization review costs
- Functional capacity evaluations

Indirect Administrative Costs

- Employee replacement, hiring/training
- Overtime
- Litigation
- Supervisory
- Lost productivity

Figure 5–5. Disability management triad.

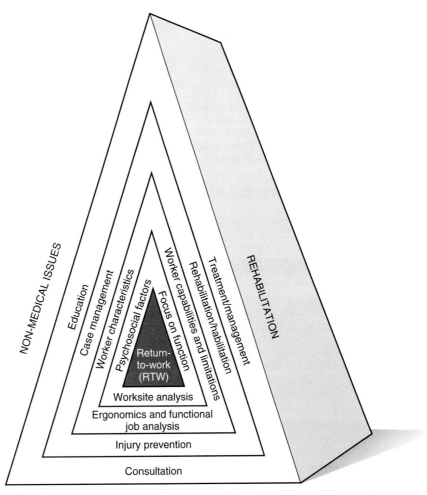

THE WORKSITE

frequency of musculoskeletal injury, the chronic nature of conditions, the degree of employer self-insurance or self-funding, and its relatively high reimbursement. Seventy-eight percent of employers consider RTW programs important in combating disability (Bell, 1999).

Rehabilitation providers can affect the cost, utilization, and human suffering associated with work-related disability through a variety of preventive interventions (Feldstein et al, 1998; Green-McKenzie et al, 1998; Martin, 1995; Reisenwitz, 1997; Roughton, 1993).

Profile of a Successful Rehabilitation Program

Each WC case, individual patient, and WC system presents threats to and opportunities for successful rehabilitation. Is there a profile for successful rehabilitation under WC? Can benchmarks for success be found in LTD cases? A Northwestern National Life (NWNL [subsequently Reliastar and now ING]) study of 9747 long-term disability claims over a 7-year period (1987 to 1993) examined trends, costs, and outcomes (Taylor et al, 1994). This study resulted in four conclusions:

Conclusion 1: Rehabilitation of disabled workers offers employers significant savings.

Conclusion 2: Companies can cut their disability costs significantly by adopting an RTW culture.

Conclusion 3: Disability case management and rehabilitation yield a high success rate in returning disabled employees to work.

Conclusion 4: RTW success rates are highest among workers with back and musculoskeletal disorders.

Specific RTW rates were as follows:

- Workers disabled with back disorders, 61%
- Musculoskeletal conditions, 60%
- Neurological conditions, 49%
- Mental conditions, 43%
- Circulatory disease, 38%
- Cardiac conditions, 33%

These data yielded savings of $35 for every $1 invested in rehabilitation. Greatest savings were found when workers returned to their previous job, at a $96 to $1 ratio. NWNL identified eight key factors that, when considered together, accounted for rehabilitation success (Table 5-6).

A Rehabilitation Triad

The complexities of WC cases demand that therapists be adept at management of psychosocial factors in the

Table 5-6 Factors Affecting Rehabilitation Success

NWNL identified eight key factors affecting rehabilitation success. They include:

Age	The optimal age range is from 25 to 45 years old. Workers in this age range are usually in good overall health, making it easier for them to recover from a disability.
Education	More education usually translates into greater employability.
Income	Moderate income at the time of disability offers more options for job placement efforts. High salaries tend to reduce the number of job options.
Work History	Experienced workers have greater value in the workplace. Specialized skills are also desirable and increase the probability of a successful return to work. A varied work history increases the number of transferable skills and allows for more options.
Motivation	A disabled worker's desire to return to the marketplace and his or her commitment to rehabilitation are critically important to a successful return to work.
Employer	Offering a light-duty position until the disabled worker is able to resume regular work or accommodating the functional skills of the disabled worker has a significant positive impact on the rehabilitation outcome.
Medical Aspects	Medical specialists must be willing to cooperate with the rehabilitation case manager to expedite vocational planning and implementation.
Local Labor Market	Low unemployment conditions equate with high demand for workers, making the disabled worker more attractive to employers.

Data from Northwestern National Life: Back to Work: Managing Disability, Recovery, and Re-employment. NWNL (now ING), Minneapolis, MN, 1994.

context of the work environment. Figure 5–5 illustrates the interdependency between a focus-on-function, psychosocial issues, and worksite analysis. Unsuccessful rehabilitation programs often fail to consider non-medical issues that serve as obstacles to a RTW. These programs generally disregard the worksite/environment to which they are attempting to return an injured employee. Critical job demands can serve as the blueprint for the design of a work rehabilitation program by identifying end points of function that must be achieved to safely RTW. This can be accomplished only after ergonomic or job analysis. Rehabilitation providers are cautioned against blind acceptance of patient-reported or employer-reported job demands, because these are commonly found by providers to vary. Ultimately, a worker's capabilities must be matched to job demands, which can be influenced by a host of psychosocial factors such as job satisfaction, first line supervisor–employee relations, mental health status, financial status, litigation, and substance abuse.

PREVENTION AND WORKERS' COMPENSATION

The prevention of work-related injuries and illnesses is the ultimate goal for many health care stakeholders. Rehabilitation providers have been relatively slow to transfer their skills, knowledge, aptitude, and experience into consultative areas devoid of treatment. Although few providers have experience in preventive services, many have the potential to perform these services.

Postoffer or Preplacement Examinations

Postoffer or preplacement examinations that establish a prospective worker's functional abilities or limitations can be effective in decreasing disability-related costs (Colacci, 1999). Once functional limitations have been identified, they can be used to identify and implement

both engineering and administrative controls rather than for dismissive purposes. Safe and appropriate worker-worksite matching can result when a worker's baseline functional levels are synchronous with critical job demands. The worker-worksite interface is a logical starting point in any loss prevention program. *Loss prevention* defines activities that focus on preventing disability. These include health and wellness, ergonomics, employee screening, training and education, industrial hygiene, and safety programs.

Employer Training and Education

Employer training and education directed at disability prevention and management is acutely needed. This intervention is especially critical at the supervisory level, where only 24% of employers report the availability of special training for supervisors (Bell, 1999). A Watson Wyatt Worldwide (1997) survey of employers indicates a lack of disability program coordination and an opportunity for provider-employer informational exchanges.

Ergonomic Analysis

Ergonomic analysis is well established as a viable approach to disability prevention and postinjury management (Anderson, 1995; Shrey & Breslin, 1992). Some occupational health providers are collaborating with employers to establish workplace or ergonomic safety committees (Daus, 1997). Daus reports a 1996 study conducted by Indiana University of Pennsylvania, wherein a 52% reduction in lost workdays followed implementation of a workplace committee.

Return-to-Work Programs

The design of aggressive, job-specific RTW programs is key to WC success. Therapists must be aware that the goal of WC is fundamentally different from that of group or general health. *Maximum medical improvement* and *maximum medical benefit* are terms under general health that imply a patient has achieved a medically stable condition. Maximum medical improvement is not an appropriate outcome in WC. The ultimate clinical outcome is a RTW or a return to gainful employment resulting from functional versus medical gains. The treatment goals of WC raise the standards by focusing on function. Design of RTW programs demand a fundamental understanding of the patient's or injured worker's critical job tasks and work environment. This is not as easy as it sounds, because providers must also be wary of various environmental or employer-based complexities. For example, knowledge of labor-management relations is equally important as clinical-based knowledge. Shrey and LaCerte's text (1995) addressing industrial-based disability is an insightful resource in this regard.

Successful worker-worksite matches are vital and may require a functional job analysis (FJA). An FJA describes an employee's job in functional terms versus vocational or competency-based terms. Once an FJA has described critical job demands, it can then be used as a blueprint for the design of a therapeutic program. Work conditioning and work hardening are two methods that can be applied in work injury management. Both require an intimate understanding of the worker-worksite interface. Discharge criteria likewise revolve around the FJA.

Reasonable Accommodations

Therapists may need to assist the attending physician, case manager, and human resources officer in the identification of reasonable accommodations. *Reasonable accommodations* is a term derived from the ADA, which guarantees all persons the right to gainful employment provided that a RTW can be effected through reasonable accommodation (ADA, 1990). Historically, many injured workers were denied reentry into the workforce until they were deemed 100%, or fully, recovered (McMahon, 1995). These workers were often denied gainful employment if they required any measure of work restrictions or limitations. The ADA ensures that federal law supersedes state WC law if policies are prohibitive of RTW for persons who desire RTW and who can be reasonably accommodated. The term *reasonable* is the operative word here, because it has different meanings to different stakeholders. An employer may view job sharing as unreasonable, whereas the attending physician believes it to be a reasonable accommodation. The number of scenarios that breed disagreement over the concept of *reasonable* are countless.

According to Title I of the ADA, *reasonable accommodation* is defined as any change in the work environment or the nature of the work that enables persons with disabilities, either demonstrated or perceived, to enjoy equal opportunity for gainful employment (Kornblau & Ellexson, 1995). Rehabilitation providers are uniquely qualified to assist employers in both engineering and administrative changes necessary to accommodate persons with disabilities. For instance, rehabilitation specialists can assist in the development of modified or transitional duty to facilitate a safe, but expedient, RTW (Feuerstein

et al, 2003). This is particularly true of therapists who covet expertise in work conditioning, work hardening, and ergonomics. Discharge criteria and reasonable accommodation selection must consider the functional status of the worker from an environmental and adaptive-equipment standpoint.

Case Management

Physical rehabilitation providers may satisfy the needs of employers, insurers, patients, and other WC stakeholders by assuming case management responsibilities. Clifton (1996) enumerated a number of roles that fall under case management, especially as it pertains to managed WC. A detailed discussion of therapists as case managers is found in Chapter 27.

Workers' Compensation Specific Outcomes Measures

Providers must operate from a different paradigm when designing WC discharge criteria and outcomes measures. Because WC is an indemnity-based system, providers must incorporate RTW status expressed as follows:

- TPD
- PPD
- TTD

The degree of work-related disability can be determined only if both the injured worker and his or her job have been jointly evaluated. Physicians and therapists who examine and treat the injured worker without analysis of the worker's job requirements are practicing without all necessary information. The disability categories listed previously can be accurately determined only through objective measures of the worker and the worksite.

Ultimately, non-medical factors can predict which workers return to work and which do not (Aronoff et al, 2000; Ensalada, 2000; Proctor et al, 2000). A host of psychosocial variables has been correlated with RTW status. Predictive variables of RTW are listed in Table 5-7.

CONCLUSION

Treatment, prevention, and management of work-related disability provide unique opportunities for physical rehabilitation providers to address an area that is generally ignored by managed care organizations and their

 Table 5-7 Predictive Variables of RTW

- Worker's age
- Worker's educational level
- Wages before injury or illness
- Job seniority
- Injury severity
- Tenure on job
- Attorney involvement
- Recent periods of unemployment

Table 5–8 Workers' Compensation Consulting Opportunities for Rehabilitation Providers

- Design transitional or modified duty program
- Identify potentially high-dollar/high-loss conditions
- Provide case management (e.g., "red flag" cases)
- Design and implement reasonable accommodations
- Design work hardening, work conditioning, and RTW programs
- Perform postoffer evaluations and functional capacity/capability evaluations
- Implement admissions and discharge criteria for physical rehabilitation cases
- Educate about cumulative trauma prevention (e.g., back school, carpal tunnel screening)
- Assist with the integration of workers' compensation and the ADA
- Perform functional job analyses that serve as a blueprint for RTW program design
- Assemble a preferred provider network of WC-literate providers who use functionally based outcomes measures tied to RTW
- Assess ergonomic needs of employees

gatekeepers. These conditions are defined by functional deficits and an assortment of psychosocial issues, not by acute medical conditions alone. From an experiential basis, no profession is better equipped to deal with the complexities of these cases than is physical rehabilitation (Table 5–8).

WC represents an insurance arena in which physical rehabilitation can carve out its rightful role across the entire injury or disability continuum. However, to do so, providers must learn more about how the WC system works. Readers are referred to the Suggested Readings to improve their knowledge of this subject.

REFERENCES

American Medical Association: Guides to the Evaluation of Permanent Impairment. Chicago, American Medical Association, 1984.

Americans with Disabilities Act of 1990. Public Law 101-338, U.S.C. 1201 b, Statute 329; July 26, 1990.

American Medical Association, Guide to the Evaluation of Permanent Impairment, Chicago: IL, American Medical Association, 1984.

Anderson D: RSI can strain the bottom line. Business and Health 16(1):44-45, 1998.

Anderson M: Ergonomics: Analyzing work from a physiological perspective. In Isernhagen SJ (ed): Comprehensive Guide to Work Injury Management. Gaithersburg, MD, Aspen, 1995, pp 3-39.

Anonymous: Workplace injuries and illnesses down to the lowest level since 1986. Facilities Design and Management 16(5):17-18, 1997.

Aronoff GM, Feldman JB, Campion TS: Management of chronic pain and control of long-term disability. Occup Med 15(4):755-770, 2000.

Beatty PW, Hagglund KJ, Neri MT: Access to health care services among people with chronic or disabling conditions: patterns and predictors. Arch Phys Med Rehabil 84(10):1417-1425, 2003.

Bell A: Experts say return-to-work plans cut disability costs. National Underwriter 103(46):13, 1999.

Bennett J, Meyer R: Avoiding workers' comp claims meltdown. Risk Management 38(5):41-45, 1991.

Boden L: Use of Medical Evidence: Low Back Permanent Partial Disability Claims in New Jersey. Workers' Compensation Research Institute (WCRI), Publication No WC-87-2, Cambridge, MA, WCRI, 1987.

Boden L, Fleischman C: Medical Costs in Workers' Compensation: Trends and Interstate Comparisons. Cambridge, MA, Workers' Compensation Research Institute, 1989.

Brostoff S: Repetitive stress injury dip found. National Underwriter 101(3):23, 1997.

Butler T, Kendra J, Grimley R et al: Can we measure the effectiveness of our organizations? Int J Health Care Q Assurance 9(5):37-38, 1996.

Butler DJ, Durbin DL, Helvacian NM: Increasing claims for soft tissue injuries in workers' compensation. J Risk Uncertain 13:73-87, 1996.

Butler RJ, Johnson WG, Baldwin ML: Managing work disability: Why first return-to-work is not a measure of success. Ind Labor Relat Rev 48: 452-469:1995.

Carey TS: Disability: How successful are we in determining disability? Neurol Clin North Am 17(1):167-178, 1999.

Carter M: Workers' comp derailment: Expectations not met. Risk Manage 38(5):22-34 1991.

Castorina JS, Rosenstock L: Physician shortage in occupational and environmental medicine. Ann Intern Med 113:983-986, 1990.

Clifton DW: Managed care and workers' compensation. In Isernhagen S (ed): The Comprehensive Guide to Work Injury Management. Gaithersburg, MD, Aspen, 1995.

Clifton DW: Managed workers' comp. Case Review 2(3):20-25, 1996.

Colacci C: Testing helps you decrease disability costs. Canadian HR Reporter 12(2):G-4, 1999.

Cross L: A bleak picture. Graphic Arts Monthly 70(6):20, 1998.

Darby C, Dervin K: Measuring Consumer Satisfaction Under Workers' Compensation Managed Care. Presented at Workers' Compensation and Managed Care: Challenges and Opportunities in a Changing Health Care System, Agency for Health Care Policy and Research (AHCPR), Chicago, July 30-August 1, 1997, www.ahcpr.gov/research/ulpwrkrs.htm, accessed June, 6, 2000.

Daus C: Pennsylvania fights the high cost of workers' compensation. Case Review 3(4); Fall 1997.

Durbin D: The cost of treating injured workers: The changing workers' compensation landscape. Benefits Q 9:9-21, 1993.

Durbin D: Attorney Involvement and Costs in High-Cost Workers' Compensation Claims. Boca Raton, FL, National Council on Compensation Insurance, 1995.

Durbin D: Workplace injuries and the role of insurance. Clin Orthop 336:18-32, 1997.

Durbin D, Appel D: The impact of fee schedules and employer choice of physician. NCCI Digest 6(30):19-38, 1991.

Durbin D, Corro D, Helvacian N: Workers' compensation medical expenditures: Price vs. quantity. J Risk Insur 63(1):13-33, 1996.

Durbin DL, Kish J: Factors affecting permanent partial disability ratings in workers' compensation. J Risk Insur 65(1):81-99, 1998.

Eccleston S: Overview of State Workers' Compensation Medical Care Initiatives. Presented at Workers' Compensation and Managed Care: Challenges and Opportunities in a Changing Health Care System, Agency for Health Care Policy and Research (AHCPR), Chicago, July 30-August 1, 1997, www.ahcpr.gov/research/ulpwrkrs.htm, accessed June 6, 2000.

Eccleston SM: Anatomy of Workers' Compensation Medical Costs and Utilization, December, WC-00-8. Cambridge, MA, Workers' Compensation Research Institute (WCRI), 2001.

Ensalada LH: The importance of illness behavior in disability management. Occup Med 15(4):739-754, 2000.

Ehrmann-Feldman D, Rossignol M, Abenhaim L et al: Physician referral to physical therapy in a cohort of workers compensated for low back pain. Phys Ther 7(2):150-156, 1996.

Feldstein A, Breen V, Dana N: Prevention of work-related disability. Am J Prev Med 14(3):33-39, 1998.

Feuerstein M, Shaw WS, Lincoln AE et al: Clinical and workplace factors associated with a return to modified duty in work-related upper extremity disorders. Pain J 102(1-2):51-61, 2003.

Fletcher M: Managed care laws test mettle: Comp programs have to keep abreast of state variations. Business Insurance, p 16, October 26, 1995.

Fletcher M: Disability management integration is growing. Bus Ins 31(46):92, 1997.

Freburger JK, Holmes GM, Carey TS: Physician referrals to physical therapy for the treatment of musculoskeletal conditions. Arch Phys Med Rehabil 84(12):1839-1849, 2003.

Galizzi M, Boden LI: What are the most important factors shaping return to work? Evidence from Wisconsin, Workers' Compensation Research Institute (WCRI). Cambridge, MA, WCRI, 1996.

Galvin DE: Employer-based disability management and rehabilitation programs. Annual Rev Rehabil 5:173-215, 1986.

Gardner J, Victor RA, Telles C et al: Cost drivers in New Jersey. Cambridge, MA, Workers Compensation Research Institute, 1994.

Granneman TW (ed): Review, regulate or reform? What works to control workers' compensation. Cambride, MA, Workers' Compensation Research Institute, 1994.

Green-McKenzie J, Parkerson J, Bernacki E: Comparison of workers' compensation costs for two cohorts of injured workers before and after the introduction of managed care. J Occup Environ Med 40(6):72, 1998.

Haig AJ, Linton P, McIntosh M et al: Aggressive early management by a specialist in physical medicine and rehabilitation: effect on lost time due to injuries in hospital employees. J Occup Med 32(3):241-244, 1990.

Harris JS, The future of workers' compensation claims: implications for occupational medicine. Occup Environ Med Report 13(3):17-19, 1999.

Hays D: Doubts arise about drop in workplace injuries. National Underwriter 102(1):6, 1998.

Hester EJ, Decelles P: Predicting Which Disabled Employees Will Return to Work: The Menninger RTW Scale. Topeka, KS, The Menninger Foundation Rehabilitation Research and Training Center for Preventing Disability Dependence, 1986.

Himmelstein J, Rest K: Working on reform. How workers' compensation medical care is affected by health care reform. Public Health Rep 111(1):12-24, 1996.

Huhn RR, Volski RV: Primary prevention programs for business and industry. Role of physical therapists. Phys Ther 65(12):1840-1844, 1985.

Isernhagen S (ed): Comprehensive Guide to Work Injury Management. Gaithersburg, MD, Aspen, 1995.

Isokowe DS, Goldstein SR, Sawyer GP et al: Workers' compensation: Business as usual may mean going out of business. National Council on Compensation Insurance Digest Risk Management 4(3):25-43, 1989.

Jette AM, Smith K, Haley SM, Davis KD: Physical therapy episodes of care for patients with low back pain. Phys Ther 74:101-115, 1994.

Kamel HK, Iqbal MA, Mogallapu R et al: Time to ambulation after hip fracture surgery: Relation to hospitalization outcomes. J Gerontol A Biol Sci Med Sci 58(11):1042-1045, 2003.

Kertesz J: Costs outweigh savings of 24-hour system study. Modern Healthcare 25(30):22, 1995.

Key GL: Industrial Therapy. St Louis, Mosby, 1995.

Kornblau BL, Ellexson MT: Reasonable accommodation and the Americans with Disabilities Act. In Isernhagen SJ (ed): The Comprehensive Guide to Work Injury Management. Gaithersburg, MD, Aspen, 1995, pp 781-798.

Krause N, Frank JW, Dasinger LK, et al: Determinants of duration of disability and return-to-work after work-related injury and illness: Challenges for future research. Am J Ind Med 40(4):464-484, 2001.

LaBarr G: Repeated trauma incidence rate drops. Occup Hazards 59(5):31, 1997.

Lankford K: Enormous employer disability costs. Life Assn News 92(1):36-37, 1997.

LaPlante MP, Carlson D: Disability in the United States: Prevalence and causes, 1992. Disability Statistics Abstract, No 7. Washington, DC, US Department of Education, National Institute on Disability and Rehabilitation Research, 1996.

Leigh JP, Markowitz SB, Fahs M et al: Occupational injury and illness in the United States. Arch Intern Med 157:1557-1568, 1997.

Lemstra M, Olszynski WP: The effectiveness of standard care, early intervention, and occupational management in workers' compensation claims. Spine J 28(3):299-304, 2003.

Lerner JR: The new direction in disability management. Bus Health 16(10):36-37, 41-45, 1998.

Levy BS: The teaching of occupational health in the United States medical schools: Five-year follow-up of an initial survey. Am J Public Health 75:79-80, 1985.

Lipow VA: Aging workers: Disability management strategies. Rehab Manag 10(1):32-34, 1997.

Lunbeck RA, Johnson JT, Lee R: Workers' Compensation: A Not-So-Parallel Universe. Boston, Hambrecht and Quist Capital Management LLC Company Report, March 20, 1997.

Margoshes B: Disability management and occupational health. Occup Med State Art Rev 13(4):693-702, 1998.

Martin KJ: Workers' compensation: Case management strategies. AAOHN J 43(5):245-250, 1995.

McMahon BT: Health insurance, workers' compensation, and the Americans with Disabilities Act. In Shrey DE, LaCerte M (eds): Principles and Practices of Disability Management in Industry. Winter Park, FL, GR Press, 1995, pp 479-498.

McNeil JM: Americans with disabilities: 1994-95. Data from the Survey of Income and Program Participation. US Bureau of the Census, Current Population Reports, P70-61. Washington, DC, US Department of Commerce, 1997.

Meerding WJ, Looman CW, Essink-Bot ML et al: Distribution and determinants of health and work status in a comprehensive population of injury patients. J Trauma 56(1):150-161, 2004.

Miller DR: A Multidisciplinary Approach to Workers' Compensation Cost Management. Presented at Infoline's 6th Annual Congress: Workers' Compensation and Managed Care, Las Vegas, March 25, 1995.

National Commission on Workmans' Compensation Laws: Report of the National Commission on Workmans' Compensation Laws. Washington, DC, National Commission on State Workmans' Compensation Laws, 1972.

National Council on Compensation Insurance (NCCI): Medical expenditures in workers' compensation: Utilization of services drives cost. Boca Raton, FL, National Council on Compensation Insurance, 1994.

National Council on Compensation Insurance (NCCI): NCCI 1996 Annual Statistical Bulletin. Boca Raton, FL, NCCI, 1996.

National Council on Compensation Insurance (NCCI): Workers' Compensation Through the Looking Glass: 1999 Workers' Compensation Issues Report, http://ncci.com, accessed September 5, 2001.

Nelson NA, Park RM, Silverstein MA et al: Cumulative trauma disorders of hand and wrist in the auto industry. Am J Public Health 82:1550-1552, 1992.

Neumark D, Johnson RW, Bresnitz FA: Costs of occupational injury and illness in Pennsylvania. J Occup Med 33:971-976, 1991.

Newman LS: Occupational illness. New Engl J Med 333(17):1128-1134, 1995.

Ozersky S: Psychiatric disabilities: The broken mind at work. J Ontario Occup Health Nurses Association Summer:12-14, 1998.

Palczynski R: Takeover of workers' comp won't cure health care ills. National Underwriter 97(24):17-19, 1993.

Ehrman-Feldman D, Rossignol M, Abenhaim L et al.: Physician referral to physical therapy in a cohort of workers' compensation for low back pain. Phys Ther 76(2):150-156,1996.

Penshorn JS, Johnson RW: The Managed Care Marketplace. Minneapolis, Piper-Jaffray, 1995.

Pozzebon S: Do Traditional health care cost containment practices really work? John Barton's Workers' Compensation Monitor, May/June, 1993.

Proctor T, Gtachel RJ, Robinson RC: Psychosocial factors and risk of pain and disability. Occup Med 15(4):803-812, 2000.

Reisenwitz EM: Absence/lost time management strategies to keep work force productive. Benefits Q 13(4):19-25, 1997.

Roberts S: Employer priorities don't match most costly worker injuries. Business Insurance 36(15 3):77, 2002.

Rosenstock L, Rest KM, Benson JA et al: Occupational and environmental medicine: Meeting the growing need for clinical services. New Engl J Med 325:924-927, 1991.

Roughton J: Workers' compensation: Program development. Professional Safety J 38(11):24-30, 1993.

Sanders SH: Risk factors for chronic, disabling low-back pain: An update for 2000. Am Pain Soc Bull 10(2), 2000.

Schultz IZ, Crook J, Meloche GR et al: Psychosocial factors predictive of occupational low back disability: Towards development of a return-to-work model. Pain J 107(1-2):77-85, 2004.

Shrey D, Breslin R: Disability management in industry: Accommodating workers with disabilities. Int J Industrial Ergonomics 9(2):183-190, 1992.

Shrey D, LaCerte M (eds): Principles and Practices of Disability Management in Industry. Winter Park, FL, GR Press, 1995.

Smail KE: Identification of the variables relevant to the recovery from post-surgical carpal tunnel syndrome. WORK J 5(4):291-299, 1995.

Smith R: Aging workers: Disability management strategies. Rehab Manag 9(1):47-49, 1996.

Smith MD: Fibromyalgia and disability. J Rheumatol 24(1):229, 1997.

Sun Tzu: The art of war. Boston, Shambhala Publications, 1991, p 88 (Translated by T Cleary).

Tate DG: Workers' disability and return to work. Am J Phys Med Rehabil 71(2):92-96, 1992.

Taylor M, Hintzman-Egan D, Farrell G: Back to Work: Managing Disability, Recovery and Re-employment. Minneapolis, Northwestern National Life, 1994.

Victor R, Fleischman C: How Choice of Provider and Recessions Affect Medical Costs in Workers' Compensation. Cambridge, MA, Workers' Compensation Research Institute, 1990.

Watson Wyatt Worldwide: Staying @ Work: Value Creation Through Integration. New York, Wyatt Watson Worldwide, 1997.

Watson Wyatt Worldwide Third Annual Report: "Staying @ Work" 1998/1999, Bethesda, MD, Watson Wyatt Worldwide, 1998/1999, www.watsonwyatt.com.

Westmorland MG, Pennock M: What prevents people with disabilities from obtaining employment? An examination of Canadian data from a national and regional perspective. WORK 5(4):255-263, 1995.

Williams DA, Feurstein M, Durbin D et al: Health care and indemnity costs across the natural history of disability in occupational low back pain. Spine J 23(21):2329-2336, 1998.

Wojcik J: Experts dispute epidemic of strain disorders. Business Insurance 31(27):59, 1997.

SUGGESTED READINGS

McGavin MF: Blueprint for Workers Comp Cost Containment. Dallas, Texas: International Risk Management Institute, Inc., 2001, www.irmi.com.

Prahl RJ: Introduction to Claims. Malvern, PA, Insurance Institute of America, 1988.

Smith B: How Insurance Works. Malvern, PA, Insurance Institute of America, 1986.

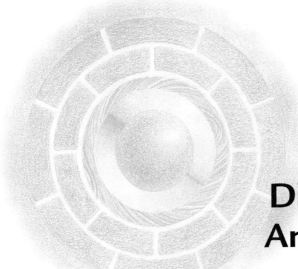

CHAPTER 6

Disability Management: An Insurer's Perspective

Mark C. Taylor, MS, CDMS, CCM

KEY POINTS

- Assessment procedures and reactivation and reconditioning programs are critical to disability management from an insurer's perspective.
- A significant benefit/cost ratio and return-on-investment can result from rehabilitation's role in disability management.
- Key features of an outstanding disability management program are similar to those of any business endeavor: effective professionals, superior communication, high expectations for success, cohesive values and approaches, and strong but malleable action planning.
- Insurers expect rehabilitation professionals to be educators in addition to being providers and managers.

Operational Definitions

Any Occupation
In long-term–disability (LTD) plans, any gainful work or service for which an employee is reasonably qualified, with consideration given to his or her training, education, and experience. A minimum income standard is not always specified, but administrative practice commonly requires 60% of *predisability earnings*.

Any-Occupation Period
The period during which disabled employees will continue to receive LTD benefits as long as they cannot perform any occupation for which they are reasonably qualified by training, education, and experience—usually 6 to 30 months. Please refer to the *own-occupation period* discussed later in this chapter.

Benefit Duration
The length of time that short-term–disability (STD) or LTD benefits will be paid to an eligible employee, as specified by the insurance contract, policy, or plan design. Federal requirements for benefit duration are contained in the Age Discrimination in Employment Act.

Claim Reserve
An amount of money set aside by an insurer to pay the total expected future cost of a disability claim. The amount may change over time given the claimant's age and expected duration of the claim.

***Diagnostic and Statistical Manual of Mental Disorders*, Fourth Edition (DSM-IV)**
A reference manual used by the medical and psychological communities to identify and classify behavioral, cognitive, and emotional conditions according to a standard numerical coding system of mental disorders.

Disability Benefit
An amount payable under a group or individual disability plan to a covered employee who meets eligibility criteria. The most common benefit percentages in STD and LTD plans are 50%, 60%, and 66⅔% of predisability income. Salary continuation plans (also designated as *STD*) often provide 80% to 100% of predisability income for the initial period of disability followed by a lower percentage for LTD (e.g., 60%).

Disability Case Management
A systematic approach to identifying, evaluating, and coordinating the delivery of disability-related services to individuals. The objective is to improve return-to-work (RTW) outcomes for employees who become disabled and to improve financial results for employers.

Duration Control Guidelines
Guidelines on the characteristic duration of different types of disabling conditions according to diagnoses, symptoms, and

Early Intervention
occupational factors. These guidelines are used to evaluate occupational and non-occupational disabilities and to determine expected recovery and return-to-work dates. Initiation of a variety of case management (medical and vocational) and stay-at-work or return-to-work efforts as soon as possible after an actual or potentially disabling event occurs. This involves communication/collaboration among employees, physicians, employers, claims administrators, and rehabilitation specialists.

Elimination Period
The number of consecutive days an employee must be disabled before LTD benefits become payable (typically 90 or 180 days); also known as the *benefit waiting period* or *qualifying period*. In some plans, employees are allowed to work during the elimination period.

Loss Control
Activities undertaken after an accident, illness, or other disabling event that are intended to reduce the future cost of a claim (e.g., case management, return-to-work programs, managed care).

Loss Prevention
Activities that focus on preventing injuries or illnesses from occurring (typically safety and wellness programs).

Preexisting Condition Limitation
Policy or plan provision that excludes or reduces disability benefits for any illness or injury for which an employee received medical treatment or consultation within a specified time period before being covered under a disability plan.

Rehabilitative Employment
Work that an individual with a disability undertakes as part of an attempt to resume regular employment in an occupation for which he or she is qualified. Earnings from such employment (often part-time work or transitional light duty) are usually offset against disability benefits as an incentive to return to regular employment. Typically, 50% of earnings are offset to provide a financial incentive for return-to-work.

Transferable Skills Analysis (TSA)
An evaluation of an employee who has been disabled to determine employability based on the worker's education, training, work history, and residual functional capacity. The results are often used to evaluate LTD benefit eligibility, determine job placement potential, and develop a vocational training plan.

Integrated Disability Program (also known as Twenty-Four Hour Program)
A program that integrates management, payment, and/or coverages for group health (medical), group disability (STD and LTD), and workers' compensation benefits. The objective is to better serve both employees and employers and to reduce administrative costs by dissolving the boundaries between occupational and non-occupational benefit programs.

THE EVOLUTION OF DISABILITY MANAGEMENT

The evolution of disability management has been dramatic in terms of the depth and breadth of the services and tools used to aid the disabled worker and employer in realizing successful outcomes following illness or injury. Case management, a subset of disability management, evolved in response to employers' desire for help in controlling escalating costs. This more expansive disability management approach embraced more tools and resources along with the expertise of a wider spectrum of health care and vocational professionals to have an even greater impact on managing disability.

The philosophy of managed care has been transformed into the concept of managed disability. The unmanageable may finally become manageable. The unfocused effort by a team of disability management professionals or lone attempts by a physician, case manager, physical therapist, or employer to effect change has progressed to coordinated programs and concerted labors that are having real impact.

What is important from an insurer's perspective? How do employers and insurers view the dynamics of disability management? What key factors do, or should, an insurer consider in using the available resources and tools of medical case management? What are the indicators for successful outcomes and the common obstacles or barriers to recovery and return-to-work? Answers to these questions offer insight for health care professionals as they work with, communicate with, and interact with each patient, insurance company or employer.

NATIONAL STATISTICS: A REVIEW

A brief review of the frequency of disability and incidence by diagnosis can define the enormity of disability, both occupational and non-occupational. The U.S. Census Bureau provided this information on work disability for civilians ages 16 to 64 years from the 2000 Census. The data support anecdotal assumptions; the likelihood of disability increases with age (Table 6-1).

The National Safety Council reported that, for 2001, 3.9 million American workers suffered from disabling injuries on the job. Work injuries cost Americans $132.1 billion in 2001. The Council also estimated that 8 million Americans suffered injuries at home in 2001—this equates to one disabling injury every 4 seconds (National Safety Council, 2001).

Claim incidence rates for LTD, as estimated by the insurance industry, are commonly 3 to 4 claims per 1000 lives (defined as the number of employees covered by the plan or policy), assuming a benefit waiting period of 180 days. Thus a corporation with 5000 employees should

 Table 6-1 National Statistics: A Review*

	Number	Percentage
Population 16 to 64 years	178,687,234	100.0
With any disability	33,153,211	18.6
With employment disability	21,287,570	11.9

*Disability Status: 2000—Census 2000 Brief.
Characteristics of the Civilian Noninstitutionalized Population by Age, Disability Status, and Type of Disability: 2000.
From US Census Bureau: Census 2000, Summary File 3, www.census.gov/hhes/www/disable/disabstat2k/table1.html, accessed January 2004.

Table 6–2 Five Impairments Most Frequently Reported under ADA*

Impairment Basis	Cumulative Total (7/26/92 to 9/30/03)	
	Number of Charges	Percentage
Orthopedic and structural impairments of back	46,693	22.8%
Mental illness	30,359	14.9%
Heart and cardiovascular impairments	7896	3.9%
Diabetes	7822	3.8%
Hearing impairment	5875	2.9%
Other	105,773	
Total	204,418	48.3% of total

*Americans with Disabilities Act (ADA) Charge Data by Impairments/Bases: July 26, 1992 to September 30, 2003.
Total ADA charges during reporting period: 204,418.
From US Equal Employment Opportunity Commission, www.eeoc.gov/stats/ada-resolutions.html, accessed January 2004.

expect 15 to 20 new claims per year. In general, the number of people who remain disabled after receiving benefits for 5 years varies from 40% to 60% (6 to 12 using the aforementioned example) based on age of the employee at the time of disability.

Table 6-2, from the Equal Employment Opportunity Commission (EEOC), reports impairments most often cited in claims filed with the EEOC for years 1992 to 2003. The most common claims were orthopedic and structural impairments (22.9%), mental illness (14.9%), heart and cardiovascular impairments (3.9%), diabetes (3.8%), and hearing impairments (2.9%).

DEFINING THE TERMS

The consulting firm William M. Mercer, Inc. and Metropolitan Life Insurance Company, in cooperation with the Washington Business Group on Health, published a glossary of terms to help employers, providers, and others share a common understanding and language. *The Language of Managed Disability* offers the following definitions (William M. Mercer Inc., 1995):

Managed disability: A comprehensive approach to integrating programs and services to help control employers' disability costs while helping employees who have been disabled return to full functionality and productive work as soon as they can. Following are key concepts in managed disability.

Partnership: Cooperation of a network of parties: employees; employers (line management, as well as disability specialists); insurers; risk managers; and occupational health, vocational, and rehabilitation specialists.

Prevention: Use of wellness programs to promote good health and safety programs to reduce accidental and occupational disabilities.

Early intervention: Initiation of a variety of case management and stay-at-work or return-to-work efforts as soon as possible after an actual or potentially disabling event occurs.

Integrated case management: Coordination of STD and LTD, health care, and workers' compensation programs to improve care delivery, streamline administration, and permit effective claims management.

Management information: Use of consolidated data on disability occurrences, costs, and outcomes to measure the effectiveness of managed disability programs.

Compliance: Active cooperation with the full spirit, not merely the letter, of all federal and state legislation pertaining to persons with disabilities.

As noted previously, case management is a key component of a managed disability model. The Case Management Society of America (2004) defines case management as follows:

"Case management is a collaborative process of assessment, planning, facilitation and advocacy for options and services to meet an individual's health needs through communication and available resources to promote quality cost-effective outcomes."

Medical management, within the context of a managed disability model, requires the coordination of primary health care with physical rehabilitation and assessment procedures. This merges the health care network's ability to provide acute care and injury management with the restorative potential of single-modality treatments such as physical and occupational therapy. For this process to be completed, opportunity for physical reactivation and reconditioning programs, as well as the assessment procedures of independent medical evaluations (IMEs) and functional capacity evaluations (FCEs), must be available.

The key to disability management is a team approach. The health care provider must have some knowledge of the employee's workplace and of the importance of the vocational and psychological aspects of disability. For many disabled workers, recovery and return-to-work is not successful without the input and influence of vocational and behavioral experts who play a major role in successful outcomes.

The primary focus for this discussion is on disability management as it pertains to occupational (workers' compensation) and non-occupational (sick pay/salary continuance, STD, and LTD) illness or injury. *Workers' compensation* programs are state-legislated systems that require employers to fund the costs of medical treatment and partial wage loss replacement for employees who endure work-related injury or illness. Federal employees, both public and private (e.g., railroad workers), are protected by a variety of federally administered laws and regulations similar to this benefit program.

Sick pay/salary continuance is typically provided for short periods of illness or injury. Often, 100% of salary is replaced with this program.

STD is an employer-sponsored plan, or an insurance policy administered by an employer or insurer, that replaces wages at a predetermined percentage of predisability earnings. Non-occupational illness or injury is the target for this employee benefit program. Earnings are generally replaced at 60% to 100% of predisability income following a waiting period (often called the *elimination period*) of 3 to 7 days. Eligibility is defined as the employee's inability to perform his or her own occupation, and in some cases, own job. These "short-term" benefits typically continue for 13, 26, or 52 weeks or until replaced by LTD payments.

LTD is also either an employer-sponsored benefit plan or an insurance product that provides partial wage replacement following an extended elimination (waiting) period of 60, 90, or 180 days. The cost of medical treatment, as with STD, is paid by the disabled worker's health insurance plan/policy.* LTD benefit eligibility is based on the employee's inability to perform the essential duties of his or her own occupation. Income replacement is commonly 60% to 70% of predisability earnings. This *own-occupation* definition of disability commonly continues for the first 2 years of benefit payments. Following this 2-year period, the definition of total disability and benefit eligibility changes, requiring that the employee be totally disabled from any gainful occupation for which he or she may be qualified, with consideration given to the claimant's training, education, experience, and residual functional capacity as a result of injury or illness. Thus this definition uses both a medical test of functionality (either behavioral, physical, or both) as a result of the disabling condition and an earnings test to evaluate a minimum income standard (a gainful employment earnings threshold is usually 60% to 80% of predisability earnings).

LTD policies or plans commonly provide partial wage replacement benefits to the worker until retirement age. Often, specific types of conditions and diagnoses are covered for a limited time period (often 2 years). These conditions and diagnoses may include mental illness (insurance jargon is "Mental/Nervous"), fibromyalgia, chronic fatigue syndrome, multiple chemical sensitivity, and other so-called "self-reported" or "subjective conditions" as defined by group insurance policies.

A glossary of terms relating to managed disability and wage replacement programs can be found later in this chapter.

THE COSTS OF EMPLOYEE INJURY AND ILLNESS

Employee benefit programs help attract and retain employees, because they aid in maintaining job satisfaction and productivity. Employers attempt to use disability

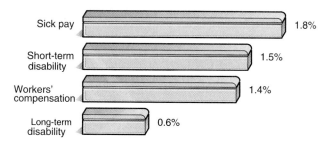

Figure 6–1. Direct costs of disability. (Reprinted with permission from Staying@Work: Improving Workforce Productivity Through Integrated Absence Management © 2002 Watson Wyatt Worldwide. For more information, visit www.watsonwyatt.com.)

management as a means to reduce the costs of disability. Figure 6–1 illustrates the average direct costs of disability by benefit type as a function of the percentage of payroll (Watson Wyatt Worldwide, 2001/2002).

This analysis by the consulting firm Watson Wyatt Worldwide was the sixth annual survey of its kind. Seventy firms, employing a median of 5200 and a total of 1.5 million full-time workers, participated in the 2001/2002 survey.

FACTORS AFFECTING SUCCESSFUL DISABILITY MANAGEMENT

Although they seem simplistic, the key features of an outstanding disability management program are similar to those of any business endeavor: effective professionals, superior communication, high expectations for success, cohesive values and approaches, and strong but malleable action planning.

From a patient treatment perspective, the health care provider can observe those traits or factors that can have a negative impact on or delay recovery to return-to-work. They include the following:

- Lack of progress in treatment
- Frequent complaints about staff, facilities, and treatment
- Patient behaviors such as frustration, agitation, or disruption
- Minimum effort or non-compliance with treatment
- Persistent focus on pain

In contrast, the positive qualities of the patient can enhance momentum toward a good outcome. The disabled worker who displays the following traits and factors makes the work of the therapist, case manager, and employer far more constructive:

- Views return-to-work as a positive and desirable goal
- Actively participates in treatment and planning decisions
- Readily transfers self-treatment techniques to the workplace and home
- Is able to modify lifestyle and abilities to match residual functioning

Although writing as a physician speaking of traumatic brain injury rehabilitation, Zasler (1994) identified important factors applicable to primary care physicians

---

*NOTE: A *plan* is generally an employer-sponsored benefit program. A *policy* is an insurance product for which both the employer and employee contribute to the cost by a payment called a *premium*.

and other health care staff relative to care, treatment, and rehabilitation:

"The physician in charge (of a) rehabilitation program should be functionally oriented, and approach patient care in a holistic manner. The well-trained physician should be able to attend to the spectrum of rehabilitation needs, as well as the medical and neurologic needs of the patient."

For employers and insurers, early intervention with a focus on functional abilities and return-to-work, as appropriate, can help a worker achieve maximum medical improvement (MMI) and return to productivity in the workplace. Key elements for successful integration of medical and vocational services should include the following:

1. A partnership between medical and vocational professionals to aid in rehabilitation planning and implementation
2. Identification of the potential for independent functioning and return-to-work early in the treatment process so that vocational case management services can be initiated quickly
3. Ongoing and frequent communication between health care professionals and disability case managers to address problems, eliminate barriers, and preserve a shared vision for successful patient rehabilitation

Specific to physical therapy and rehabilitation, what skills and competencies are insurers looking for in a therapist or clinic treating their claimants or injured workers? An obvious answer is the restoration of strength, flexibility, and movement. However, in addition, education is of key importance. A review of the underlying pathological condition and prevention techniques can help the employee transition back to work and reduce the likelihood of recurrent disability. This knowledge can also help with future self-treatment and present or future problem solving.

In a reconditioning program that has a dual focus, the area of injury and the entire body are both valuable to the employer. Appropriate documentation of functional capacity is also essential. Specific delineation of physical restrictions and functional abilities should be made in collaboration with the treating or consulting physician. Detailed knowledge of the patient's occupation from a review of the job description and/or job analysis can be used for assessment against the worker's physical capabilities. This information can be used to simulate work conditions when evaluating work capacity or to constitute the focus of a work hardening program. This has immediate and relevant application to return-to-work planning.

The employer and case manager from any workers' compensation and STD or LTD program want return-to-work to be a component and outcome of the treatment plan. The focus of medical rehabilitation should be the elimination of or a reduction in the severity of disability, to allow return-to-work. Treatment plans should concentrate on occupational tasks and help identify and address barriers to functional recovery. This process aids the patient in a more timely rehabilitation and more positive experience in the disability system. Thus a resumption of productivity and job satisfaction will result. Return-to-work can take several paths to success—work readiness through work hardening programs, transitional employment (initial return-to-work to less physically or emotionally demanding work that progresses to regular work activity), and other means or accommodations to realize a successful return to productive work.

Is the health care marketplace enlightened, from an insurer's perspective? At this time, the answer is a qualified *no*. Although occupational and physical therapists, occupational medicine physicians, and physiatrists most often have good knowledge of the world of work and the needs of insurers and employers, many primary care physicians do not. Yet, there are pockets of innovation in the health care community. In Canada, the Alberta Medical Association issued a position statement in 1994 stating that, "Prolonged absence from work may be detrimental to a patient, and returning to work as soon a possible without endangering the patient's health or safety should be encouraged. An early return-to-work after an illness or injury (work-related or otherwise) benefits a patient socially and financially. It also preserves a skilled and stable workforce for the employer" (Corbet et al, 1994).

This ad hoc committee of the Alberta Medical Association also described the role of the physician in return-to-work planning. Again, this opinion has transferability to all health care professionals who treat disabled workers. The position statement is reviewed here in part:

1. Planning for return-to-work should begin early in the disability period.
2. The physician should become familiar with the essential physical demands and health and safety hazards of the patient's work and, in particular, any additional risks to the patient, co-workers, or the public because of the medical condition or prescribed medications. The patient should be asked about the essential demands and hazards of the work. A written job description, including available work modifications, can then be requested from the employer for clarification. Occupational health professionals and disability claims managers can also help obtain this information.
3. The physician has a responsibility to both the patient and to society (in terms of endangering the safety of others; the public interest may supersede that of the patient).
4. When the physician believes the patient has sufficiently recovered and can safely participate in a trial return-to-work, the patient should be clearly informed. When providing a written note to the employer, the physician should consider task limitations, (work) schedule modifications, environmental restrictions, and medical aids or personal protective equipment.
5. Because a supervisor, safety officer, or nurse (or case manager) will determine whether suitable work is available, the physician should be as specific as possible when describing work modifications. If a physician's recommendations cannot be accommodated, it is reasonable for the physician to expect a response from the employer identifying the minimum level of capacity that can be accommodated.

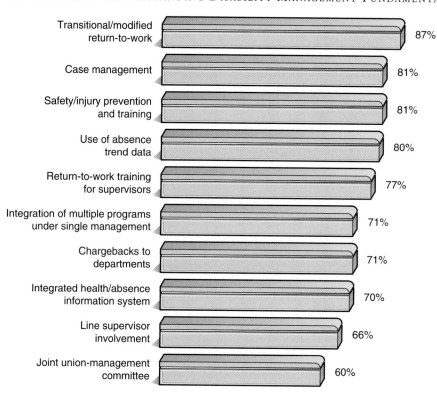

Figure 6–2. Ten most effective cost-cutting programs. (Reprinted with permission from Staying@Work: Improving Workforce Productivity Through Integrated Absence Management © 2002 Watson Wyatt Worldwide. For more information, visit www.watsonwyatt.com.)

6. Depending on the nature of the medical condition and the work available, a trial return-to-work may extend over weeks or months. When dealing with complex cases, the physician should use the special skills of other health care professionals, including the occupational health staff of the patient's employer. Formal analysis of job demands and hazards, work capacity assessment, and structured rehabilitation programs may be necessary in some cases.

As noted previously, a team approach is necessary for success in disability management. The subjective nature of disability offers great opportunity for understanding the needs of the claimant and employer. The value of education across disciplines on the roles and goals of each participant in the disability management process should be highlighted. Furthermore, considering the inexact nature of injury, illness, and disability, there are a multitude of factors, many difficult to quantify (motivation, pain behavior, job demands versus physical capacity), suggesting that negotiation can play a significant role in the process. Discussion, understanding, and compromise can be beneficial in reaching a mutually satisfactory outcome.

From an employer's perspective, the five most effective disability management activities in terms of cost reduction, as determined by the Watson Wyatt Worldwide Survey, are (1) transitional and modified return-to-work programs, (2) case management, (3) safety/injury prevention and training, (4) use of absence trend data, and (5) return-to-work training for supervisors. The survey results can be seen in Figure 6-2.

Health care professionals should be enthusiastic participants in the aforementioned disability management activities. Both physicians and physical therapists can be closely involved in transitional and modified return-to-work, because they are important team players in case management. Potential exists for both disciplines to offer expertise and services for safety and prevention procedures. The role of the physician in the IME is readily apparent.

Figure 6-3 shows the prevalence of various activities available to employers, according to the Watson Wyatt Worldwide survey (2001/2002).

FACTORS AFFECTING THE INDIVIDUAL WORKER

To address factors that impact individuals unable to work because of disabling conditions, Northwestern National Life Insurance Company (NWNL) and now ING Employee Benefits conducted a study to identify trends, costs, and outcomes related to LTD (Taylor et al, 1994). Included in this study were 9,747 incurred LTD claims, covering both insured and self-funded employers, that were administered by the insurer from January 1987 through December 1993. The major findings emerged from a more detailed analysis of 2501 claims referred for case management and rehabilitation. The study showed that employers and insurers could reduce disability costs and return more employees to work by fostering a return-to-work culture and using effective disability management strategies.

CHAPTER 6 DISABILITY MANAGEMENT: AN INSURER'S PERSPECTIVE **97**

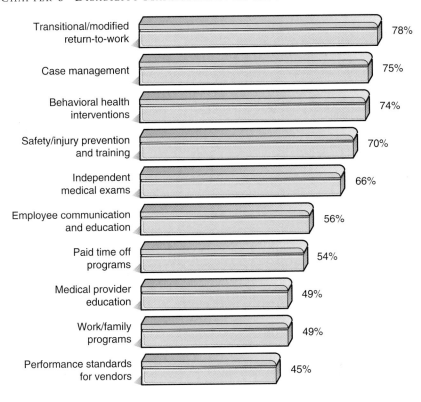

Figure 6–3. Ten most prevalent absence management programs. (Reprinted with permission from Staying@Work: Improving Workforce Productivity Through Integrated Absence Management © 2002 Watson Wyatt Worldwide. For more information, visit www.watsonwyatt.com.)

The insurer identified key factors that affect successful rehabilitation of the disabled worker. An optimal employee profile included the following:

Age: The optimum age range for successful rehabilitation is from 25 to 45 years old. Workers in this range are usually in good overall health, making it easier for them to recover from disability.

Education: More education usually translates to greater employability.

Income: Moderate income at the time of disability offers more options for job placement efforts. High salaries tend to reduce the number of job options.

Work history: Experienced workers have greater value in the workplace. Specialized skills are also desirable and increase the probability of a successful return-to-work. A varied work history increases the number of transferable skills and allows more options for vocational rehabilitation and job placement.

Motivation: A disabled worker's desire to return to the marketplace and his or her commitment to rehabilitation are critically important to a successful return-to-work.

The NWNL study (1994) discovered that returning disabled workers to work, especially to the same employer and same job, yields significant savings for employers and insurers.

Reserve savings (a financial liability that an insurer must set aside to meet future claims and other obligations, as calculated under a state insurance code) for returning disabled workers to the same employer/same job averaged $96 for every $1 spent on rehabilitation expenses (this included only rehabilitation expenses external to the insurer). The savings decreased to $46 for every $1 spent when employees returned to a new job with the same employer and to $38 for every $1 spent if workers found a new job with a new employer (Figure 6–4).

A CLOSER LOOK AT AN INSURER'S CLAIM MANAGEMENT OPERATION

A basic understanding of the procedures of a typical insurance company's claim operation can provide insight to help the health care professional in his or her understanding of the claims process. For simplicity, Figure 6–5 is based on an LTD claim operation. For this model, the claim analyst and the disabled worker are at the center, surrounded by other key participants in claim management and a description of their primary duties. In addition, an outline of many of the tools of managed disability is also provided.

When dealing with insurance companies, providers find it difficult to escape the use of claim forms. For purposes of this review, two of the forms most likely to be seen and used by health care professionals are offered as exhibits for analysis. One is the attending physician statement (APS). The APS is used with every initial LTD claim application. This form is also sent to the attending physician and other treating physicians periodically during the

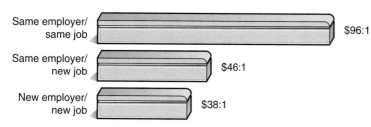

Same employer/same job $96:1

Same employer/new job $46:1

New employer/new job $38:1

Figure 6–4. Returning disabled workers to the same employer and same job yields the greatest savings to insurers and employers. (Data from Taylor M et al: Back to Work: Managing Disability, Recovery and Re-employment. Minneapolis, MN, Northwestern National Life Insurance Company, 1994.)

length of the patient's eligibility for benefit payments. Figure 6–6 is a composite taken from the forms of various disability insurers' APSs.

The APS attempts to gather as much information as possible, albeit in a truncated manner, to reduce the completion time for the physicians yet maximize the amount of information that can be gathered on two pages. Often, the claims analyst or medical case manager sends a follow-up communication to the physician to ask for a narrative report or to answer diagnosis-specific questions.

To delineate functional capacity, insurers typically use the physical capacity evaluation form before, or in lieu of,

a formal FCE performed by a physical therapist. The treating physician completes the physical capacity evaluation form, sometimes with consultation from an occupational or physical therapist. This form attempts to objectify the patient's residual physical abilities and limitations following illness or injury. In many cases, the physical capacity evaluation is used as a gross screening device to identify the claimant's ability to perform sedentary, light, medium, or heavy work activity based on the U.S. Department of Labor's definitions of strength demands. This form can be used to evaluate specific job targets and return-to-work options, or it can lead the insurer toward further evaluation

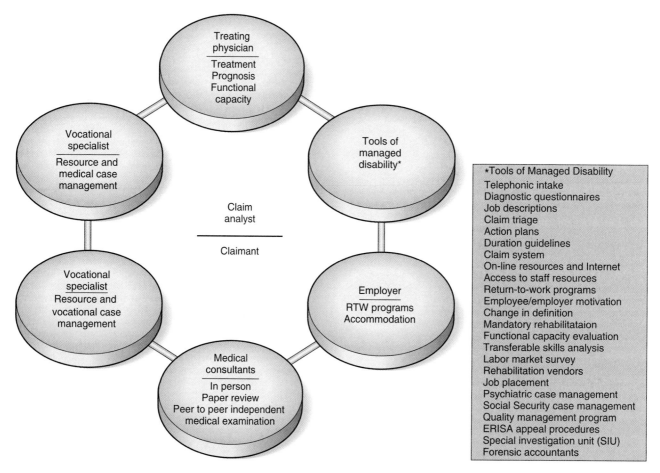

Figure 6–5. Disability management process elements.

Attending Physician's Statement

Name of Patient_____ DOB____/____/____

SS#_____ Height_____ Weight_____lbs

1) History

Patient's symptoms result from:

Employment [ ]   Illness [ ]   Pregnancy [ ]   MVA [ ]

Date symptoms first appeared ____/____/____   First visit to you for this condition ____/____/____

Most recent visit ____/____/____   Next scheduled visit ____/____/____

If hospital confined, date(s) _____

Has patient undergone surgery? Yes [ ]   No [ ]   If yes, date(s) _____

Procedure and result _____

_____

If no, is surgery planned? Yes [ ]   No [ ]   If yes, date ____/____/____

Procedure _____

2) Diagnosis

Diagnosis _____ ICD-9_____ Secondary diagnosis _____ ICD-9_____

DSM IV Axis 1 – V (GAF): _____

Subjective complaints _____

_____

Objective findings (include X-ray, lab, clinical) **Attach medical records**

Has the patient had the same or similar condition? Yes [ ]   No [ ]

If yes, what year(s)? _____   Describe _____

_____

3) Treatment

Describe the treatment plan for your patient's return to work or return to prior level of functioning?_____

_____

Please list medications with dosage and frequency of use_____

_____

Frequency with which you see patient: Weekly [ ]   Monthly [ ]   Other [ ]

Describe _____

Has patient been referred to other physicians or therapy programs? (PT, OT, psychotherapy, etc)

Yes [ ]   No [ ]   If yes, please ID provider. Describe type of therapy _____

Name of physician/therapist _____ Phone _____

_____ Phone _____

_____ Phone _____

Figure 6–6. Attending physician's statement.

Continued

4) Prognosis

Terminal ☐   Poor ☐   Good ☐   Excellent ☐

Has the patient reached maximum medical improvement? Yes ☐   No ☐

If no, how soon do you expect fundamental changes in the patient's medical condition?

1 – 2 months ☐   3 – 4 months ☐   5 – 6 months ☐   More than 6 months ☐

5) Physical capabilities

Have you have reviewed Patient's job description? Yes ☐   No ☐   Patient's self-report of job tasks Yes ☐   No ☐

Please explain how the patient's condition affects his/her ability to work and why _____

_____

_____
_____

Please describe how the patient's condition affects the ability to perform activities of daily living _____

_____

If you have knowledge of the patient's job, would modifications enable the patient to work? Can you identify any? _____

_____

Would you recommend vocational/rehabilitation services? Yes ☐   No ☐

When would you expect a return to employment? _____   Part-time _____   Full-time _____

6) Level of Impairment
Physical impairment (if applicable)

☐ Class 1. No limitation of functional capacity/capable of heavy work.

☐ Class 2. Slight limitation of functional capacity/capable of medium manual work.

☐ Class 3. Moderate limitation of functional capacity/ capable of light work.

☐ Class 4. Marked limitation of functional capacity/ capable of sedentary work.

☐ Class 5. Severe limitation of functional capacity/ incapable of sedentary work.

Mental/nervous impairment

☐ Class 1. No limitation: able to function under stress and engage in interpersonal relationships.

☐ Class 2. Slight limitation: able to function in most stress situations and engage in most interpersonal relationships.

☐ Class 3. Moderate limitation: able to engage in only limited stress and limited interpersonal relationships.

☐ Class 4. Marked limitation: unable to engage in stress or interpersonal relationships.

☐ Class 5. Severe limitation: has significant loss of psychological, physiological, personal and social adjustment.

Cardiac funtional capacity – American Heart Association:

Class 1. No limitation ☐   Class 2. Slight limitation ☐   Class 3. Marked limitation ☐   Class 4. Complete limitation ☐

Do you believe your patient is competent to endorse checks and direct the use of the proceeds thereof? Yes ☐   No ☐

Physician's Name: _____   **Degree/Specialty:** _____

Address: _____

Telephone: (   ) _____   **Fax (   )** _____

Signature _____   **Date:** _____ / _____ / _____

Figure 6–6. (*cont'd*)

of the physical demands of return-to-work targets. The physical capacity evaluation form is used to determine possible worksite accommodations, whether these accommodations include job restructuring (changes in job tasks or work hours) or job modification (changes in the physical requirements of a job), and it may be a precursor to a formal FCE.

Figure 6-7 shows the physical capacity evaluation form commonly sent to the attending physician to estimate the patient's physical capacities.

Insurers use a formal FCE when the claimant, his or her physician, and sometimes, the physical therapist are uncertain regarding the claimant's physical capacity for work. At times, the attending physician prescribes an FCE. In other situations, an FCE is used in an attempt to examine patients whose self-report of functional limitations appears to exceed objective evidence of disability.

The insurance claim analyst or case manager typically sends medical records and other information to the FCE provider that offers insight into the patient's injury, illness,

Physical Capacities Evaluation

Return to:

Patient	Group Number	Date of Birth	Date Disabled

Please complete the following items based on your most recent clinical evaluation, diagnostic testing and other pertinent information.

I. Date of last examination ____________________

II. Patent can work full-time? Yes ☐ No ☐
If not full-time, patient can work part-time? Yes ☐ No ☐ (If "yes," hours per day: ______ days per week: ________)

III. In a work day, patient can stand/walk:
(Hours at one time) ☐ 0–2 ☐ 2–4 ☐ 4–6 ☐ 6–8 ☐ 8–10
(TOTAL hours during day) ☐ 0–2 ☐ 2–4 ☐ 4–6 ☐ 6–8 ☐ 8–10

In a work day, patient can sit:
(Hours at one time) ☐ 0–2 ☐ 2–4 ☐ 4–6 ☐ 6–8 ☐ 8–10
(TOTAL hours during day) ☐ 0–2 ☐ 2–4 ☐ 4–6 ☐ 6–8 ☐ 8–10

IV. Patient can lift/carry:	Minimally 0–2.5 hrs.	Occasionally 2.5–5.5 hrs.	Frequently 5.5 hrs.+	Continuously
Up to 10 pounds	☐	☐	☐	☐
11–20 pounds	☐	☐	☐	☐
21–50 pounds	☐	☐	☐	☐
51–100 pounds	☐	☐	☐	☐

V. Patient is able to:	Minimally	Occasionally	Frequently	Continuously
A. Stoop (bend at waist)	☐	☐	☐	☐
B. Kneel (coming to rest on knees)	☐	☐	☐	☐
C. Ascend, descend ladder	☐	☐	☐	☐
D. Ascend, descend stairs	☐	☐	☐	☐
E. Push/pull	☐	☐	☐	☐
F. Reach above shoulder level	☐	☐	☐	☐
G. Crawl	☐	☐	☐	☐

VI. Use of hands for repetitive action:	Minimally	Occasionally	Frequently	Continuously
Manual dexterity (hold, grasp, turn)	☐	☐	☐	☐
Finger dexterity (pinch, pick, use keyboard)	☐	☐	☐	☐

VII. Is a formal Functional Capacity Evaluation necessary? Yes ☐ No ☐

Remarks

Other special medical considerations/functional limitations

VIII. Do you believe these physical capacities to be permanent? ____________________

______________________________ ______________
Physician's Signature Date

______________________________ (______) ______________
Address Phone

Figure 6-7. Physical capacity evaluation.

and physical abilities. In many cases, the goal is to determine whether the claimant has the ability to perform and sustain part-time or full-time work to sedentary or light physical demands. The ability to perform medium to heavy work is evaluated less frequently. In some instances, a job description and the physical demands of a particular job or group of jobs may be given to the physical therapist to address physical capacity in preparation for vocational exploration and job placement.

Although many physical therapy clinics use standardized tests to assess functionality, an insurer may ask for work simulation as a part of an FCE to address duties and physical demands specific to a particular job. The length of an FCE is important to many disability management specialists. A single 4-hour assessment does not always provide an accurate gauge of the ability of the disabled worker to sustain work activity at a prescribed pace and strength level. Two half-day sessions are common. Two-, or even four-, day evaluations, although more expensive, are viewed by many as better indicators of functionality.

In addition to being a profile of functionality, the FCE can also be used to determine the need for physical reactivation, work conditioning, or job accommodation options that will allow a resumption of job duties in the future. The physical therapist should address overall functional capacity and the level of effort (maximum or sub-par) exhibited by the patient during the evaluation, as appropriate. Observations of behaviors, including pain complaints, documentation of motivation, cooperation, and involvement in the process, are constructive. All questions from the referring party (usually a case manager or claim analyst) should be answered. These will likely include an estimate of the optimum work hours the claimant can perform, the extent to which the current functional capacity is permanent, suggestions for reconditioning or job accommodations, and whether the demonstrated capabilities fit the worker's job demands. A schedule for gradual return-to-work may also be addressed, beginning with part-time work and increasing to full-time work over a prescribed timeline of a few weeks to a few months. In this situation, the gradual return-to-work is used as a reconditioning program or is done concurrently (part-time work with formal physical therapy before or after work).

MEDICAL MANAGEMENT, PREVENTION, WELLNESS, AND EARLY INTERVENTION

Medical management is a form of case management by which the insurer/employer, or a designated representative for either, evaluates the medical status, treatment, and prognosis of the disabled worker. For most types of employee benefits, the claimant is obligated to meet certain requirements of the insurance policy to maintain benefit eligibility. Usually, the worker must be under the regular care and attendance of a physician for treatment. Benefit policies require that treatment be aimed at maximizing recovery to realize the ability to return-to-work, as appropriate and possible. The worker's failure to comply with the attending physician's treatment plan can sometimes result in suspension or denial of benefits until reasonable treatment resumes. Sustained non-compliance can lead to termination of benefit eligibility.

After gathering medical information and completing one or more discussions on the telephone to address follow-up issues or questions with the claimant, the claim analyst will refer the claimant (disabled worker) to a nurse case manager or insurance company physician consultant for review and assessment. Either medical professional may use written communication with the treating physician to gain additional insight and information on treatment issues. The nurse or physician may also conduct a peer-to-peer telephone consultation with the treating doctor to further discuss issues or to attempt, in a collaborative manner, to guide the doctor and patient toward more suitable treatment. On an extra contractual basis and if a financial barrier exists, the insurer may provide partial funding to the claimant for more appropriate treatment.

If the opinions of the insurer and treating physician differ to a significant degree and they cannot reach consensus on a reasonable action plan, the insurer may complete an IME. The IME physician is generally a board-certified specialist who has some familiarity with occupational issues as they relate to treatment, recovery, and return-to-work. The following are some common referral questions asked of the IME physician:

1. What is the diagnosis of the patient's injury or illness?
2. Does the patient require additional diagnostic testing? If so, can you list specific tests to consider?
3. Is the patient under appropriate care and treatment for the identified condition or syndrome? Are prescribed medications appropriate for the disease or injury? If so, are they being used at therapeutic levels? Do you recommend additional or alternative treatment to further aid in recovery and return-to-work?
4. Are any secondary issues, either medical or nonmedical, significantly affecting treatment or the lack of movement toward recovery?
5. Can the patient perform work activity at the Sedentary, Light, or Medium work levels? (NOTE: It is important to define these strength categories for the physician.) Please complete the attached physical evaluation form for this purpose.
6. Would a formal FCE, administered by a registered physical therapist, be more appropriate to ascertain residual capacity?
7. Has the patient realized MMI? If not, can you estimate when this may occur?
8. If the patient has reached MMI, what is his or her impairment rating? Please use the American Medical Association's *Guides to the Evaluation of Permanent Impairment* or identify your method of analysis. (NOTE: This question is for cases involving workers' compensation.)

Occasionally, the insurer will agree to use the IME to gain a second opinion for the patient. In this example, the patient may not have the appropriate medical coverage or financial resources to pursue another evaluation. In addition, the treating physician may be in full agreement to proceed with the IME and may even recommend a physician to conduct the examination. Insurers use an IME for only a small percentage of all claims, but it is a valuable tool for medical assessment.

Early intervention is a concept by which case management is initiated early in the life of a claim, sometimes shortly after injury or illness but before benefit eligibility has been determined. Disease management, ergonomics, physical therapy, vocational counseling, job site accommodations, or the use of assistive devices to aid in work performance are a few of the tools of disability management that are used to keep a worker on the job or to dramatically reduce the duration of disability. From a physical rehabilitation viewpoint, onsite assessment of job tasks, ergonomic issues, and therapy targeted at improvement of functioning as it relates to work duties is of key importance. Early intervention is a concept well known to workers' compensation insurers. Many STD and LTD insurers are still developing this process. Prevention and wellness programs have become much more popular as employers and insurers have begun to realize the high cost of lost time and disability. Generally employer sponsored, these programs often take a holistic approach to injury and illness prevention, with a goal of improving the quality of life of a company's workforce. Fitness, nutrition, weight loss programs, blood pressure screening, and other health status appraisals are common components. The importance of worksite ergonomics and job fitness cannot be understated as forms of prevention. Training in proper body mechanics and lifting techniques and improvements in strength and flexibility are extremely valuable means to maintain productive and healthy workers.

To make gains in productivity and job satisfaction and to reduce the frequency and duration of illness and injury, the payer of services in a managed disability environment is cognizant of the importance of a team approach to assist workers in maintaining a healthy workplace and to minimize the impact of disability. Health care specialists, disability case managers, employer representatives, and claim professionals must continue to understand their roles in this process. Effective outcomes can be realized only when reasonable action plans are implemented that use the myriad tools of disability management to aid the disabled worker in recovery and return-to-work.

REFERENCES

American Psychiatric Association: Diagnostic and Statistical Manual of Mental Disorders: DSM-IV, 4th ed. Washington, DC, American Psychiatric Association, 1994.

Case Management Society of America, Little Rock, AR, www.cmsa.org, accessed January 2004.

Corbet K, Brox D, Cheng J et al: Position statement: Early return to work after illness or injury. Alberta, Ad Hoc Committee on Return to Work after Illness or Injury (of the Health Issues Council), Alberta Medical Association, February 1994.

National Safety Council: Report on Injuries in America, 2001, www.nsc.org/library/rept2000_072803.htm, accessed January 2004.

Taylor M, Hintzman-Egan D, Farrell G: Back to Work: Managing Disability, Recovery and Re-employment. Minneapolis, Northwestern National Life Insurance Company, 1994.

US Census Bureau: Census 2000, Summary File 3, www.census.gov/hhes/www/disable/disabstat2k/table1.html, accessed January 2004.

Watson Wyatt Worldwide Sixth Annual Survey Report: "Staying @ Work: Improving Workforce Productivity Through Integrated Absence Management" 2001/2002. Bethesda, MD, Watson Wyatt Worldwide, 2002, p 3, www.watsonwyatt.com, accessed January 2004.

William M. Mercer, Inc (New York, NY): The Language of Managed Disability. New York, William M. Mercer, Inc., and Mt. Prospect, IL, Incorporated and Metropolitan Life Insurance Company, 1995.

Zasler ND: TBI rehabilitation program assessment. Putting a yardstick to duality and efficacy. Contin Care 13(4):30-34, 36, 50, 1994.

CHAPTER *7*

Confounding Obstacles to Disability Management

David W. Clifton, Jr., PT

"To view disability strictly as a biological phenomenon is to categorize it as a medical entity and to ignore the complexity of factors that in combination determine whether a physical or mental impairment will progress to a functional limitation and then to disability (the inability to perform expected social and personal roles and tasks)."

- Pope & Tarlov, 1991

"In the arena of disability management and rehabilitation of chronically ill, injured and disabled workers, one steps into a maelstrom of public and private sector policies as well as policy preferences of organized groups...i.e., the business community, labor organizations, professional associations and disability consumer groups."

- Galvin, 1986

KEY POINTS

- For rehabilitation providers to optimize clinical outcomes, they must recognize and address non-clinical factors (e.g., psychosocial) associated with disability.
- Each rehabilitation case presents a unique constellation of obstacles to recovery. Rehabilitation providers can unwittingly become enablers of disability through a failure to recognize and address psychosocial issues. This is chiefly done by a continued focus on pathological conditions and impairments.
- To delay rehabilitation is to compromise rehabilitation. A lapse in time from injury or illness to referral for physical rehabilitation is one of the most prevalent and costly obstacles to recovery.

Operational Definitions

Biophysical   Those aspects of a treatment episode that focus on anatomical, biological, and physiological findings; variables that are either patient-specific or condition-specific (e.g., range of motion, edema, muscle performance, physical function).

Environmental   Those worksite variables that factor into disability management decisions, especially as they relate to matching the worker to the worksite (e.g., unsafe worksites, critical job demands, vocational skills and aptitudes, productivity measures).

Psychosomatic   The degree to which disability experiences are related to internal psychological factors.

Somatopsychological   The degree to which disability experiences are related to social and environmental factors that are external to the individual.

Subjective Disabilities Disabilities in which clinical examination, laboratory findings, or imaging studies fail to produce reasonable explanation for a person's symptoms or disability-related behavior.

CHALLENGES TO DISABILITY MANAGEMENT

To be successful in disability management, providers must command a greater understanding of the system in which their particular services are embedded, as well as a better understanding of the patient's perspective (Bongers et al, 1993; Gard et al, 1998; Tan et al, 1997; Vierling, 2001). However, at least one author (Sanders, 2000) contends that the health care system is too preoccupied with psychosocial issues and has abandoned care itself.

This chapter addresses some of the most common challenges or obstacles to disability management confronted by rehabilitation providers. Although these issues are discussed individually, providers should be mindful of the interrelationships that may exist between various obstacles to recovery. These issues can have a profound impact on the design, implementation, and outcome of a rehabilitation program, especially for clinicians who have limited training, education, and experience with psychosocial aspects of health care delivery.

THE BIOMEDICAL MODEL OF HEALTH CARE

The health care system in the United States heavily relies on a biomedical perspective of pain and illness. This paradigm overlooks the contribution of environmental influences on symptom behavior and care seeking (Cahill, 1996; Devereux et al, 1999; Fordyce, 1997; Thorbjornsson et al, 2000). Providers who are educated and trained under the medical model of care often ignore the effect of environmental factors on human functioning. The medical model ensures that an underlying pathological condition exists to explain a person's symptoms, dysfunction, or disability. This model typically is predicated on laboratory or imaging proof of an organic basis for a problem. This patient-centric or disease-centric approach often ignores the social or contextual factors associated with disability. Regrettably, exploration of social or contextual factors may occur only after an exhaustive examination of biomedical causation yields nothing tangible, poor clinical outcomes, or subjective disabilities. Subjective disabilities are those in which clinical examination, laboratory findings, or imaging studies fail to produce reasonable explanation for a person's symptoms or disability-related behavior. Subjective or poorly understood conditions are often points of contention between various stakeholders, especially those involved in medicolegal cases. It has been long established that physical findings are pinpointed as the cause of patient symptoms in only 12% to 15% of all back injury cases (McGill, 1968; Partridge & Duthie, 1968).

Subjective disabilities include chronic pain syndromes, fibromyalgia, post-traumatic stress disorder (PTSD), psychiatric claims, and other diagnoses for which specific diagnostic tests are either lacking or are of questionable validity or reliability (Beger, 1997). However, the absence of a clinical finding or negative test result does not necessarily imply the absence of a problem. Chronic illnesses and injuries serve to focus attention on the potential power and impact of these "extradermal" influences (Fordyce, 1997). Clinical skills, although vital to successful rehabilitation, may be less important than are case management techniques and consideration of external or non-clinical variables (Gates et al, 1989).

Shortcomings of a Biophysical or Biomedical Approach to Disability

Our current system of health care delivery may inadvertently contribute to the development of chronic disabilities. For example, consider a patient whose symptoms include pain of unknown origin. The fragmented design of health care leads to a series of diagnostic workups that require the patient to navigate a medical maze in search of an organic basis for pain. The deeper the patient gets into the system, the more expensive the tests and the more specialized the providers become. This journey may entrench the patient in a "sickness" model that, until now, was absent. In worst-case scenarios, the expenditure of human and financial resources can lead a reasonably healthy patient to perceive that his or her problem is beyond indentification via diagnostic tests and clinical examination.

Because many view the American health care system as the world's most developed, expectations may be higher for a cure or at least the diagnosis of a problem. When a diagnosis is not forthcoming, patients may assume that their problem is extremely rare or complex. This should not sound like a fictional or rare account to those who have dealt with chronic disability and its causes.

To the contrary, employers or insurers may conclude that a negative test battery disproves the presence of a problem and the medical necessity for treatment. Both perceptions may be misguided. Pain by definition is a subjective phenomenon that cannot be measured through diagnostic tests (Monsein & Clift, 1995). It is unfortunate that, over time, perceptions may become realities, and ultimately, barriers to recovery. The biomedical focus may serve to delay rehabilitation that addresses psychosocial, psychosomatic, and somatopsychological elements of disability.

A disability management and physical rehabilitation text is incomplete without a discussion of non-biophysical barriers to recovery. A number of terms will be used interchangeably throughout this chapter to describe the variables that fall outside of the physical function domain. These include psychosocial, non-biophysical, biomedical, non-medical, and non-clinical variables. These non-physical variables can dictate the degree of rehabilitation success more significantly than biophysical variables can (Burton et al, 1995).

Rehabilitation providers are highly equipped with an abundance of skills and knowledge in the treatment and management of impairment and disability. However, efforts are likely to be of limited success if the principal focus is on biophysical aspects of a case. Clinicians are expert at examining and treating various biophysical impairments such as range of motion or muscle performance deficits. However, experienced providers recognize that to engage in a holistic approach to disability prevention and management, practitioners must consider numerous confounding non-clinical obstacles.

Disability Perceptions Across Stakeholders

One's perception of a patient's disability dynamics may or may not be synchronous with the views of others. For instance, the definition of a disability itself is subject to various interpretations depending on a given stakeholder's paradigm (Jette, 1994). Figure 7–1 illustrates this point. An attorney may view disability from a legal context without a full appreciation or understanding of the clinical or psychosocial aspects involved. Rehabilitation specialists may principally use physical functioning as a measure of disability. A psychologist may more heavily weigh a person's emotional response to a physical injury.

Employers may focus on job tasks and productivity concerns when addressing disability. The patient or injured worker may define disability through the prism of pain, whereas cost may be a principal focus of insurers or payers. Disability assessments vary significantly among physicians for similar conditions and tend to focus on impairment, a medical appraisal, versus disability, a legal and/or administrative judgment (Brand & Lehmann, 1983).

Overview of Psychosocial Obstacles

Confounding obstacles to disability management have been recognized by clinicians for decades (Berkowitz, 1980; Better, 1979; Carpenter, 1985; Eaton, 1979; Fathallah et al, 1996; Micek & Bitter, 1974; Spratt et al, 1990; Tuck, 1983).

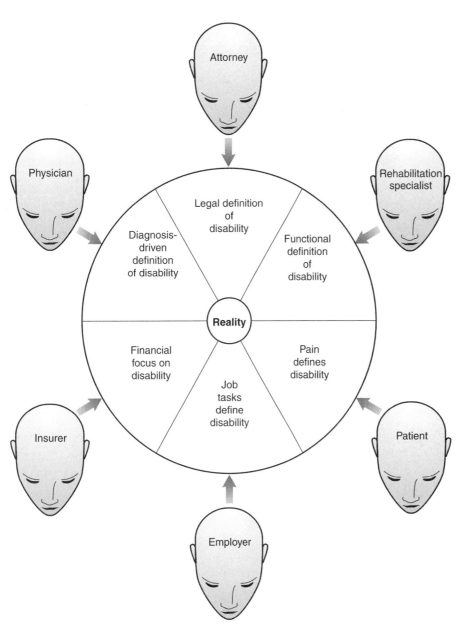

Figure 7–1. Health care stakeholder perceptions of disability status.

These obstacles generally fall within the following three primary domains (Figure 7–2):

1. Individual: psychological, biomedical, functional, health history, pain tolerance and response to injury, cultural preferences, support network
2. Environmental: jobsite, tools, equipment, supervisors, job accommodations, modified duty
3. Societal: legal system, health benefits, labeling by others

Each rehabilitation case presents a unique set of variables that can result in opportunities or threats to successful disability management. Rehabilitation providers must deal with many confounding obstacles that may fall outside of their traditional clinical training, education, and practice competencies (Clifton, 1992; Proctor et al, 2000). For instance, one study identified 42 psychological and socioeconomic variables have been shown to be related to chronically disabled persons with low back pain (Polatin et al, 1989). An employee's work load, degree of autonomy,

role ambiguity, and co-worker relations can lead to work-related psychological disorders in the absence of significant organic problems (Sauter et al, 1990; Eisenstat & Felner; 1984; Iglen, 1990).

These and many other variables must be considered when planning and executing a rehabilitation program. It is shortsighted to assume that physical rehabilitation success is ensured through the application of diagnostic and clinical competencies only (Tan et al, 1997). Clinical skills and knowledge alone are of limited value in the emerging health care marketplace. Today's clinicians are bombarded with unprecedented change and information overload. Although many advances in clinical diagnostics have been developed over the past several decades, no appreciable improvement in clinical outcome measures for certain conditions has been achieved. This is partly due to relative neglect of the psychosocial components of disability (Burton et al, 1995).

Predictive models that correlate medical, psychological, and functional variables to rehabilitation success or

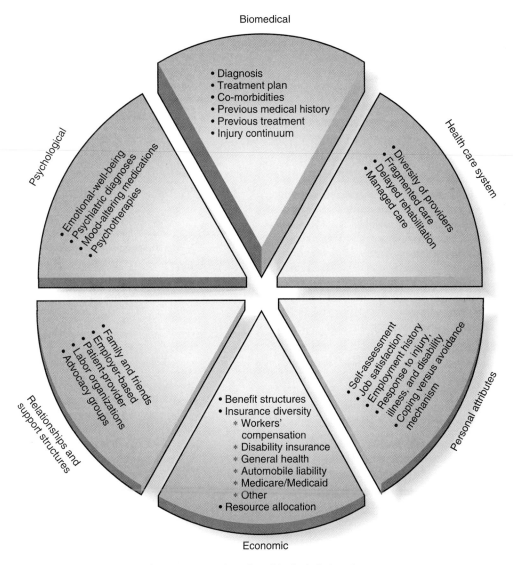

Figure 7–2. Domains of non-biophysical obstacles.

Table 7–1 Prediction of Outcome Disability Scores

Conventional Clinical Measures	Psychosocial Measures
7% across all patients	32% across all patients
10% across acute cases	59% across acute cases

Data from Burton AK et al: Psychosocial predictors of outcome in acute and subacute low back trouble. Spine 20(2):722-728, 1995.

failure have evolved. (Polatin et al, 1989; Tate et al, 1994). One predictive model purports to correctly identify those variables associated with successful rehabilitation 70% of the time (Polatin et al, 1989). Correlations between an individual's anthropometry and return-to-work (RTW) likelihood have even been established. Anthropometry can determine the availability and viability of reasonable accommodations under the Americans with Disabilities Act of 1990 (ADA) (Das & Sengupta, 1995; Goswami, 1997; Jarosz, 1996).

Early identification of psychosocial problems is important in understanding and preventing the progression of conditions into chronic problems or disabilities (Burton et al, 1995; Ensalada, 2000). Table 7–1 illustrates the predictive ability of psychosocial data when compared with conventional clinical data. These data, generated through multiple regression analyses, suggest that psychosocial measures are more predictive of 1-year disability rates than are conventional clinical measures.

Conventional clinical measures include the following system-based tests: musculoskeletal, neurological, pulmonary, cardiac, and integumentary. Specific measures may include range of motion, muscle performance, nerve root tests, balance assessment, edema, VO_2 max, vital signs, and other biophysical assessments.

Psychosocial variables can be assessed through a battery of instruments designed to explore pain behaviors, fear-avoidance beliefs, coping strategies, and work activity elements. Conventional clinical measures successfully predicted outcome disability scores in only 7% of all patients and in only 10% of patients with acute-stage back injury (Burton et al, 1995).

Psychosocial measures were significantly more predictive, at 32% across all patients and 59% in acute cases. These data suggest that persisting symptoms in persons with low back conditions, especially in those with a previous history of back injury, may result more from psychosocial influences than from medical or biophysical issues (Burton et al, 1995).

Early identification of psychosocial problems during the acute stage of irritability may potentially prevent some conditions from reaching the chronic stage. Rehabilitation providers are encouraged to design early intervention strategies based on results of a multivariate analysis of psychosocial variables. A sampling of non-biophysical variables associated with disability management is displayed in Table 7–2.

Impairment and Disability

A cursory review of a disablement model is appropriate here, because the relationship between impairment and disability is pertinent to any discussion of confounding obstacles to disability management. The presence of a disease or injury does not guarantee impairment, nor do all impairments necessarily lead to disability. For example, not all persons with Type II or late-onset diabetes develop blindness or require amputation of a limb secondary to vascular insufficiency. Therefore an assumption of disability is flawed.

Physicians play a dominant role in the acute stage of injury or illness, especially as gatekeepers in managed care organizations. Identification and treatment of pathological abnormalities is the principal focus at this stage of irritability. If a condition progresses into the subacute stage, rehabilitation services become more involved. Delayed rehabilitation is often a reason that some patients are not seen during the acute phase. Essentially, the pathology paradigm of physicians (versus the functional paradigm) delays referral to rehabilitation providers. Although they involve physicians and rehabilitation, chronic cases often demand increasing services of social workers, psychologists, case managers, and vocational counseling experts (Aronoff et al, 2000).

A Disability Continuum

Figure 7–3 depicts a hypothetical continuum from injury → pathology → disability. This schematic demonstrates a condition as it progresses along the continuum toward disability. The complexity of a case increases because of the introduction of psychological and social variables, which are potential obstacles to recovery. It is important, however, to recognize that disability development may not be linear in nature and that not all injuries or illnesses result in disability. The continuum illustrates a generalization of when, from a temporal standpoint, professionals intervene in the disability management process. It is important to understand that this model is dynamic and allows for provider-service flexibility. Providers are not locked into any point of intervention but are free to provide services at any point along the continuum.

A Sampler of Psychosocial Variables: Obstacles to Recovery

Studies have demonstrated poor positive correlations between organic pathology and impairment or disability (Alaranta et al, 1994; Battie et al, 1990; Biering-Sorensen, 1984; Mellin, 1986). In contrast, positive correlations between psychosocial involvement and disability development have been well demonstrated (Anthony, 1994; Brodwin, 1993; Fitzgerald, 1992; Marinelli, 1977; Martin, 1990; Rutman, 1994; Waddell et al, 1980). For instance, Bigos et al (1991) were the first to use the Minnesota Multiphasic Personality Inventory (MMPI) premorbidly to determine predictors of acute low back pain. These researchers reported a statistically significant predictive power of work perceptions and psychological factors for reports of acute low back pain among industrial workers. These data support a psychosocial-based versus an injury-based model. For example, low job satisfaction has been shown to be highly predictive of delayed return-to-work (Froom et al, 2001). Krause et al (1997) demonstrated strong associations between workplace environment and the incidence of disability-based retirement. Poor working conditions include employee communication difficulties and lack of support from management.

Table 7–2 Non-Medical Variables Associated with Disability Management

Study	Variable	Conclusion
Kennedy, 1974	Education Public assistance Employment status at referral	Successful RTW is associated with higher educational levels and absence of public assistance
Krauft & Bolton, 1976	Public assistance Family support Mental disability	RTW is less successful with presence of public assistance or mental condition
Schechter, 1981	Disability severity Education Gender Financial status	Mild disability, higher educational level, male gender, and greater financial needs are all associated with RTW
Better, 1979	SSI and SSDI Gender Marital status	Non-beneficiaries of SSDI and SSI have greater likelihood of RTW; females are more likely to RTW than males; non-married employees are more likely to RTW than married employees
Hester & Decelles, 1986	Support level Education Occupation Wage replacement Disability severity Employment status Gender Age Residence Marital status	All of these and other factors are significantly associated with RTW
Brown et al, 1991	Vocational evaluations Medical evaluations	Correlation between impairment and vocational or economic loss is low; medical evaluations have only a poor association with disability settlement amount, but vocational evaluations have a high correlation
Akabas, 1979 Davis, 1983 Galvin, 1986 Niemeyer et al, 1994 Pati, 1985	Time to rehabilitation referral	Early intervention is associated with successful rehabilitation, reduced severity, and decreased reinjury rates
Burton et al, 1995 Polatin et al, 1989	Role of psychological conditions	Psychological behavior is correlated with RTW
Taylor & Bonfiglio, 1992	Psychological issues	Psychological issues are predictive of success or failure in functional restorative program; rehabilitation is most effective in the absence of psychological issues
Block, 1980 Gil et al, 1987 Lipton & Marbach, 1984 Newby, 1996	Family dynamics	Family-patient psychosocial dimensions correlate with chronic illness
DiFabio et al, 1995 Mayer et al, 1987 Reilly et al, 1989	Patient's attitude	Patient's positive attitude and motivation promotes successful rehabilitation
Williams et al, 1998	Job satisfaction	Job satisfaction insulates against development of chronic disability; job dissatisfaction may be a consequence rather than a predictor of pain
Burton et al, 1995	Multiple psychosocial factors	Disability depends on psychosocial domain
Frederickson, 1988	Litigation	RTW occurs in 80% of workers without legal claims, but in less than 40% with legal claims
Moffroid et al, 1993	Preinjury employment status	Job attachment to a preinjury employer has a strong relationship with RTW after rehabilitation

RTW, Return-to-work; *SSDI*, Social Security Disability Insurance; *SSI*, Social Security Insurance; *ADA*, Americans with Disabilities Act of 1990; *DM*, disability management; *HR*, human resource; *MMI*, Maximum Medical Improvement; *MMPI*, Minnesota Multiphasic Personality Inventory; *NIDMAR*, National Institute for Disability Management & Research; *NCCI*, National Council on Compensation Insurance; *WHO*, World Health Organization.

The effect of financial compensation on movement along the disability continuum toward a return to gainful employment also has been studied (Ambrosius et al, 1995; Tate, 1992; Fowler, 1969). The degree of financial compensation can affect the disability status of a beneficiary, especially under workers' compensation, Social Security, or other disability programs. Dereberg and Tullis (1983) contend that chronicity in compensable injury cases should be considered psychogenic unless a failure to recover can be explained by a normal response to physiological insult. Kennedy (1997) opines that once a patient with orthopedic problems initiates litigation, he or she becomes invested in permanent disability, and "the slide down the slippery slope of a lifetime of disability has begun."

Disability Management Programs Directed at Non-Clinical Barriers

The design and duration of a disability management program that includes comprehensive rehabilitation can have a direct impact on clinical efficacy. Comprehensive functional restoration programs that use an interdisciplinary model to address and ameliorate non-clinical barriers to recovery have been effective (Polatin et al, 1997). A number

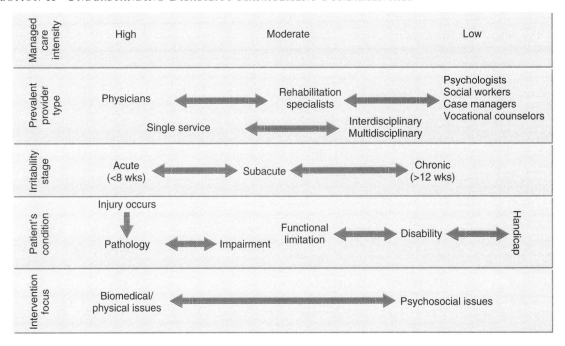

Figure 7–3. Health care disability continuum.

of studies have shown that aggressive multi-disciplinary programs achieve impressive return-to-work rates (Bendix et al, 1995; Cleary et al, 1995; Niemeyer et al, 1994). Effective programs combine physical therapy, occupational therapy, case management, and behavioral therapies (Hazard et al, 1989). Unfortunately, outcome data tend to be restricted to the chronic stage of disability.

Chronic injury and illness are nearly synonymous with the involvement of psychosocial issues, yet providers often avoid discussing obstacles to recovery, citing reasons such as time constraints (Keith, 1998). Satisfaction with the degree of attention dedicated to psychosocial problems is infrequently measured (Hall & Dornan, 1990). One means of facilitating a greater degree of attention to these issues is to reconstruct patient evaluation forms to display categories for non-biophysical variables such as those contained in Figure 7–2. This will ensure that therapists, at a minimum, will examine the associative or causative relationship of psychosocial issues with disability. Programs can then be designed that address these needs as well as physical function.

Typically, physical rehabilitation data collection largely focuses on biophysical issues, despite the suggestion that non-biophysical variables may actually be more predictive, or in this case restrictive, of disability-related outcomes.

Building a Consensus: NIDMAR's Standards

If DM is to effectively manage non-medical/non-biophysical or psychosocial issues, the real challenge is to reach a consensus among divergent stakeholders, each of whom has his or her own bias. The National Institute of Disability Management and Research (NIDMAR) developed the first-ever consensus-based "National Occupational Standards in Disability Management" (NIDMAR, 1999). This Canadian effort involved the collaboration of labor,

business, workers' compensation boards, insurance carriers, government entities, rehabilitation providers, disability professionals, and other stakeholder groups. These standards recognize that DM requires an understanding of many complex issues that span the following: accident/injury prevention, injury/illness knowledge, labor relations, benefit structures, economics, labor contracts, information management, service delivery, and conflict resolution. NIDMAR's standards are critical of current DM efforts that fail to take into account non-medical disability management factors in the workplace. For post-acute conditions, the workplace is considered the therapeutic environment of choice rather than the clinical setting, which tends to focus on medically based issues. NIDMAR standards are equally critical of labor's and management's abdication of responsibility for DM, which historically has involved relinquishment of control and responsibility to insurance companies, claims managers, workers' compensation boards, physicians, rehabilitation professionals, case managers, and others.

There are several causes for delayed rehabilitation, including the sheer size and complexity of the American health care system, managed care "gatekeepers," and fragmentation of services. Table 7–3 contains a more extensive listing of delayed rehabilitation causes. A legal tort system that rewards injured persons based on the extent and duration of injury or illness is clearly a disincentive for a referral to efficacious rehabilitation.

Neglected Disability and Early Intervention

It is a longstanding dictum in the rehabilitation profession that "to delay rehabilitation is to compromise rehabilitation" (Galvin, 1986; Hood & Downs, 1985; National Council on Compensation Insurance [NCCI], 1989). An NCCI study (NCCI, 1989) of 624 rehabilitation cases in the Michigan workers' compensation system demonstrated that 60% of

Table 7–3 Causes of Delayed Rehabilitation

- Managed care's emphasis on primary care and non-referral to specialists (e.g., rehabilitation)
- Overuse of palliative modalities
- Litigation
- Reimbursement structures (e.g., workers' compensation, full medical, indemnity)
- Non-availability of modified, transitional, or light duty positions
- Health benefits reduction specific to rehabilitation
- Uninsured/underinsured population
- Primary care physicians' poor understanding of rehabilitation's role and offerings
- Rehabilitation sector's poor job of producing and disseminating outcomes data
- Increased financial burden on patients (e.g., higher co-payments, higher deductibles)
- Incomplete or poor diagnostic workups
- "Dueling doctors" with opposing viewpoints (e.g., company doctor versus plaintiff doctor)
- Aggressive competition from alternative caregivers
- Biomedical focus on pathological conditions and impairments instead of disability issues
- Erroneous assumptions (e.g., "It will get better on its own.")
- Passivity of individuals and the principle of least effort
- Presence of psychosocial elements
- Patients' lack of understanding or distrust of health care system
- Failure of other interventions (e.g., surgery, medication, chiropractic, nerve blocks)

injured workers referred in the first 90 days after injury returned to work, whereas only 29% of those referred after two years did so.

Neglected disability has been recognized for decades as disability that is permitted to persist and worsen until multiple physical, psychological, and/or social problems complicate the initial disability (Akabas et al, 1979). The results of delayed rehabilitation or neglected disability, including high costs and poor functional outcomes (e.g., RTW rates), are well documented (Dereberg & Tullis, 1983; NCCI, 1989; Taylor et al, 1994). A neglected disability involves one of the following: delayed rehabilitation, application of palliative modalities only, medical care without a focus on worksite demands, absence of modified or transitional duty, and a failure to address various psychosocial elements of a case.

Early intervention is associated with successful rehabilitation outcomes, diminished severity, lower costs, and decreased reinjury or recidivism rates (Davis, 1983; Galvin, 1986; Niemeyer et al, 1994; Pati, 1985).

Early intervention programs can potentially minimize or eliminate non-medical obstacles to recovery. Earlier intervention can be accomplished through a number of mechanisms, including the following:

- Use of rehabilitation specialists (e.g., physical and occupational therapists in a triage capacity). Direct access in physical therapy is now available in a majority of states. Physical therapists are trained to screen patients and to recognize when to refer them elsewhere, if necessary. Direct access should significantly reduce the delay built into the current system, especially for patients with musculoskeletal conditions, which are rarely life threatening events. Currently, a patient is examined by a primary care physician, then is referred to a specialist,

typically an orthopedist who then makes a referral for therapy. By the time this process plays itself out, a chronic condition can result. Chronic conditions are virtually synonymous with psychosocial issues.

- It is critical to educate primary care physicians (PCPs) concerning the value of rehabilitation and most notably, clinical outcome measures expressed in functional terms.
- Involvement of therapists as preferred providers on workers' compensation panels would facilitate earlier referral for rehabilitation *before* the onset of many psychosocial variables.
- Participation in injury and illness prevention programs, wellness centers, and ergonomic committees as required by the Occupational Safety and Health Administration and some state workers' compensation laws.

Chapter 27 explores these and other areas in greater detail.

Effect of Litigation on Disability Management

The definition of *disability* is derived from two primary sources: the medical and the legal communities. There is often divergence of opinion regarding the presence and degree of disability among individual patients. For example, a PCP may focus on a pathological condition or impairment and equate it to disability. The rehabilitation specialist may focus on functionality as a determinant of disability and may possess a different view of a patient's disability status. In the legal context, a plaintiff attorney representing his or her client may loosely apply the label of "disability" to seek a higher disability payment. These generalizations may or may not be with merit; however, there is some evidence to support the aforementioned tendencies. Plaintiff or patient-secured attorneys may project a worst-case scenario: to project permanent disability and to minimize the value of rehabilitation potential (Kennedy, 1997).

The defense attorney (who represents the employer and/or insurer) may minimize the effect of disability. This is especially true in workers' compensation systems, which, unlike other health care environments, are legal, not medical, systems. Some have suggested that in workers' compensation, essentially, the claimant expert exaggerates, whereas the defense expert understates disability (Boden, 1987). Studies strongly suggest that litigation has a direct effect on the assessment of disability and rehabilitation outcomes (Blake & Garrett, 1997; NCCI, 1989).

One study of particular interest demonstrated that two groups (one without litigation, the other with litigation) shared significant improvements in measures of impairment (e.g., lumbar flexibility, trunk muscle endurance, pain) and disability (e.g., exercise, fitness) (Blake & Garrett, 1997). However, the participants in the litigation group scored themselves higher in terms of handicap (using the Sickness Impact Profile, which defines the impact of the condition on the patient's quality of life). A perception of disability can directly affect clinical outcomes, specifically, return-to-work rates. RTW rates are consistently higher for non-litigation cases than for those with litigation (Frederickson, 1988; NCCI, 1989).

A confounding dichotomy results when providers interact with lawyers and litigation. The provider's role is to support full recovery, whereas the plaintiff attorney's role may be to project a worst-case scenario of permanent disability and an ultimate lack of rehabilitation potential, to maximize a financial verdict (Kennedy, 1997). The employer or insurance company attorney may desire an earlier RTW than the provider deems judicious. However, readers should understand that these statements are generalizations only and that each medicolegal case has its own unique characteristics.

Rehabilitation Providers

These competing influences often compound the challenge of functional restoration, because the "legal client" may portray a disability in one manner, whereas the "medical patient" may portray it in another manner. In effect, the goals of rehabilitation and those of the legal system can be at odds. Thus what may have begun as a manageable problem now becomes an investment in "permanent disability, and the slide down the slippery slope of a lifetime disability" (Kennedy, 1997).

Joint Labor-Management Empowerment

The American health care system is principally an employer-driven system. Employers finance more than 82% of total health care (American Management Association, 1995). Employee-employer relationships can substantially affect the success of a rehabilitation or disability management program (Shrey & Lacerte, 1995). Employers' attitudes toward their workers can have a profound effect on the cost, prevalence, and severity of disability in the workforce. Team-based organizations are more likely to offer support of employees' psychosocial needs than are "line n' staff" hierarchical organizations (Breton & Largent, 1996). A line n' staff model tends to be hierarchal with one layer reporting to and, in many cases, taking marching orders from another management level. Line n' staff organizations consider titles to be very important. Ideas and innovations are generally passed downward in these organizations. Those in the upper echelon of management are expected to be the visionaries who provide directives to their underlings. Team-based organizations tend to be ego-less as they fully encourage innovation at every level and do not place a premium on titles.

Rehabilitation providers have three principal means of gauging employers' attitudes regarding disability prevention and management: through employers directly, through intermediaries (e.g., managed care organizations), or via their patients or injured workers. Providers who manage workers' compensation injuries enjoy relatively greater direct access to employers than do those serving managed care beneficiaries. In either case, it is essential that providers understand the corporate culture in which the injured party worked. Corporations assume or create a corporate identity or culture that has direct bearing on how injured workers are managed or mismanaged.

Many psychosocial variables can be managed through joint empowerment of labor and management, provided certain obstacles can be overcome (NIDMR, 1999;

Mills, 1995; Shrey & Lacerte, 1995). A "culture-work-health" model of interdependency prevails in American industry (Peterson & Wilson, 1998). This model is based on a belief that the culture employees bring to the company, as well as the culture created by the company, provides a context in which issues of control and helplessness affect individuals and the corporation. There may be subcultures within the same employer, according to occupational categories. Workers from different occupational categories may not understand each other or may have cross-purposes. For instance, the medical department may have a different agenda than does the human resources department. This essentially means that employers rarely have interdepartmental consensus on how disability should be managed. Dysfunctional organizations create environments that invite or foster disability through depersonalization of workers and oppressive tactics (Brotherton, 1991). These corporations share the following attributes: They provide few opportunities for advancement, offer a minimum of information, place profits over people, possess poor communications, and fail to view workers as their greatest assets. These companies allow the costs associated with a failure to prevent or to manage disability and may present providers with great obstacles in the design, implementation, and outcomes of rehabilitation programs. For example, these corporations may not be receptive to transitional or modified duty programs, ergonomic analysis, or reasonable accommodations that may effect a safe and/or earlier RTW.

An escalation in merger and acquisition activity occurred in the 1990s, which was of unparalleled magnitude. During this period, even those companies that attempted to balance economic interests with humanitarian concern became victims of poor management. According to a study conducted by the American Management Association and Cigna Corporation, many employers learned that the money saved from downsizing their staff was soon offset by higher disability rates and costs (Anonymous, 1997) (Table 7-4).

Companies that fail to address employees' attainment of psychosocial needs experience increases in health claims (Eisenstat & Felner, 1984; Ilgen, 1990; James, 1992). Employers with disability management policies that demonstrate concern for their employees are associated with more favorable outcomes (Hunt & Habek, 1993). These organizations seek to understand the

 Table 7-4 Environmental Factors Versus Behavioral Factors

Environmental Factors	Behavioral Factors
Workload	Co-worker relations
Role ambiguity	Degree of worker control/autonomy
Unsafe worksite	Unsafe behaviors
Task repetition	Individual values and beliefs
Benefit structures	Motivational levels
Organization structure	Skill, knowledge, and aptitude
Communication systems	Communication styles
Employee performance measures	Worker attitudes

Data from Shrey DE, Lacerte M (eds): Principles and Practices of Disability Management in Industry. Winter Park, FL, GR Press, 1995.

physical and psychosocial reasons for disability and demonstrate a top-down approach. They have commitment from upper management and first-line supervisors. Their lines of communication are well established, and they engage in a constructive, not a punitive, mode of problem identification and solution. Some companies form disability management teams that comprise both management and workers (Cotter & Williams, 1997).

In general, larger employers have disability management strategies that foster collaborative employee-employer relationships that are more difficult to achieve in smaller organizations (Cheadle et al, 1994). Smaller companies commonly lack the flexibility of larger companies in terms of accommodating disabled workers through modified duty or reasonable accommodations (Table 7–5).

A complex "push-pull" system exists at some companies relative to employee placement after injury (Krute & Treital, 1981). From one viewpoint, the system pushes disabled persons out of employment partly due to a lack of job accommodations. A counterforce may be simultaneously in effect by "pulling" the employee back to work, often prematurely before they are ready or without reasonable accommodation. This push-pull phenomenon is best exemplified by the tension between the medical and human resources departments in larger companies.

Medical units typically want an injured employee to RTW as quickly as possible. To facilitate an RTW, physicians may place various "restrictions" on the worker's activities (e.g., the employee cannot lift more than 50 pounds or sit longer than 30 minutes). Conversely, the human resources director may not want an injured employee to RTW until he or she is 100%; otherwise, reasonable accommodations must be considered under the ADA. For human resources directors in unionized situations, a medical department's insistence on RTW presents a conundrum because of a number of factors including: seniority, collective bargaining issues, and balancing "Maximum Medical Improvement" (MMI) with ADA compliance. MMI describes an injured person when his or her condition has stabilized and treatment has achieved its optimum effect or has reached the level that constitutes maintenance care. MMI does not describe a person's functional abilities or candidacy

for RTW. In fact, it may be specious to equate MMI with RTW status.

In general, employers who are sensitive to the needs of injured workers are more successful in disability management. For example, employers who have a job reserved for the injured employee enhance the likelihood of RTW (Moffroid et al, 1993; Wilson et al, 1994). Workers who have job attachment to the preaccident employer have a more than 200% greater chance of RTW than do those who require post-rehabilitation job search assistance (Voaklander et al, 1995).

Conversely, employers who are perceived to be less than caring or even callused toward their workers as compared with "responsible employers" incur poor rehabilitation results. Employees who rate their supervisors poorly are less likely to RTW in a timely manner (Bigos et al, 1986). This has proven to be one of the more predictive psychosocial variables in the clinical literature. Employability can align employer, employee, and provider interests if parties co-establish treatment goals and posttreatment management. Designing reasonable accommodations that facilitate a safe but expeditious RTW may satisfy the needs of those involved. According to the Job Accommodation Network (JAN), 50% of reasonable accommodations cost less than $50, whereas an additional 20% of reasonable accommodations cost less than $500 (Miller, 1996; JAN, 2003). The alternative, a non-working employee, is more costly by comparison. The estimated cost to a company for one missed workday is $13,000 in lost productivity alone (Matthes, 1992).

Providers are encouraged to explore opportunities to interact with labor organizations and unions. This must begin by first understanding how organized labor operates. In unionized companies, employee benefit schemes are often negotiated through a collective bargaining process. Providers need to understand the scope of these benefits, especially as they relate to RTW programs. Unfortunately, labor organizations, like employers, can impede a disability management plan. Labor organizations that encourage their members to consume full health benefits (e.g., indemnity benefits, lost wage replacement) provide disincentives to rehabilitation program compliance (Mills, 1995). Employees may view indemnity benefits as an entitlement of guaranteed financial security rather than as a temporary bridge between disability and a RTW. Figure 7–4 depicts an injured employee between the health care team and employer team. The term *team* implies a unified approach to disability management; however, this may not be the case. Each team member may possess a different view of his or her role, the appropriate intervention, and worker expectations. A collaborative model of disability management demands a partnership between all members of the health care team and employer team. This requires shared goals, clear communication, and a commitment to serve the needs of injured parties rather than the teams' own needs. This is a challenge because of different, and perhaps opposite, views of the injured worker. Rehabilitation providers may refer to the injured worker as their "client." This implies that the provider serves the client. Employers may view the injured worker as one who serves their needs, a completely opposite paradigm (Table 7–6).

 Table 7–5 Employer-Related Obstacles to Disability Management

- Failure to accommodate work environment
- Employer ignorance, prejudices, and perceptions concerning persons with disabilities
- Absence of or poor vocational rehabilitation and counseling
- Union or labor organization policies
- Job dissatisfaction
- First-line supervisor attitudes
- Lack of modified, transitional, or light duty position
- Interdepartmental tension
- Managed care intrusiveness in the employer-employee relationship
- Failure of providers to communicate directly with employers
- Non-alignment of goals between employee, employer, provider, and managed care organization

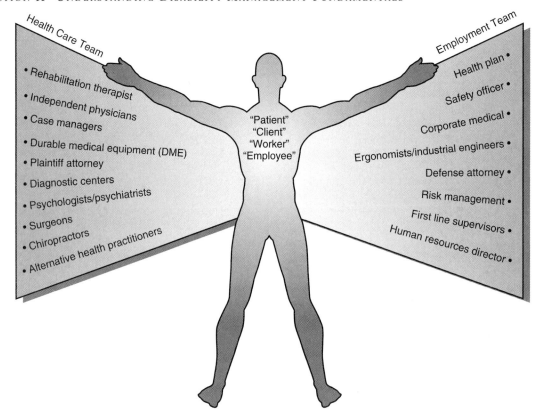

Figure 7–4. Health care team and employer team: Friend or foe.

The Employee's Perspective

A constellation of non-medical factors accounts for why some patients or workers respond to disability management better than others. Patients with similar or identical conditions can have dramatically different functional outcomes. This partially accounts for why the application of standardized treatment guidelines is so challenging. Although diagnostic frameworks and case definitions can be standardized, psychosocial factors are less amenable to standardized measures.

Some pioneering researchers have packaged psychosocial factors into assessment instruments that provide some degree of utility (Hester & Decelles, 1986). Despite these attempts, this area of disability management requires research that is much more dedicated.

 Table 7–6 Most Common Strategies Used by Employers to Facilitate Return-to-Work

Strategy	Percentage of Employers Using Strategy
Redesign of job station	27%
Sensitization of supervisors	18%
Sensitization of employees	19%
Adaptation of training	16%
Installation of ramp or elevating devices	5%
Use of interpreter	4%

Data from Westmorland MG, Pennock M: What prevents people with disabilities from obtaining employment? An examination of Canadian data from a national and regional perspective. WORK 5(4):255-263, 1995.

Multivariate analyses have yielded some interesting relationships that may be of use to the rehabilitation provider. For example, workers with longer disability periods shared the following non-medical attributes (Galizzi & Boden, 1996):

1. Short job tenure (less than 6 months)
2. Recent periods of unemployment
3. Switched employers preinjury and postinjury
4. Employed by smaller employers
5. Attorney presence

Numerous factors, including occupation, education, work-related demands, and the presence of chronic diseases, have been correlated to varying disability levels (Astrand, 1987; Bigos et al, 1992; Frederickson et al, 1988; Kearney, 1997; Moffroid et al, 1993; Williams et al, 1998; Wilson et al, 1994). Psychosocial factors have been found to be predictive of success or failure in response to a conservative functional restorative program (Polatin et al, 1989). Findings have included the following:

1. Lower initial self-report of pain intensity correlates with a higher degree of successful outcome.
2. Self-report of depression (Beck Depression Inventory) is predictive of success or failure.
3. Physical rehabilitation efforts are most effective in the absence of major psychological overlay.
4. Increased preinjury employment time increases the likelihood of successful rehabilitation.
5. Multiple surgeries correlate with poor rehabilitation results.

An individual's motivational level and degree of program compliance has been correlated with rehabilitation outcomes by numerous researchers over the years (DiFabio et al, 1995; Mayer et al, 1987; Reilly et al, 1989). These data are valuable for rehabilitation providers who wish to design and implement restorative programs that look beyond clinical presentation and take into account non-biophysical factors.

PROVIDER'S PERSPECTIVE

Providers of disability management services should be cognizant of variables associated with disability amelioration or a lack of such variable. For instance, abnormal illness behavior is one of the most challenging obstacles confronting rehabilitation providers. Unlike many medical interventions, restorative programs demand a fully active patient who is compliant with his or her program and is highly motivated. However, this is often not the case when dealing with chronic illnesses and injuries, multiple traumas, or psychosocial elements superimposed over physical impairments and disabilities. Legions of studies have noted that a significant percentage of patients have abnormal or disruptive responses to common afflictions (Burton et al, 1995; DiFabio et al, 1995; Henderson, 1987; Matheson, 1988; Mayer et al, 1987; Polatin, 1989; Reilly et al, 1989; Taylor & Bonfiglio, 1992; Waddell et al, 1980). Therefore psychosocial evaluations are useful adjuncts to physical rehabilitation in identifying those complications and contributing factors specific to preexisting personality traits, traumatic neuroses, secondary gain issues, symptom magnification or minimization, and malingering behaviors (Killian, 1988). Clinical depression and escape and avoidance behaviors are associated with persons suffering from reported high levels of pain (McCracken et al, 1998). Patient educational levels have been shown to have a high correlation to propensity for recovery (Schechter, 1997). Table 7–3 (see p. 111) provides a brief summary of several variables associated with rehabilitation outcomes. Job satisfaction is one of the most predictive variables of who returns to work and who does not (Bigos et al, 1992; Niemcryck et al, 1987; Williams et al, 1998).

Employment duration has a correlation to disability disposition (Astrand, 1987; Galizzi & Boden, 1996; Kelsey et al, 1979). A plethora of literature examines the role of patient-family dynamics in disability management (Altman et al, 1999; Block, 1981; Gil et al, 1987; Lipton & Marbach, 1984; Newby, 1996). Providers, to be effective, must examine the entire family unit (particularly with regard to support structures) to more fully understand the nature of disability and its likely prognosis.

Likewise, employers need to understand program parameters and how these parameters may be perceived by certain employee populations (Alvarez & Lambert, 1997). Language and communication are frequently overlooked barriers to successful disability management. Language barriers threaten the provider-patient communication model and can have a disastrous effect on who develops disability. It is estimated that by 2050, one in five persons in the United States will be of Hispanic descent (Ruiz, 1996). The need for bilingual rehabilitation providers is certain to grow in concordance with these data. Speaking a patient's language means more than just understanding the spoken tongue. It means understanding what his or her motivating factors are and how to modify aberrant behavior.

Selected literature describes the relationship between disability and financial gain, especially under government programs, workers' compensation, and disability insurance (Frueh et al, 1997; Rainville et al, 1997). Patients who remain "disabled" for monetary reasons require different skill sets that may go beyond clinical competency.

Patient behaviors may be influenced by drug and substance abuse, both in and out of the workplace. This represents another example of a variable that can have a greater effect on disability than the original injury or illness itself. This issue presents an extreme challenge to rehabilitation providers, because substance abuse crosses every socioeconomic, educational, ethnic, racial, and age threshold. This pervasiveness offers enormous challenges to the rehabilitation provider in terms of problem and resource identification. The problem is magnified, because it can involve the abuse of both illicit and prescription drugs for chronic pain. It is estimated that at least 10% of all American workers are addicted to drugs or alcohol (Wrich, 1988). Another 10% to 15% of workers have a family member who is addicted. Substance abuse is only one illustration that health maintenance and disability management are products of a complex array of failures, many of which fall outside the traditional province of health care (Pope & Tarlov, 1991).

Skilled clinical interviews are essential in establishing a focus on disability rather than pain alone. Regrettably, a great deal of rehabilitation clinical documentation dwells on pain. Providers, to be effective disability managers, must look beyond signs and symptoms and even beyond the patients themselves. This may require de-medicalization of problems that contribute to the development of disability. Patient profiles that are more comprehensive and that incorporate the biomedical and social models are also needed. These models can be combined only by providers reaching out to employers, even when HMOs serve as intermediaries. Providers must educate employers about real versus perceived barriers to gainful employment. First and foremost, employer perceptions that employees who are disabled cannot be productive must be obliterated. A new paradigm that focuses on returning the worker to gainful employment must supplant a patient-focused disability management plan. For example, employers may require education concerning reasonable accommodations as not only the right thing to do, but the financially prudent approach as well.

Providers may also wish to learn more about corporate structure to more fully understand how to engage both the employee and his or her employer in productive behaviors. Rehabilitation providers may serve as a vital link in this capacity. Serving in an intermediary role can help close the gap between the tip of the organizational pyramid (upper management) and the base (employees) (Semler, 1989). Rehabilitation providers can be especially helpful to employers by teaching them how to effectively prevent illness and injury, skills essential to managing an aging workforce.

Readers are advised to read Chapter 3 for an in-depth discussion of specific disability management strategies.

Rehabilitation Provider Recommendations

To ensure successful rehabilitation and disability management, each stakeholder in the health care process must gain something that he or she values. This principle can be easily forsaken when parties view the disability recovery process through their own prism without consideration of the myriad of issues commonly found in physical rehabilitation cases.

- Make frequent onsite visits to employer sites
- Offer to provide "brown bag" lunch presentations to claims adjusters, case managers, and attorneys regarding the value of rehabilitation and its role in disability management
- Meet with organized labor officials to ascertain their members' concerns
- Co-develop transitional or modified duty programs along with other reasonable accommodations
- Attend conferences and educational programs presented by other stakeholders, especially employers since it is they who finance over eighty percent of health care
- Revise clinical evaluation forms to reflect the importance of collecting non-biophysical or psychosocial data
- Read literature produced by other stakeholder groups, especially employers, insurers, case managers, vocational counselors, disability managers, and employee benefit managers
- Facilitate focus-group sessions or colloquia that are interdisciplinary
- Participate in collaborative rehabilitation programs
- Learn a second language and be mindful of cultural differences in response to disability

This chapter has addressed a relatively small sampling of variables that can serve as obstacles to disability management. Rehabilitation programs, to be effective in addressing the myriad of confounding obstacles, must incorporate worksite-based disability management, not simply clinical "treatment" (Brooker, 2000).

Disability Management Benefits

A comprehensive DM program offers benefits that transcend the individual worker or patient. These include:

- Retention of qualified, trained workers
- Reduction in the human cost of disability
- Enhancement of worker involvement in RTW planning
- Illness and injury reduction (e.g., prevalence and cost)
- Decreased incidence of accidents and severity of disability
- Promotion of prevention, early intervention and optimal health outcomes
- Reduction of work disruptions and unnecessary lost-time
- Maximization of employer resources
- Facilitation workplace (versus clinic-based) control of disability issues
- Enhancement of employee morale
- Reduction in the adversarial nature of disability and litigation
- Increased corporate competitiveness and financial solvency
- Coordination in the management of external service providers

Disability is a functional concept, hence providers should focus on a patient's abilities rather than his or her disabilities. Placing an emphasis on pain alone can lead to prolonged inactivity and reinforcement of the "sick role" and ultimately enable disability (Waddell 1986). Margoshes (1998) provides the following basic principles that will assist providers in facilitating full functionality and productive work.

- Prevent exacerbation and aggravation
- Focus on functional ability, not pain
- Establish realistic goals and RTW expectations
- Identify functional limitations and abilities
- Assess medical and psychosocial disability factors
- Communicate effectively with all parties
- Consider vocational rehabilitation when indicated
- Practice recurrence management

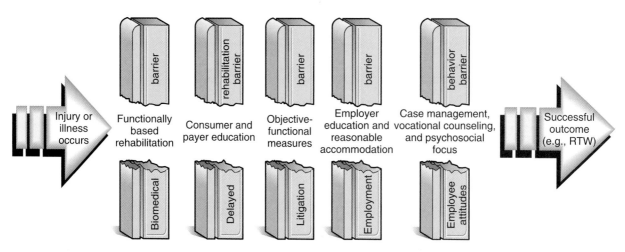

Figure 7–5. Barriers to successful physical rehabilitation and disability management.

Rehabilitation professionals who offer work conditioning, work hardening, functional job analysis, ergonomics, modified duty or transitional work design, reasonable accommodation, case management, employee and employer education, and prevention programs will be well-positioned to take the lead in tomorrow's disability management of both occupationally based and non-occupationally based disability.

These programs will be substantially geared for an aging population for the foreseeable future (Sommerfield, 1978; Anonymous, 2002). In doing so, stakeholders must delicately balance "a curious mixture of humanitarian concern and economic rationality" in a "community context" (Clifton, 1992) (Figure 7–5). When this balance is achieved, the aforementioned benefits can result for employers and employees and solidify rehabilitation's role in the future (NIDMAR, 1999).

REFERENCES

Akabas SH, Gottlieb A, Yasser R: Preventive rehabilitation: Untapped horizon for vocational rehabilitation. Am Rehabil 5(2):20-24, 1979.

Alaranta H, Rytokoski U, Rissanen A et al: Intensive physical and psychosocial training program for patients with chronic low back pain. A controlled clinical trial. Spine 19:1339-1349, 1994.

Altman BM, Cooper PF, Cunningham PJ: The case of disability in the family: Impact on health care utilization and expenditures for nondisabled members. Milbank Q 77(1):39-75, 1999.

Alvarez M, Lambert J: The impact of cultural differences on disability management programs. Employment Relations Today 23(4):37-49, 1997.

American Management Association: Employer-Provided Health Care: Options, Costs and Quality. Survey in cooperation with Fortis, Inc. New York, American Management Association, 1995.

Anonymous: Downsizing and disability go together. Business & Health 15:10, 1997.

Anonymous: Employers face health and safety concerns for older workers. Human Resource Focus (HR Focus) 79(7):S2-S3, 2002.

Anthony WA: Characteristics of people with psychiatric disabilities that are predictive of entry into the rehabilitation process and successful employment. Psychosocial Rehabil J 17(3):3-13, 1994.

Aronoff GM Feldman JB, Campion TS: Management of chronic pain and control of long-term disability. Occup Med 15(4):755-770, 2000.

Astrand N: Medical, psychological and social factors associated with back abnormalities and self-reported back pain. Br J Med 44: 327-336, 1987.

Battie MC, Bigos SJ, Fisher D et al: The role of spinal flexibility in back pain complaint in industry: A prospective study. Spine 15: 768-773, 1990.

Beger CS: The importance of subjective claims management. Benefits Q 13(4):41-45, 1997.

Bendix AF, Bendix T, Ostenfeld S et al: Active treatment programs for patients with chronic low back pain: A prospective randomized, observer-blinded study. Eur Spine J 4:148-152, 1995.

Berkowitz M: Work disincentives and rehabilitation. National Rehabilitation Information Center (NARIC) Publication No 02673. Falls Church, VA, Institute for Information Studies, 1980.

Better SR: Overcoming Disincentives to the Rehabilitation of SSI and SSDI Beneficiaries. Monograph #5, NARIC Publication No 50114. Birmingham, AL, Union of Alabama Medical Rehabilitation Research and Training Center, 1979, p 141.

Biering-Sorensen F: Physical measurement as risk indicators for low-back trouble over one-year period. Spine 9:106-119, 1984.

Bigos S, Battie M, Spengler DM et al: A longitudinal prospective study of industrial back injury reporting. Clin Orthop 279:21-34, 1992.

Bigos SJ, Battie MC, Spengler DM: A prospective study of work perceptions and psychological factors affecting the report of back injury. Spine 16(1):1-6, 1991.

Bigos S, Spengler D, Martin N et al: Back injuries in industry: A retrospective study. Part III: Employee related factors. Spine J 11: 252-256, 1986.

Blake C, Garrett M: Impact of litigation on quality of life outcomes in patients with chronic low back pain. Irish J Med Sci 166(3):124-126, 1997.

Block AR, Kremer EF, Gaylor M: Behavioral treatment of chronic pain: The spouse as a discriminative cue for pain. Pain J 9(2):243-252, 1980.

Block AR: An investigation of the response of the spouse to chronic pain behavior. Psychosom Med 43:415-422, 1981.

Boden L: Use of Medical Evidence: Low-Back Permanent Partial Disability Claims in New Jersey. Cambridge, MA, Workers' Compensation Research Institute (WCRI), WC-87-2, 1987.

Bongers PM, de Winter CR, Kompier MA et al: Psychological factors at work and musculoskeletal disease. Scand J Work Environ Health 19:297-312, 1993.

Brand RA, Lehmann TR: Low-back impairment ratings of orthopaedic surgeons. Spine 8(1):75-78, 1983.

Braverman B: The model of human occupation and prediction at work: Review of related empirical research. WORK 12:25-35, 1999.

Breton D, Largent C: The Paradigm Conspiracy. Center City, MN, Hazelton, 1996.

Brodwin MG: Medical, Psychosocial and Vocational Aspects of Disability. Athens, GA, Elliott and Fitzpatrick, 1993.

Brooker AS, Clarke J, Sinclair S et al: Effective disability management and return-to-work practices. In Sullivan T (ed): Injury and the New World of Work. Vancouver, UBC Press, 2000.

Brotherton C: The onward march of the neurotic organization. Work and Stress 5(2):71-76, 1991.

Brown CD, Woodard D, McDaniel RS: Differences in workers' compensation settlements using vocational or medical impairment ratings. Natl Assn Rehab Professionals in Private Sector (NARPPS) Dec:239-243, 1991.

Burton AK, Tillotson KM, Main CJ et al: Psychosocial predictors of outcome in acute and subacute low back trouble. Spine 20(2):722-728, 1995.

Cahill J: Psychological aspects of intervention in occupational health. Am J Ind Med 29:308-313, 1996.

Carpenter ES: Roadblocks to rehabilitation. Business & Health 3(2): 22-24, 1985.

Cheadle A, Franklin G, Wolhagen C et al: Factors influencing the duration of work-related disability: A population-based study of Washington state workers' compensation. Am J Public Health 84:190-196, 1994.

Cleary L, Thombs DL, Daniel EL: Occupational low back disability: Effective strategies for reducing lost work time. Am Assn Occup Health Nurses (AAOHN) J 43:87-94, 1995.

Clifton DW: Critical issues for determining successful work hardening outcomes. Phys Ther Pract 1(3):52-60, 1992.

Cotter D, Williams C: Managing health-related absences. Compensation & Benefits Rev 29(3):58-64, 1997.

Das B, Sengupta AK: Computer-aided human modeling programs for workstation design. Ergonomics 38(9):1958-1972, 1995.

Davis DH: Bridging the claims dollar gap through rehabilitation. Risk Management March:3-8, 1983.

Dereberg VJ, Tullis WH: Delayed recovery in the patient with a work compensable injury. J Occup Med 25(11):829-835, 1983.

Devereux JJ, Buckle PW, Vlachonikolis IG: Interactions between physical and psychosocial risk factors at work increase the risk of back disorders: An epidemiological approach. Occup Environ Med 56: 343-353, 1999.

DiFabio RP, Mackey G, Holte JB: Disability and functional status in patients with low back pain receiving workers' compensation. A described study with implication for the efficacy of physical therapy. Phys Ther 75:180-193, 1995.

Eaton MW: Obstacles to vocational rehabilitation of individuals receiving workers' compensation. J Rehabil 45(2):59-63, 1979.

Eisenstat R, Felner R: Toward a differential view of burnout: Personal and organizational mediators of job satisfaction and stress. Am J Community Psychol 12(4):411-430, 1984.

Ensalada LH: The importance of illness behavior in disability management. Occup Med 15(4):739-754, 2000.

Fathallah FA et al: The role of psychosocial factors in occupational musculoskeletal disorders. In Proceedings of the Human Factors and Ergonomics Society 40th Annual Meeting, Philadelphia, September 2-6, 1996.

Fitzgerald TE: Psychosocial aspects of work-related musculoskeletal disability. In Quick JC, Murphy LR, Hurrell JJ (eds): Stress and Well-Being at Work. Washington, DC, American Psychological Association, 1992.

Fowler DR, Mayfield DG: Effect of disability compensation. Arch Environ Health 19(5):719-725, 1969.

Froom P, Melamed S, Nativ T et al: Low job satisfaction predicts delayed return to work after laparoscopic cholecystectomy. J Occup Environ Med 43(7):657-662, 2001.

Frueh BC, Gold PB, de-Arellano MA: Symptom overreporting in combat veterans evaluated for PTSD: Differentiation on the basis of compensation seeking status. J Personality Assessment 68(2):369-384, 1997.

Galizzi M, Boden LI: What Are the Most Important Factors Shaping Return to Work? Evidence from Wisconsin. Cambridge, MA, Workers' Compensation Research Institute, 1996.

Galvin DE: Employer-based Disability Management and Rehabilitation Initiatives. A Rehabilitation Research Review. NARC National Institute of Handicapped Research. Washington, DC, US Department of Education, 1986.

Gard G, Sandberg AC: Motivating factors for return to work. Physiother Res Int 3(2):100-108, 1998.

Gates LB, Yecheskel T, Akabas SH: Optimizing return to work among newly disabled workers: A new approach toward cost containment. Benefits Q 5(2);19-27, 1989.

Gil KM, Keefe FJ, Crisson JE et al: Social support and pain behavior. Pain 29(2):209-217, 1987.

Goswami A: Anthropometry of people with disability. In Kumar S (ed): Perspectives in Rehabilitation Ergonomics. Bristol, PA, Taylor & Francis, 1997.

Hall JA, Dornan M: Meta-analysis of satisfaction with medical care: Description of research domain and analysis of overall satisfaction level. Soc Sci Med 30:811-818, 1990.

Hammonds W, Brena SF, Unikel IP: Compensation for work related injuries and rehabilitation of patients with chronic pain. Southern Med J 71(6):646-666, 1978.

Hazard RG, Fenwick JW, Kalisch SM: Functional restoration with behavioral support. Spine 14:157-161, 1989.

Henderson AS: The etiology of abnormal illness behavior. Psychiatr Med 5(1):25-28, 1987.

Hester EJ, Decelles P: Predicting Which Disabled Employees Will Return to Work: The Menninger RTW Scale. Topeka, KS, The Menninger Foundation Rehabilitation Research and Training Center on Preventing Disability Dependence, 1986.

Hood LE, Downs JD: Return to work: A literature review. Topeka, KS, The Menninger Foundation, 1985.

Hunt A, Habek R: The Michigan Disability Prevention Study. Kalamazoo, MI, W.E. Upjohn Institute for Employment Research, 1993.

Ilgen D: Health issues at work: Opportunities for individual/organizational psychology. Am Psychol 45(2):273-283, 1990.

James L: Psychological climate and affect: A test of a hierarchical dynamic model. In Cranny CJ, Smith PC, Stone EF (eds): Job Satisfaction: How People Feel About Their Jobs and How It Affects Their Performance. New York, Lexington Books, 1992.

Jarosz E: Determination of the workspace of wheelchair users. Int J Indust Ergo 17:123-133, 1996.

Job Accommodation Network (JAN), www.jan.wvu.edu/media/CTD.html, accessed November 17, 2003.

Karjalainen K, Malmivaara A, van Tulder M et al: Multidisciplinary biopsychological rehabilitation of subacute low back pain in working-age adults: A systematic review within the framework of the Cochrane Collaboration Back Review Group. Spine 26(3):262-269, 2001.

Kearney JR: The work incapacity and reintegration study: Results of the initial survey conducted in the United States. Soc Secur Bull 60(3):21-32, 1997.

Keith RA: Patient satisfaction and rehabilitation services. Arch Phys Med Rehabil 79:1122-1128, 1998.

Kelsey J, White A III, Pastides H et al: The impact of musculoskeletal disorders on the population of the United States. J Bone Joint Surg 61A:959-964, 1979.

Kennedy WA: Permanent disability: The legacy of tort litigation. Clin Orthop 336:67-71, 1997.

Killian L: Psychological barriers to recovery in work injury. In Isernhagen S (ed): Work Injury: Management and Prevention, 2nd ed. Gaithersburg, MD, Aspen, 1988.

Krause N, Lynch GA, Cohen RD et al: Predictors of disability retirement. Scand J Work Environ Health 23(6):403-413, 1997.

Krute A, Treital R: Reintegration of the Severely Disabled into the Work Force: United States Experience. Social Security and Disability: Issues and Policy Research, Studies and Research #17. Geneva, International Society Social Security Association, 1981.

Lipton JA, Marbach JJ: Ethnicity and the pain experience. Soc Sci Med 19(12):1279-1298, 1984.

Marinelli RP (ed): The Psychological and Social Impact of Physical Disability. New York, Springer, 1977.

Margoshes B: Disability management and occupational health. Occupational Medicine: State of the Art Reviews 13 (4):693-703, 1998.

Martin ED: Rehabilitation and Disability Case Studies. Springfield, IL, Charles C Thomas, 1990.

Matheson LN: Symptom magnification syndrome. In Isernhagen S (ed): Work Injury: Management and Prevention, 1st ed. Gaithersburg, MD, Aspen, 1988.

Matthes K: Companies have the ability to manage disability. Human Resource Focus 69(4):3, 1992.

Mayer TG, Gatchel RJ, Mayer H et al: A prospective two-year study of functional restoration in industrial low back injury. An objective assessment procedure. JAMA 258:1763-1767, 1987.

McCracken LM, Faber SD, Janeck AS: Pain-related anxiety predicts non-specific physical complaints in persons with chronic pain. Behav Res Ther 36(6):621-630, 1998.

McGill CM: Industrial back problems: A control program. J Occup Med 10:174-178, 1968.

Mellin G: Chronic low back pain in men 54-63 years of age: Correlations of physical measurements with the degree of trouble and progress after treatment. Spine 11:421-426, 1986.

Micek LA, Bitter JA: Service delivery approaches for difficult rehabilitation clients. Rehabil Lit 35(9):258-263, 271, 1974.

Miller M: The ADA offers unique opportunities for physical and occupational therapists. WORK 6(1):47-52, 1996.

Mills D: Building joint labor-management initiatives for worksite disability management. In Shrey DE, Lacerte M (eds): Principles and Practices of Disability Management in Industry. Winter Park, FL, GR Press, 1995, pp 225-243.

Moffroid MT, Aja D, Haugh LD et al: Efficacy of a part-time work hardening program for persons with low-back pain. WORK 3: 14-20, 1993.

Monsein M, Clift RB: Pain and return to work: Turning the corner. In Isernhagen SJ (ed): The Comprehensive Guide to Work Injury Management. Gaithersburg, MD, Aspen, 1995, pp. 543-556.

National Council on Compensation Insurance (NCCI): Making rehabilitation work. 4(4):89-99, Boca Raton, FL, December 1989.

Newby NM: Chronic illness and the family life-cycle. J Adv Nurs 23: 786-791, 1996.

Niemcryck S, Jenkins C, Rose R et al: The prospective impact of psychosocial variables on rates of illness and injury in professional employees. J Occup Med 29:645-652, 1987.

Niemeyer LO, Jacobs K, Reynolds-Lynch K et al: Work hardening: Past, present, and future—The work programs special interest section, national work hardening outcome study. Am J Occup Ther 48:327-339, 1994.

Partridge RE, Duthie JJR: Rheumatism in dockers and civil servants: A comparison of heavy manual and sedentary workers. Ann Rheum Dis 27:559, 1968.

Pati G: Economics of rehabilitation in the work place. J Rehabil 51(4):220-230, 1985.

Peterson M, Wilson J: A culture-work-health model: A theoretical conceptualization. Am J Health Behav 22(5):378-390, 1998.

Polatin P, Gatchel R, Barnes D et al: A psychosociomedical prediction model of response to treatment by chronically disabled workers with low back pain. Spine J 14(9):956-961, 1989.

Polatin PB, Cox B, Gatchel et al: A prospective study of Waddell signs in patients with chronic low back pain. When they may not be predictive. Spine J 22(14):1618-1621, 1997.

Polatin P, Gatchel R, Barnes D et al: A psychosociomedical prediction model of response to treatment by chronically disabled workers with low-back pain. Spine J 14(9):956-961, 1989.

Pope AM, Tarlov AR: Disability in America: Toward a National Agenda for Prevention. Washington, DC, National Academy Press, 1991, p 36.

Proctor T, Gatchel RJ, Robinson RC et al: Psychosocial factors and risk of pain and disability. Occup Med 15(4):803-812, 2000.

Rainville J, Sobel JB, Hartigan C et al: The effect of compensation involvement on the reporting of pain and disability by patients referred for rehabilitation of chronic low back pain. Spine 22(17): 2016-2024, 1997.

Reilly K, Lovejoy B, Williams R: Differences between a supervised and independent strength and conditioning program with chronic low back syndromes. J Occup Med 31:547-550, 1989.

Ruiz I: Recommendations for working with interpreters. WORK 6(1): 41-46, 1996.

Rutman I: How psychiatric disability expresses itself as a barrier to employment. Psychosocial Rehabil J 17(3):15-36, 1994.

Sanders SH: Risk factors for chronic, disabling low-back pain: An update for 2000. Am Pain Soc Bull 10(2):, March/April 2000, www.ampainsoc.org/pub/bulletin/mar00/clin1.htm, accessed January 28, 2002.

Sauter SL, Murphy LR, Hurrell JJ: Prevention of work-related psychological disorders: A national strategy proposed by the National Institute for Occupational Safety and Health (NIOSH). Am Psychol 45(10):1146-1158, 1990.

Schechter ES: Work while receiving disability insurance benefits: Additional findings from the New Beneficiary Followup Survey. Soc Secur Bull 60(1):3-17, 1997.

Semler R: Managing without managers. Harvard Bus Rev 89(5): 76-89, 1989.

Shrey DE, Lacerte M (eds): Principles and Practices of Disability Management in Industry. Winter Park, FL, GR Press, 1995.

Sommerfield J: Dealing with the aging workforce. Harvard Bus Rev 56(6):81-92, 1978.

Spratt KF, Lehmann TR, Weinstein JN et al: A new approach to low back examination: Behavioral assessment of mechanical signs. Spine 15:96-102, 1990.

Tan V, Cheatle MD, Mackin S et al: Goal setting as a predictor of return-to-work in a population of chronic musculoskeletal pain patients. Int J Neurosci 92(3-4):161-170, 1997.

Tate D, Forchheimer M, Maynard F et al: Predicting depression and psychological stress in persons with spinal cord injury based on indicators of handicap. Am J Phys Med Rehab 73(3):175-183, 1994.

Taylor M, Hintzman-Egan D, Farrell G: Back to Work: Managing Disability, Recovery and Re-employment. Minneapolis, MN, Northwestern National Life Insurance Company, 1994.

Taylor RS, Bonfiglio RP: Industrial rehabilitation medicine. 4. Assessment of the outcome of treatment in industrial medicine, program development, documentation, and testimony. Arch Phys Med Rehabil 73(5-S):S369-S373, 1992.

Thorbjornsson CB, Alfredsson L, Fredriksson K et al: Physical and psychosocial factors in low back pain during a 24-year period. A nested case-control analysis. Spine 25(3):369-375, 2000.

Tuck M: Psychological and sociological aspect of industrial injury. J Rehabil 49(3):20-25, 1983.

Vierling LE: Return to work dynamics: A perspective on the three R's. Topics in Case Management January/February 2001, pp 46-48.

Voaklander DC, Beaulne AP, Lessard RA: Factors related to outcome following a work hardening program. J Occup Rehabil 5(2):71-85, 1995.

Waddell G, McCullough JA, Kunnel E et al: Non-organic physical signs in low-back pain. Spine 5(2):117-125, 1980.

Waddell G: A new clinical model for the treatment of low-back pain. Spine 12:632-644, 1986.

Walls RT: Disincentives in vocational rehabilitation: Cash and in-kind benefits from other programs. Rehabilitation Counseling Bulletin 26(1):37-46, Eric Doc. No. EJ268049, (NARIC call no. J1523), 1982.

Westmorland MG, Pennock M: What prevents people with disabilities from obtaining employment? An examination of Canadian data from a national and regional perspective. WORK 5(4):255-263, 1995.

Williams RA, Pruitt SD, Doctor JN et al: The contribution of job satisfaction to the transition from acute to chronic low back pain. Arch Phys Med 79:366-373, 1998.

Wilson S, Haws C, Naccarato P et al: Functional activities versus work hardening in the rehabilitation of the injured worker. WORK 4:366-373, 1994.

Wrich JT: Beyond drug testing: Coping with drugs at work. Harvard Bus Rev 66(1):2-8, 1988.

SUGGESTED READINGS

Fordyce WE: Behavioral Methods for Chronic Pain and Illness. St Louis, Mosby, 1976.

Grahn B, Stigmar K, Ekdahl C: Motivation for change in patients with prolonged musculoskeletal disorders: A qualitative two-year follow-up study. Physiother Res Int 4(3):170-189, 1999.

Guccione AA: Physical therapy diagnosis and the relationships between impairments and function. Phys Ther 74:499-504, 1991.

Jette AM: Physical disablement concepts for physical therapy research and practice. Phys Ther 74:380-386, 1994.

Nagi S: Some conceptual issues in disability and rehabilitation. In Sussman M (ed): Sociology and Rehabilitation. Washington, DC, American Sociological Association, 1965, pp 100-113.

National Institute of Disability Management and Research (NIDMR): National Occupational Standards in Disability Management, www.nidmar.ca/standards, accessed October 23, 2000.

World Health Organization (WHO): ICIDH-2: International Classification of Functioning, Disability and Health: Final Draft, Full Version. Geneva, WHO, 2001.

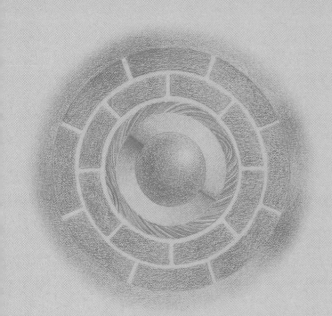

Disability Assessment

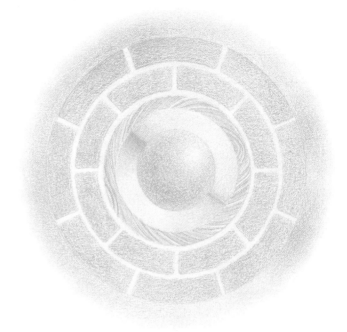

CHAPTER 8

Disability Determinations

Elizabeth Genovese, MD, MBA

"Physicians involved in determination of work capacity need to appreciate the difference between a pathologic process (disease or impairment); its functional ramifications (disability); and the handicapping environment of the disabled person."

- Steven Scheer, MD, 1995

KEY POINTS

- Independent medical examinations (IMEs) are different from second opinions in that no patient-physician relationship exists.
- No justification exists for the examiner to use the claimant's self-reported capacities as the basis for a determination regarding disability if these capacities are not supported by the physical examination.
- When investigating multifactorial conditions, the examiner often discovers that heredity, lifestyle, and overall health status are at least as important as occupational and traumatic factors in the development of disease or the extent of disability. In some instances they are the only real cause of disease and/or disability

---

Operational Definitions

Causality	The association between a medical condition and a given exposure leads one to believe that the condition would not have occurred in the absence of the exposure.
Maximum Medical Improvement	A point after which a patient is not expected as a result of medical intervention to demonstrate a significant change in objective presentation, subjective complaints, or both.
Permanency	Patient status that occurs when impairment is unlikely to change substantially or by more than 3% in the next year.
Prognosis	The examiner's expectation or forecast of the progress of a disease or injury in terms of impairment or disability involvement.

INDEPENDENT MEDICAL EVALUATIONS VERSUS SECOND OPINIONS

IMEs are fundamentally different from traditional second opinion examinations. No physician-patient relationship is usually believed to exist and the patient (better described as the "claimant") is not entitled to a copy of the report, but can request one from the referral source. The independent medical examiner ideally should have no personal or professional relationship with any of the physicians treating the claimants or with the claimants' attorneys, and should act as a subcontractor for the insurance company or employer involved. Although examiners are always requested to provide a diagnosis or diagnoses, IMEs virtually always require the examiner to comment on impairment and disability. Independent examiners often must reach conclusions regarding permanency, maximum medical improvement (MMI), and prognosis, including the need for future treatment and the likelihood that treatment will return claimants to their premorbid status. Causality and the reasonableness and necessity of treatment may also need to be addressed. Such an assessment requires a far more thorough review of the records than the examiner would ordinarily need to perform.

As a consequence, the independent examiner needs to have an orientation and set of "skills," as it were, that differ markedly from those needed for "usual" patient care. These skills will be described in depth later in this chapter.

These skills can best be applied to an individual evaluation when the independent examiner understands the pertinent issues that need to be addressed. IMEs are requested by attorneys; employers; the Social Security Administration; and by worker's compensation, long-term disability, motor vehicle, short-term disability, general liability, and life insurance carriers or their agents. The best examinations are often performed by those who thoroughly understand the unique needs of each referral source.

Social Security

The Social Security Administration (SSA) administers the largest combined disability program in the United States. SSA consists of two components: Social Security Disability Insurance (SSDI: Title II of P.L.74-271) and Supplemental Security Income (SSI: Title XVI). SSDI is the system under which injured or disabled workers and their families receive income when a worker is unable to work for at least a year as the result of a physical or mental impairment. SSI is primarily "need-based" and is intended to provide a minimum income level for needy, blind, or disabled adults (and for disabled and blind children) who are younger than 65 years of age and are not covered under other programs.

Children are classified as disabled if they have an objectively defined condition that causes interference with normal growth and development. In adults, disability is defined as the inability to engage in any "substantial gainful activity" by reason of a medically determinable physical or mental impairment, or combination of impairments, that can be expected to result in death or has lasted or can be expected to last for a continuous period of not less than 12 months (Social Security Act [a]). The impairment (or a combination of impairments) is then classified as disabling if it is severe enough to significantly limit an individual's physical or mental ability to do basic work activities; if it meets or equals a previously "listed" impairment; if it prevents an individual from doing "past relevant work"; or, after an assessment of residual functional ability, precludes the performance of "substantial gainful work," taking into consideration the applicant's age, education, skills, and work experience.

An individual is deemed to have a "medically determinable impairment" if he or she is blind or if he or she has objectively (determined through physical examination or diagnostic testing) demonstrable anatomical, physiological, or psychological abnormality. Exceptions are made for conditions in which the diagnosis is predominantly based on symptoms, such as chronic fatigue syndrome or chronic pain, or when impairment is the result of the combined effect of several well-documented diagnoses, none of which would cause significant impairment in isolation.

When the medical evidence of record is not sufficient to support disability, the claim is either denied (in which case the claimant can ask for reconsideration and then a hearing, which are the first steps in the appeals process) or a consultative examination is requested. The examiner must be able to provide the SSA with data about the claimant that will either confirm the existence of a disabling "listed impairment" (or an impairment of similar severity) or provide other information supporting the presence of a disabling condition. Decisions made regarding the qualifications of a claimant for SSI or SSDI do not have to be consistent with determinations made for other disability carriers. The SSA differs from these carriers in using the availability of employment within the claimant's geographic area as one of the criteria for disability payments [Social Security Act (b)].

Workers' Compensation Carriers

Workers' compensation (WC) laws differ in every state (the federal government has yet another set of rules). The laws are similar, however, in providing the employer with immunity from liability claims in return for guaranteeing medical care and wage-replacement payments to persons with work-related injuries. The wage replacement lasts until claimants return to their original job, a job with modified duties with the same employer, or another job with a different employer. Medical care is payable by the insurer until the claimant no longer requires any treatment that can be attributed, either directly or indirectly, to the compensable event.

Independent medical examiners for WC carriers are often asked to provide a diagnosis; comment on various aspects of causality; and assess whether a claimant has reached MMI, the permanency of impairment, and the reasonableness and necessity of current and future medical treatment. In some states the examiner will have to provide an "impairment rating" using the *Guides to the Evaluation of Permanent Impairment* or an equivalent standard (American Medical Association [AMA], 1993).

The main objective of the referral source, however, is usually to obtain clearance for the employee to return to his or her previous job, preferably without restrictions. If the employee is not capable of doing so, a release to a less-demanding job is acceptable as well. Ability to get to and from work is of limited, if any, relevance. An accurate determination regarding ability to work can only occur when the examiner feels able to provide an accurate functional assessment. Although ostensibly this can be achieved simply by asking the claimant to describe his or her functional capacities, the claimant is not necessarily motivated to be entirely truthful in doing so. As a consequence, determining a claimant's "true" abilities requires the examiner to assess his or her physical status, degree of disability, and credibility. Many examiners find this difficult.

Motor Vehicle Insurers

Individuals involved in motor vehicle accidents are sent for IMEs only when they appear to have injuries, treatment, and/or disability in excess of what one would expect. The type of insurance coverage that the claimant possesses is also a factor, because policies may have limitations in coverage of medical costs, may or may not include wage-loss benefits, and vary in the degree to which a claimant can recover for pain and suffering or a permanent loss of function.

The examiner thus may be asked to use treatment records, diagnostic test results, and information regarding the mechanism of the accident and damage to the vehicle(s) involved to reach conclusions regarding causality, impairment, and disability (especially if there is an ongoing wage-loss claim). If the examiner needs to assess whether the claimant sustained a "serious" or "permanent" impairment of bodily function, or is experiencing any residual "pain and suffering," it is necessary to both ascertain impairment and assess what activities performed before the accident (other than work) have now ostensibly been abandoned. Motor vehicle insurers are also generally quite interested in past and future treatment requirements and may request a record review as part of the IME.

Group Health (Long- and Short-Term Disability Carriers)

This group of insurers has no interest in causality, unless it can be used as a basis for subrogation of benefits (decreasing their financial exposure through the application of wage-loss payments from another source) because their policies require wage-loss replacement regardless of "fault." An elimination period must lapse before policies take effect, and the definition of disability can vary over time, as does coverage for certain conditions (especially psychiatric). As a consequence, these insurers are predominantly interested in the degree to which a claimant is impaired and the extent to which loss of function from the impairment translates into disability.

Short-term insurers ostensibly need only to know if claimants are physically capable of performing their occupations, but in general they assess whether the claimant can do his or her specific job. An "occupation" is distinct from a "job." Used to define work capacity, an occupation does not make any allowance for interpersonal stressors as a source of disability or instances in which a specific "job" may require an employee to perform at a physical or mental level that exceeds the "formal" definition of his or occupation in the Dictionary of Occupational Titles (U.S. Department of Labor, 1991).

This issue is relevant in that long-term disability insurers initially base their determination about claim payment on whether a claimant can work in his or her original occupation, not in his or her specific job. Furthermore, after 1 to 5 years, many of these policies switch from a definition of disability as the inability to perform in "a given occupation" to the inability to work in "any occupation" commensurate with an individual's previous income and educational training. IMEs may be requested at any time, but they are most commonly used on or before the change from a given occupation to "any occupation." The disability insurer is then primarily interested in discovering whether a claimant has the residual physical (and mental) capacities to work in an occupation appropriate to his or her skills and education. The need for further treatment is only relevant to the degree that it affects the ability to work and the prognosis. The existence of jobs in the area where a claimant lives and the ability to drive to and from work are not relevant to the insurer (these factors are considered by administrators of SSDI).

Virtually all claimants sent for IMEs by disability carriers believe themselves to be totally disabled or, at the very least, are invested in presenting themselves as such.

Hence the examiner is not justified in using the claimant's self-described capacities as the basis for the determination regarding disability if these are not supported by the physical examination. Although formal functional testing is of value in WC and other evaluations, it is of particular benefit in this venue.

Employers

Employers may be self-insured for WC and/or disability and may request IMEs to ascertain an employee's ability to work. They also may need an IME to assess whether a "qualified individual with a disability," as defined by the Americans with Disabilities Act (ADA), is able to perform the "essential functions" (fundamental duties) of a given job. Under the ADA, an individual is disabled if he or she has an impairment or record of an impairment that has substantially limited one or more major life activities or if the individual is "regarded as having a disability" (ADA, 1990).

To perform this type of evaluation, the examiner must have an accurate job analysis that specifically lists which job functions are essential and which are marginal, as well as a thorough knowledge of the ADA. He or she then must assess whether the claimant is simultaneously both disabled and qualified and, if so, indicate what reasonable accommodations the employer needs to make to permit the claimant to perform in the position sought. These determinations are necessary for newly hired employees, but they also are often required (and far more problematic) when a newly impaired employee wishes to return to a previously held position.

The ADA and WC law may conflict in those situations when a physician indicates that a claimant is permanently restricted. This situation can be interpreted as a disability and may require an employer to attempt accommodation in situations in which this would otherwise not occur. Likewise, in instances in which an employee has limitations that do not preclude performing the essential functions of a given job, a disability insurer might choose to deny the claim although both the employer and employee agree that the employee should seek disability benefits. The "lesson" to be learned is that the independent examiner is wise to consider not only the specifics of a given insurer's needs, but also how these needs interact with other disability and compensation systems before he or she issues a report that will become part of the legal documentation in a file.

The Family Medical Leave Act (1993) entitles employees to as long as 3 months of unpaid leave for their medical care or that of a family member. An employer will sometimes request an IME when the leave is mandated by illness of the employee if doubt exists that the leave is needed and if it is difficult to hold the employee's job vacant while he or she is absent. Employers also will request IMEs when an employee takes sick days sporadically rather than consecutively, because this type of absence is often highly inconvenient for them. As is the case for ADA examination, the examiner must have a good understanding of the disease process or processes and, when the employee is ill, the degree to which his or her illness truly requires leave or an alteration in schedule.

Miscellaneous

The rehabilitation professionals and lawyers who work for insurers may request IMEs. IMEs are also needed as part of the analysis of medical malpractice, product liability, and other "personal injury" claims. The examination can be used to establish a claimant's current condition and future treatment needs and also to assess whether a claimant's representation of his or her injury and subsequent clinical course appears credible and consistent with medical knowledge regarding the conditions involved.

DISABILITY VERSUS IMPAIRMENT

Virtually all IMEs require the examiner to assess whether there is any impairment or disability. The *Guides to the Evaluation of Permanent Impairment* (AMA, 1993) is used by many state WC boards to apply numerical ratings to the degree of impairment exhibited by claimants. This publication defines impairment as the "loss, loss of use, or derangement of any body part, system, or function." Although claimants' self-reports are of some relevance, especially in the case of psychological problems or a bona fide "chronic pain syndrome," impairment represents the objective effects of a disease process on bodily function and should not be cited unless substantive support exists for the examiner's determination.

Although other impairment rating systems exist, those of the AMA are most widely used. The most recent version of the *Guide* is the fifth edition (AMA, 2000). Impairment ratings are not required by WC laws in all states, and not all states use the same edition of the *Guide*. Some significant differences exist between editions. For example, the second edition allows the use of numerical ratings for psychiatric disability, but later versions do not. The fourth edition rates spinal injuries by diagnosis and certain physical findings regardless of whether MMI has been reached. All versions of the *Guide* divide the body into organ systems to rate the percentage of an individual's impairment. If impairment exists in more than one system, the examiner needs to "combine" impairments, adjusting for existing impairment before assessing the contribution of the second medical condition to the individual's impairment. No science exists behind the numbers used in the *Guide*. Ratings are nonetheless very consistent internally.

Disability is defined by the AMA as "an alteration of an individual's capacity to meet personal, social, or occupational demands, or statutory or regulatory requirements because of an impairment." The disability hence "arises out of the interaction between impairment and external requirements, especially those of a person's occupation" and represents the gap between what a person *can* do and what the person *needs* or *wants* to do" (AMA, 1993).

Disability is not the same as impairment. A violinist with a finger injury may be disabled occupationally but have little impairment. Conversely, a computer programmer who becomes paraplegic has substantive impairment but virtually no occupational disability. Determination of disability should be based solely on objective findings, unless the examiner suspects that concomitant psychological pathology (e.g., "chronic pain syndrome") is a contributing factor. One of the greatest challenges for the examiner is to accurately differentiate those with true disability from those who feign disability for personal gain. This often requires the use of ancillary services such as functional capacity evaluations (FCEs), psychological testing, and surveillance.

Maximum Medical Improvement and Permanency

All patient evaluations require the examiner to formulate a diagnosis. IMEs, also will require the examiner to comment on MMI and permanency, both of which differ from prognosis. Prognosis is defined as the expectation that a patient will recover to the point at which his or her degree of impairment and disability is roughly equivalent to that which existed before the accident or exposure under evaluation after "permanency" has been reached.

The AMA's *Guide to the Evaluation of Permanent Impairment* (1993) defines permanency as occurring when impairment is "unlikely to change substantially and by more than 3% in the next year with or without treatment." Claimants with a permanent impairment usually have reached MMI, which is said to exist if medical intervention is not expected to produce a significant change in the claimant's objective presentation, subjective complaints, or both. Claimants who have reached MMI, however, do not necessarily have a permanent impairment. They may improve independently of treatment solely on the basis of the natural history of the disease process. The conclusion that a patient has reached MMI does not preclude further treatment, but does imply that this treatment will only be for "maintenance" purposes.

Causality

Often examiners need to state which diagnoses are related to the injury in question (if liability/compensation are involved) and, preferably explain, why. These diagnoses are to be differentiated from new-onset (but unrelated) diagnoses, preexisting conditions, and those diagnoses that represent a worsening of a preexisting condition unrelated to the injury/exposure in question.

Unless it has already been accepted by the insurer, an assessment of causality as part of the IME is presumptive (i.e., routinely accepted on the basis of case law or legislation) or has been established through litigation. Causality must always be addressed when the referral source has significant doubts regarding the legitimacy of a patient's complaints as they relate to the initial injury (or alleged injury). Even in the presence of a clear causal relationship between an accident and subsequent physical pathology, the examiner may need to state whether an exacerbation, recurrence, or aggravation of a previous condition occurred and apportion liability accordingly.

Causality is imputed when the association between a medical condition and a given exposure (physical, biological, or chemical) suggests that the condition would not have occurred in the absence of the exposure. For a causal relationship to exist, a clear temporal relationship should exist between the exposure/injury and the claimant's illness/complaints. Even in the presence of a temporal relationship, the presumption of causality needs to be biologically plausible.

Plausibility is established by the presence of studies that show a statistically significant association between the medical condition and the exposure; specificity of the association for the injury (i.e., the absence of other factors, especially preexisting disease, that could have caused/contributed to the problem); and a duration, intensity, and/or mechanism of exposure/injury sufficient to cause the illness/injury in question. It is often necessary to apportion or assess to what extent a given factor or exposure under evaluation was a contributing cause of a medical condition that is classically multifactorial in etiology. When investigating multifactorial conditions, the examiner often discovers that heredity, lifestyle, and overall health status are at least as important as occupational and traumatic factors in the development of disease or the extent of disability. Sometimes these factors are the only real cause of disease. Under these circumstances, apportionment requires the examiner to not only understand the biological plausibility of the alleged association between the exposure/injury and the disease, but also to know the claimant's past medical history and the "usual" natural history of the medical condition.

Apportionment requires an understanding of the terms "precipitation," "acceleration," "exacerbation," "aggravation," and "recurrence." Precipitation implies that the injury or exposure caused a disease process for which the claimant was at risk but had not (and possibly would have never) become manifest. In acceleration the exposure hastens, or is claimed to hasten, the course of the disease (i.e., the disease would have eventually become symptomatic, but in this case it did so more rapidly). When an exposure accelerates the manifestation of a given disease process, it is not necessarily any worse than it would have been in the absence of the exposure. This situation differs from aggravation, which is the permanent worsening of a previous condition by a particular event or exposure.

Exacerbation is the transient worsening of a previous condition by an injury or illness, with the expectation that the situation will eventually return to baseline. A recurrence is similar to an exacerbation but usually involves the reappearance of signs or symptoms attributable to a previous injury with minimal or no provocation. A detailed description of the alleged "new" injury is mandatory when recurrence is suspected, although it should be obtained in all circumstances in which the causal link between a medical condition and an exposure is less than clear.

ELEMENTS OF THE INDEPENDENT MEDICAL EXAMINATION

The History

The examiner should begin by obtaining the claimant's own version of how he or she was injured or taken ill, including all body parts allegedly affected at the time. Discrepancies between this history and information in the medical record may be useful in the assessment of the claimant's credibility. The history from the time of injury to the present should be recorded chronologically, including the names of all physicians and chiropractors who have provided treatment, especially during the first weeks after the loss. The claimant should be asked to describe the nature and outcome of all diagnostic testing and treatments performed. This history allows the examiner to determine whether any information has been omitted without which one cannot assess whether MMI has occurred, if there are missing records, and whether previous treatment was reasonable and necessary. A consistently poor response to seemingly appropriate treatment should alert the examiner to the possibility that the diagnosis is incorrect or the claimant is magnifying symptoms.

The "past medical history" must be thorough. The examiner must ascertain whether the claimant has a previous history of similar complaints or injuries, by whom the claimant was treated, and the clinical course of the complaint. All previous chronic conditions should be noted and subsequently listed in the "diagnoses/impression" section of the report. Some of these conditions, such as arthritis, gout, and other connective tissue disease, and medications the claimant is using may have relevance to the claimant's current complaints and physical findings. Chronic conditions that are primarily subjective in nature may give insight into the claimant's psyche. A history of mental illness or alcohol or drug abuse should be considered a "red flag" because chronic pain disproportionate to objective findings is particularly prevalent in these individuals.

Family history should be obtained, with a focus on the disease processes under evaluation and mental illness. Work history should be obtained. If claimants are on modified duty or not working, the examiner should ask what portions of their former jobs they could perform. Information about previous occupations is relevant to long-term disability determinations and in planning for vocational rehabilitation. This information may also be of relevance in determining apportionment. Social history is relevant but not always obtainable. When available, it can tell the examiner a great deal about the incentives or disincentives under which the claimant is operating. Poor prognostic factors include the involvement of an attorney or a history of substance abuse or antisocial behavior.

The examiner should request that claimants list all painful body parts and quantify the pain he or she usually experiences in each area on a scale of 0 to 10 (with 0 representing "no pain" and 10 "unbearable pain"). The ancillary use of pain diagrams and questionnaires such as the Oswestry (Fairbank, 1980), the Ransford (Ransford, 1976), the Roland-Morris (Roland & Morris, 1983), or SF-36 (Ware, 1982), to name a few, may be appropriate.

The examiner should definitely inquire about work, household, and recreational activities, both before and after the injury. It is critical to compare information obtained from the claimant's direct history with medical records and findings from the physical examination. One can also compare these answers with answers provided on any ancillary pain questionnaires that the claimant was asked to complete. Discrepancies should lead the examiner to question the claimant's credibility.

Physical Examination

The physical examination should focus primarily, but not exclusively, on the medical problems that led to the need for the IME, and thoroughly evaluate the alleged "source(s)" of disability and impairment. Musculoskeletal examinations should include a description of strength, range of motion, sensory abnormalities, neurological findings including atrophy (the examiner should measure the affected limb and compare with the other), and tenderness or spasm (the examiner should differentiate between the two). The examiner should clearly document whether sensory complaints and pain symptoms follow a rational dermatomal or radicular pathway. Other areas should be briefly examined for completeness and to observe the claimant's behaviors (e.g., the ability to turn the head during an ophthalmologic examination but not during range of motion testing of the cervical spine). The examiner should also look for inconsistencies between different elements of the physical examination, between the physical examination and the history, and between the history and the "usual" anatomy and pathophysiology of the claimant's condition that might shed light on his or her "true" status.

The IME differs from a "usual "examination in requiring the examining physician to question, and attempt to evaluate, the validity of subjective complaints. The examiner should observe the claimant's overall attitude (e.g., pleasant, hostile), posture, gait, and the use of ambulatory aids to determine whether these are consistent with subjective complaints and objective findings/testing. The examiner should assess whether a claimant who states he or she has difficulty with sitting, standing, or various body positions manages to perform the biomechanical equivalent of these positions during the examination. Differences in the gait and mobility of the claimants in the examining room, waiting room, on exiting the building, and when getting into their cars should also be noted. The examiner should note whether complaints of weakness or abnormal positioning of an extremity are accompanied by objective evidence of weakness or disuse such as atrophy, wasting, or differential patterns of shoe wear and sensory loss/paresthesias are consistent with what the examiner would expect anatomically. The presence of tan lines or calluses inconsistent with the claimant's history, and scars (especially if the claimant does not tell the examiner what caused them during the history) should also be noted.

The examiner can use a number of simple "tests" to assess whether the claimant's symptoms are consistent with what one would expect to find objectively. Waddell's signs (Waddell, 1980) are the best known of these tests and are used in the examination of the low back. A total of five areas are rated:

"Simulation" (axial loading and trunk rotation)
"Regional symptoms" (sensory abnormalities and weakness)
"Tenderness" (should be neither superficial nor non-anatomical)
"Distraction testing" (abnormalities with straight leg raising should also be present if the leg is raised to the same extent when the claimant is sitting—also referred to as the "Flip" or "Michele" test, and difficulty with bending should consistently be present when the claimant is asked to do something that is physiologically equivalent)
"Overreaction"

A point (up to a maximum of five) is given whenever the response in one or more of these areas is non-physiological. The Hoover test also assesses the examinee's degree of effort. The examiner places a hand under the contralateral heel while asking the claimant to perform straight leg raising. Downward pressure should be felt on the hand; if not, effort is questionable. The cogwheel muscle release test provides a means of assessing the claimant's sincerity of effort. A cogwheel or ratcheting release of a muscle during manual muscle testing may indicate that the examinee is trying to simulate weakness. "Psychological list" is a postural test of an examinee. Psychological list is assessed if the claimant is leaning to one side when standing or walking, as can occur in disk disease. When the list is genuine, it will persist when the claimant bends forward in an attempt to touch the floor with his or her fingertips. A list that disappears with forward bending may suggest a non-organic finding. The use of additional pain diagrams and rating systems can provide even more information or, at the very least, scores that allow the examiner to quantify the consistency and validity of claimants' pain behaviors, but are best used as part of a complete FCE.

If the examiner chooses to purchase a few pieces of equipment, some additional testing can be used as a supplement to the physical examination and pain diagrams to screen further for functional overlay. The examiner can use goniometers of different sizes to measure range of motion of joints. Measurements of the spine are done with inclinometers. No more than a 10% difference should exist between trials. Computerized models are easier to use but are obviously more expensive. Measurements with both goniometry and dynamometry should also make physiological "sense" and be consistent with what the claimant achieves spontaneously.

The Jamar dynamometer is used for tests of grip strength that, when invalid, suggest functional overlay even in claimants who are seen with problems in areas other than the upper extremities. Overall grip strength has been shown to fall within certain norms based on age and sex (Mathiowetz et al, 1985). Unusually low readings for a given diagnosis hence are suspect. In the five-position grip-strength test the claimant is asked to grip the dynamometer as hard as possible in position two (one is the tightest), and then to squeeze as hard as possible in all five positions (Stokes, 1983; Niebuhr & Marion, 1987). Maximum grip strength in position two should be the same with both maneuvers. The strength in all five positions should also follow a bell curve; if not, the effort was submaximal. Rapid-exchange grip testing is yet another way of assessing validity of effort (Hildreth et al, 1989). After the examiner has ascertained the position at which the claimant achieves maximum grip strength, the claimant is asked to shift the dynamometer from hand to hand using this position, squeezing as hard as possible (usually 8 to 10 repetitions). In healthy individuals, strength falls to approximately 85% of the maximum grip. When maximum effort is not put forth during initial grip testing, the grip strength will remain the same or increase. Pinch strength (key, tip, and palmar) is usually used only with hand injuries (and by hand surgeons) (Mathiowetz et al, 1985). Trials should vary by no more than 0% to 15%; more than 20% is considered invalid. Lift testing is generally reserved for FCEs and can be quite sophisticated (Harber & Soo Hoo, 1984; Mayer et al, 1988, Pt I; Mayer et al, 1988, Pt. II; Chaffin, 1975). Nonetheless, the motivated examiner can design customized forms of lift testing to have the claimant perform during the IME. The results can then be interpreted by using the principles on which FCE validity determinations are based.

Record Review

All relevant records should generally be sent to the examiner to review in conjunction with an IME. If the examiner is asked to provide only a "snapshot" picture of the claimant's current diagnosis, residuals, and employability, no need usually exists to spend a great deal of time reviewing these records. When causality or the necessity of previous treatment is to be addressed, it is mandatory for the examiner to review the records in detail. Although often omitted, the record review should include notes from physical therapists, nurses, and other "ancillary" health service providers, because they often are less likely to consider the legal aspects of a patient's care when providing information about complaints, motivation, response to treatment, physical examination, or past medical history. Any missing records should be requested. If possible, examiners should avoid making any definite conclusions regarding issues that might be affected by information in these records until they become available.

Diagnostic Testing

The examiner should review all available diagnostic tests if within his or her area of expertise. Tests differ in their sensitivity and specificity and, in particular, exhibit a decrease in positive predictive value as the prevalence of disease decreases in the population screened. In practical terms, this translates to a high false-positive rate when tests are performed in the absence of strong clinical indicators. Treating physicians also have a tendency to "over read" tests if this is to the benefit of the claimant. Hence conclusions regarding such conditions as "disk herniations" in magnetic resonance images, "radiculopathy" or "carpal tunnel syndrome" on electromyography (EMG) images, should not be based solely on statements in physician progress notes. Such conclusions sometimes cannot even be based on the interpretation of the radiologist or electromyographer. If test results do not seem to "match" the claimant's clinical presentation, the examiner should state this and either request hard copies of the actual data for review or request that these be reviewed by another expert.

Diagnoses

The examiner should list all diagnoses. When the claimant alleges sequelae from an injury or exposure, the examiner must clearly indicate which are related, which are unrelated, and which ones cannot be determined on the basis of currently available information.

Objective findings should be compared with the history and "working diagnoses." If a claimant has symptoms without objective findings, it is reasonable to ask whether an occult diagnosis has been missed or a "soft-tissue" condition of a nature that would not necessarily present with objective findings.

Unfortunately, many claimants magnify their symptoms. This situation has been formally described by Matheson (1988), who has defined "symptom magnification syndrome" as "a conscious or unconscious self-destructive, socially reinforced behavioral response pattern consisting of reports or displays of symptoms which function to control the life circumstances of the sufferer." Symptom magnification is used to achieve primary or secondary gain. Primary gain refers to the unconscious relief of psychological stress through physical symptoms. Secondary gain occurs when illness leads to benefits to the patient such as attention, money, and decreased responsibility that would not have been available in the absence of illness behavior. "Malingering" is volitional symptom magnification, and the term implies that all symptoms are consciously fabricated, although many claimants are more appropriately classified as "partial malingerers" (i.e., individuals who are consciously exaggerating symptoms that are or were present in order to achieve secondary gain) (Resnick, 1990).

One should suspect symptom magnification when symptoms are vague, ill-defined, overdramatized, inconsistent, or not in conformity with signs and symptoms known to occur. Symptom magnification is also likely to be present when the results of physical and mental status examinations and other data are inconsistent with complaints. The presence of "Waddell's signs" (Waddell, 1980) during the physical examination, invalid results with grip or lift testing, and exaggerated responses to questions in pain questionnaires may all be cited as evidence of symptom magnification. The examiner should consequently evaluate the history, pain questionnaires, and results of validity testing performed during the physical examination to determine whether the claimant appears to be magnifying the symptom and, if so, whether this is representative of psychological factors (these factors often cannot be ascertained without additional testing) or of full or partial malingering. If the former, the examiner will later need to assess whether the claimant's dysfunctional behaviors (usually representative of preexisting psychopathology) are so severe as to lead to a state of effective disability. If exaggeration is so flagrant and inconsistent as to be clearly representative of malingering, in the absence of objective findings the examiner should state that the claimant has recovered from any injury or illness and can return to work. If magnification exists in the presence of objective findings, the examiner needs to "tease out" the true impact of the findings (impairment) on the claimant's function instead of simply taking the disability at face value.

The examiner should remember that the IME was scheduled because the referral source wanted an objective evidence-based evaluation of the claimant's status. It may be useful to compare the "medical model," under which examiners generally operate, with the "functional model," under which examiners need to operate when performing IMEs.

Under the medical model, examiners assume an organic basis for symptoms, assume they are missing something when nothing is found on physical examination, have a tendency to treat symptomatic patients indefinitely, and are loath to state that someone is malingering.

Under a functional model, however, the claimant has the responsibility to provide a valid representation of his or her status that is devoid of symptom exaggeration, non-organic signs, or attempts to mislead the examiner. The examiner is then mandated to base all decisions on objective data. Examiners should consequently never give a claimant's physiological diagnoses unless supportive objective data exists or, in the case of diagnoses that are primarily subjective, unless absolutely no evidence exists of symptom magnification. In other words, in the absence of objective findings, examiners should use terms such as "low back pain," "neck pain," and "headache" as diagnoses rather than characterize these complaints as resulting from a lumbar sprain, radiculopathy, herniated disk, or postconcussion syndrome, indicating that this is indeed the case. When evidence exists of symptom magnification (also referred to as "embellishment" or "functional overlay"), this should be an additional diagnosis. In those situations in which the claimant asserts that he or she has sustained injury as the result of an accident or exposure, the examiner is obliged to state which diagnoses are causally related to the event under investigation. As stated previously, examiners should not "accept" causality unless it is consistent with the mechanism of injury and supported by the records. It is perfectly acceptable, and actually preferable, for the examiner to request additional information and defer making any definitive conclusions until it becomes available.

Estimating Physical Capacities

Disability assessment is a critical part of most IMEs, and is generally accompanied by the completion of an "estimated physical capacities form." One should begin the assessment of physical capacities by asking the claimant his or her tolerance for various activities. Although one can take claimants' symptoms into account when reaching a determination, it is inappropriate to base determinations of disability solely on statements by claimants (or the treating physician), because in many situations their goal may be to maximize an impairment or disability rating. As a consequence, it is best to first determine capacities on the basis of the examination and other objective data. Objective findings include abnormalities on physical examination, including evidence of degenerative disease, vascular disease, and poor muscle tone. These findings also include any abnormalities on diagnostic testing that might be of physiological relevance, including evidence of disease processes unrelated to the injury or exposure being evaluated. The claimant's baseline height, weight, build, and level of conditioning are not "abnormal" findings, but they are still objective pieces of information that allow the independent examiner to assess physical capacities.

Age, flexibility, body habitus, degenerative disease, and other anatomical factors will influence the ability of claimants to perform activities such as sitting, standing, walking, squatting, bending, climbing, driving, or using the hands and feet. Because it is difficult to assess to what extent a given person can do so "continuously" (66% to 100% of an 8-hr workday or shift), "frequently" (33% to 66%), or "occasionally" (1% to 33%) in an 8-hour day, it is often easiest to simply state that "no restrictions" exist if no clearly limiting abnormalities can be found. In the presence of potentially limiting abnormalities, the examiner can only use his or her experience with similar patients to estimate the degree to which function will be affected.

Weight, sex, body habitus, and level of conditioning are all factors that affect the ability of individuals to lift. A body of research exists that allows the examiner to extrapolate the ability to lift during an 8-hour period from performance during specific static and dynamic lifting maneuvers (Snook, 1978; Mayer et al, 1988, Pt I; Mital et al, 1986). This information can be used to then state whether a claimant can do "sedentary," "light," "medium," "heavy," or "very heavy" work (Table 8-1). Information of this nature, however, is not usually available during an independent examination. The examiner thus has no recourse but to estimate these abilities, a difficult task when the referral source wishes a claimant to be cleared

Table 8-1 Physical Demand Characteristics

Physical Demand Level	Occasional 0% to 33%	Frequent 34% to 66%	Constant 67% to 100%	Approximate Energy Required
Sedentary	10 lbs	Negligible	Negligible	1 to 1.5 METS
Light	20 lbs	10 lbs*	Negligible†	2 to 3 METS
Medium	20-50 lbs	10-25 lbs	10 lbs	3.5 to 5.5 METS
Medium heavy	75 lbs	25-35 lbs	10-15 lbs	6 to 7.5 METS
Heavy	50-100 lbs	35-50 lbs	15-20 lbs	
Very heavy	100+ lbs	lbs	20-50 lbs	

METS, Metabolic rate expressed as energy consumption.

*Walk/stand and/or push/pull arm or leg controls.

†Push/pull arm or leg controls while sitting.

From variation of U.S. Department of Labor: Dictionary of Occupational Titles, 4th ed, revised supplement, U.S. Department of Labor, Employment and Training Administration, Appendix C, Washington, DC, Department of Labor, 1991.

to do more than light to light-medium work. When it is mandatory for the examiner to provide an accurate estimate of a claimant's ability to perform various activities, the best way to do so is by ordering an FCE.

The presence of symptom magnification complicates disability assessment, because no exists justification for basing an assessment of physical capacities on a claimant's self-reported activities and limitations if one questions the credibility of these statements. In general, examiners should base the assessment of physical capacities on what most individuals with similar physical and diagnostic study findings could do, rather than on the claimant's description of his or her limitations. The examiner should indicate what behaviors of the claimant were exaggerated or inconsistent. As stated previously, the claimant is responsible for providing an accurate and valid description of symptoms. Consequently, in those cases where claimants appear to be consciously exaggerating symptoms, the examiner really has no option but to conclude that they have wholly recovered (or they would not need to exaggerate) and complete the capacities form accordingly. If the examiner believes that limitations may still exist, or is uncertain as to whether the claimant is exaggerating symptoms, an FCE may be helpful. Surveillance is another alternative because, when "successful," it often provides a great deal of information about claimants' activities that would not have ordinarily been available.

Functional Capacities Evaluations

FCEs are used to establish whether individuals, in the absence or presence of an impairment or alleged impairment, can do specific tasks, especially those relevant to past or future occupational activities. Although examiners use the term "capacity" to describe results, the FCE actually tells more about a person's current ability than about his or her maximum potential, because ascertaining the latter requires knowledge that the therapist often does not have about motivational factors and the status of any existing medical conditions.

During FCEs, examiners assess whether objective testing substantiates the claimant's self-defined capabilities. They enable the examiner to ascertain the ability to carry out various functions that are not amenable to evaluation during a standard physical examination. Comprehensive FCEs therefore evaluate flexibility, strength, general conditioning, and the ability of claimants to perform various job specific tasks. Quantifying the amount of work that can safely be performed can then be used to: (a) return a person to a former job, (b) establish what type of alternative employment he or she may be capable of performing, or (c) assess whether someone is "fit for duty" [i.e., can safely meet the essential functions of his or her job (used when a claimant is returning to a strenuous job after a medical leave or applying for a job that requires a high degree of physical fitness)].

Functional capacity tests can also (but do not always) incorporate various "validity tests" to assess whether a patient is attempting, either consciously or unconsciously, to manipulate the data. In those situations when an FCE is valid, the abilities and restrictions it provides can be used by the independent examiner as a guide to completion of the estimated physical capacities form. When it is invalid, or only marginally valid, the examiner needs to carefully compare the raw data in the FCE with that from the history, physical examination, diagnostic testing, records, and any clandestine surveillance that may have been performed to assess to what degree the claimant's pain behaviors were uniformly consistent (suggestive of a chronic pain disorder) or inconsistent (suggestive of intentional misrepresentation). If the FCE alone or in combination with other data leads the examiner to doubt the claimant's credibility, the examiner must be willing to state this clearly to the referral source, disregard subjective claims of disability, and complete the estimated physical capacities form solely on the basis of objective indices of impairment.

CONCLUSION

In general, IMEs are ordered to get an accurate sense of whether a claimant's self-described restrictions can be documented as valid and, in personal injury cases, consistent with one or more previous injuries or exposures. Strong clinical skills are necessary but not sufficient for the examiner, as he or she must use and be comfortable in using and applying a wide range of ancillary tests and aids that focus more on functional evaluation and credibility assessment than on establishing a diagnosis or treatment plan. The extent to which an examiner can provide an accurate, supportable claimant assessment will determine the degree to which he or she establishes credibility in this area.

REFERENCES

American Medical Association: Guides to the Evaluation of Permanent Impairment, 4th ed. Chicago, American Medical Association, 1993.

American Medical Association: Guides to the Evaluation of Permanent Impairment, 5th ed. Chicago, American Medical Association, 2000.

American with Disabilities Act, Public Law No. 101-336, 1990.

Chaffin DB: Ergonomics guide to the assessment of human static strength. Am Ind Hyg Assoc J 36(7):505-511, 1975.

Fairbank JCT: The Oswestry low back pain disability questionnaire. Physiotherapy 66(8):271-273, 1980.

Family Medical Leave Act, Public Law No. 103-3, 1993.

Harber P, Soo Hoo K: Static ergonomic strength testing in evaluating occupational back pain. J Occup Med 26(12):877-884, 1984.

Hildreth DH et al: Detection of submaximal effort by use of the rapid exchange grip. J Hand Surg 14A:42-45, 1989.

Matheson LN: Symptom magnification syndrome. In Isernhagen SJ (ed): Work Injury: Management and Prevention. Rockville, MD, Aspen, 1988, pp 257-282.

Mathiowetz P et al: Grip and pinch strength: Normative data for adults. Arch Phys Med Rehabil 66:69-72, 1985.

Mayer TG et al: Progressive isoinertial lifting evaluation. I. A standardized protocol and normative database. Spine 13(9):993-997, 1988.

Mayer TG et al: Progressive isoinertial lifting evaluation. II. A comparison with isokinetic lifting in a disabled chronic low-back pain industrial population. Spine 13(9):998-1002, 1988.

Mital A et al: Reliability of repetitive dynamic strengths as a screening tool for manual lifting tasks. Clin Biomech 1:125-129, 1986.

Niebuhr BR, Marion R: Detecting sincerity of effort when measuring grip strength. Am J Phys Med 66(1):16-23, 1987.

Ransford AO, Cairns D, Mooney V: The pain drawing as an aid to the psychological evaluation of patients with low back pain. Spine 1:127-134, 1976.

Resnick PJ: The detection of malingered mental illness. American Psychiatric Association, 143rd Annual Meeting, New York, May 12-17, 1990.

Roland M, Morris R: A study of the natural history of back pain. Part I: development of a reliable and sensitive measure of disability in low-back pain. Spine 8(2):141-144, 1983.

Scheer S: The role of the physician in disability management. In Shrey DE, Lacerte M (eds): Principles and Practices of Disability Management in Industry. Winter Park, FL, GR Press, 1995, p 175.

Snook S: The design of manual handling tasks. Ergonomics 21:963-985, 1978.

Social Security Act (a)—20 CFR—part 404:1520–1568.

Social Security Act (b) (Section 223 (d)[1] [A].

Stokes HM: The seriously uninjured hand—weakness of grip. J Occup Med 25(9):683-684, 1983.

US Department of Labor: Dictionary of Occupational Titles, 4th ed. Washington, DC, US Department of Labor, 1991.

Waddell G et al: Non-organic physical signs in low back pain. Spine 5:117–125, 1980.

Ware JE and Rand Corporation: Short Form 36 Health Survey. Boston, Medical Outcomes Trust, 1982.

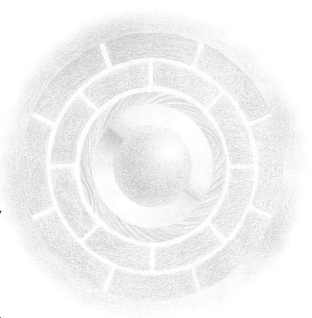

CHAPTER 9

Functional Capability Evaluation

David W. Clifton, Jr., PT, and
Ruth Ann Burnett, BSN, CRRN, CCM, CDMS

Once the injured worker moves beyond the acute stage of rehabilitation, the workplace should be considered the therapeutic environment of choice.

- Donald E. Shrey, PhD, CRC, 1995

KEY POINTS

- Medical or clinical assessment of the link between impairment and disability is insufficient when used alone.
- Functional capability evaluations (FCEs) play a vital role in disability determination and return-to-work (RTW) decision making.
- Functional capacity is an untestable construct, but functional capability or ability can be both qualified and quantified.
- Analysis of the worksite is often the critical missing link or element essential to a safe and appropriate worker-worksite match.
- FCE providers must consider non-physical or psychosocial influences on physical disability and RTW determination.

Operational Definitions

Functional Capability Evaluation (FCE)	FCE is an independent, impartial, and objective assessment of both a person's functional capabilities and limitations.
Independent Medical Examination (IME)	An impartial medical examination provided by a physician, typically at the request of an employer, insurer, or attorney. IMEs are used to determine maximum medical improvement (MMI) or benefit (MMB); disability status; or RTW status, including work restrictions and limitations.
Impairment	A disruption of normal anatomical or physiological function that may or may not lead to disability.
Disability	A relative term used to describe any restriction or lack of ability to perform an activity in the manner or within the range considered to be normal. Disability can be defined from a medical, economic, social, employment, or legal perspective.

FUNCTIONAL CAPABILITY EVALUATIONS

Functional evaluation is an integral component of disability prevention, treatment, and management programs. FCEs serve a vital role in returning injured workers to function and gainful employment (Randolph, 2000; Isernhagen, 1993; Owens & Buckholtz, 1995). The FCE is considered an objective assessment of an individual's physical capabilities. Why is an "objective" assessment required? The actual physical capabilities of an individual are not easily assessed, because the assessment may be influenced by lack of motivation, secondary gain, finances, the desire for workplace productivity, or a lack of knowledge of injury and/or illness and recovery/physical abilities.

The awareness that medicine is not an exact science and that physical ability varies in each individual gives rise to the need for an objective examination and evaluation of physical capabilities to allow an unbiased assessment of functional capabilities.

It is important to remember that the level and extent of medical recovery and return to functional capability will vary on the bases of the individual's age, premorbid condition, severity of the medical diagnosis, the type and aggressiveness of the medical treatment plan, and the individual's perception of his or her own well-being. Physical and mental functional assessment serves as a linchpin in

Table 9–1 Common Abbreviations Associated with Functional Testing

FCE	Functional capability or capacity evaluation
FCA	Functional capability or capacity assessment
WCA	Work capacity assessment
WCE	Work capacity evaluation
FJA	Functional job analysis
OCE	Occupational capacity evaluation
JCE	Job capacity evaluation
IME	Independent medical examination
FAE	Functional abilities evaluation
PCE	Physical capacities evaluation

Table 9–2 Psychophysical Versus Kinesiophysical Approaches to Functional Capacity Evaluation

Psychophysical	Kinesiophysical
Tested subjects determine maximum levels.	Clinician determines maximum levels on the basis of pain behaviors, biomechanics, fatigue observations, and compensatory behaviors.
Accuracy of results is tied to injured person's effort.	Accuracy of results is tied to clinician's skills and competence.
Maximum function is defined by safe ability.	Maximum function is defined by safe movement patterns.

Data from Isernhagen SJ: Functional capacity evaluation: Rationale, procedure, utility of the kinesiophysical approach. J Occup Rehabil 2(3):1257-1258, 1992.

disability determination under various health benefit programs, including workers' compensation (WC), group health, automobile liability, short-term and long-term disability, and Social Security.

The need for FCEs was identified in the 1980s by workers' compensation systems (American Physical Therapy Association, 1998). The FCE was deemed a WC claims management tool to provide information on the physical abilities of workers. This tool was and continues to be used as a foundation for safely returning workers to the workplace after they have experienced illness or injury and medical recovery. A number of terms are associated with FCEs and the process of worker-worksite matching (Table 9–1).

Several approaches exist to evaluation of physical function. Most FCEs incorporate combinations of patient or evaluee self-reports of pain and function, medical or clinical assessment, and actual functional testing. FCEs differ from other disability assessment strategies by virtue of actual functional assessment (Fishbain, 2000).

The American Medical Association states, "The effect of the patient's impairment on his or her ability to perform meaningful tasks is the focus of functional capacity evaluation" (Matheson, 1996). A more accurate description replaces the term "patient" with evaluee, client, subject, claimant, or worker, because no treatment relationship typically exists that is comparable to the traditional doctor-patient or therapist-patient relationship. FCEs are ideally independent and impartial assessments devoid of treatment. The FCE serves as a learning tool but does not technically constitute treatment.

Models of Functional Capability Evaluations: Psychophysical Versus Kinesiophysical

In an effort to reduce the number of persons on its disability logs through the use of FCEs, the Social Security Administration (SSA) sponsored a study that identified more than 700 FCE models (Rucker et al, 1996). Although there is tremendous diversity in FCE models, FCEs can be categorized as psychosocially based or kinesiophysically based. Table 9–2 compares and contrasts these general models. In the psychophysical model, the claimant terminates each functional task at his or her own discretion.

In the kinesiophysical model, the evaluator terminates each functional task on the basis of his or her clinical observations and objective findings and not based on the claimant's subjective reporting, pain reports, or fatigue complaints.

In reality, many FCEs probably blend elements of these two models. For instance, purveyors of the kinesiophysical approach still analyze evaluee self-reports and observations of pain, fear avoidance, and perceived exertional level. Both FCE models place safety first as a priority; however, advocates of the kinesiophysical approach contend that it has more inherent safety when compared with the psychophysical approach (Isernhagen, 1992; Smith, 1994). The kinesiophysical model requires evaluators with medical knowledge, in particular, kinesiology, biomechanics, anatomy, physiology, and illness/injury behavior. A knowledge of ergonomics enhances both FCE models and the ability to craft functional job analyses that enhance the worker-worksite match. Evaluators under both models should be adept at identifying psychosocial or non-physical variables that affect an individual's disability status. Readers are encouraged to refer to Chapter 7 for a more detailed exploration of these issues. Identification and management of psychosocial issues need to be accomplished to offer a truly comprehensive assessment of disability status, especially prognostic indicators.

A kinesiophysical approach is defined by a number of parameters (Isernhagen, 1992). It establishes a safe framework within which maximum functional effort can occur. This approach differentiates functional limitations that are caused by physical limitations versus injured employee self-limitation resulting from pain, fear, anxiety, or avoidance behavior. It identifies physical reasons for activity limitations, thus facilitating engineering or administrative controls or modifications. The FCE can serve as a blueprint for a rehabilitation program. It narrows the gap between actual functional performance and the evaluee's own perception of function.

A psychophysical approach to FCEs empowers the evaluee with more decision-making authority, particularly the end point of each functional task assessment (e.g. lifting, carrying, and pulling) (Key, 1995). Key cautions that regardless of how the end point is determined (by the evaluee or evaluator), it should be consistent from evaluee to evaluee or case to case. Specific evaluee instructions provided during a psychosocial FCE may include the following (Key, 1995):

1. Stop when you can't do any more.
2. Stop when it starts to hurt.

3. Stop when you feel pain.
4. Stop when the pain gets so bad you cannot do any more.
5. Stop when you think you should stop.
6. Stop when you first start to feel anything.
7. Stop when I tell you to stop.
8. Stop after you have done as much as you possibly can.

No infallible method exists to determine an end point when a manual task is performed (Key, 1995). Like rehabilitation, functional testing remains an art and not a science, although its methodology can have scientific underpinnings. Tests and assessment tools in and of themselves are neither good nor bad. A test's disposition is determined by how the data generated by the test are analyzed and applied. Communication between the evaluator and evaluee, the evaluee and employer, the evaluator and employer, the evaluee and insurance company, and the evaluator and insurance company determines whether an appropriate worker-worksite pairing results.

Functional "Capacity" or "Capability" Evaluation?

The literature is replete with numerous terms ascribed to physical function testing. These terms can be found in Table 9–1. A lack of standardized terminology within the disability management community hampers consistent functional assessment across treatment settings, conditions, and disciplines (Abel-Moty et al, 1996) (see Table 9–1). In this chapter, the term functional "capability" evaluation is preferred to the conventional label of functional "capacity" evaluation. This choice is based on the notion that capacity is by definition an untestable construct, and

that what evaluators truly assess is capability. On the other hand, evaluators estimate or predict functional capacity. The term "capacity" implies potential, whereas "capability" implies demonstrable actions or results. This difference is depicted in Figure 9–1.

What is a Functional Capability Evaluation?

An FCE is an independent, impartial, and objective assessment of a person's functional capabilities as well as his or her limitations. FCEs strive to describe the relationship or correlation of disease/injury to impairment, impairment to disability, and disability to handicap. Readers are encouraged to refer to Chapter 1 for a more detailed analysis of disablement models.

FCEs can be job-specific, general, or baseline in design (American Occupational Therapy Association, 2001; Frings-Dresen & Sluiter, 2003). A job-specific FCE attempts to identify an injured worker's functional capabilities for the following purposes:

- RTW to a previous job.
- RTW at a current job.
- Vocational exploration, training, and counseling directed at identifying a prospective job for placement purposes.

A number of indications exist for FCE (Table 9–3).

An FCE focuses on a work-related goal and not necessarily on an individual's aptitudes, interests, job competencies, or temperament (American Occupational Therapy Association, 2001). Baseline or general FCEs attempt to identify correlations between an injured worker's self-reports of pain/dysfunction and actual function without specific work goals in mind. These FCEs may be used to identify a

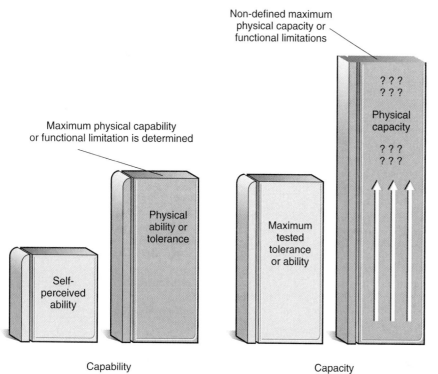

Figure 9–1. Functional capability versus functional capacity.

Table 9-3   Indications for a Functional Capabilities Evaluation

1. Determination of residual functional capabilities to perform a previous or other occupation.
2. Determination of presence of disability following injury, disease, or insult.
3. Determine severity of disability.
4. Identify the need for reasonable accommodation and job modifications.
5. Determine the need for future treatment (e.g. rehabilitation).
6. Correlate subjective complaints with objective functional measures.
7. Determine loss of earning capacity.
8. Litigation resolution.
9. Assess consistency of effort, worker behaviors, and symptom magnification/minimization.
10. Augment the data secured through an independent medical examination.
11. Inclusion in preemployment or, more appropriately, postoffer screening.

claimant's degree of disability for disability insurance benefit purposes or medico-legal issues (e.g., professional liability/malpractice) or to assist in the identification and/or design of an alternative treatment/management program.

Worksite Assessment: The Other Half of the Functional Assessment Formula

An injured worker's functionality occupies one-half of the disability assessment formula. Worksite or environmental assessment represents the other half of the formula necessary to facilitate a safe, appropriate and timely RTW or worker-worksite match. Figure 9-2 illustrates the link between these two pieces of the disability puzzle. Worker attributes include functional capabilities, limitations, training, education, aptitudes, skill sets, motivation, and interests. Worksite integrants include a functional job analysis (FJA), ergonomic analysis, and requisite job modifications or accommodations necessary for a safe worker-worksite match. Job modifications can be described as engineering-based or administratively based. Examples of engineering controls include job redesign, tool design, the use of assistive equipment, and personal protection equipment. Administrative controls include job rotation or sharing, rest breaks, pacing skills, warm-ups, and instruction in policies and procedures.

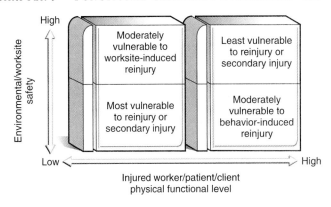

Figure 9-3. A relative model of worker functional levels from a safety perspective.

The safety of the work environment may affect the worker's performance as profoundly as injury rates. Clearly, unsafe work environments lead to more frequent and severe injuries than safer environments. Figure 9-3 depicts the relationship between environmental/worksite safety and the functional level of workers.

Medical/Clinical Assessment of Function

Many disability determinations are determined through medical/clinical examinations versus actual functional assessment. Disability determinations are often embedded within independent medical examinations (IMEs). Refer to Chapter 8 for a more detailed discussion of IMEs. IMEs are commonly performed for a host of musculoskeletal conditions (Kraus, 1997). Physicians routinely complete physical capacity reports or forms during an IME, but often with a degree of trepidation (LaCerte and Desjardins, 1995). In most cases, physicians rely on medical judgment and extrapolate data (rightly or wrongly) for the purpose of disability determination. This medical-only assessment can consequently lead to premature RTW, protracted treatment that reinforces the sick role, or a failure to adequately identify job restrictions, accommodations, and modifications. LaCerte and Desjardins assert that occupational and physical therapists are more appropriately credentialed to perform disability assessments through functional or work capacity evaluations. A therapist is more likely than a physician to have knowledge of job modifications and reasonable accommodations.

Although common, a medical approach to disability determination can be seriously flawed (Wyman, 1999). Physicians are trained and experienced in the identification and treatment of pathologies, both anatomical and physiological. Disablement models, however, do not necessarily equate pathology with impairment, impairment with disability, or disability with handicap (Nagi, 1993; Jette, 1999; World Health Organization, 1993). Johnson states that physicians often use a "best guess scenario" when conducting assessments of residual function or disability (Johnson, 1996). Substantial variations are reported when physicians assess impairment and its relationship to disability (Boden, 1987). A California-based study of disability ratings by different independent medical examination physicians demonstrated differences in disability

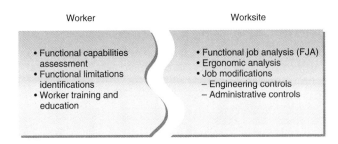

Figure 9-2. Worker-worksite matching. The key to all functional capability evaluations.

appraisal of 0% to 70% in the same cases (Clark et al, 1988). Extreme disability rating variations commonly result between plaintiff or claimant/worker-secured physicians and defense or workers' compensation insurer physicians (Boden, 1987). Boden asserts that claimant experts usually tend to exaggerate the degree of disability, and defense experts usually tend to understate the degree of disability. This "dueling doctor" phenomenon has been shown to significantly delay the claims resolution process, create an adversarial environment, and drive costs upward (Boden, 1987). Because the FCE is important in bringing objectivity to decision making as it relates to return to work planning or determining and planning for one's future lifestyle, the FCE must be performed by a professional who is knowledgeable and experienced in physiology, musculoskeletal anatomy, the cardiopulmonary system, the neuromuscular system, and the integumentary system. Evaluators must also consider the dynamics and probability of physical ability as it relates to specific diagnoses and the aging process. In some instances a physician may provide an assessment of physical function on the basis of his or her medical knowledge, the symptoms and general condition of the claimant, what the claimant verbalizes, and/or a general physical examination of the claimant. All of these factors provide good information in assessing the medical status of a claimant; however, more information and expertise in physical function is required to provide an overall assessment of functional ability.

It is equally critical to assess the non-biological or psychosocial issues that may affect the individual's own assessment of his or her disability as well as the opinion of others (Shaw et al, 2001; Vowles & Gross, 2003; Fritz & George, 2002; Krause et al, 2001; Livneh, 2001). Linking impairment to disability is a fundamental purpose of many FCEs. This link is difficult if not impossible to achieve through a purely medical examination. The examiner cannot equate impairment with disability without first measuring function and effort (Richman, 1997). Functional assessment often falls on the shoulders of primary care physicians, however, who are untrained in disability decision making, particularly when it requires functional versus medical testing (Owens, 1999). Because medical limitations are assessed in relationship to work demands, physicians are doubly challenged. Through no fault of their own, relatively few physicians covet skill sets and knowledge related to the critical demands of job tasks. Richman (1997) outlines the goals of an IME, which include identifying other types of investigations (e.g., FCEs). IMEs usually result in the estimation of function/ability or dysfunction/disability and do not assess actual function, especially job-specific disability.

An FCE should be a coordinated effort among the evaluee, treating physician, physical therapist, the source that requested the FCE (in many instances, an insurance carrier), and in some cases the evaluee's attorney. Communication and cooperation among these parties minimize the potential for an adversarial tone during the FCE process. In the case of multiple stakeholders who are concerned about the outcome of the FCE, communication, coordination, and cooperation must occur among the stakeholders to ensure the intent, goals, objectiveness, and professionalism that are the foundation of the FCE process.

Combined Use of Independent Medical Examinations and Functional Capability Evaluations

Growing support exists for the use of a linked IME/FCE model (Wyman, 1999; Richman, 2000; SSA, 2001). When combined, the expertise of different musculoskeletal professionals produces a more reliable disability determination. A physician's expertise in pathology identification coupled with a therapist's functional expertise results in a comprehensive assessment of the patient along any point of the injury/disability continuum, from injury to chronicity. This combination is especially critical in those cases in which the injured worker must perform at a "medium" or above category. Some physicians may be reluctant to release these workers for RTW without solid evidence of actual versus estimated physical and mental functioning. Therapist involvement can also contribute worksite-specific data collected through on-site visits and the crafting of an FJA. FJAs can serve as the blueprints for actual functional testing. Martin asserts that FCEs remove the subjectivity of some medical decisions and advocates the combined use of IMEs and FCEs for disability determination (Martin, 2000). When FCEs are performed before an IME, more objective and defensible data and opinions result. This, however, assumes an FCE that is standardized and has established validity and reliability.

FCE STANDARDS

A wide variety of functional evaluation protocols (more than 700 according to the SSA) exists within the disability assessment field (Lechner et al, 1991; King et al, 1998). Matheson et al (2001) describe a new database: the "Functional Assessment Measures Database," that comprises 4200 different measures used in the functional assessment of persons with disability across life spans. This database contains 3033 scales found in 633 measures linked to at least one functional assessment construct. This database appears to be the most comprehensive analysis to date of the clinical literature on functional assessment. Future study may reveal those prognosticators that may have utility in functional assessment of disability.

Some degree of standardization exists despite the sheer number and diversity of FCEs. Most FCE protocols address evaluee responses across three distinct domains: biomechanical, cardiopulmonary, and psychophysical (Table 9–4).

Many FCEs have been predominantly designed and marketed by proprietary or for-profit entities. This situation does not in itself invalidate these protocols; however, prudent providers should be aware of the potential for bias. King et al (1998) define standardization as the development of a clear set of procedures for the administration and scoring of tests. An absence of FCE standardization existed throughout most of the 1970s and 1980s and into the early 1990s. During this period a number of proprietors promoted their own versions of the FCE, but these protocols were in general not substantiated or supported by the clinical literature from a reliability/validity perspective. Further, the intended protocols were often modified

Table 9–4   Evaluee Responses to Functional Testing by Domain

Domain	Observed Response During Activity
Biomechanical	Abnormal postures, movement patterns, material handling techniques
Cardiopulmonary	Vital sign monitoring, heart rate, blood pressure, breathing pace, and pattern
Psychophysical	Perceived exertional levels, pain behaviors, anxiety, fear, avoidance behavior, depression, poor motivation, sincerity of effort

by users. At times the purchaser's FCE barely resembled the developer's.

Professional Associations' Role in FCE Guidelines

Professional associations and groups have recently begun to address the need for functional capacity/capability standards. The physical therapy profession has taken a leading role in defining and establishing the professional practice standards for performing FCEs. The physical therapy profession helped to develop relative functional tests to assess the ability of workers to perform functions as described in the selected characteristics of occupations defined in the Dictionary of Occupational Titles (American Physical Therapy Association, 1998).

During the 1990s a number of professional associations, specialty medical societies, and government agencies/entities developed FCE standards or guidelines (California APTA, 1996; Maryland APTA, 1993; APTA, 1997; AOTA, 1998; SSA, 1996).

Physical therapists in Maryland were among the first in the country to address the need for standardization (Hart et al, 1994). Hart et al (1994) identified the following basic components of a functional capacity evaluation:

1. History
2. Physical impairment
   a. Joint range of motion
   b. Muscular function
   c. Neurological status
   d. Movement patterns
   e. Endurance
3. Worker behavior and/or symptom magnification behaviors
4. Evaluee's perception of his or her disability
5. Significant functional abilities/limitations
6. Physical abilities as compared to physical demands of the job
7. Problem list
8. Recommendations
   a. Interpretation of test results
   b. Goals of treatment
   c. Plan of care

The California Functional Capacity Evaluation Guidelines for Physical Therapists is substantially patterned after the Maryland guides that preceded them (California, 1993).

The SSA has concluded that objective functional assessment can and should be a component of the disability determination process (SSA, 1996). The SSA assigns the following three essential uses to objective functional assessment:

1. Initial screening of applicants and determination of disability severity
2. Supplementation/substantiation of objective clinical disability assessment
3. Determination of residual functional capabilities to perform a) prior occupation b) other occupation

The SSA has embarked on an aggressive path to de-list beneficiaries from its ever swelling disability roster. Table 9–5 portrays the SSA's "Stage Model of Disability Determination."

The Social Security agency recognizes that functional assessments facilitate the integration of factors that reside beyond the domain of the medical or physical. Functional assessments incorporate environmental variance, coping mechanisms, and social supports.

Components of an FCE

Despite the plethora of FCE protocols, a consensus appears to exist regarding the following basic components of an FCE:

- Informed consent of the client
- Objective tests and measures designed to assess function or lack of function
- Subjective data collection from client or worker through history taking and evaluee self-reports
- Musculoskeletal screening and cardiovascular assessment

Secondary elements include work task simulation, consistency or sincerity of effort testing, and pain assessment.

Table 9–5   Social Security Administration's Stage Model of Disability Determination

Stage of Disability Determination Process	Applicability of Functional Assessment
Step 1: Engage in substantial gainful activity.	Not applicable
Step 2: Determine severity of impairment.	Administration of global multidimensional FA screening instrument
Step 3: Determine whether impairment meets or equals listing in regulations.	FA supplement to medical determination
Step 4: Determine residual functional capacity to perform past work.	Comparison of domain-specific FA findings and follow-up with occupational standards and/or generally established norms of social functioning. Note: Functional domains include movement, mobility, mental, medical/health status, social support networks, and activities of daily living
Step 5: Determine residual functioning capacity to perform other work.	Same as step 4

These may be primary components in some FCEs depending on the purpose of the assessment. For instance, all work-related functional capacity/capability evaluations, otherwise known as work capacity/capability evaluations, strive to assess the worker's functional traits as they relate to a current or prospective job position.

The Role of Functional Job Analysis

An FJA may be an equally important component of an FCE. In some FCEs or work capability evaluations, the FJA serves as the blueprint for testing. Figure 9–4 depicts the vital role that FJAs play in the work disablement arena. FJAs describe the critical job demands of a given occupation. Measurements and observations related to the effective performance of a job are described. These may include repetitive tasks, object weights, work surface heights, walking/carrying distances, awkward postures, ambient temperature, forceful exertions, vibration, task durations, and safety precautions.

FJAs used as integral components of functional assessment have a number of advantages. An FJA can be instrumental to a physician during the conduct of an IME. The effectiveness of an IME can be enhanced through a written, verbal, or videotaped FJA. Worker-worksite matches may be more accurate and defensible from a legal perspective. Videotaped FJAs are particularly useful because an examining physician who has not visited a worksite must rely on others for accurate descriptions. A videotaped FJA of another worker performing the job of the subject provides both qualitative and quantitative information. FJAs are often crafted by case managers or rehabilitation specialists; therefore they provide a means for physical or occupational therapists to meet employers face-to-face. Such a meeting may lead to the development of a business relationship that benefits both parties.

Methods-Time-Measurement

Methods-time-measurement (MTM) is a fundamental element of matching FJAs to FCEs, namely through physical function testing. MTM as a work measurement methodology has been around since the early 1950s. The MTM Association for Standards and Research is an international association dedicated to a range of services designed to support multiple aspects of industrial engineering. (MTM Association, 2004). MTM involves techniques that facilitate the analysis of task performance during a prescribed time period. In MTM, critical job tasks are broken down into component parts for functional analysis. These components are then compiled to reflect a work shift typically, an 8-hour workday. For instance, a truck driver may load his tractor trailer for 2 hours, then drive for 3 hours, arrive at his destination and unload for 3 hours, return to his rig and return to his depot. An FCE of this man would entail a combination of driving skills and manual materials handling. The U.S. Department of Labor description of task frequency as occasionally, frequently, and constantly exemplifies the MTM approach to functional assessment (Table 9–6).

It is logical to assume that functional performance degrades over time for a number of reasons, including fatigue and boredom. Peak performance measured through an FCE of 2 hours length cannot therefore be accurately compared with an FCE of 8 hours length. The degradation curve is depicted in Figure 9–5.

Disadvantages of FJAs may include additional expense to an employer or client. The claims resolution process may be slowed down when an FJA is added, although one could argue that the FJA may accelerate the RTW decision making through credible evidence that does not require as much debate. Case managers may welcome therapists performing the FJA. Last, FJAs may be most practical in own-job FCEs or with injured workers who are returning to their previous job.

Evaluator consensus supports FCEs that are designed through a combination of biomechanical, physiological, and psychological assessments (King et al, 1998; Lechner et al, 1991; Andrews, 1998; Velozo, 1993). There is widespread use of the Department of Labor's Critical Job Tasks (U.S. Department of Labor, 1991). Refer to Table 9–7 (p. 140) for a listing. Despite efforts to standardize FCEs, these assessments ultimately suffer the same disadvantage as do clinical assessments: neither is adequately standardized. As a result, both remain more of an art than a science (Mather, 1993).

The SSA contends that although functional assessments can provide more consistent data than clinical assessments, clinical assessments will continue to provide richer individualized data than standardized FCEs

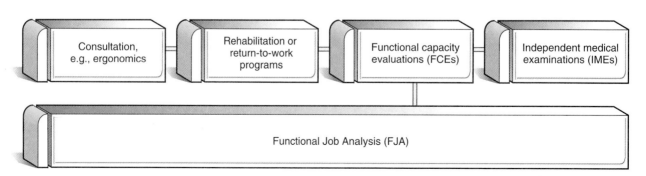

Figure 9–4. Functional job analysis: FJA's as a foundation for other disability prevention, management, and assessment services.

Table 9–6   Department of Labor Motion-Time-Methods Approach to Functional Assessment

Rating for Material Handling by Strength and Energy Required	Never	Rarely (1%-5% of 8-hr shift)	Occasionally (0%-33% of shift)	Frequently (34%-66%)	Constantly (> 67%-100% of shift)
Sedentary: 1.5 to 2.1 METS	Worker is never to perform tasks		10 lb	Negligible	Negligible
Light: 2.2 to 3.5 METS			20 lbs	10 lbs	Negligible
Medium: 3.6 to 6.3 METS			20 to 50 lbs	10 to 25 lbs	10 lbs
Heavy: 6.4 to 7.5 METS			50 to 100 lbs	25 to 100 lbs	10 to 20 lbs
Very heavy: >7.5 METS			100 + lbs	50 to 100 lbs	20 to 50 lbs
level of effort	Unsafe— contraindicated	Maximum effort	Heavy effort	Moderate effort	Light effort

METS, Metabolic units.
Data from US Department of Labor: Dictionary of Occupation Titles, 4th ed., revised supplement, Washington, DC, U.S. Department. of Labor Employment and Training Administration, Appendix C, 1991; and Isernhagen SJ: Contemporary issues in functional capacity evaluation. In Isernhagen SJ (ed): The Comprehensive Guide to Work Injury Management. Gaithersburg, MD, Aspen, 1995, p 413.

(Rucker et al, 1996). Some FCE evaluators would certainly argue this point.

Indications for a Functional Capability Evaluation

FCEs are quite versatile in their application; this characteristic begins to explain the difficulty in standardizing FCEs. Functional assessment can be conducted at any point along the disability continuum from prevention or preinjury to the posttreatment chronic stage.

Admission criteria for an FCE generally include two elements: a medically stable client and the informed consent of the client.

Providers of FCEs are advised to consider the National Institute of Occupational Safety and Health's *Work Practices Guide for Manual Lifting* (1981) when considering the design and implementation of an FCE protocol. This document has been endorsed by a number of

FCE experts (King et al, 1998; Isernhagen, 1988; Miller, 1991).

The National Institute of Occupational Safety and Health provides criteria in the form of questions that can be applied to FCEs:

- Is the test safe to administer?
- Does the test give reliable results?
- Is the test valid and specific to job requirements for predicting a safe level of work?
- Is the test valid specific to work-related abilities?
- Is the test practical to administer?
- Does the test predict the risk of future injury or illness?

The American Physical Therapy Association's *Occupational Health Guidelines Testing Functional Capacity* outlines the following indications for an FCE:

1. The client reaches a point at which he or she is not making functional gains with treatment.

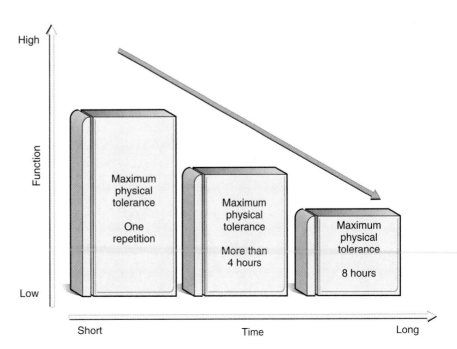

Figure 9–5. Degradation curve: Repetitions over time.

Table 9–7 Critical Job Tasks

- Lifting
- Pushing
- Pulling
- Climbing
- Standing
- Sitting
- Walking
- Balancing
- Stooping
- Carrying
- Kneeling
- Crouching
- Crawling
- Reaching
- Handling
- Finger manipulation
- Depth perception
- Feeling
- Hearing
- Talking
- Vision

2. The client has not returned to full duty or modified duty.
3. The client demonstrates physical deconditioning, with a resulting decrease in job-related functional abilities.
4. The client displays discrepancy between subjective complaints and objective findings.
5. A need exists for objective functional information before disability determination, loss of earning capacity, or litigation resolution.
6. A need exists for objective functional information on which future rehabilitation or vocational plans may be based

Providers of FCEs need to consider other issues before completing the assessment. Clinical, legal, or vocational considerations may need to be examined by the FCE evaluator. For instance, can the FCE disturb the client's condition, especially if he or she is not beyond the normal time frame for tissue healing? Is a physical or occupational therapist the most credentialed provider to address patient motivation, sincerity of effort, testing, and behavior that is potentially illustrative of symptom magnification? Or should a psychologist or psychiatrist address these issues? From a vocational perspective, should an FCE be completed if there is no job availability?

Functional capacity/capability evaluation components or subsets lend some degree of reliability and validity to the overall disability assessment process (Jebsen et al, 1969; Tiffen, 1968; Alpert et al, 1991). Although selected components of an FCE may be validated by peer-reviewed literature, a relative paucity exists of research data that address global FCE standards (King et al, 1998; Lechner et al, 1991; Isernhagen, 1992).

On the other hand, it is acknowledged that no single FCE protocol can address the diversity of conditions, client/worker needs, aggravating circumstances, mitigating issues, and medico-legal scenarios that exist (King et al, 1998; Miller, 1991; Hart, 1993; Isernhagen, 1992). The lack of standardization makes head-to-head FCE comparisons difficult.

Standardization may indeed reduce the degree of customization that is critical to offering a worker-specific or worksite-specific assessment. For the sake of this discussion, standardization is the attempt to establish consistent policies and procedures within a given testing protocol designed to ensure intertester and intratester reliability. The term "standardization" as used in this chapter is not intended to imply that all tests should have the same or similar components. Some contend that FCEs need to reflect the precise work demands of each employee's job (Frings-Dresen & Sluiter, 2003). This is a logical conclusion given that few jobs or worksites have identical attributes.

Some FCE evaluators contend that although jobs may differ from one FCE to another, consistency should be ensured in the design methodology and assessment administration (King et al, 1998).

An FCE constitutes a set of objective tests and activities packaged together to individually and collectively assess an individual's work-related capabilities, limitations, or disabilities. An FCE may not be indicated, however, if it will not add anything new or substantive to the disability assessment process or if it is to be completed by a poorly credentialed evaluator. Likewise, an FCE may not be indicated if it is poorly timed, even though its design may be appropriate.

Contraindications and Precautions of Functional Capability Evaluations

Conducting FCEs presents a variety of challenges that cross political, economic, legal, medical, research, and social spheres (Velozo, 1994; Mather, 1993; Turk et al, 1988). The complexity of uses and applications for FCE data demand that a degree of caution be demonstrated both when selecting and utilizing a testing protocol. There are no hard fast rules involved.

Instead, a common sense approach should be exercised in both the selection of candidates for an FCE and in its administration. Not all persons are candidates for FCEs despite the myriad of testing protocols. The safety and health of the client must be first and foremost in the evaluator's mind. Although technically no patient-provider relationship is involved in FCEs, professional ethics should mandate a "do no harm" policy.

Candidates for FCEs must be medically stable and free of any significant cardiovascular, pulmonary, neurological, or systemic problems. Persons with these conditions may be precisely the group that requires an FCE. This situation creates a paradox for the evaluator, who needs to balance the risks and benefits of an FCE. Tests that compromise a person's safety and health, both physical and mental, are to be avoided. This too represents a challenge to the evaluator even in cases in which the person was screened and deemed a legitimate FCE candidate. An FCE is by its very design provocative. This is particularly true in workers' compensation cases, in which the injured worker may allege that a specific task is the cause of his or her disability. For example, lifting is one of the activities most often cited by injured workers as the cause of low back pain. Asking a client to simulate the very task that he or she perceives caused the initial insult may lead to fear, anxiety, or avoidance behavior.

A variety of other obstacles exist to FCE performance. These include illiteracy; diminished hearing, sight or cognition; the presence of a language barrier; and limited verbal communication abilities. Suppose that a client meets the FCE admission criteria on the basis of their primary medical condition, but suffers from one of the aforementioned problems. Does the evaluator still conduct the FCE? Does he or she provide a means of accommodation (e.g., an interpreter) before beginning testing? Or are these barriers sufficient grounds for contraindication of an FCE despite medical stability?

It is important to remember that an FCE is not curative. The FCE will address functional capabilities and communicate these in terms of limitations on functionality. The limitations may be temporary or permanent. Regardless of the temporary or permanent nature of the limitations, a more positive way of communicating the functional status of an individual is to refer to this status as the "abilities" of the individual. The Americans with Disabilities Act of 1990 uses the term "abilities." This term helps to focus on the return of individuals to the workplace in positions that fit the individual's physical abilities.

Mental illness and emotional instability must be carefully assessed before an FCE is conducted. Organic problems that have had insufficient tissue-healing time are another potential contraindication (Hart et al, 1994).

If the lack of or loss of physical function is affected by a psychological/condition, a medical specialist with knowledge and licensure to assess conditions of this type must address the issues. The FCE does not assess psychological illness. The functional ability evaluator must be cognizant of his or her professional role and refrain from making diagnoses outside of his or her professional scope.

The ultimate litmus test that FCE providers should consider can be framed in the question, "Would the performance of the FCE compromise this client's mental, emotional or physical health and welfare beyond the information or benefit that can be gained from testing?" Each FCE evaluator must ask himself or herself this question on a case-by-case basis. Although helpful, the adoption of standardized criteria for FCE testing may be insufficient in lieu of sound clinical judgment.

Providers are again reminded that disability is a legal and/or administrative issue, not a medical one. The admission criteria therefore may need to vary from that of treatment-driven decisions.

Providers should be mindful of potential conflicts of interest that may arise in the course of considering an FCE. One low back consensus document makes a very clear point, "No doctor involved in the treatment of a patient with chronic pain, irrespective of the cause, should be involved in assessing impairment or disability in the same patient" (Coetzer, 2001). The bottom line is that an FCE is an independent, impartial, functional assessment that should be conducted and submitted in a non-adversarial manner. Evaluators should have no preconceived notions about a person's functional ability or disability status.

Reliability and Validity Concerns of Functional Capability Evaluations

The predictive validity of FCE results are influenced by a number of variables that researchers have addressed over the past several decades (Smith et al, 1986). Some contend that when FCE test criteria are unrelated to job performance or involve subjective evaluation criteria, the validity of results is questionable (Pransky & Dempsey, 2004). Perhaps, no other issue raises the question of FCEs' validity to a higher degree than that of sincerity of effort and submaximal effort testing (Baker, 1998; Berryhill et al, 1993; Simonsen, 1996). FCE evaluators claim that the results provide evidence for a relationship between self-reported disability, depression, anxiety, and the evaluee's physical performance (Kaplan et al, 1996). Inconsistencies in subjects' performance across multiple sessions of safe maximum lifting determinations have been shown to be a significant source of variability in FCE measurement (Gross & Battie, 2002). A survey of FCE evaluators suggests that they view themselves as the assessment instrument central to the credibility of an assessment (Innes & Straker, 2003). This implies that evaluator observational skills versus measurement skills are of greatest importance. However, this injects a degree of subjectivity into the assessment process. Allen et al report that the reasoning behind occupational therapists' recommendations in FCE reports is frequently not stated (Allen et al, 2004). Gross et al (2004) found that one individual test embedded in a comprehensive FCE was as predictive of functional performance as the entire floor-to-waist lift protocol.

An FCE may at times be more a measure of what the subject is willing to do than of what the subject is capable of doing. Although many FCE tests are performed to suggest the presence of maximal or submaximal effort, it remains unclear whether these tests actually do what they purport to do (Lemstra et al, 2004). Co-efficient of variation (COV) is the most commonly used tool to assess the consistency of an evaluee's effort (Schechtman, 1999; Matheson, 1996; Lechner et al, 1998; Robinson et al, 1993). A COV is calculated by conducting a series of tests and retests with use of the same task. The standard deviation of a set of at least three trials is divided by the average of the scores and expressed as a percentage (Matheson, 1996). An acceptable COV for FCEs ranges from 10% to 18%, depending on the test and author. Despite the use of COV test batteries, evaluation of motivation continues to be a conundrum, especially when psychological or psychiatric conditions are involved (Owens, 1999). Physical functioning is predicated on the degree of a subject's motivation and resultant effort. Therefore it begs the question: Is a maximum functional output the product of physical limitation and/or psychological attributes, namely, motivation? Some have suggested that the presence and strength of psychosocial variables obviate the need for physical performance assessment, especially in persons with chronic pain (Ruan et al, 2001).

Acceptable maximum effort testing was introduced as a quantitative measurement of static strength and is commonly used during FCEs to determine the validity of effort (Khalil et al, 1987). Hand dynamometer tests are a prime example of this testing method. A number of evaluators have used this method to determine sincerity of effort (Niebuhr & Marion, 1987; Janda et al, 1987; Robinson et al, 1993; King, 1998; Hildreth & Lister, 1989). The COV between repetitive dynamometry gripping is used as a gauge of sincerity of effort. When the COV exceeds the established acceptable range (e.g., 10% to 18%), evaluators may conclude that the subject underachieved.

Despite its common use in FCEs, this technique remains controversial (Menard & Hoens, 1994). Although acceptable maximum effort testing can be an appropriate measure in healthy populations, safety and liability issues potentially challenge its use as a standard with impaired populations.

Matheson (1996) cautions that the reliability of an FCE can be compromised by internal and/or external threats. Examples of external threats include the FCE protocol, and equipment and administration reliability. Internal threats center around evaluee behaviors including fear, motivation, and pain avoidance.

Reliability and validity are considered the two most important features of a well-designed FCE (Lechner et al, 1991). FCE reliability has been examined by a number of researchers (Innes et al, 1999; Lechner et al, 1991; Schechtman, 1999; Mather, 1993; Lechner et al, 1994; King et al, 1998). Jette (1999) concedes that reliability preservation may not always be possible, because it demands a balance between practical and pragmatic concerns. This situation may be especially true of FCEs because of the many variables present in every RTW or disability assessment decision. Providers of FCEs are advised to select functional tests that have widespread use, have been described in peer-reviewed journals, and possess content validity. The content validity of FCE measurements can be assessed on the basis of the clinician's reasoned professional judgment about the degree to which a given functional measure correlates with job demands (King et al, 1998). Validity is established if the functional measure closely correlates with critical job demands. This can best be accomplished by using an FJA as a test template. Although this approach may not achieve empirical evidence status, it does meet the requirements of a logic-based methodology.

A discussion of validity of effort is incomplete without at least a cursory review of subject self-reporting. Self-reporting by an injured worker about their disability status is an integral component of an FCE. This step has both its advantages and disadvantages. One could conclude that injured individuals are in the best position to articulate functional levels, especially in association with pain. Validity and reliability of this information must be established, however, if it is to be meaningful. Although practical, efficient, and appealing at times, self-reporting mechanisms would be difficult to scientifically justify because of the probability of false-positives (Jette, 1999). Subject self-reports must therefore be corroborated by functional measures and clinical examination.

Diseases or conditions that are diagnosed solely on the basis of clinical findings and physical abnormalities are not necessarily associated with the cause of a resultant disability. Deyo and Phillips (1996) cite examples of conditions that in themselves do not equate to disability.

For instance, fully functioning persons can have bone spurs, spondylolysis, Schmorl's nodules, disk vacuum signs, increased lumbar lordosis, transitional vertebrae, and narrowing of vertebral spaces without suffering from low-back–generated disability (Deyo, 1991). Reciprocally, persons with no demonstrable organic condition can express significant degrees of disability. Again does the responsibility for making these distinctions rest with a physical or occupational therapist or psychologist? Readers are reminded that the individual who coined the term "symptom magnification," Leonard Matheson, PhD, is a licensed psychologist, not a physical or occupational therapist.

Two of the greatest challenges in disability management concern decisions about which disability assessment tools to use and when to use them. For instance, *"When should an independent medical examination be employed?" "An FCE?" "When is a psychological, psychiatric, or neuropsychiatric examination preferable to an orthopedic IME?"* Other questions can arise as a result of an FCE: *"Should positive findings of insincere or submaximal effort lead to examination of a claimant's mental status?" "Are physical or occupational therapists qualified to make determinations about 'symptom magnification'"?* These and other questions must be addressed on a case-by-case basis and, even then, there are no easy answers.

FCEs can be considered incomplete if they do not address mental function in addition to physical function. Goetzel et al (1998) studied more than 46,000 employees during a 3-year period to discern the effects of depression and stress on function. The health expenditures of individuals who suffer from depression are 70% greater than non-depressed individuals. The health care costs of persons under mental stress are 46% higher than persons without this impairment. Interestingly, although more common in females, depression tends to be more severe in males (Dewa et al, 2002). Overall, disability claims for mental health continue to increase; between 1989 and 1994, a mere 5 years, claims doubled. It is only logical to conclude that because many persons who undergo FCEs are in the chronic stages of illness/injury, mental health issues such as depression and stress must be acknowledged and, if possible, factored into testing protocols. Although physical and occupational therapists focus principally on physical function, these providers must recognize the challenge presented by mental dysfunction in disability determination (Anthony, 1994; Dawson & Chipman, 1995; McGurrin, 1994; Stapleton & Livermore, 1995).

The Functional Capability Evaluation Report

The FCE report represents tangible evidence of an evaluee's physical, cognitive, and psychosocial functioning. Some, however, are critical of clinical reports submitted to insurance companies for the purpose of disability assessment, contending that these seldom present objective opinions or findings and, in fact, that most dwell on subjective complaints (Coetzer, 2001).

Some persons may assume that any FCE report requested by an insurance company or employer will favor a RTW, and that those requested by the injured worker's attorney will favor full disability and inability to RTW.

These attitudes are fairly common within the field of workers' compensation, which tends to be more litigious and adversarial than other lines of insurance. It must be noted that workers' compensation is not a medical system (like some other insurance lines), but rather a legal system that is governed statutorily.

Miller (1991) points out the need for timely, clear, logical, and easy-to-read reports because of the variety of persons involved, especially non-medical persons.

Objective data can remove the emotion from decision-making and is therefore of paramount importance in disability determination. A liberal use of charts, graphs, tables, diagrams, and other graphics is beneficial for the expression of objective measures that depict complicated data. Because clarity is ultimately what an FCE referral source is seeking, reports must contain definitive language. Wise (1992) recommends that evaluators avoid the use of vague or non-definitive terms such as "possibly," "appears to be," and "seems to be."

Providers are advised to add the following elements as appendices to the main body or text of the FCE report:

- A list of operational definitions with literature citations is preferable. Examples of terms that may require definition include *impairment, disability, validity, reliability,* and *consistency of effort.*
- Validity and reliability data.
- Literature references to support the text.
- FCE standards used by the provider, with references.
- The evaluator's curriculum vitae with an emphasis on functional assessment, FJA, and ergonomics experience.
- A list of all written records that were reviewed before or during the FCE. Examples include diagnostic studies, IME reports, and physical and occupational therapy records.

Specific issues that require definitive documentation within the body of an FCE report include the following:

- Correlation of impairments to disability
- Matching of worker's function with the functional job analysis
- Linkage of medical with vocational issues
- The correlation between pain and function
- Specific work restrictions, job limitations, and reasonable accommodations under the Americans with Disabilities Act of 1990
- Correlation of the results of the IME and the FCE

If any clinical or legal records (e.g., depositions) were reviewed in conjunction with the FCE, the examiner should note when they were reviewed: before, during, or after FCE. The potential always exists for an allegation of bias when medical records, depositions, or IME reports are examined before the FCE. Professional evaluators, however, are capable of providing independent judgments that are not influenced by other variables. The evaluator should also be prepared to explain any inconsistencies that were noted in the FCE, and be prepared to provide a rationale that falls within the scope of his or her practice. If no apparent reason or rationale exists for the inconsistencies, the evaluator should be prepared to make statements to that effect. In this case, evaluators simply report their results without arriving at any conclusions.

The examiner should avoid speculation and stick to the facts, record direct observations, and use quotation marks when referencing subjective complaints emanating from the test subject.

The examiner should note any persons who were present during the FCE (e.g., spouse, attorneys, and assistants). The examiner should also record whether or not the FCE was videotaped. FCE components should be documented in real time, and the examiner should consider having the test subject sign off on his or her attendance. Parties entitled to a copy of the report should also be noted.

Use of the term "patient" should be avoided, because it implies a treatment intervention and a doctor-patient or therapist-patient relationship. This may have significant liability consequences. Preferred terms may include test subject, evaluee, employee, claimant, or client. The examiner should not assume that readers of the reports will understand FCE jargon, abbreviations, or acronyms. Technical terms should be spelled out before they are abbreviated. The examiner should refer to the operational definitions and appendix items.

Unless the evaluator is specifically requested to comment on whether or not the evaluee can return to work, he or she should not comment on this matter. If requested to comment on the ability to return to work, the evaluator must have knowledge of the specific duties of the job, number of hours the evaluee is expected to work, and the environment (e.g., temperature, air quality, type of flooring) of the workplace. These factors must all be considered, along with the physical ability of the evaluee, to determine the ability to return to work.

Insurance companies have professional medical and vocational staff members who are responsible for assessing the ability of individuals to return to work. These professionals base their decisions on medical and vocational information. The FCE is a valuable tool in helping the professionals make return to work decisions.

Clearly delineate testing/assessment from that which is subjectively reported by the evaluee. Examples of appropriate versus inappropriate verbiage are found in Examples "A" and "B."

Example A

Inappropriate wording	"A 20-lb box caused the employee's low back pain." Appropriate wording: "The employee states that lifting a 20-lb box caused her low back pain."
Explanation	Examiner was not present during alleged injury. To describe the event would be highly speculative.

Example B

Inappropriate wording	"The patient fatigued during the carrying task."
Appropriate wording	"The patient reported fatigue during the carrying task."
Explanation	An evaluator cannot feel an employee's fatigue although clinical observations can suggest it. A more accurate citation directly quotes the patient.

Provided confidentiality provisions are not breached, a second person (preferably a layperson) should be asked to read the FCE report. The report should be edited to

Table 9-8 Terms and Phrases to Avoid in Functional Capability Evaluation Reports

- Malingering/malingerer/faking
- Appears as if
- Could have
- Should have
- Probably can
- Apparently
- Seemed to
- Patient (use evaluee or claimant instead)
- Manipulated test
- Insincere effort
- Game playing
- Absolutely
- Never
- Unequivocally
- Unconditionally

remove contradictory statements, redundant comments, and misspellings to enhance its clarity and readability.

The examiner should indicate whether or not an FJA was used as a blueprint for assessment. A copy of the FJA should be attached o the FCE report. Whether or not a musculoskeletal examination/screening preceded the actual FCE should be indicated; if so, it should be attached to the FCE report.

Professionally crafted reports avoid terms that are ambiguous, speculative, inflammatory, or slanderous (Table 9-8). FCE evaluators must refrain from making medical diagnoses, slandering the client/evaluee, and offering speculation without objective support. A rule of thumb during FCEs is to state the facts and avoid editorializing. The FCE report should remain within the scope of practice of the evaluator. Last, evaluators should understand that an individual's disability might be fluid and unstable. Terms that imply absolutes should be carefully considered, especially as regards the impact of non-biological or psychosocial aspects on disability. This recommendation does not imply that reports should be "wishy-washy," indecisive, or devoid of objective professional opinions.

O*NET: Occupational Information Network

A new and improved resource is available to FCE evaluators and others involved in disability assessment. O*NET is a comprehensive database that describes worker attributes and various job characteristics. The O*NET officially replaces the long-standing *Dictionary of Occupational Titles* and is sponsored and administered by the federal Department of Labor (2004). O*NET was developed to assist individuals in career counseling, education, employment and vocational training activities. The O*NET has extensive applications that include the following:

- Alignment of educational and job training curricula with current workplace needs.
- Creation of occupational clusters based on knowledge, skills, and abilities.
- Development of job descriptions.
- Facilitation of employee training and retraining.

- Development of assessment tools to identify worker attributes.
- Identification of criteria to guide selection and placement decisions.
- Creation of skills-match profiles.
- Improvement of vocational and career counseling.

O*NET is an invaluable resource for medical, rehabilitation, human resource, and vocational professionals who strive to keep employees on the job and return those with disabilities to gainful employment. Specific to this chapter, O*NET may be useful to rehabilitation providers in the development of functional job analyses that are supported up by a federal agency, the Department of Labor.

Additional Resources

Rehabilitation providers should be aware of additional resources that can assist in the design and implementation of worker and worksite assessment. Table 9-9 provides a partial listing.

 Table 9-9 Support Documents for Functional Capacity Evaluation Design and Administration

- U.S. Department of Labor: Occupational Safety and Health Administration, Ergonomics Program and Management Guidelines for Meat Packing Plants, 1990.
- Equal Employment Opportunities Commission: Americans with Disabilities Act: Handbook, US Equal Employment Opportunities Commission, Washington, DC, 1992.
- Equal Employment Opportunities Commission: Americans with Disabilities Act: Technical Assistance Manual. US Equal Employment Opportunity Commission, Washington, DC, 1992.
- US Department of Labor, Employment and Training Administration: Handbook for Analyzing Jobs. Washington, DC, US Government Printing Office, 1972.
- American Educational Research Association, American Psychological Association, National Council on Measurement in Education Standards for Education and Psychological Testing, Washington, DC, American Psychological Association, 1985.
- American Medical Association: Guideline to the Evaluation of Permanent Impairment, 4th ed. Department of Preventive and Environmental Medicine, Chicago, American Medical Association, 1995.
- US Department of Labor, Employment and Training Administration. Selected characteristics defined in the Dictionary of Occupational Titles, US Department of Labor, Washington DC, US Government Printing Office, 1981.
- National Institute for Occupational Safety and Health: Work Practices Guide for Manual Lifting, US Public Health Service Publication No. 81-122, Washington DC, US Government Printing Office, 1981.
- World Health Organization: International Classification of Impairments, Disabilities, and Handicaps: A Manual of Classification Relating to the Consequences of Disease. Geneva, World Health Organization, 1980.
- American Physical Therapy Association: Guidelines for Evaluating Functional Capacity. Alexandria, VA, American Physical Therapy Association, 1998.
- O*Net, Occupational Information Network (this document replaces the Dictionary of Occupational Titles), http://www.onetcenter.org/overview, accessed October 3, 2002.

From Helewa A, Walker JM (eds): Critical Evaluation of Research in Physical Rehabilitation. Philadelphia, W.B. Saunders, 2000.
Deyo RA, Phillips WR. Low back pain: A primary care challenge. Spine 21(24):2826-2832, 2996.

REFERENCES

Abel-Moty E, Compton R, Steele-Rosomoff R: Process analysis of functional capacity assessment. J Back Musculoskeletal Rehab 6:223-236, 1996.

Allen S, Rainwater A, Newbold A et al: Functional capacity evaluation reports for clients with personal injury claims: A content analysis. Occup Ther Int 11(2): 82-95, 2004.

Alpert J et al: The reliability and validity of two new tests of maximum lifting capacity. J Occup Rehabil 1(1):13-29, 1991.

Alpert J: Functional capacity evaluation guidelines for physical therapists, California Chapter of the American Physical Therapy Association, Alexandria, VA, 1996.

American Occupational Therapy Inc: Functional capacity evaluation, Consumer Fact Sheets, http://www.aota.org, accessed July 10, 2001.

Andrews D, Norman R: A current review of functional capacity evaluation. Proceedings of the 30th Annual Conference of the Human Factors Association of Canada, 1998.

Anthony WA: Characteristics of people with psychiatric disabilities that are predictive of entry into the rehabilitative process and successful employment. Psychosocial Rehabil 17(3):3-13, 1994.

Baker JC: Burden of proof in detection of submaximal effort. Work J 10:63-70, 1998.

Berryhill R et al: Horizontal strength changes: An ergonometric measure for determining validity of effort in impairment evaluations. J Disabil 3(1-4):143-148, 1993.

Boden LI: Use of medical evidence in low-back permanent partial disability claims in New Jersey. Cambridge, MA, Workers' Compensation Research Institute, 1987.

Clark WL, Haldeman S, Johnson P et al: Back impairment and disability determination: Another attempt at objective, reliable rating. SPINE J 13:332-341, 1988.

Coetzer P: Disability assessment of lower backache (2001 Consensus Document). South Africa Orthopaedic Association, Society Neurosurgeons of South Africa, Life Offices Association of South Africa, http://www.loa.co.za/asslowerback.htm, accessed September 5, 2001.

Dawson DR, Chipman M: The disablement experienced by traumatically brain injured adults living in the community. Brain Inj 9:339-353, 1995.

Dewa CS, Goering P, Lin E: Depression-related short-term disability in an employed population. Occup Environ Med 44(7):628-633, 2002.

Deyo RA, Phillips WR. Low back pain: A primary care challenge. Spine 21(24):2826-2832, 1996.

Fishbain DA: Functional capacity evaluation. Phys Ther 80(1):110-112, 2000.

Frings-Dresen MH, Sluiter JK: Development of a job-specific FCE protocol: The work demands of hospital nurses as an example. J Occup Rehabil 13(4):233-248, 2003.

Fritz JM, George SZ: Identifying psychosocial variables in patients with acute work-related back pain: The importance of fear-avoidance beliefs. Phys Ther 82(10):973-983, 2002.

Goetzal RZ, Anderson DR, Whitmer RW: The relationship between modifiable health risks and health care expenditures. Occup Environ Med 40:843-854, 1998.

Gross DP, Battie MC: Reliability of safe maximum lifting determinations of a functional capacity evaluation. Phys Ther 82(4):364-371, 2002.

Gross DP, Battie MC, Cassidy JD: The prognostic value of functional capacity evaluation in patients with chronic low back pain: Part 1: Timely return to work. Spine 29(8):914-919, 2004.

Hart DL, Isernhagen SJ, Matheson LN: Guidelines for functional capacity evaluation of people with medical conditions. J Orthop Sports Phys Ther 18:682-686, 1993.

Hart DL, Berlin S, Brager PE et al: Development of clinical standards in industrial rehabilitation. J Orthop Sports Phys Ther 19(5):232-241, 1994.

Helewa A, Walker JM (eds): Critical Evaluation of Research in Physical Rehabilitation. Philadelphia, WB Saunders, 2000.

Hildreth DH, Lister GD: Detector of submaximal effort by use of the rapid exchange grip. J Hand Surg14A:742-745, 1989.

Innes E, Straker L: Workplace assessments and functional capacity evaluations: Current beliefs of therapists in Australia. Work 20(3): 225-236, 2003.

Isernhagen SJ: Functional capacity evaluation: Rationale, procedure, utility of the kinesiophysical approach. J Occup Rehabil 2(3):157-168, 1992.

Isernhagen SJ: Functional capacity evaluation. In Isernhagen SJ (ed): Work Injury Management and Prevention. Rockville, MD, Aspen Publishers, 1988, pp 139-174.

Janda DH, Geringer SR, Hankin FM et al: Objective evaluation of grip strength. J Occup Med 22:332-336, 1987.

Jebsen RH et al: An objective and standardized test of hand function. Arch Phys Med Rehabil 50:311, 1969.

Jette AM: Desired characteristics of instruments to measure functional capacity to work. In Measuring Functional Capacity and Work Requirements, 1999, http://www.nap.edu/readingroom/books, accessed July 10, 2001.

Johnson EW: Editorial: residual functional capacity. J Back Musculoskeletal Rehabil 6:219-220, 1996.

Kaplan GM, Wurtele SK, Gillis D: Maximal effort during functional capacity evaluations: An examination of psychological factors. Arch Phys Med Rehabil 77(2):161-164, 1996.

Khalil TM, Goldberg ML, Asfour SS et al: Acceptable maximal effort (AME), A psychophysical measure of strength in back pain patients. Spine 12:372-376, 1987.

King PM, Tuckwell N, Barrett TE: A critical review of functional capacity evaluations, Low Back Pain Special Series. Phys Ther 78(8):852-866, 1998.

King PM: Analysis of approaches to the detection of sincerity of effort through grip strength measurement. Work 10:9-13, 1998.

Key GL: Functional Capacity Evaluation in Industrial Therapy. St Louis, Mosby, 1995, pp 220-253.

Kraus J: The independent medical examination and the functional capacity evaluation. Occup Med 12(3):525-556, 1997.

Krause N, Dasinger LK, Deegan LJ et al: Psychosocial job factors and return-to-work after compensated low back injury: A disability phase-specific analysis. Am J Industrial Med 40(4):374-392, 2001.

LaCerte M, Desjardins L: Evaluation of work disability from a worker-work environment perspective. In Shrey DE, La Certe M (eds): Principles and Practices of Disability Management in Industry. Winter Park, FL, 1995, pp207-221.

Lechner DE, Bradburg SF, Bradley LA: Detecting sincerity of effort: A summary of methods and approaches. Phys Ther 78:867-888, 1998.

Lechner D, Roth D, Straaton K: Functional capacity evaluation in work disability. Work 1(3):37-47, 1991.

Lechner DE, Jackson JR, Roth D: Reliability and validity of a newly developed test of physical work performance. J Occup Med 36:9:997-1004, 1994.

Lemstra M, Olszynski WP, Enright W: The sensitivity and specificity of functional capacity evaluations in determining maximal effort: A randomized trial. Spine 29(9):953-959, 2004.

Livneh H: Psychosocial adaptation to chronic illness and disability: A conceptual framework. Rehabil Couns Bull 44(3):151-160, 2001.

Martin SE: Functional capacity evaluations, The Physical Medicine Review. Physical Medicine Research Foundation (PMRF), 3-11, 2000.

Mather JH: The problem of functional assessment: Political and economic perspectives. Am J Occup Ther 47:240-246, 1993.

Matheson LN: Functional capacity evaluation. In Demter SL, Andersson GBJ, Smith GM (eds): Disability Evaluation. St Louis, Mosby, and the American Medical Association, 2002, pp 168-187.

Matheson LN: Work capacity evaluation for occupational therapists. Orange, CA, Rehabilitation Institute of Southern California, 1982.

Matheson LN: Evaluation of lifting and lowering capacity. Vocational Work Adjustment Bull Fall:107-111, 1986.

Matheson LN: How do you know he tried his best? The reliability crisis in industrial rehabilitation. Indust Rehabil Q1(1):1-11, 1988.

Matheson LN, Kaskutas V, McCowans et al: Development of a database of functional assessment measures related to work disability. J Occup Environ Health 44(7):628-633, 2001.

Menard MR, Hoens AM: Objective evaluation of functional capacity: Medical, occupational, and legal settings. J Orthop Sports Phys Ther 19(5):249-260, 1994.

Miller M: Functional assessments: A vital component of work injury management. Work 1:6-10, 1991.

McGurrin MC: An overview of the effectiveness of traditional vocational rehabilitation services in the treatment of long-term mental illness. Psychosocial Rehabil 17(3):37-56, 1994.

MTM Association for Standards and Research, Des Plaines, IL, http://www:MTM.org, accessed June 28, 2004.

Nagi SZ: Disability concepts revisited. In Pope AM, Tarlov AR (eds): Disability in America: Toward a National Agenda. Washington, DC, National Academy Press, 1993, pp 309-327.

Niebuhr BR, Marion R: Detecting sincerity of effort when measuring grip strength. Am J Phys Med 66:16-23, 1987.

National Institute for Occupational Safety and Health: Work Practices Guide for Manual Lifting, US Public Health Service Publication No. 81-122, Washington, DC, US Government Printing Office, 1981.

Owens P: The use of functional capacity measures in public and private programs in the United States and in other countries. In Measuring Functional Capacity and Work Requirements, Washington, DC, National Academy Press, 1991, http://www.nap.edu/readingroom/books, accessed July 10, 2001.

Owens LA, Buckholtz RL: Functional capacity assessment: Worker evaluation strategies, and the disability management process. In Shrey DE & Lacerte M (eds): Principles and Practices of Disability Management in Industry. Winter Park, FL, GR Press, 1995, pp 269-301.

Pransky GS, Dempsey PG: Practical aspects of functional capacity evaluations. J Occup Rehabil 14(3):217-229, 2004.

Randolph DC: Use of functional employment testing to facilitate safe job placement. Occup Med 15(4):813-821, 2000.

Richman J: Focusing on abilities. Phys Med Rehabil Foundation Rev Summer:5-7, 1997.

Rucker KS, Wehman P, Kregel J: Analysis of functional assessment instruments for disability/rehabilitation programs, Social Security Administration, Washington, DC, SSA Contract No. 600-95-21914, Department of Physical and Medical Rehabilitation, Medical College of Virginia, Virginia Commonwealth University, July 18,1996.

Robinson ME, Geisser ME, Hanson CS et al: Detecting submaximal efforts in grip strength testing with the coefficient of variation. J Occup Rehabil 3:45-50, 1993.

Ruan CM, Haig AJ, Geisser ME et al: Functional capacity evaluations in persons with spinal disorders: Predicting poor outcomes on the Functional Assessment Screening Test (FAST). J Occup Rehabil 11(2):119-132, 2001.

Schechtman O: Is the coefficient of variation a valid measure for detecting sincerity of effort or grip strength? Work J 13:163-169, 1999.

Shaw WS, Pransky G, Fitzgerald TE: Early prognosis for low back disability: Intervention strategies for health care providers. Disabil Rehabil 23:18, 815-828, 2001.

Shrey DE: Worksite disability management in industrial rehabilitation: An overview. In Shrey DE, LaCerte M (eds): Principles and Practices of Disability Management in Industry. Winter Park, FL, GR Press, 1995, p 8.

Simonsen JC: Validation of sincerity of effort. J Back Musculoskel Rehabil 6:289-295, 1996.

Smith RL: Therapist's ability to identify safe maximum lifting in low back pain patients during functional capacity evaluation. J Orthop Sports Phys Ther 19(5):277-281, 1994.

Smith SL, Cunningham S, Weinberg R: The predictive validity of the functional capacities evaluation. Am J Occup Ther 40(8):564-567, 1986.

Social Security Administration: 2001: Measuring Functional Capacity and Work Requirements: Recurring Themes and Issues, http://www.hap.edu/readingroom/books/mfc/ch7.html, accessed October 15, 2001.

Stapleton D, Livermore G: Impairment trends in applications and awards from SSA's disability programs. Paper presented at the Social Security Administration's Disability Programs: Explanations of recent growth and implications for disability policy, Washington, DC, July 20-21, 1995.

Tiffen J: Purdue Pegboard Examiner's Manual. Science Research Associates, Chicago, 1968.

Turk DC, Rudy TE, Stieg RL: The disability determination dilemma: Toward a multiaxial solution. Pain (34):217-229, 1988.

US Department of Labor: Dictionary of Occupational Titles, 4th ed, Revised supplement. US Department of Labor, Employment and Training Administration, Appendix C, 1991.

US Department of Labor: O*Net, http://www.onetcenter.org/overview.htm, accessed June 27, 2004.

Velozo CA: Work evaluations: Critique of the art of functional assessment of work. Am J Occup Ther 47(3):203-209, 1993.

Velozo CA: Should occupational therapy choose a single functional outcome measure? Am J Occup Ther 48(10):946-947, 1994.

Vowles KE, Gross RT: Work-related beliefs about injury and physical capability for work in individuals with chronic pain. Pain J 101(3):291-298, 2003.

Wise D: The functional capacity evaluation summary report. Orthop Phys Ther Clin North Am 1(1):99-104, 1992.

World Health Organization: International Classification of Impairments, Disabilities and Handicaps: A Manual Relating to the Consequences of Disease, Vol. 41, 1993 reprint, Geneva, World Health Organization, original publication, 1980.

Wyman DO: Evaluating patients for return-to-work. Am Fam Phys 59(4):844-848, 1999.

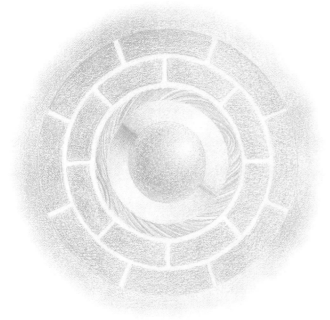

## CHAPTER 10

Utilization Review and Management

David W. Clifton, Jr., PT

"Terms like 'wasteful,' 'ineffective,' 'inappropriate,' 'of unproven effectiveness,' 'unnecessary,' and even 'irrational' are used loosely and interchangeably in the literature that is critical of current medical practice."

- Blustein J & Marmer TR, 1992

KEY POINTS

- Peer review is not synonymous with utilization review (UR) or utilization management (UM).
- UR is not synonymous with UM.
- UR, UM, and case management are all components of a comprehensive disability management program.
- Medical necessity and reasonable care determinations constitute core features of UR/UM.
- Both UR/UM compare and contrast an individual case or treatment episode with standards of care established through a variety of means, including curriculum, practice guidelines/standards, clinical literature, peer consensus, professional associations, and government agencies.
- Appropriate UR/UM decisions are made on the basis of objective evidence shared among stakeholders, not cloaked in a "black box " approach, defined by non-disclosure of review criteria.

Operational Definitions

Medical Necessity	Health care services that conform to acceptable treatment guidelines/standards and are appropriate to the patient's condition, location of service, and benefit plan.
Peer Review	A process in which one clinician (reviewer) examines the proposed or rendered treatment of another clinician (provider) of similar education, licensure, and experience. Peer review compares/contrasts individual treatment with community standards of care.
"Red Flags"	Issues related to a given case that give payers reason or cause to have a case reviewed. The presence of red flags does not in and of itself imply that care is medically unnecessary, unreasonable, or inappropriate.
Utilization Management	A proactive approach to care management that involves early communications with providers (e.g., precertification of service) that can alter the course of treatment as well as result in cost savings.
Utilization Review	A concurrent or retrospective approach to care management that typically involves a medical record review and does little to alter the course of clinical treatment.

OVERVIEW OF UTILIZATION REVIEW AND MANAGEMENT

UR and UM are universal components of any comprehensive disability management program. Virtually every provider at one time or another has had a medical record reviewed, fielded a question from a claims adjuster, received a visit from a case manager, or had a bill denied because of an external review process. Medical providers' knowledge and understanding of UR/UM principles and methodologies are often limited and reflect isolated experiences. Providers may possess a natural reflex to resent and thwart UR/UM interventions, partly due to a lack of understanding of the process. This response is especially likely if practice autonomy is threatened or the utilization process interferes with the provider-patient relationship.

Although UR/UM constantly evolve, the continued existence of some form of care analysis is certain. A thorough understanding of UR/UM can assist providers in becoming more effective disability managers, protecting their financial interests, ensuring practice autonomy, and representing their patients in an advocacy role. These are the goals of this chapter.

WHAT IS UTILIZATION REVIEW?

UR is "the process of assessing medical care services to assure quality, medical necessity, and appropriateness in terms of level of care and locus of treatment (Webber & Goldbeck, 1984). A sound UR program examines both overutilization and underutilization.

The initial boost for UR began in 1972 when Medicare mandated that each state select a "professional standards review organization." A second generation of UR resulted in "peer review organizations" (PROs). These organizations became the successors of professional standards review organizations in 1982 through the establishment of the Tax Equity and Fiscal Responsibility Act (TEFRA). These early Medicare-based peer review groups enjoyed little provider support because they were enacted by the federal government to control costs, not necessarily to improve the quality of care.

In 1983 Congress enacted the Medicare prospective payment system that changed the mission of PROs from exclusively looking at overutilization or costs to assessing quality of care issues as well. This paradigm shift represented construction of a major bridge between utilization "review" and utilization "management." Ironically, medical societies themselves became PROs under Medicare. PROs are now known as QIOs, or quality improvement organizations.

UR and UM both target healthcare costs, but they use different methodologies at different points along the injury and illness continuum (Figure 10-1). The earliest UR programs focused on hospital-associated costs and have intensified scrutiny of outpatient services only in the past decade or so (Feldstein et al, 1988). This scrutiny is partly the result of reduced hospital length of stay (LOS) and the concomitant surge in outpatient services.

UR fundamentally involves focused medical record review. This review is accomplished through a retrospective or concurrent analysis. The payer retains a UR agent or conducts an internal audit to establish whether or not services were medically necessary and reasonable.

Retrospective review is conducted after treatment has concluded and typically does not involve reviewer-provider dialogue. Given its forensic nature, this form of UR does little or nothing to influence the course of treatment. Retrospective review can result in a sentinel effect on providers, however, when they learn that their services are on the payer's radar screen. Since retrospective review does not alter the treatment course, it tends to focus primarily on the cost of services. A reviewer's opinion may encourage the payer to either deny (partially or fully) or accept the provider's reimbursement request. However, final reimbursement decisions always reside with the payer, not the reviewer.

Concurrent review involves review of medical records while care continues. Concurrent review is typically triggered by the presence of one or more "red flags." Red flags are also referred to in the UR business as "edits," "screens," or "thresholds." Peer review red flags are intended to serve as a means of identifying those cases that should be considered for a peer review. Red flags attempt to identify cases that appear inconsistent with some aspect of the community standard of care. Results of the actual peer review should be derived through an evidence-based approach. Red flags are varied and typically fall within a given category.

Categories and Examples of Red Flags

1. *Provider credentials:* protracted physical therapy is rendered by supportive personnel without evidence of physical therapist supervision.
2. *Treatment cost:* the per-visit cost of rehabilitation exceeds the usual-customary-reasonable (UCR) amount, or the total case cost exceeds an expected range.
3. *Clinical intervention:* the selected intervention is inappropriate for the patient's condition (e.g., extended use of palliative modalities of unproven efficacy in chronic low back treatment).
4. *Length of stay (LOS):* the total number of visits exceeds the expected duration of service for a condition (e.g., 68 visits for lumbar strain, compared with 6 to 12 visits across all providers).

Figure 10-1. Injury or illness continuum.

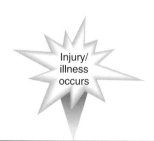

Injury/ illness occurs

Prevention	Treatment/management	Forensics
• Injury	• Clinical care	• Retrospective review
• Illness	• Preauthorization	• Independent medical evaluations
• Impairment	• Concurrent review	• Disability determinations
• Disability	• Case management	• Medicolegal services

Table 10–1 Rehabilitation Red Flags

1. Paucity or absence of medical documentation.
2. Patient fails to make significant, functional progress in a predictable or reasonable time frame.
3. Provider fails to document functional improvement, focusing on pain only.
4. Treatment did not require "skilled services."
5. The frequency of treatment was excessive for the condition and its severity.
6. Treatment was not specific to the patient's admitting diagnosis(es)
7. Extended use of "palliative" modalities beyond acceptable norms.
8. Services were "maintenance" in nature.
9. The patient's condition plateaued.
10. Non-supervision of supportive or assistive personnel.
11. Absence or vagueness of treatment goals.
12. Treatment continues unmodified for protracted period.
13. Poor or low patient compliance.
14. Unexplained significant lapse in treatment (e.g., > 2weeks).
15. Treatment commence without any evidence of an initial evaluation.
16. Reevaluation of the patient's condition is not done on a regular basis (e.g., 30-day intervals).
17. Evidence of concurrent treatment between providers, (e.g., physical therapy).
18. Duplication of services between similar or different providers.
19. Duplication of treatment interventions (e.g., use of two heating agents).
20. Excessive fees relative to the usual customary and reasonable standards.

5. *Treatment setting:* provision of inpatient therapy for a condition that is routinely managed via home care or outpatient therapy.
6. *Clinical documentation:* a paucity of weekly visit notes that justify ongoing service.

Unlike retrospective review, concurrent review can partially influence the course, duration, and cost of health care services. A provider may redirect, expand, or reduce his or her treatment after a concurrent review. Reviewers may suggest an alternate treatment pathway that is grounded in the clinical literature and represents a community standard of care. Some providers welcome this input and others are offended by the apparent intrusion into the provider-patient relationship (Table 10–1).

Preauthorization of services

Preauthorization or precertification of service falls under the utilization management label, not utilization review. Preauthorization of service occurs after a patient has been evaluated, but before hands-on care is rendered. Preauthorization can be conducted through several mechanisms. Providers can directly contact a payer through interactive voice response (IVR). IVR requires a provider to navigate a series of computer-based or telephone-based queries to determine whether proposed care falls within pre-established guidelines. When care meets coverage criteria, an affirmative response is given. When proposed services are inconsistent with established guidelines, care may be denied or provisionally certified or the case is referred for additional review. Cases that have attributes falling outside of accepted ranges may be routed to a reviewer with a medical background. This typically includes nurses, physicians, and therapists. Telefax and electronic mail transmission of preauthorization requests represent additional vehicles.

Contractual Obligations

The following section does not constitute legal advice but rather general information that may assist providers in understanding how reimbursement decisions are made and by whom. When in doubt, consult with a qualified legal representative.

It is helpful to understand the contractual relationships that exist between the patient, the payer, and the UR organization (URO). A patient may have a contractual relationship with his or her employer for the provision of health care benefits. In cases such as workers' compensation, benefits are required by state law. The employer may have a contractual relationship with an insurance company or managed care organization (MCO) for the provision of general health, disability, or life insurance benefits. The patient and provider may have two contractual relationships between them: a business relationship and professional or clinical relationship. Last, the URO may be retained by the employer, insurance company, or managed care firm. Self-insured or self-funded employers may directly contract with UROs without the intercession of an insurance company. These relationships determine the responsibilities of each party and dictate with which entities a health care provider can discuss a specific issue. For instance, generally it is not an accepted practice for a URO to communicate directly with the patient. It is critical for providers to understand that UROs do not technically deny reimbursement of services; they simply provide a recommendation to the insurer or MCO. These latter entities then determine whether to pay a particular provider. If they agree with the URO that care was medically unnecessary, inappropriate, or unreasonable for a given condition, they may elect to partially or completely deny reimbursement. The insurer or MCO is not bound by a reviewer's professional opinion, however.

Providers are often in the position of defending their care for reimbursement purposes. They must be mindful of the proper appeal mechanisms to carry the right message to the right party.

Finally, UROs generally have no formal contract with either the patient or the provider unless they also serve as the payer. Many MCOs have an internal UR program and do not use external or third-party reviewers (Figure 10–2 and Table 10–2).

Utilization Review Versus Utilization Management

The mechanisms of UR and UM substantially differ and are contrasted in Table 10–3. Perhaps the greatest distinction centers on time. UR tends to be forensic or after the fact. and UM often begins with preauthorization of care. This process is also known as precertification or preadmission authorization.

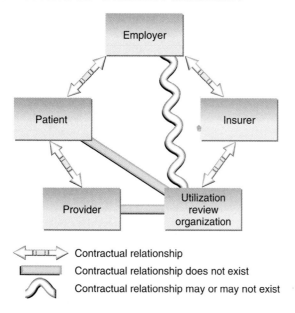

⟨▭▭▷ Contractual relationship

▭▭ Contractual relationship does not exist

⋀⋀ Contractual relationship may or may not exist

Figure 10–2. Patient–provider–payee relationship.

Table 10–3 Utilization Review Versus Utilization Management Comparison

Utilization Review	Utilization Management
Primarily retrospective	Primarily prospective
Little/no provider profiling	Frequent provider profiling
No direction of care	Direction of care
Weak/no case management	Strong case management
Focus on cost	Focus on "value" or cost benefit
Income-driven (overutilization)	Outcome-driven (overutilization and underutilization
Primarily written record review	Telephonic/live case management
Case-by-case review	Case-by-case pattern analysis
Review criteria kept in "black box"	Disclosure of review criteria
No participation in practice guideline development	Collaboration in practice guideline development
Minimal dialogue with provider	Frequent reviewer-provider dialogue

Data from Clifton DW: A shift toward utilization management. PT Magazine 3(6):32-35, 1995a.

Provider Profiling

Provider profiling is another major distinction between UR and UM. Provider profiling is the act of comparing the services of an individual provider with aggregate data collected from a comparative group of providers. An individual provider's treatment and cost data are compared with that of a group across zip codes, treatment settings, or conditions. A URO or payer may also compare the individual therapist's data to their so-called "preferred provider group."

Provider organizations such as independent practitioner associations or outcome measurement entities may compare individual with group data as part of a peer review or quality assurance program.

UR is generally devoid of provider profiling because clinical data have been provided after the fact or post-treatment. When providers submit data after the commencement of services as in a medical record review, provider information tends to show great variability. This variability challenges any attempts at meaningful comparisons after concurrent or retrospective review. On the contrary, UM generates multiaxial comparisons of data that are useful for comparison between providers. These data may include clinical and financial information. For instance, a provider's average treatment visit number for a specific ICD-9 diagnostic code may be compared with aggregate data collected on a group of providers.

Outcome measures, or daily visit costs, are other parameters that can be used in provider profiling.

Figure 10–3 depicts a provider-profiling construct based on a pattern analysis of two parameters: medical costs and duration of care in visits. Providers who fall in the lower left quadrant A of this schematic may be considered as the most desirable from a cost standpoint because both their costs and visit number are lowest. These providers may be invited by payers to participate in "preferred provider" networks that are principally cost-driven. Many workers' compensation preferred provider organizations (PPOs) operate within this cost-based paradigm, typically through fee discounts (e.g., 15% discount from the UCR fees).

The least desirable providers from a cost/visit standpoint are those located in the upper right quadrant C of the schematic," because both visit count and costs are highest for this group. These providers are most likely to undergo intensive UR or preauthorization and are not likely participants in preferred networks.

Providers in the left quadrant B may be viewed as "centers of excellence" because although their fees are relatively high, they are more efficient, at least in terms of disability duration. Their LOS in visit duration is significantly lower. Providers in quadrant D may be desirable to payers from a medical cost per visit standpoint, but in reality their aggregate cost may be driven higher by extended treatment.

Notably absent from this two-dimensional model is the clinical outcome achieved by all providers. When outcomes

Table 10–2 Party Responsibilities

Patient	Provider	Payer	Reviewer
Make co-payments	Render medically necessary, reasonable, and appropriate care	Provide health care benefits which are medically necessary, reasonable, and appropriate	Provide an unbiased independent opinion about medically necessary, reasonable, and appropriate care
Meet deductibles	Maintain adequate records and provide them to payer or payer agent (e.g., a URO)	Deny medically unnecessary, unreasonable, and inappropriate care	Apply clinical literature and community standards to specific cases

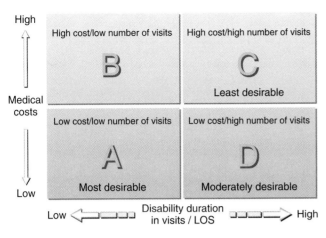

Figure 10–3. Provider profiling quadrant.

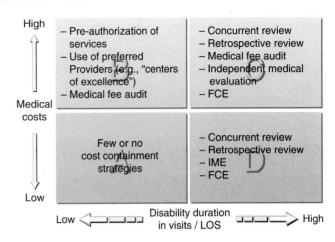

Figure 10–4. UR/UM application quadrant.

are factored into the equation, provider reassignment to different quadrants is probable. This three-dimensional model can be labeled "days, dollars, and disability." This model is discussed later in the chapter.

UM facilitates the collection of more reliable outcome measures when entry-level data elements are standardized. UR, on the other hand, involves a "catch as catch can" approach to data collection. Clinical documentation under UR is typically fragmented, non-standardized, and not easily compared on a provider-to-provider basis. Retrospective record review is devoid of the data standardization enjoyed by prospective strategies that require specific data elements to successfully navigate the preauthorization gauntlet. The development of accepted treatment protocols and review criteria foster pattern analysis because of the uniformity of data element collection. Accurate data collection, analysis, and application reduce the likelihood of the "black box" approach to care review often alleged during UR. A "black box" approach describes reviews in which the reviewer or URO fails to explain the methodology of data collection, analysis, and application or the review criteria that these data generated. A "black box" approach to review can occur when an individual record undergoes an evidence-based review to determine whether services were medically necessary and reasonable, or when care is precertified on the basis of a pattern analysis of similar cases.

Pattern analysis, unlike individual record review, involves data analysis across groups (e.g., patient or provider). Pattern analysis allows payers and providers alike to establish critical pathways of care or "best practices" "on the basis of standardized data submitted by "preferred providers." These data can then be shared with network providers so that treatment expectations are better understood. Although UR can involve an evidence-based approach, it typically only looks at one case at a time unlike the pattern analysis of UM (Figure 10–4).

WHAT IS UTILIZATION MANAGEMENT?

"UM is defined as the evaluation of quality, outcomes, and efficiency of services (Carpenter, 1992). UM addresses quality and cost or "value purchasing." UM is proactive and deliberately attempts to alter the course of care before or during delivery to assure quality and appropriate outcomes. UM tends to be more intrusive on the provider-patient relationship than UR. As a result it can serve as both a sword and shield to providers. UM is a shield when it leads to good outcomes without compromising provider incomes. When a provider has their care preauthorized, UM conceivably serves as a risk management tool from both a financial and legal perspective. Preauthorization of services avoids retroactive denial of care after providers have expended both human and capital resources.

When a provider's reimbursement is scaled back or completely denied, however, UM becomes a sword. UM decisions may result in non-authorized treatment, or reduce provider revenue. Under a worst case scenario UM may lead to termination of a provider from a payer's network.

'DAYS, DOLLARS, AND DISABILITY'

UR and UM are increasingly used in the private sector as cost containment measures. Two elements have been fundamental drivers of UR/UM: the high cost of health care and treatment overutilization. In recent years, outcomes measurements have entered the picture. These three factors have been referred to as "days, dollars, and disability" (Clifton, 1997). This triad represents the most salient issues that must be addressed to execute a comprehensive disability management system (Table 10–4).

Utilization rates, or "days," refer to the number of visits, LOS, or intensity of service required during an episode of care. Many persons equate high cost to a high number of visits or protracted LOS, when in reality the intensity of the service fundamentally drives cost, especially in a fee-for-service environment. Intensity of service involves the number of interventions provided during a visit.

"Dollars" obviously describes the costs associated with a unit of care or visit. Aggregate costs for a diagnostic category, treatment setting, or provider group are often considered in the development of reimbursement or coverage policies by payers. Dollars are managed through a variety of mechanisms that range from direct rate setting to indirect reductions associated with visit controls.

Table 10-4 Days, Dollars, and Disability

Days	Dollars	Disability
Provider selection	Co-payments/ deductibles	Insured selection
	Fee discounts	
	Fee schedules	
	Fee audits	
Capitation	Capitation	
Single service		
Global		
Case rates	Case rates	Case rates
Episodic rates	Episodic rates	Episodic rates
Facility benchmarking	Facility benchmarking	Facility benchmarking
Precertification	Precertification	
Concurrent review	Concurrent review	Concurrent review
	Retrospective review	
	Code rebundling	
		Disability ratings examinations
		Independent medical examinations
		Functional capacity evaluations
		Clinical outcomes

Data from Clifton DW: Days, dollars and disability: The three dimensions of utilization. Case Review 3(3):81-85, 1997.

Treatment and diagnostic codes or both can be rebundled or collapsed, thereby restricting reimbursement. This occurs when the payer or auditing firm combines codes that are believed to be too similar to warrant additional reimbursements.

"Disability" refers to the individual's degree of functioning as a result of a therapeutic intervention. Disability status is frequently influenced by non-medical issues such as psychosocial or economic factors. These are covered in great detail in Chapter 7. Key issues or terms contained within each component of the triad are defined in the glossary section of the Appendix. The number of days associated with care can be controlled primarily through provider behaviors. The initial selection of preferred providers may be predicated on their willingness to accept specific treatment time frames and reimbursement levels. These time frames are further influenced by the reimbursement structure of care. Capitation or case rate reimbursement clearly places a premium on provider treatment efficiency. The more efficiently a provider manages the patient from admission to discharge, the greater the profitability of a given case. Clinical outcome data tied to visit number allows payers to profile providers and benchmark facilities. For instance, a provider or facility can be compared with community standards when ICD-9 diagnostic codes are attached to visit number. Although this is an imperfect system for gauging quality of care, it nevertheless is a common approach.

Disability rates can be controlled through insured selection and placement procedures after injury or illness. Disability duration or length can also be indirectly influenced through reimbursement structures such as episodic or case rates. A person's disability status is determined through independent medical examinations, functional capacity evaluations, or disability ratings examinations.

PREVALENCE OF UTILIZATION REVIEW/UTILIZATION MANAGEMENT

At least 300 private sector UR organizations, 50 Medicare PROs, and hundreds of managed care plans conduct UR (GAO, 1992). Treatment variation has been acknowledged for years as a prime driver of rising health care costs (Chassin et al, 1986; Lewis, 1969; Roos & Roos, 1982; Wennberg & Gittlesohn, 1982). Treatment variation has a number of progenitors, including severity indices, insurance coverage, technology investments, patient population differences, medical staff availability, different regional costs of doing business, and a host of other variables too numerous to mention. Certain regions of the country have much higher or lower utilization rates, costs or disability payouts than others. A seminal study conducted by the RAND corporation found significant variation within 123 medical and surgical procedures in 13 metropolitan locations (Chassin et al, 1986). In extreme instances, utilization rates for certain procedures were three times higher in some areas when compared with others.

In a supplier-driven or demand-creation system, providers are in a position to determine cost, utilization, and disability rates regardless of patient elements. For instance, a relationship may exist between carpal tunnel release procedures and a new surgeon in town. This situation raises an obvious question. *Is the carpal tunnel release rate indicative of the patient population's clinical needs or the surgeon's financial needs?* Although this question may seem to take a cynical view of treatment, associations such as these have been established secondary to data analysis.

Paradoxically, treatment variation may be viewed by providers as a necessary extension of the art of medicine. However, treatment variation in the view of payers may demand explanation and, ultimately, standardization. It cannot be debated that UM interventions are directly driven by a lack of professional norms for appropriate care and treatment variation (Wolff & Schlesinger, 1999). UR and UM will continue to flourish if providers collectively fail to use evidence-based treatment interventions. The introduction of new technologies, whether good or bad, encourages scrutiny until techniques becomes the "gold standard." Even then some degree of review will take place of providers who may abuse or misuse a proven technique. Providers need to appreciate that not only so-called "questionable" treatments or diagnoses receive scrutiny, but also well-established ones. Table 10-5 provides a sample listing of rehabilitation conditions that often warrant scrutiny. This listing includes both controversial and non-controversial conditions. Insurance companies and UROs often include legitimate conditions that unequivocally require rehabilitation in "red flag" lists that trigger review.

For example, conventional wisdom holds that persons with reconstructed anterior cruciate ligaments (ACLs) will require protracted treatment. A typical treatment protocol could include different stages of treatment during a period of 9 to 12 months, especially for elite athletes or those who must return to "heavy duty."

Figure 10-5 illustrates a grouping of hypothetical ACL cases before and after UR. Both the median cost and visit values have been reduced secondary to UR strategies.

Table 10-5	Commonly Reviewed Medical Conditions

Low back pain
Whiplash associated disorders
Traumatic brain injury
Carpal tunnel syndrome
Reflex sympathetic dystrophy
Thoracic outlet syndrome
Fibromyalgia, myositis, fibromyositis
Chronic fatigue syndrome
Temporomandibular joint dysfunction or disorder
Posttraumatic stress disorder
Headache syndromes
Spinal subluxation
Sprains and strains
Fractures
Contusions
Postural syndromes

Despite recent advances in surgical technique, rehabilitation processes, and donor graft selection, few would argue that significant rehabilitation is medically necessary and reasonable. Imagine for a moment a patient entering a facility known to consistently exceed treatment norms both in cost and duration. Despite a legitimate diagnosis and anticipated protracted course of therapy, the case may be precertified and undergo a concurrent or retrospective record review because of the facility's reputation and history.

This level of scrutiny in a capitated plan would in all likelihood not be required, but under workers' compensation and fee-for-service it may be mandated. UR has been described as a "rationalization of clinical practice" through two mechanisms: reducing variance in clinical procedures so that they fall within professional norms, and pushing the entire distribution of clinical practices to the left of central tendency (Gold et al, 1995). These mechanisms are known as the "standardization" strategy that is used by

reviewers and providers alike to reduce practice variation and to profile providers (Figure 10-5, *A*) and Figure 10-5, *B*, depicts this shift in a hypothetical ACL diagnosis.

Virtually all of the 60 million enrollees in prepaid (capitated) plans are covered by external review to some degree (Gold et al, 1995). In some benefit structures waste or unnecessary care can consume as much as 25% of total costs (Berman, 1991).

Physical rehabilitation has risen high on the radar screens of many insurers and UROs and will continue to do so with the aging of the population and the chronic conditions that call for these services. A number of high-profile studies and stories have heightened interest in standardization of physical rehabilitation practices (National Council on Compensation Insurance, 1994; Workers' Compensation Research Institute, 1994; Government Accounting Office, 1994; Miller, 1994; Office of Inspector General, 1994).

In prepaid programs based on capitation, the shift in UR/UM is from overutilization to underutilization. Providers are more prone to undertreat when they are financially rewarded for "doing less compared with fee-for-service," which rewards "doing more" (Clifton 1996b). This situation is regrettable, because it is ethical to treat all cases equally regardless of reimbursement schemes. We are dealing with a sector that has become big business, however.

A Government Accounting Office report of 1995 concerning alleged overutilization and fraudulent billing practices under Medicare partly contributed to the largest-ever federal fraud and abuse initiative, "Operation Restore Trust" (Government Accounting Office, 1995).

Reports such as this have led to vigorous initiatives geared at balancing costs and benefits. A plethora of UM strategies have emerged in an attempt to reduce treatment variation or to standardize care. Additionally, these

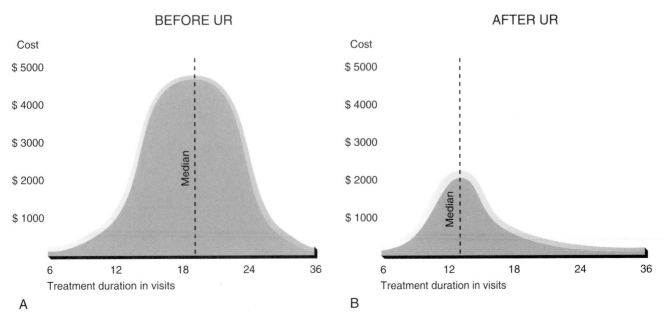

Figure 10-5. A and **B,** Hypothetical clinical practice shifts due to utilization review.

Table 10-6   Most Commonly Used Utilization Management Strategies

- Insured selection
- Insured co-payments/deductible
- Provider selection: credentialing/recredentialing
- Fee discounts
- Capitation
- Case or episodic rates
- Disease state management
- Provider profiling
- Facility benchmarking
- Case management
- Disability examinations
- Independent medical examinations
- Medical fee audits
- Provider withholds
- Preauthorization or precertification
- Prospective-concurrent-retrospective review
- Code rebundling or collapsing
- Functional capacity evaluations
- Collaboration in development of practice guidelines or treatment protocols
- Provider education
- Patient/consumer education

strategies have been used on a case-specific basis to trim costs (Table 10-6).

KEY CONCEPTS IN UR/UM

"Peer Review"

The terms "peer review" and "UR" are often used as synonyms by those in the provider, payer, and UR sectors. These terms may or may not be interchangeable, depending on program design. Some may think of a voluntary, blinded, institution-based (e.g., a hospital) assessment of a practitioner's performance when they hear "peer review." In this context, peer review is "a process that examines and evaluates the standards of care among staff members of similar levels of experience" (Wainwright et al, 1992). Institutionally based or internal review is not ordinarily used for reimbursement purposes, however, but principally for continuous quality improvement.

For the sake of this discussion, "peer review" involves an external review process in which the payer retains a reviewer to assess the care given by a similar or similarly licensed and experienced practitioner. Throughout most of the 1970s and 1980s, the UR industry did not engage in a "like reviewing like" process (e.g., an occupational therapist reviewing an occupational therapist). As a result, many claims were denied with no review of the pertinent patient and treatment data by a qualified professional. Regrettably, under this system many claims were denied without due process. This strategy was used during the era of UR when little regulation and few professional standards existed. Now a majority of states require a "true peer review" process before a claim can be denied.

Levels of Review

Some payers, case management firms, and UROs continue to use administrative staff or nurses for Level I or II

screening, but secure the opinion of a peer before officially denying a claim at Level III or IV. Level I screening is a stage during which a submitted claim form is reviewed to determine whether it is a "clean claim." A clean claim is one in which the patient is determined to be insured, the documentation is complete, and the provider is a preferred or network provider. In Level II a nurse typically reviews the clinical records and compares them with "screens" or "red flag" lists. Screens are specific thresholds used to determine whether care is medically necessary and reasonable. These screens or "red flags" may include utilization data (e.g., number of visits, LOS), specific treatment interventions (e.g., experimental, non-efficacious), dollar amounts (e.g., costs exceeding the UCR range), or they may contain specific provider information. Claims are not denied at levels I or II or until a peer review process has occurred (Level III) (Table 10-7).

Many states have enacted external review committees (Level IV) to review cases that have been appealed by providers after denial. These committees are typically formed under the auspices of a state health or insurance department or agency. Figure 10-6 illustrates the flow of a case through various UR levels including the appeal processes.

Providers who demand a true peer review should be prepared for the consequences. Although no unequivocal evidence exists to prove it, peers potentially can be more demanding of their peers during case review. Some logical explanations for this observation are suggested in the following list:

1. Peers understand the body of literature and the "wool cannot be pulled over their eyes."
2. Peers know the tough questions to ask.
3. A peer may take personal and professional pride in their field and thus hold a provider to a higher standard than a non-peer.
4. The reviewer may be a practicing provider and because of their review work, he or she is closer to the literature and optimal practice.
5. Peer reviewers may overcompensate for the perception of payers that the "fox is guarding the chicken coop" or that they may "rubber stamp" their colleagues' care.

Some merit exists, however, in the argument that a peer may actually be softer on a colleague. It would be interesting to generate research with external and internal reviewers reviewing the same claims.

Table 10-7   Levels of Review

	Care approvals	Care denials	Non-medical staff	Medical staff
Level I	✓		✓	✓
Level II	✓			✓
Level III	✓	✓		✓
Level IV	✓	✓		✓

NOTE: Level III is typically a function of a utilization review organization (URO). Level IV is external to the URO and typically a statutory mechanism, independent panel of reviewers or adjudicators.

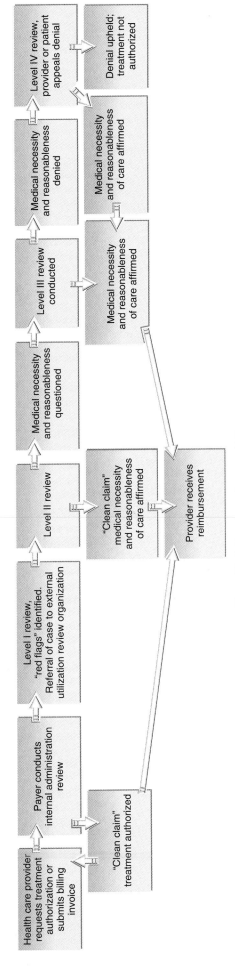

Figure 10-6. Flowchart of a general UR process.

Medical Necessity

Medical necessity is at the very core of UR and UM activities. The determination of the medical necessity and appropriateness of care is more critical than interventions that focus solely on cost containment (Berman, 1991; Geisel, 1989; Jacobson et al, 1997). Cost-containment mechanisms include provider fee schedules, code rebundling, repricing of claims, capitation payments, provider discounts, and case or episodic rates.

"Medical necessity" is a highly controversial concept that elicits both positive and negative responses. This term has both a medical and a legal connotation, and as such it is hotly debated by multiple health care stakeholders. For instance, the patient may perceive that any care that helps his or her problem is medically necessary even if it is "experimental" or expensive. Payers may view experimental care as medically unnecessary. Providers may believe that any care that is supported by clinical literature and community practice standards must be medically necessary, regardless of what a patient's health insurance benefits cover.

Consequently, "medical necessity" is an ambiguous term and subject to numerous confusing and often contradictory medical and legal interpretations (Gold, 1999; Charles, 1997). One highly regarded health care attorney refers to "medical necessity" as "a woefully inadequate phrase to describe an appropriate standard or performance" (Gosfield, 1991).

Table 10-8 illustrates the different domains from which interpretations of medical necessity emanate. Providers are advised to attempt to understand the paradigm from which a given health care stakeholder views medically necessary care.

The following definition of medical necessity may be useful to providers who wish to understand the standards against which their services are be compared. As previously stated, no universally accepted definition exists because of the various medical and legal interpretations of the term. For the purpose of this chapter, the following definition is provided.

Medically necessary care constitutes any service or supply used to identify or treat illness or injury which is appropriate to the patient's diagnosis, consistent with the location of the service, and with the level or intensity of care provided. The service should be widely accepted by the practicing peer group as a community standard of care and should be based on scientific criteria. The service may not be of an experimental, investigative, or research nature and it should be reasonably safe to administer.

 Table 10–8   Domains of "Medical Necessity"

Domain	Perception
Medical	Whatever is supported by clinical literature, prevailing practice, or curriculum
Legal	Case law, regulations, legislation
Benefit structure	Health insurance policy language
Financial	UCR fees, high outlier costs
Patient	Whatever works, at any cost
Societal	Whatever society can afford, but with equal access for all

Reasonable and Appropriate Care

Once the medical necessity for service is established, it must then be determined whether the care is reasonable and appropriate. These two terms have a diverse meaning, because they too describe value from a clinical point of view, the individual's or patient's perspective, and the viewpoint of society at large (Sharpe, 1996). Medical necessity establishes that the medical condition or diagnosis does indeed warrant treatment. The reasonable and appropriate care approach looks at other issues. Generally speaking, reasonable and appropriate treatment share the following attributes:

Reasonable and Appropriate Treatment Attributes

- Medical necessity for care has been established.
- Patient/client is covered under the insurance benefit.
- Treatment is consistent with the diagnosis.
- Treatment is consistent with peer or community standards.
- Treatment falls within a UCR fee range.
- Treatment is provided by an appropriately trained and credentialed person(s).
- Interventions were appropriate to the irritability stage of the illness/injury (e.g., acute-subacute-chronic).
- Treatment is rendered or proposed at the most appropriate locus.
- Frequency and duration of services is consistent with norms or exceptions explained by the clinical documentation.
- Clinical documentation supports treatment.
- Therapy goals are realistic and achievable.
- Care is restorative, not maintenance, in nature.
- Patient is in compliance with the program.
- Outcomes are appropriate to the diagnosis, goals, and treatment interventions.

Figure 10–7 depicts the critical thinking process that is required of both providers and reviewers if they are to establish the medical necessity of and reasonableness of care, and ultimately, reduce treatment variation.

The proof of medical necessity and reasonableness of care may be more a matter of sound documentation than of a medical litmus test per se (Figure 10–8).

Function is the keystone of rehabilitation clinical documentation if one is to satisfy the medical necessity and reasonable standards of care. Clinical records are subjected to intense scrutiny by reviewers during both retrospective and concurrent review. Peer reviewers routinely see substandard documentation that fails to support the initiation or continuation of services. This situation is unfortunate, especially in those cases in which the diagnosis or condition warrants care and the reviewer intuitively knows that rehabilitation is justifiable. The dictum for reviewing clinical documentation is that "if it is not documented, then it was not done." This philosophy of review flows from the traditional Medicare paradigm. In today's managed care environment, this philosophy has been expanded: "If it is documented poorly, it is non-reimbursable."

Table 10–9 provides a sampling of documentation entries received in the course of conducting physical rehabilitation peer review.

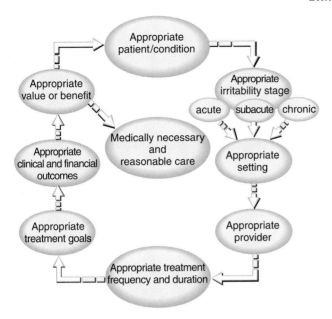

Figure 10–7. Medical necessity and reasonable care algorithm.

From Clifton DW: You be the reviewer! PT Magazine 4(7):34-37, 1996a.

Table 10–9   Sampler of Poor Rehabilitation Clinical Documentation

- "Knee some what swollen"
- "Slight discomfort"
- "ROM is 50% of normal"
- "Soft ultrasound"
- "Hard ultrasound"
- "Weak-firm-hard electrical stimulation"
- "Has made nice progress"
- "Still a lot of pain"
- "Gradual good progress"
- "Slow steady progress"
- "Patient has fair endurance to exercise"
- "40% strength achieved"
- "Patient reports that he is 20% better"
- "Problem is resolving" or "problem is resolved"
- "Limited in all planes"
- "Function limited by tightness"

An all-time favorite entry:

S: Cat died, patient upset
O: Ultrasound, massage, electrical stimulation
A: Doing better
P: Continue until maximum benefit achieved

ROM, Range of motion.

Sound clinical documentation is especially vital as patient's progress slows or becomes intermittent. This situation routinely occurs when tissues begin to achieve a state of healing or the condition leaves the acute phase of irritability. Figure 10-9 depicts a typical soft-tissue recovery curve.

This schematic shows rapid improvement in a patient's condition during the first 6 weeks. Progress then begins to taper off. This situation is known by a few terms: "patient plateaus," "maximum medical benefit," "maximum medical improvement," and "maintenance care." Provider justification of continued services is exponentially more difficult, because progress is relatively insignificant when compared with earlier gains. At this point in recovery a peer review is frequently triggered.

Medical Review Criteria

Medical review criteria or review sets represent quantitative and qualitative data used to guide the review process and lead to decisions about medical necessity, reasonableness, and appropriateness of care. Review criteria can be prospectively applied before actual care, concurrently or retrospectively. The Institute of Medicine gives the following definition of medical review criteria: "systematically developed statements that can be used to assess the appropriateness of specific health care decisions, services, and outcomes." (Institute of Medicine, 1990).

Figure 10–8. Documentation: The foundation of care.

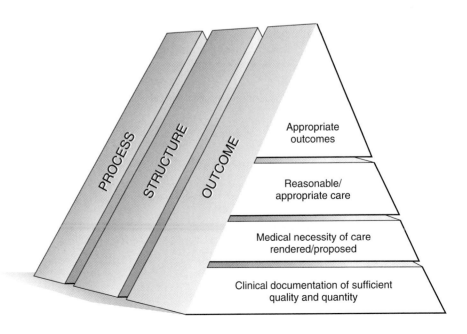

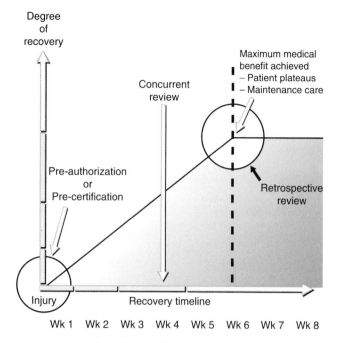

Degree of recovery

Concurrent review

Maximum medical benefit achieved
– Patient plateaus
– Maintenance care

Pre-authorization or Pre-certification

Retrospective review

Injury

Recovery timeline

Wk 1 Wk 2 Wk 3 Wk 4 Wk 5 Wk 6 Wk 7 Wk 8

Figure 10–9. Soft-tissue injury curve.

 Table 10–10 Sample Disability Duration Table

Example 1: By diagnosis/condition

Service	Rehabilitation
Condition	Sprains of joints, muscle strains
Frequency	3 times per week
Duration	2 weeks

Example 2: By procedure

Procedure	Functional activities
Time to produce outcome	2 to 4 treatments
Frequency	2 to 3 times per week
Duration	4 to 6 sessions

These instruments can but do not necessarily mirror clinical practice guidelines. Review criteria are typically either diagnosis-driven or procedure-driven. Examples of quantitative criteria include the number of visits for specific conditions, commonly referred to as "treatment" or "disability duration tables" and UCR fee schedules. These edits or screens as they are also known, compare a specific case with a normative database for similar diagnoses or treatment interventions. Some disability tables simply state an acceptable range or number of visits in a specific time frame or are treatment-based, assigning a specific number of applications per intervention. Comprehensive tables provide evaluation details, treatment protocols or plans, and criteria for additional visits. Disability or treatment tables can be poorly constructed, non-reflective of peer consensus, non-specific, and punitive in design (Clifton & Burcham, 1997). Medical review criteria are not typically used to make final reimbursement decisions. Rather they are guidelines developed to provide customary ranges for treatment and therefore should not be considered as absolutes. Review criteria are designed by a plethora of entities, including-third party administrators, insurance companies, provider organizations, government entities, professional societies, employee benefits firms, UROs, and health care software companies.

Well-designed tables have a primary goal of improving care and clinical outcomes. Criteria sets are developed through a number of methodologies including a retrospective analysis of closed or captive claims, literature searches, peer consensus documents, and controlled clinical trials. It is common for clinical practice guidelines to be amended for application by non-providers. Criteria are often written to conform to an 80/20 rule in which 80% of all reviewed cases pass through the screens, but only 20% actually undergo intense review (Clifton, 1995) (Table 10–10).

Some may view review criteria as "cookbook medicine" and others may appreciate them as guideposts. Concerns about criteria can be obviated through collaborative development involving providers and payers. Full disclosure also tends to quell protests among providers.

Providers owe it to themselves and their patients or clients to ask a series of specific questions when care is denied after the application of medical review criteria such as disability or treatment duration tables.

Provider Questions for Utilization Review Organizations

1. How were the disability duration table numbers derived? Are they based on a retroanalysis of claims data, peer consensus, a case manager's personal experience, or are they arbitrary?
2. How many cases make up your database?
3. Are cases adjusted for patient populations, severity, or provider type?
4. Which measures of central tendency or dispersion were used? Mean? Mode? Median?
5. Were other variables taken into consideration when denying care? Co-morbidities? Secondary diagnoses? Irritability stage? Psychosocial issues?
6. How do I appeal the denial?
7. Was a "peer review" ever conducted? If so, by whom? In which specialty? What body of knowledge or review criteria was used?

Satisfactory responses should be forthcoming; if they are not, an immediate appeal or reconsideration should be requested. Most state laws allow for the provider or patient to initiate the appeal process. A strong trend exists toward publication of the appeal process in the body of the denial or UR report.

Providers should be forewarned that some claims adjusters and case managers use these devices without a case-by-case or evidence-based record review. Disability or treatment duration tables are incredibly varied and no universal implement is in use (Clifton, 1997a). Again, tables should only be used to affirm payment of a particular treatment. Claims denial demands a more comprehensive approach and may include a medical record review, evidence-based judgments, and a telephonic review/consult with the provider or an independent examination of the patient. Disability duration tables alone cannot provide the objective evidence on which to base a claims denial. Unlike quantitative criteria such as disability tables, qualitative review criteria address issues such as provider credentials, locus of care, documentation requirements, and treatment protocols. Qualitative criteria tend to be proprietary medical review standards applied by a payer or URO.

SAMPLING OF REVIEW CRITERIA DEVELOPERS

- American Medical Association
- Appropriateness evaluation protocol
- Blue Cross/Blue Shield
- Government agencies [e.g., the Agency for Health Care Policy and Research (now the Agency for Health Care Quality and Research [AHCQR]), Health Care Financing Agency (HCFA), and the National Institutes of Health]
- Interqual
- Intensity of service, severity of illness, and discharge screens—appropriateness
- Milliman and Robertson
- National Health Services
- National Medical Audit
- Optimed
- Pace Company/Pace Healthplan Management
- State workers' compensation systems
- Value Health Sciences
- Workability/CORE

Some of these criteria sets were developed with input from physical rehabilitation providers or their professional associations, but it is safe to conclude that a significant number were not. Some criteria sets have their genesis in purely actuarial analysis.

Review Criteria Disclosure

A vociferous complaint that providers often have about UROs involves the "black box" approach to claims review. Under this scenario, review criteria are made available to the reviewer only and are essentially off limits to the provider or patient. In defense of this secrecy, UROs often claim they are unable to share review criteria with providers because of the proprietary nature and development costs of this information. Or they may assert that if review criteria are disclosed to providers, providers will "game" the system or "upcode" to maximize reimbursement. To some this may appear to be a cynical view, to others, good business practice.

One could argue that on the contrary, when providers are aware of review criteria, they responsibly mete out appropriate amounts of care. This is especially true if providers know that radar exists in the form of peer review. In fact, many independent provider networks operate on a full disclosure basis to standardize care. These networks operate quality assurance UR committees or panels. Still others may suspect that when asked to reveal their medical review criteria, UROs and case management firms have none to show or use arbitrary and indefensible data.

For review criteria to be meaningful, they must be accepted by the target group, especially if quality assurance is a desired goal. Readers are directed to Chapter 11 for a discussion of a precertification program under workers' compensation.

Review criteria must undergo rigors similar to practice standards. A logical first step may involve an analysis of the clinical literature to identify acceptable treatment guidelines. This analysis is done with the understanding that a lag period will always exist between clinical research and clinical practice. In fact, this lag time may even be desirable so that treatment protocols can be refined during time and undergo beta-site or pilot testing.

Peer consensus can fill in some of the gaps in knowledge that invariably exist. Grimshaw et al (1995) discuss the practical implications for guideline development and the role of peer review guidelines.

Review criteria evolve from the practice guideline development processes of different factions, including provider associations, proprietary healthcare software firms, academic institutions, UROs, disability management firms, benefit administrators, and government entities. Each group possesses unique motives and methodologies concerning review criteria. Various accreditation and certification bodies (e.g., Utilization Review and Accreditation Commission) may offer some guidance concerning criteria development and application. Provider certification and accreditation bodies (e.g., Commission for Accreditation of Rehabilitation Facilities [CARF] and National Committee for Quality Assurance [NCQA]) have something to offer as well. Certain states have promulgated practice guidelines under workers' compensation (e.g., Rhode Island, Texas, and Massachusetts). These guidelines have been amended for use as review criteria and serve as a platform for dialogue between payers and providers.

Despite the availability of review criteria, especially automated criteria, a peer reviewer must rely on his or her clinical experience, intuition, sense of fairness, and common sense when reviewing claims. The review process is not unlike the critical thinking process that a master clinician uses when making treatment decisions in concert with diagnostic technology applications. Clinical judgment is rightfully factored into and, in some cases, trumps the result of a diagnostic test. Similarly, review criteria although of some utility, falls well short of sound case-by-case analysis of claims.

The AHCQR was created as an extension of the U.S. Public Health Service. This subsidiary is charged with facilitating guideline development and conducting review/revision of these guidelines. AHCQR convenes panels of experts to develop these guidelines, which have generated enormous debate concerning their application. Providers or professional associations may argue that AHCQR guidelines should not be used for UR purposes, but this application is imminent, particularly if other data sources are sparse. It is a virtual certainty that any treatment guideline developed by a federal government agency will be used in some form or fashion by payers and UROs. This usage is consistent with AHCQR's own mission (Bigos et al, 1994). To date, AHCQR clinical practice guidelines for adult acute low back problems and post-stroke rehabilitation have gained significant traction within the rehabilitation community as well as the UR sector.

Regardless of the source of review criteria or developmental methodologies, a fair degree of alignment should exist between practice guidelines or treatment protocols and medical review criteria. Collaboration and disclosure between providers and reviewers represents the future of UR/UM.

Review Ethics

Health care providers pledge to uphold ethical standards embodied by their professional organizations. Ethical standards are grounded in the uniqueness of the patient-provider relationship. This relationship does not exist when claims adjusters or UR agents examine a medical record. A patient-provider relationship does not exist even when an independent medical examination or functional capacity evaluation is performed. UR organizations have only recently begun to standardize their practices. This standardization represents a voluntary process, however, that is not regulated by statutory or professional membership standards. UROs are far more diverse in their composition than are hospitals, clinics, and other health care provider organizations. Some UROs are without onsite medical staff altogether.

Table 10–11 presents 20 guiding principles for peer review or UR. The author developed this list while serving as president of a UR and disability management organization.

Critical Analysis of Utilization Review

Ironically, substantial variation exists within the very industry charged with managing variation in the provider community, the UR sector. UR and management organizations have not to date embraced a universal system for evaluating the medical necessity and reasonableness of medical services, and it is extremely unlikely that one will ever emerge, given the enormous complexity of today's health care system. Therefore it remains of utmost importance that each and every case is evaluated on its own merits before a denial decision is made. An evidence-based approach entails comparing the facts of a given case with the community standard of care and the clinical literature.

Variation exists even within federal government sponsored programs designed to offer standardized benefits regardless of one's state of residence (e.g., Medicare). One study of claims processed by six different Part B carriers in 1993 demonstrated enormous variation among those charged with reducing treatment variation (Government Accounting Office, 1994) (Table 10–12).

This exhaustive study addressed the consistency of denial rates for the 71 most utilized and costly services. These services involved 576 million Part B claims submitted by 780,000 physicians and 136,000 suppliers. A total of 112 million Part B denials were issued, wholly or partly accounting for $17 billion in billings. This amount represented 18% of all Part B billings. "Sizable" differences were found across carriers with respect to denial rates for similar or identical services screened for 58 of 71 services. The chiropractic rate of denial was most profoundly variable, at a range of 18 to 174 denials per 1000 services. A number of reasons for denial variation are postulated, including differences in medical policies between carriers. Provider differences in billing practices were also cited as causal factors. Different regions of the country may have different degrees or patterns of fraud and abuse among providers. Aberrant billing practices by as few as two or three providers are considered to contribute to variation.

Table 10–11   Twenty Guiding Principles of Peer-Based Utilization Review

1. When in doubt, err in favor of the patient, who has often lost control of his or her medical and legal destiny.
2. The service provider has the burden of proof in supporting medical necessity and reasonable and appropriate care.
3. All reasonable attempts should be made to ensure a "like reviewing like" process.
4. A case-by-case evidentiary process should be used in peer review.
5. Optimal care may not be reasonable or feasible in every case, but should be the goal. However, reviewers should focus on a range between minimally acceptable and optimal service.
6. Peer reviewers should be as current as possible in their understanding of clinical literature, curricula and prevailing practice guidelines. They should appreciate and accept that a lag exists between clinical research and practice.
7. On request, the provider the patient are entitled to fair and expeditious appeals.
8. There are essentially two levels of proof of medical necessity, reasonableness, and appropriateness.
   a. service must result in significant sustainable progress.
   b. the clinical documentation must support the intensity of care.
9. Reviewers should appreciate and accept that there may be legitimate regional variations in practice.
10. Reviewers must recognize that not all patients possess equal reparative powers, functional abilities, or pain thresholds.
11. Reviewers should focus on both cost and quality.
12. Reviewers should focus on both overutilization and underutilization.
13. Reviewers should be as objective as possible regardless of how or by whom they are reimbursed for their services.
14. Reviewers should review and revise their criteria at least once a year.
15. Reviewers should avail their services to any party including payers, providers, and patients.
16. Reviewers should explain the rationale for any denials in the body of their report and be prepared to provide supportive materials substantiating their recommendations and opinions.
17. Like providers, reviewers subscribe to strict patient confidentiality and non-disclosure.
18. The peer review process should serve to educate multiple stakeholders.
19. On request, the provider of health care services should have the opportunity to dialogue with the reviewer and/or submit additional documentation.
20. The review process should be non-adversarial.

Table 10–12 Reasons for Denial of Medicare Part B Claims

30%	Duplicate claim
14%	Service not covered
10%	Incomplete documentation
9%	Care not medically necessary
8%	Ineligible claimant
6%	Medicare a secondary insurer
1%	Claim filing deadline exceeded
16%	Other

Data from Government Accounting Office: Medicare Part B: Inconsistent Denial Rates for Medical Necessity Across Six Carriers. GAO/T-PEMD-94-17, Gaithersburg, MD, US Government Accounting Office, 1994.

Last, it is purported that some providers still continued to bill the program despite medical necessity denials. Regardless of the cause, this report emphasizes the need for standardization in Medicare review procedures. One postscript to this study is that some carrier representatives supported the need for development of national parameters for medical necessity determinations given that Medicare is a federal and not a state program. Yet Medicare policy directed carriers to develop medical necessity policies that reflected local standards of care. In reality, carriers have historically had extreme latitude and the system has been pockmarked with inconsistencies, contradictions, and at times mindless policies. It can be disconcerting to think that many commercial carriers of private sector lines of insurance look to this program for the lead in UR/UM issues. Although carriers have made strides in this regard, inconsistency and variation still dominate the adjudication of Medicare claims even at the hearing officer and administrative law judge levels.

Not all standardization is good or has a sound basis, however. Using a broad-brush approach, HCFA (now known as the Centers for Medicaid and Medicare), which oversees Medicare, categorically denied as medically necessary a number of treatment interventions. One such initiative directly impacted rehabilitation when the HCFA, despite mountains of clinical evidence supporting the technique, categorically denied the use of electrical stimulation in wound care. This universal denial is in direct contradiction to a sacred covenant of the UR/UM industry: case-by-case consideration before denial of medical necessity. This initial decision (which has since been repealed) was also in direct contradiction to the findings of another federal agency. The Agency for Healthcare Policy and Research (now known as Agency for Healthcare Quality and Research) determined in 1995 that electrical stimulation was an effective intervention for a number of conditions: decubitus ulcers, stage III and stage IV pressure ulcers, and recalcitrant stage II ulcers. It is worthy to note that the HCFA followed the advice of its technical advisory committee, which is made up of physicians but no physical rehabilitation providers or experts in electrical stimulation and wound care.

Several lessons are to be learned from this shortsighted approach. First, if an opinion exists, facts must be found to support it. Second, not all attempts to standardize medical necessity determinations are worthy or effective. Third, it is incumbent on providers to contribute to the database of knowledge so that practice standards, outcomes measures, and case studies are readily available to support individual treatment or to rebuke those who embrace arbitrary and, in some cases, capricious standards of review. Providers must also discard treatment interventions that are unsupportable in favor of those with adequate support. Last, open frank dialogue among all stakeholders must ensue if meaningful review criteria are to result.

Utilization Review/Utilization Management Effects on Cost, Length of Stay, and Quality

The net effect of UR/UM on health care costs is hotly debated, but the fact that it continues to persist suggests that it is driving some value to those who use it. Some data are available that show cost savings associated with UR/UM activity (Feldstein et al, 1988; Faulkner & Gray, 1995). Predictably, many proprietary UROs tout cost savings and benefit-cost ratios in marketing and collateral literature. Across all patient populations, provider groups, insurance lines, and treatment settings the range in savings is between 10% and 20%. These data are "soft" and deserve more study. It is also not known whether the actual cost of UR/UM services is factored into these estimates. During the 1970s and 1980s a fair number of UROs received payment from insurers or employers on a contingent fee basis or as a percentage of savings. This remuneration model has been substantially diminished by provider protest and the enactment of national review guidelines and state regulations discouraging such practices.

LOS is another important measure of health care quality, cost and usage. Although the term was initially coined to describe hospital days or stays, it has been expanded to describe the number of visits rendered on an outpatient basis. Data from the 1992 National Health Interview Survey conducted by the Congressional Budget Office yielded the following data:

- Health maintenance organizations (HMOs) (both staff and group models) reduced utilization by an average of 19.6%.
- Independent practitioner associations reduced utilization by 0.8%.
- All HMOs reduced utilization on average by 7.5%. (National Health Interview Survey, 1992).

Conducted every 10 years, this survey supports some earlier contentions. One, independent practitioner associations with internal review processes versus external reviews may be softer on their network members. Also, the nearly 20% reduction for staff and group HMOs is consistent with data reported by external review organizations.

LOS is a surrogate measure of cost because of the presumption that more visits means more costs, which may not be the case in a prepaid system. LOS has been associated with quality indicators (Thomas, 1997). This study sampled between 3752 and 12,871 hospital cases across 13 clinical conditions, including some that routinely receive rehabilitation services. In all of the 13 conditions examined, cases that received poor quality care had significantly longer risk-adjusted LOS than cases whose care was of acceptable quality. This finding confirms the commonly held belief within the URO community that longer LOS is not only more expensive, but of poorer quality.

LOS has been described as the "invisible anvil that hangs above every hospital bed and clinic treatment room," because in virtually every treatment setting LOS has dropped by nearly two-thirds since the early 1990s (Reynolds, 1996).

The following is a list of situations that are either causes or consequences of lower LOS:

- Earlier discharge planning
- Rise in the number of case managers
- Detailed "payer diaries" maintained by providers to track benefit structures, limitations, coverages, durable medical equipment (DME) policies
- Heightened need for more patient educational services
- Increase in trend toward patient self-care
- More group therapy
- Increased use of professional home rehabilitation
- Increased use of "extenders of care"
- Staff downsizing or restructuring
- Increased use of "care maps" written in lay terms
- Poorer quality of care

A severe paucity of research remains specific to LOS and visit frequency regarding physical rehabilitation efficacy. A survey of the results of hospital-based treatment of acute orthopedic conditions found no significant difference or reduction in overall LOS for patients treated at 7 days per week versus those treated at a frequency of 5 days per week (Holden & Daniele, 1987). A fair question is, why is so much rehabilitation therapy given on a 3 times-per-week (TIW) basis? The clinical or pathological rationale for this standard remains a mystery. Perhaps a TIW frequency works best in a 5-day workweek because it affords equal spacing of visits, with a day off in between. Payers and UROs legitimately have the right to an explanation for this universal practice.

More important than UR's/UM's reports of cost or utilization savings are its effects on quality. Here again mixed and "soft" data exist. Providers are often quick to point out that managed care has eroded quality, and payers are quick to respond that only the fat has been trimmed from the pudgy healthcare waistline. The jury is still out regarding the effect of UR/UM on health care quality, although some authors report an absence of negative effects on quality (Robinson & Casalino, 1995). Other sources report concern about erosion of quality in managed care environments (Miller & Luft, 1994; Ware et al, 1996).

Rehabilitation providers can effect positive changes within the UR sector through a number of mechanisms. First and foremost should be the acceptance that some form of UR and management is necessary to curb medically unnecessary and unreasonable services. Providers are encouraged to participate more fully in the UR and management sector especially, in the development of review criteria sets. More providers are required during the review process to ensure that a true "like reviewing like" process is guaranteed. Providers must better educate payers and review agents about their profession's interventions, core competencies, provider credentials, and outcomes measures. The following list provides suggestions for greater contact with those who make reimbursement and coverage decisions:

- Read payer literature (refer to the Appendix for listings).
- Attend payer and URO conferences.
- Participate at the professional association level (e.g., insurance symposia).
- Become a peer reviewer for a provider organization, URO or payer.
- Stay current with clinical literature.
- Become knowledgeable concerning health policy, legislative, and regulatory initiatives.
- Understand your profession's code of ethics, documentation standards, practice guidelines, and position statements.

A fair and effective peer review process can occur when health care stakeholders work together but self-police. Legitimacy of this process is further enhanced through the shared development and disclosure of review criteria.

REFERENCES

Berman H: Taking charge of workers' compensation costs. Compensation and Benefits Rev 24(3):69, 1992.

Bigos S, Bowyer O, Braen G, et al: Acute Low Back Problems in Adults. Clinical Practice Guideline No. 14, Rockville, MD, Agency for Health Care Policy And Research, Public Health Services, US Department of Health and Human Services, AHCPR publication 95-0642, 1994.

Blustein J, Marmer TR: Cutting waste by making rules: Promises, pitfalls, and realistic prospects. University of Pennsylvania Law Rev 140(5):1546, 1992.

CARF, The Rehabilitation Accreditation Commission, Tucson, AZ, http://www.carf.org, accessed June 15, 2004.

Carpenter MA: UR: A perspective on the future. American Association of Preferred Provider Organizations (AAPPO) J May/June:11-16, 1992.

Charles C, Lomas J, Giacomini M: Medical necessity in Canadian health policy: Four meanings and ... a funeral? Milbank Q 75(3):365-394, 1997.

Chassin MR, Brook RH, Park RE, et al: Variations in the use of medical and surgical services by the Medicare population. New Engl J Med 314(5):285-290, 1986.

Clifton DW: A shift toward utilization management. PT Magazine 3(6):32-35, 1995a.

Clifton DW: Review criteria: Cookbook medicine or professional tool? PT Magazine 3(9):37-40, 1995b.

Clifton DW: You be the reviewer! PT Magazine 4(7):34-37, 1996a.

Clifton DW: Underutilization: The new monster? PT Magazine 4(11):25-27, 1996b.

Clifton DW: Days, dollars and disability: The three dimensions of utilization. Case Rev 3(3):81-85, 1997a.

Clifton DW: Disability duration tables: A range of examples. PT Magazine 5(11):34-39, 1997b.

Clifton DW: Utilization management in long-term care. Rehab Management 1998.

Clifton DW, Burcham M: Disability duration tables: Borders or barriers? PT Magazine 5(9):36-39, 1997.

Congressional Budget Office: 1992 National Health Interview Survey, Washington, DC, 1994.

Feldstein PJ, Wickizer TM, Wheeler JRC: Private cost containment: The effects of utilization review programs on health care use and expenditures. New Engl J Med 318(20):1310-1314, 1988.

Florida Workers' Compensation Law, I7, 440.13, Bulletin No. 154:3.

Frank AO, DeSouza LH, McAuley JH, et al: A cross-sectional survey of the clinical and psychological features of low back pain and consequent work handicap: Use of the Quebec Task Force Classification. Int J Clin Pract 54(10):639-644, 2000.

General Accounting Office: Tighter rules needed to curtail overcharges for therapy in nursing homes. Washington, DC, HEHS 95-23, Office of Health, Education, and Human Services, 1995.

General Accounting Office: Utilization review: Information on external review organizations. GAO/HRD-93-22FS, Washington, DC, General Accounting Office, 1992.

Geisel J: No simple solution for outpatient costs. Bus Insur April:21, 1989.

Gold M, Hurley R, Lake T, Berenson R: Arrangements between managed care plans and physicians. Selected External Research Series, No. 3, Washington, D.C., Physician Payment Review Commission, 1995.

Gold M: The changing U.S. health care system. Milbank Q 77(1):3-37, 1999.

Gommick M: Medicare patients: Geographic differences in hospital discharge rates and multiple stays. Soc Serv Bul 40:22-41, 1977.

Gosfield A: Value purchasing and effectiveness: Legal implications. In Gosfield A (ed): Health Law Handbook. Deerfield, IL, Clark Boardman Company, 1991, p 186.

Government Accounting Office: Medicare Part B: Inconsistent Denial Rates for Medical Necessity Across Six Carriers, GAO/T-PEMD-94-17, Gaithersburg, MD, US Government Accounting Office, 1994.

Grimshaw J, Eccles M, Russell I: Developing clinically valid practice guidelines. J Eval Clin Pract 1(1):37-48, 1995.

Holden MK, Daniele CA: Comparison of seven and five-day physical therapy coverage in patients with acute orthopedic disorders. Phys Ther 67:1240-1246, 1987.

Institute of Medicine: Clinical Practice Guidelines: Directions for a New Program. Washington, DC, National Academy Press, 1990.

Jacobson D, et al: Defining and implementing medical necessity in Washington State and Oregon. Inquiry 34:143-154, 1997.

Lewis CE: Variations in the incidence of surgery. New Engl J Med 281:880-884, 1969.

Manning WG, Leibowitz A, Goldberg GA, et al: A controlled trial of the effect of a prepaid group practice on use of services. New Engl J Med 310(23):1505-1510, 1984.

Miller L: One bum knee meets five physical therapists. The Wall Street Journal, September 22, 1994;B1, B6.

Miller RH, Luft HS: Managed care plan performance since 1980. JAMA May 18:1512-1519, 1994.

Milstein A: Managing utilization management: A purchaser's view. Health Affairs 16(3):87-90, 1997.

National Committee for Quality Assurance: http://www.ncqa.org, accessed June 15, 2004.

National Council on Compensation Insurance: Medical expenditures in workers' compensation: Utilization of services drives cost. Boca Raton, FL, National Council on Compensation Insurance, 1994.

Office of Inspector General: Physical therapy in physicians' offices. Washington, DC, US Department of Health and Human Services, publication number OEI-o2-90-00590, 1994.

Reynolds J: LOS: SOS? PT Magazine 4(2):38-46, 1996.

Robinson JC, Casalino LP: The growth of medical groups paid through capitation in California. New Engl J Med 333(25):1684-1687, 1995.

Roos NP, Roos LL: Surgical rate variations: Do they reflect the health or socioeconomic characteristics of the population. Med Care 20:945-958, 1982.

Sharpe VA: Appropriateness in patient care: A new conceptual framework. Milbank Q 74(1): 200-207, 1996.

Thomas JW: Is patient length of stay related to quality of care? Hosp Health Serv Adm 42(4):489-508, 1997.

Vibbert S (ed): Medical utilization review directory, New York, Faulkner and Gray Healthcare Information Center, 1993.

Wainwright S, Crandall G, Brodovsky W: Patient care in focus: Peer review. Clinical Management 12(5):30-37, 1992.

Ware JE et al: Differences in 4-year health outcomes for elderly and poor: Chronically ill patients treated in HMO and fee-for-service systems. JAMA 276(13):1039-1047, 1996.

Webber A, Goldbeck A: Utilization review. In Fox P, Goldbeck W, Spies J (eds): Healthcare Cost Management: Private Sector Initiatives. Ann Arbor, MI, Health Administration Press, 1984.

Wennberg J, Gittlesohn A: Variations in medical care among small areas. Sci Am 246(4):120-135, 1982.

Wolff N, Scheslinger M: Risk, motives, and style of utilization review: A cross-condition comparison. Soc Sci Med 47(7):911-926, 1999.

Workers' Compensation Research Institute: Cost Drivers In New Jersey, WCRI Research Brief, 10(7):5, 1994.

SUGGESTED READINGS

Jacobson PD: Legal challenges to managed care cost containment programs: An initial assessment. Health Affairs, The People to People Health Foundation 18(4):69-85, 1999.

Milstein A: Managing utilization: A purchaser's view. Health Affairs 16(3):87-90, 1995.

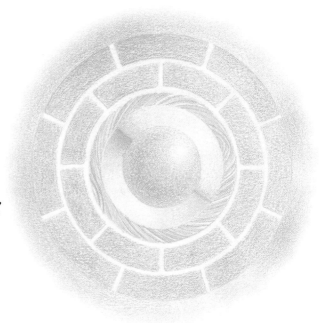

CHAPTER 11

Descriptive Study of Physical Therapy Case Management

Jan Stephen Tecklin, MS, PT

🌀 KEY POINTS

- Utilization review and management can be conducted in a non-adversarial manner when reviewers and providers engage in data disclosure, reciprocal education, and use an evidence-based approach for clinical decision making.
- A reduction in workers' compensation visits does not necessarily lead to a diminution in clinical outcomes.
- A precertification of care program provides benefits to both payers and providers. Payers are assured that services are medically necessary and reasonable and providers can avoid retrospective denial-of-service claims after the expenditure of human and capital resources.
- A precertification program in which reviewers and providers collaborate in a non-adversarial model can potentially result in benefit to patients.
- A true peer–to–peer program, wherein "likes review likes" (PT reviews PT, OT reviews OT), can overcome obstacles frequently associated with utilization review and case management.

◢ Operational Definitions

Disability Duration Tables	Tables that link visit number or length of stay (LOS) to a patient's diagnosis, condition, or a specific treatment intervention.
Overutilization	Health care services (either rendered or proposed) that do not significantly enhance clinical outcomes but result in higher costs; overutilized services are generally inconsistent with accepted treatment guidelines or standards relative to a diagnosis.
Precertification	The process of seeking advance approval of health care services before treatment is rendered but after an initial evaluation has been conducted; also known as preauthorization.

INTRODUCTION

Workers' compensation programs in the United States were developed to protect both workers and employers. Workers receive medical coverage, replacement of lost wages, and protection against dismissal should they suffer work-related injury or illness. Employers are protected against liability lawsuits. Workers' compensation laws fall under state jurisdiction and therefore vary, but most have common features, including absence of co-payment by injured workers; no deductible payments; payment for various types of disability; vocational rehabilitation expenses; and unlimited medical coverage, often referred to as "first-to-last dollar coverage" (Bednar et al, 1998). Many states offer access to a physician of the employee's choice, and rehabilitation is one of the major objectives for all states (Durbin, 1997; Robinson et al, 1997). The percentage of medical costs as a portion of workers' compensation costs reached the point in 1993 where medical benefits paid out represented 41.9% of all workers' compensation dollars compared to only 35% in 1984 (Burton, 1996). In addition to medical costs, indemnity costs include payments for replacement of lost wages, legal expenses, and total or partial permanent disability, whereas administrative costs are also borne by the insurance companies that insure workers. A managed care pilot program for workers' compensation in Florida found that indemnity costs were 17.9% of total costs per case, whereas administrative costs were 19.5% (WCRI, 1993).

The National Council on Compensation Insurance (NCCI) stated that workers' compensation costs rose during the early 1990s at 14% per year, almost twice the annual rise in general medical costs (National Council on Compensation Insurance Digest, 1992). As increases in reimbursement for general medical care have slowed over the past decade due to varying approaches to managed care, cost-shifting to workers' compensation has occurred (Curtis, 1994; Butler et al, 1997). That is, the relative lack of restrictions on reimbursement has been a factor in the increase of the average workers' compensation medical claim from $1750 in 1980 to $6600 in 1990 (Hager, 1992). For example, carpal tunnel surgery performed under worker's compensation claims was approximately three times more costly than it was when workers had similar surgery without a workers' compensation claim. More astonishing is that workers' compensation surgeries for carpal tunnel syndrome were approximately *five times more costly* than non–workers' compensation surgeries (Palmer & Hanrahan, 1995). Hager (1992) suggested several other reasons for this growth, including increased legal costs to the insurer, provider fraud, and an expansion of definitions of job-related injuries. The expansion of job-related, compensable injuries is most clearly seen in cumulative trauma injuries (e.g., in carpal tunnel syndrome and psychological-stress cases) (Durbin, 1997; deCarteret, 1994). Berman (1991) attributed these escalating medical costs, driven in part by physical therapy, to preventable injuries, inappropriate treatment, undirected care, and poor or absent planning for return to work. Jette et al (1994) supported some of Berman's assertions by showing that physical therapy episodes for low back injury covered by workers' compensation were 36%, or $164 per case, more expensive than those covered under other insurances. It appears that higher costs are related more to overutilization than to higher charges for various physical therapy procedures. Durbin (1997) shows that therapeutic exercise is used more than twice as frequently, and hot packs and ultrasound almost three times as frequently, in workers' compensation cases when compared to group health cases for similar body part injuries.

In an effort to reduce rising costs and provide for improved case direction and planning, managed care and utilization management (UM) techniques have been introduced into the workers' compensation arena (WCRI, 1993; WCRI, 1994a). The cost-containment measures used include limited initial provider choice and change, hospital and medical fee schedules, utilization review, and bill audits (Curtis, 1994). However, because workers' compensation programs are regulated by law and are often interpreted to favor the employee, they have lagged behind other health insurance products in the implementation of managed care and utilization review procedures. This time lag for workers' compensation has resulted in meager data regarding managed care approaches. Daiker (1995) indicated that various methods of managing care in workers' compensation have increased implementation dramatically from 1991 to 1992. She noted that various managed care networks increased by 30%, utilization review increased over 40%, precertification of cases tripled, and case management more than doubled. She also noted that managed care in workers' compensation is designed to reduce costs in both medical pricing and utilization of various services. Friedlieb (1994) studied the effects of practice guidelines on the cost of treatment for low back pain in almost 1800 cases, including a large percentage of work injuries. Practice guidelines were developed using a variety of utilization review techniques including literature review, data analysis, and expert consensus. Inappropriate requests for diagnostic or therapeutic procedures were identified in 168 of the 1796 cases, resulting in a net savings of $398,960. A managed care pilot project in the state of Washington showed that the mean unadjusted medical cost per injury was 21.5% lower in a managed-care group when compared to a fee-for-service group (Cheadle et al, 1999). Gill (1995) stressed that, under managed care, workers' compensation programs should include ergonomic assessment, functional job description development, on-the-job safety instruction, and new payment models including capitation, negotiated fees, and rehabilitation fee schedules. McGrail et al (1995) demonstrated an 18% reduction in medical and indemnity costs after instituting a managed-care program for workers in a large medical institution. The managed care included a preferred provider organization, medical case management, and an ergonomics program to reduce workplace injuries. An extensive MEDLINE search failed to find any published studies regarding precertification of physical therapy for workers' compensation or any other patient group. Precertification studies have primarily centered around pharmaceuticals (Smalley et al, 1995).

A Workers' Compensation Research Institute (WCRI) report on rapidly escalating medical costs in New Jersey workers' compensation programs demonstrated that the escalation "was due largely to increased utilization, especially of chiropractors and physical therapy services" (WCRI, 1994b). In response to this finding, the New Jersey Manufacturers Insurance Company (NJM) implemented a UM program for physical therapy based upon two approaches—establishment of a per visit fee for all physical therapy providers and precertification of all cases by experienced physical therapists. The UM program was developed and administered by Disability Management Associates of Springfield, Pennsylvania.

THE PROGRAM

Philosophical Positions

In developing this program, it was important to posit several philosophical attitudes related to interaction with both providers and payers.

Non-Adversarial

The first of these attitudes was employed in our dealings with physical therapy providers. We attempted to approach treatment issues on a non-adversarial basis; that is, the reviewers perceived themselves as consultant case managers as opposed to naysayers whose goal is usually to reduce reimbursement at almost any cost. The providers first viewed this notion with some skepticism, but over several months of the program's existence, we earned the respect of the vast majority of physical therapists. Many of the providers would periodically contact DMA reviewers to help them with particularly confounding cases.

Peer-to-Peer

The second position was that physical therapists, rather than other health care practitioners, would deal with all case-content–related issues. Many peer review programs employ nurses and, in many instances, untrained clerical personnel to serve as reviewers of practitioners. Although nurses surely have a broad overview of care, a true peer—another experienced physical therapist—can best decide issues of utilization for physical therapy cases (Rasmussen, 1990). The issue of true peer-to-peer review has been incorporated into statutory requirements by individual states.

Educational

The program was developed to provide a two-way educational process; that is, the reviewers regularly offered relevant citations and article reprints about utilization and appropriate treatment approaches from evidence-based articles in peer-reviewed journals to practitioners. Conversely, the practitioners educated the reviewers about specific treatment approaches and protocols that they used in daily practice. We believe this approach added to the non-adversarial aspect of the program and provided a means of rebuttal for the practitioners.

Disability Durations

Rather than develop a list of numbers of visits and durations to serve as a template for precertification, we asked providers to identify their expected number of visits and the expected duration for each case. They provided this information with the knowledge that recertification could be requested and would be evaluated based upon objective progress. At a later point in the program, we instituted a series of disability durations for non-complex soft tissue cases. These durations will not be discussed in this chapter, but they were based upon the initial findings from the 3500 cases described later in this chapter.

Cost Reductions

This UM program was instituted to achieve cost reductions for the insurer. Nonetheless, reviewers were completely unfettered in their case management. There was neither explicit nor implicit pressure from the insurer to save money for its own sake. Cases were managed and visits were precertified based entirely upon their merits. As described later in this chapter, objective documentation of the need for and benefits from physical therapy were required in every case.

Determination of Utilization

Consistent with the Code of Ethics of the American Physical Therapy Association, the program functioned under the principle that physical therapists were the professionals to ultimately determine utilization (that is, physician referral for a specific visit frequency and duration should only have provided a guideline to the physical therapist). Ultimately, it was the physical therapist's knowledge, skill, and experience (and not a physician's referral) that determined how long any patient benefited from ongoing intervention.

Precertification Procedure

All previous NJM physical therapy providers, specifically excluding those centers identified as physician-owned, were invited to submit their credentials via questionnaire to be considered for inclusion in the "preferred provider network" (Dept. of Health and Human Services, 1994). The network included approximately 160 outpatient physical therapy practices throughout New Jersey, including both corporately owned and individually owned practices. Priority for inclusion in the network was determined by NJM and based upon the insurer's prior dealings with the physical therapy provider and geographic coverage of the state.

Procedures for precertification of care by preferred providers under the workers' compensation UM program are presented in Table 11-1. The DMA reviewers were all licensed physical therapists with an average of more than 20 years of practice experience and from 5 to 12 years of experience in utilization review. The reviewers examined material provided by the centers and recommended action for each case, but when recommendation for a case was in question, reviewers decided to err on the side of the patient and recommend provision of care. NJM held the final authority and fiscal responsibility for care decisions.

Program Analysis

Data for analysis were provided by NJM. Descriptive statistics were used to examine various features of the population treated, including cost of medical care and physical therapy, lapse in time between injury and the start of physical therapy, length (in weeks) of treatment, visits requested by the provider, visits precertified, visits actually used for care, canceled visits, and "no-show" visits. No-show visits were instances in which the patient neither came for an appointed visit nor called to either reschedule or cancel. Data pertaining to days lost from work and the related indemnity cost for reimbursed wages were also collected. Percentages of various categories for work-related outcomes were also examined for a subset of patients for whom these outcomes were available.

This chapter examines data for all 3516 completed cases in this UM program from February 14, 1994, the start of precertification, through October 31, 1995. The latter date was chosen to coincide with a change in the process used to certify all subsequent cases. We also compared the data from the UM program to three other groups of data to which we had access:

1. NJM workers' compensation physical therapy cases for the first 3 months of 1993, 1 year prior to the UM program. Comparisons were made of medical and physical therapy costs and the number of physical therapy visits: the three major economic variables of interest.
2. Caremark Orthopedic Services Division; Schaumburg, IL (subsequently acquired by HealthSouth; Birmingham, AL).
3. Focus on Therapeutic Outcomes; Knoxville, TN.

Table 11-1 Precertification process for worker compensation cases insured by The New Jersey Manufacturer Insurance Companies

Process Steps

1. Upon referral by physician, required by law in New Jersey, the patient or employer makes an appointment for initial evaluation at an NJM-identified physical therapy center.
2. The physical therapist evaluates the patient and determines if treatment is necessary.
3. Given the decision to treat, the physical therapist submits a copy of the initial evaluation and a precertification intake form by fax to Disability Management Associates (DMA).
4. The intake form and initial evaluation provide information to DMA regarding the injury, its mechanism, objective findings, functional work-related deficits, a plan of care including suggested frequency and duration of visits, and treatment goals. In addition, various demographics are provided by the physical therapist.
5. Within 48 hours, a licensed physical therapist employed by DMA will review the information provided and either accept, modify, or reject the request. Rejection is most commonly a result of absent or inadequate objective and functional data.
6. The DMA therapist's decision is reported back to the provider therapist via fax with an indication of the frequency of visits and duration of care. In addition, noted reasons for rejection are accompanied by means to remedy the rejection, if possible.
7. If, upon completion of the allotted number of visits, the provider therapist believes that additional treatment is necessary, the process above (2 through 6) is repeated with a recertification intake form that is similar to the precertification form but also includes the following: (1) the number of visits previously certified, (2) the number of visits actually used, (3) the number of canceled visits, and (4) the number of no-show visits.
8. The process continues until the patient is discharged from care or until the DMA physical therapist declines to recertify additional care, in which case a rationale is provided.
9. Upon discharge from physical therapy, a Discharge Summary Form is completed by the treating therapist and forwarded to DMA.

The cases in Groups 2 and 3 were similar to the NJM cases for two reasons: All cases were from outpatient centers that included urban and suburban populations, and all centers in these groups regularly treated individuals with workers' compensation claims.

Program Results

The means for number and percentage of cases reviewed, reimbursement for physical therapy, and number of visits for NJM, CM, and FOTO are presented by body part in Table 11-2.

Cost per Case

The overall mean cost per case for physical therapy was $981 ± 9.20 for NJM versus $1401 and $1164 reported in the CM and FOTO databases, respectively. The total NJM medical costs per case were $7581 ± 254.41, which resulted in physical therapy accounting for 12.9% of the medical costs.

Compared with the NJM cases from early 1993, the UM cases were associated with markedly reduced costs for physical therapy. The mean cost for physical therapy was $2563 for the 406 cases in 1993 versus $981 for

Table 11-2 Number and Percentage of Cases, Physical Therapy Cost, and Number of Visits by Body Part Injured for Three* Databases

Injury site	No. of cases			% of Cases			PT $$			Visits		
	NJM	FOTO	CM	NJM	FOTO	CM	NJM	FOTO	CM	NJM	FOTO	CM
Lumbar	1374	505	3599	39.08	13.83	27.00	866	1279	1243	12.4	12	12
Multiple sites	444			12.63			1168			15.6		
Knee	368	1158	2081	10.47	31.71	15.60	1075	1096	1649	15.4	12	15
Arm/shoulder	238	846	1848	6.77	23.17	13.86	1144	1211	1839	16.9	11	15
Finger	203			5.77			1147			16.0		
Wrist	175			4.98			972			13.2		
Hand	172			4.89			967			12.9		
Ankle	146			4.15			947			11.9		
Leg	119			3.38			1156			16.5		
Neck	75	203	1103	2.13	5.64	8.27	850	1176	1210	12.2	11	12
Elbow	73			2.08			917			12.6		
Thumb	50			1.42			830			12.0		
Hip	27			0.77			1000			14.1		
Burns	17			0.48			882			13.2		
Ribs	15			0.43			640			8.9		
Toe	7			0.20			679			10.0		
Groin	7			0.20			606			8.7		
Chest	6			0.17			483			12.0		

*Data for FOTO and CM did not include all body parts.

the 3516 cases beginning in 1994, which represents a 61.7% decrease in physical therapy cost per case. These figures also represent a large decrease in percentage of medical costs represented by physical therapy. The percentage decreased from 17.3% for the 1993 cases versus 12.9% of medical costs for the UM cases. Other factors for which data were unavailable, such as severity of injury, injury mechanism, specific diagnoses, ergonomic factors, and environmental conditions, could have played a role in the differences in costs. However, there is no reason to expect that those items would have changed markedly in a two-year period, and UM, although not the singular cause, was the most likely factor in this reduction of costs.

The mean reimbursement per visit for NJM cases was $71.09 versus $107.76 and $116.41 for CM and FOTO providers respectively. A mean of $89.67 ± 1.39 was reimbursed per visit for the 406 NJM cases in 1993. One reason the precertified NJM cases cost 70% and 84.3% of the CM and FOTO costs, respectively, can be traced to NJM having established per visit fee schedules with each physical therapy network provider as part of the UM program. The modal fee negotiated by NJM with physical therapy providers was $65 per visit. Some providers negotiated for higher fees and additional payment when two or more body parts were treated.

Visits per Case

Physical therapists requested a mean of 28.1 ± 0.72 visits per case. Several reasons could account for this request, which represents an unusually high number when compared to other databases. First, the New Jersey requirement for physician *prescription*, including frequency and duration of visits, rather than *referral* has resulted in the common practice of physical therapists, who were requesting precertification of care, merely noting the frequency and duration stated on the physician's prescription rather than making their own determinations. In many cases, the reviewers noted that physician prescriptions for physical therapy far exceeded guidelines promulgated both by providers of care and by payers. These guidelines, commonly referred to as disability durations, were collected by the American Physical Therapy Association (APTA) Workers' Compensation Focus group and included several insurers (MetLife, Aetna, and Medicare), several APTA Chapters (Kentucky, Michigan, and New Hampshire), and a draft of guidelines from the Texas Workers' Compensation Commission (Workers' Compensation Focus Group, 1994). The lack of widespread physician and physical therapist knowledge of these guidelines was likely one reason for large numbers of requested visits. In addition, the 1993 NJM cases show that providers were accustomed to reimbursement for an average of almost 30 visits per case. Providers probably expected this pattern of reimbursement to continue even with the new precertification program in place.

One could speculate that planned overutilization by physical therapists resulted in requests for large numbers of visits. Physical therapists in locally-owned centers depend wholly upon patient visits for their livelihood and may request and use more than necessary. Therapists in corporate centers may similarly request more visits than

necessary in an effort to maintain the corporate "bottom line" philosophy which may include quotas for daily treatment or billing. None of these positions is consistent with the APTA Guide for Professional Conduct that states:

Principle 3: Section 3.3 Provision of Services

B. Provision of services for personal financial gain rather than for the need of the individual receiving the services is unethical.

C. When physical therapists judge that an individual will no longer benefit from their services, they shall so inform the individual receiving the services. Physical therapists shall avoid overutilization of their services (APTA, 1999).

I must note that nothing in this program attempted to identify overutilization, and the mere request for precertified visits does not constitute overutilization. Surely, for more involved cases, large numbers of visits over long periods of time are required for good patient outcomes, and the availability of an adequate number of precertified visits for particularly difficult cases reduced the administrative time, effort, and expense of repeated requests for recertification.

Of the 28.1 visits requested per case, 18.2 ± 0.31, or 64.8%, of the visits were precertified by the reviewers. From those 18.2 visits that were precertified, only 13.8 ± 0.24 were actually used. This figure represents 75.8% of precertified visits but only 49.1% of visits originally requested—a significant decrease in visits at each step in the precertification process.

The program was particularly interested in a comparison of large, corporate-owned practices to the overall mean values for economic data. There was little difference in utilization patterns between the corporate-owned centers and the overall group of practices. Values for physical therapy expenditure per case, numbers of visits requested, visits precertified, and visits actually used were essentially the same with no obvious evidence of corporate overutilization when compared with the smaller "mom and pop"–type practices.

The number of visits precertified by the reviewers was based upon figures compiled from previously cited sources of disability durations (Workers' Compensation Focus Group, 1994). As might be expected, guidelines developed by physical therapists were more liberal than those developed by the insurers. In an attempt to consider the position of each group, we used figures at a midpoint between the high and low numbers proposed. In addition to decreasing the number of visits based upon disability-duration guidelines, a large number of cases were denied care due to inadequate initial documentation of the need for physical therapy. Upon receipt of proper documentation, care was usually precertified.

The figure of 13.8 visits used per case was consistent with the two national databases, CM having shown 13 visits and FOTO having shown 10 visits for similar populations. The reduction in visits per case, from the mean of 29.5 visits for 1993 NJM cases to 13.8 visits after the institution of UM activities, was notable. Of great interest to the reviewers was the 50.9% reduction in visits actually used compared to the original request of 28.1 visits during precertification. One can only speculate about why such a marked decrease in number of visits occurred after the original request. Again, the onus could be placed upon the physician for overprescribing or upon the physical therapist for over-requesting. One possible explanation of the reduction in actual visits was the "sentinel" effect. That is, the physical therapists were aware of the UM program and accurately expected their treatment regimens to be reviewed by a peer with similar credentials—in essence a sentinel. The mere expectation that a review may occur has been shown to have a significant impact upon utilization data for diagnostic and surgical services (Rosenberg et al, 1995). It is likely that a similar effect occurred in this program.

Notably, the data appear to refute the possibility of overt or planned overutilization by physical therapists. Although a mean of 18.2 visits were precertified per case and available for use, patients were seen for only 13.8 visits. Had overutilization for profit been a motive of the physical therapists, the number of visits used should have approached the 18.2 visits precertified, but this was not the finding.

Patient Adherence

Another interesting finding in the UM program pertained to patient adherence. The mean number of no-shows was 0.8 plus or minus .06 per case, and the visit cancellation rate was 1.3 plus or minus .08 per case. Compared with a mean of 13.8 actual visits per case, the missed visits represented 15.2%, or almost one out of seven actual visits. Despite more than 90% of therapists requesting three visits per week, the mean visit frequency was 2.1 visits per week, slightly more than two-thirds of the request. The dearth of information regarding patient adherence in workers' compensation physical therapy makes it is difficult to compare this figure with others. FOTO data reported 31.3% of patients below an acceptable level of treatment with session adherence, but it did not include specific numbers of visits missed. Nonetheless, one could speculate that missing as many visits as seen here could have delayed rehabilitation and return to work, thereby increasing indemnity costs for replacement of lost wages.

Time-Lapse Until Treatment

Early implementation of physical therapy has been shown to have a strong predictive effect on return to work within a 60-day period (Ehrman-Feldman et al, 1996). Unfortunately, the time-lapse data was not available for all cases due to a lack of stringent reporting requirements in this category. For 631 cases in which time-lapse before treatment was reported, the time from injury to the start of physical therapy was a surprisingly long 109.4 ± 8.5 days, or 15.6 weeks. However, 46 of the 631 cases for which start of therapy dates are available did not begin physical therapy until more than one year after the injury and clearly skewed the mean for this value. When a mean is skewed by outliers, the median is often a more useful statistical indicator of central tendency. The median interval from injury to start of therapy for these 631 cases was 35 days, or 5 weeks—a much more reasonable time period. Several reasons were identified for these delays.

First, many workers were reported to have ignored the initial injuries and continued to work. Physicians saw other patients and either did not refer for physical therapy or first referred to other health personnel such as chiropractors and massage therapists. Some cases represented either chronic problems or re-injury, and other patients may have been managed medically for a period then referred for surgical consultation and intervention, with physical therapy commencing only after surgery.

Physical therapy began within 1 year of injury in 585 cases. The mean interval from injury to treatment was only 9.2 weeks. Similarly examining the median for this group, we find a 30-day time period before instituting treatment. Because New Jersey requires physician prescription, there was a reduced likelihood of patients reaching physical therapy as early in the course of care as may be seen in those states with direct access.

Days Lost From Work

A mean of 117 days or 16.7 weeks per case were lost from work across the NJM population. The mean cost for wage replacement, as calculated at NJM, was $295 per week (Worthington, 1996) thereby amounting to approximately $4926.50 per case, i.e., 16.7 weeks times $295. Adding the wage replacement figure to the medical reimbursement results in a substantial cost of $12,507.48 per case. This figure includes neither administrative nor legal costs of the workers' compensation program nor costs of full or partial permanent disability payments. Access to those latter figures was unavailable.

Work-Related Outcome

Work-related outcome data were available for 629 of the 3516 cases reviewed. As with time data, the reporting requirement for this information was not stringent in the first phase of the program. Among those 629 cases, 276 or 43.7% of them immediately returned to their previous jobs without restrictions upon discharge from physical therapy while 60 or 9.5% returned immediately to the same job with various restrictions. This total of 53.2% returning to work immediately upon cessation of physical therapy is comparable to the CM database in which 52.8% and the FOTO data in which 53.4%, respectively, returned to the same job. Less than 1% of the 629 NJM cases returned to different jobs or had vocational counseling. Eighty-four cases (13.3%) resulted in patients dropping out of therapy, and slightly over 2% transferred to a different treatment facility for ongoing care, usually to a site where work conditioning was available. Less than 1% of cases were in litigation, and 181, or 28.7%, had some other outcome, with discharge from medical care and surgical intervention being the two most common reasons for discontinuance of physical therapy.

PROGRAM ANALYSIS

A comparison between the visit data from the UM cases versus the 1993 NJM cases demonstrated a marked decrease in mean and median visits per case during the UM program. The mean of 13.8 reimbursed visits during the program was less than one-half of the 29.5 visits during the prior period. An even greater decrease was seen for the median number of visits, which dropped from 23 in 1993 to 9 during the UM program. Similar reductions were seen in costs. The 1993 mean cost for physical therapy was $2563 per case versus $981 under the UM program. It appears that compared to the 1993 cases, although smaller in number than the UM group, the UM methods were associated with a large diminution in both the number of visits and the dollars spent for physical therapy. Interestingly, despite these significant reductions, the return-to-work data for the UM program were consistent with the two national databases used for comparison. That is, a major reduction in visits and costs had no obvious impact upon return-to-work outcomes for the workers. Savings generated by the UM program for one major indemnity cost, salary replacement, have been identified and are closely tied to the rapidity of return to work.

Because an insurer instituted this program, the outcome data collected comprised treatment cost, utilization measures, and return to work status. These outcomes do not negate the importance of more traditional physical therapy outcome measures of reduction in impairments and work-related functional gains. Rather, this program examines the perspective of the payers—can we achieve cost savings without reducing the work-related outcomes? Himmelstein and Pransky (1996) state that outcomes such as medical and indemnity costs, time lost from work, and outpatient utilization are good quality indicators in the worker's compensation arena. The New Jersey workers' compensation statute provides a powerful incentive for return to work because employers and insurers can unilaterally end benefits in a number of instances. Most notable is the ability to stop benefits when workers are given medical release to full duty but do not return to work (WCRI, 1994b). NJM patients returned to their previous jobs immediately upon discharge from physical therapy without restrictions in 43.7% of cases and returned with restrictions in another 9.5% of cases. This total of 53.2% immediate return to previous jobs is remarkably similar to the CM return to work figure of 52.8% and to data from FOTO showing 53.4% return to the same job with 28.2% working without restriction and 25.2% with some restrictions. The three databases are also consistent with a study of long-term follow-up of individuals with chronic low back pain treated in a multidisciplinary setting in which there was a 49% "good job outcome" after 1½ to 2 years. Although not all of the subjects in the study by Lanes et al (1995) represented workers' compensation claims, the return to work rate seen in the UM program was very similar to those subjects who were covered by workers' compensation. DiFabio et al (1995) found that 75% of workers' compensation claimants with low back pain returned to some level of work at discharge from physical therapy without regard to patient compliance or leg symptoms. Sanderson et al (1995) found that Oswestry Disability Scores were better, i.e. showed less disability, for claims in which the claimant was employed rather than unemployed. Therefore, safe return to employed status should be considered an important goal for physical therapists in an effort to help reduce the claimants' self-perception of disability. A study by

Hall et al (1994) supports this goal and suggests that physical therapists can significantly influence the probability of a successful return to unrestricted work by formally recommending such a return to the patient. In instances where a restricted return to work was recommended, there was an increased probability of failure of this return.

Lubow (1995) stated that as many as 70% of California workers' compensation cases with lost time from work went into litigation. Given this figure, it was surprising to find only three cases, representing less than 0.5%, with reported outcomes in litigation in this population. However, litigation under workers' compensation is more difficult in New Jersey.

Numerous cases reported in the category of "other" on the discharge summaries were discharged from medical care and thereby from ongoing physical therapy with or without the prior knowledge of the physical therapist; a fact that was made clear in the commentaries on the discharge summaries. The large group of patients listed as "other" also included those undergoing surgical intervention. This group was often referred back to the same physical therapy center for postoperative rehabilitation. When the latter scenario occurred, the postoperative treatment was viewed as an additional set of data for that case.

SUGGESTIONS FOR FUTURE STUDY

Retrospective analyses such as this often suffer from both inadequate categorization and organization of data and the inability to revise data collection procedures when problems occur. Weaknesses in this program analysis included lack of specificity of diagnoses, no attempt to account for severity of injury, and limited size of a comparison group from cases prior to the UM program. Subsequent studies should attempt to categorize both providers and cases by demographics, mechanisms of injury, geographic location, and other related characteristics.

Future studies of the economic impact of physical therapy and workers' compensation should include some improved scheme for grouping the injuries by diagnostic category. The categories here are based entirely upon body part injured and thereby included in one category such disparate clinical problems as anterior cruciate ligament reconstruction versus knee strain, and lumbar strain versus surgical repair of a herniated disc. Perhaps a scheme by which to identify severity of injury, as suggested by Delitto et al (1995) would have also made the results more useful to the clinician.

Future programs of physical therapy for workers' compensation injuries could also include an examination of the role of oversight. The "sentinel effect" may or may not have been active in this project, but it has been shown to reduce utilization and costs in a fee-for-service health plan (Worthington). Such a finding in physical therapy could support or refute the administrative cost of this type of UM program in comparison to savings of treatment and indemnity costs.

Finally, the findings suggesting the efficacy of UM techniques would have been strengthened by an analysis that included a group of cases larger than the 406 included from

1993 prior to the UM program. Unfortunately, such data were unavailable, and had they been available, the time involved in collecting the information would have been prohibitive because the data collection system at NJM was upgraded for the utilization management program.

CONCLUSIONS AND SUMMARY

This UM program of fee negotiation and precertification of treatment for physical therapy, provided to a population of 3516 injured workers in New Jersey, found that low back injury is the most common reason for referral to physical therapy, followed by multiple site injuries and then knee injuries. An average of 13.8 visits at a mean cost of $71.09 each were reimbursed per case, despite requested precertification for greater than twice that number. UM was associated with lower costs per case and per visit than that found in two other databases. Finally, there were fewer visits per case with markedly lower costs per case and per visit for a population of injured workers when compared with data collected by the same insurer prior to initiating the UM program. Despite the savings to the insurer, the return-to-work rate of 53.2% to the same job, which is a major goal for rehabilitation under worker's compensation, was remarkably similar to the other databases.

ACKNOWLEDGMENTS

I would like to acknowledge the encouragement and assistance of David Clifton, PT, in the development and implementation of this project. Al Amato, PT, was generous in providing the Focus on Therapeutic Outcome data for my use. Several individuals at New Jersey Manufacturers Insurance (NJM) were instrumental in this project, including Richard Worthington, Edward Palsho, Donald Lash, and Jerry Crossley.

REFERENCES

American Physical Therapy Assn: Guide for professional conduct. Alexandria, Va, 1999.

Bednar JM, Baesher-Griffith P, Osterman AL: Workers compensation. Effect of state law on treatment cost and work status. Clin Orthop (351):74-77, 1998.

Berman H: Taking charge of workers compensation costs. Employee Benefit News (10):35-37, 1991.

Burton JF. Workers' compensation benefits and costs: Significant developments in the early 1990s. In Burton JF, Schmidle TP (eds): 1996 Workers' Compensation Yearbook. Horsham, PA 1996, LRP Publications.

Butler RJ, Hartwig, RP, Gardner H: HMOs, moral hazard and cost shifting in workers' compensation. J Health Econ 16:191-206, 1997.

Cheadle A, Wickizer TM, Franklin G, et al: Evaluation of the Washington State Workers' Compensation Pilot Project II: Medical and disability costs. Med Care 37: 982-983, 1999.

Curtis NM: Managed care and workers' compensation. Hand Clinics 2:373-377, 1994.

Daiker B: Managed care in workers' compensation. AAOHN J 43(8): 422-427, 1995.

deCarteret JC: Occupational stress claims: Effects on workers' compensation. AAOHN J 42:494-498, 1994.

Delitto A, Erhard EE, Bowling RW: A treatment-based classification approach to low back syndrome: Identifying and staging patients for conservative treatment. Phys Ther 75:470–489, 1995.

Department of Health and Human Services, Office of Inspector General: Physical Therapy in Physician's Offices. (Report No. OEI-02-90-00590), 1994.

DiFabio RP, Mackey G, Holte JB: Disability and functional status in patients with low back pain receiving workers' compensation: A descriptive study with implications for the efficacy of physical therapy. Phys Ther 75:180-193, 1995.

Durbin D: Workplace injuries and the role of insurance: Claims costs, outcomes, and incentives. Clin Orthop 336: 94-106, 1997.

Ehrmann-Feldman D, Rossignol M, Abenhaim L, Gobeille D: Physician referral to physical therapy in a cohort of workers compensated for low back pain. Phys Ther 76:150-156, 1996.

Friedlieb OP: The impact of managed care on the diagnosis and treatment of low back pain: A preliminary report. Am J Med Qual 9(1):24-29, 1994.

Gill HS: The changing nature of ambulatory rehabilitation programs and services in a managed care environment. Arch Phys Med Rehabil 76(12):SC10-15, 1995.

Hager W: Harnessing the forces of change. National Council on Compensation Insurance Digest 3:1-19, 1992.

Hall H, McIntosh G, Melles T, et al: Effects of discharge recommendations on outcome. Spine 19:2033-2037, 1994.

Himmelstein J, Pransky G: Measuring and improving the quality of workers' compensation medical care. In Burton JF, Schmidle TP (eds): 1996 Workers' Compensation Yearbook. Horsham, PA, LRP Publications, 1996.

Jette AM, Smith K, Haley SM, Davis KD: Physical therapy episodes of care for patients with low back pain. Phys Ther 74:101-115, 1994.

Lanes TC, Gauron EF, Spratt KF, et al: Long-term follow-up of patients with chronic back pain treated in a multidisciplinary rehabilitation program. Spine 20:801-806, 1995.

Lubow HW: Integrating managed care and workers' compensation: What has happened, what can happen. Health Care Innovations May/June:17-34, 1995.

McGrail MP, Tsai SP, Bernacki EJ: A comprehensive initiative to manage the incidence and cost of occupational injury and illness. J Occup Environ Med 37(11):1263-1268, 1995.

National Council on Compensation Insurance Digest. Medical portion of comp reaches 44%. Boca Raton, Fl, National Council on Compensation Insurance, 1992.

Palmer DH, Hanrahan LP: Social and economic costs of carpal tunnel surgery. Instr Course Lect 44:167-172, 1995.

Rasmussen B: Claims reviews and PTs. Clinical Management 10:12, 1990.

Robinson JP, Rondinelli RD, Scheer SJ, Weinstein SM: Industrial rehabilitation medicine. 1. Why is industrial rehabilitation medicine unique? Arch Phys Med Rehabil 78: S3-S9, 1997.

Rosenberg SN, Allen DR, Handte JS, et al: Effect of utilization review in a fee-for-service health insurance plan. N Engl J Med 333:1326-1330, 1995.

Sanderson PL, Todd BD, Holt GR, Getty CJ: Compensation, work status, and disability in low back pain patients. Spine 20:554-556, 1995.

Smalley WE, Griffin MR, Fought RL, et al: Effect of a prior authorization requirement on the use of nonsteroidal antiinflammatory drugs by Medicaid patients. New Engl J Med 332:1612-1617, 1995.

Workers' Compensation Focus Group: Summary of Top 15 Rehabilitation Diagnoses. Alexandria, VA, American Physical Therapy Association, 1994.

Workers' Compensation Research Institute: Review, regulate, or reform? What works to control workers' compensation medical costs. WCRI Research Brief 10(8):1-5, 1994.

Workers' Compensation Research Institute: Cost drivers in New Jersey. WCRI Research Brief 10(7):1-8, 1994.

Workers' Compensation Research Institute: Cost savings provided by studied managed care. WCRI Research Brief 9(9):1-3, 1993.

Worthington R. Personal communication, West Trenton, NJ, New Jersey Manufacturers Insurance Companies, March 1996.

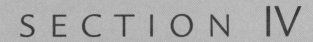

SECTION IV

Health Information Management

## CHAPTER 12

Information Technology in Disability Management

David W. Clifton, Jr., PT

"Conventional wisdom now holds that the health care system will be transformed over the next few decades into a paperless clinical enterprise that will permit clinicians to synthesize and apply the sum of human medical knowledge at the patient's bedside through the medium of advanced information technology."

- Anonymous, 1996

KEY POINTS

- Information technology has fundamentally changed how health care services are delivered through evidence-based practice and clinical decision-support systems.
- Today's clinicians must apply data and information for both business and clinical purposes (compound integration).
- Technology does not supplant the need for clinical decision making, it simply serves to enhance it.
- A plethora of health care stakeholders collect, analyze, and apply data for their own unique purposes. Stakeholders include regulatory agencies, payers, providers, consumer groups, utilization review organizations, and the legal community.

Operational Definitions

Client-Server Architecture	The ability of multiple personal computers (PCs), known as clients, to link with more powerful computers, known as servers.
Compound Integration	The integration of data management for different applications (e.g., business and clinical applications).
Clinical Decision Support Systems (DSS)	The development of databases to assist clinicians in making treatment decisions; also known as clinical decision support (CDS). CDS applies rules to clinical and demographic data. These rules address intervention selection, episodic care cost, and expected outcomes and ultimately strive to reduce treatment variation.
Intranets	Computer linkages that allow large or multi-site organizations to share data in both an input and output direction. Storage of computerized patient records in a central depository is a common intranet application.
Artificial Intelligence	Computer technologies that attempt to mimic human thought processes.
Data Mining	The ability of an information technology (IT) system to reveal new uses of information from existing large data repositories.
Enterprise Financial System	A computer-based system that allows a health care organization with multiple sites to unify a variety of functions, including patient registration and scheduling, billing and accounts receivables

	collection, cost reporting, and contract management.
Expert or Rules-Based Systems	Systems in which preprogrammed rules (e.g., clinical treatment guidelines and protocols) are embedded, allowing a degree of artificial intelligence.
Interface Engine	Software that facilitates the exchange of data between different applications or computer systems in real time (e.g., Point "A" transmits to "B," then on to "C").
Web Browser	A software application that serves as a user interface between a computer on one end and servers that contain data on the other end. Browsers interpret hypertext markup language (HTML), which is the common language of the World Wide Web (www). Microsoft's Internet Explorer and America OnLine's (AOL) Netscape Navigator are two of the dominate browsers available.

INFORMATION TECHNOLOGY'S ROLE IN PHYSICAL REHABILITATION

Information technology (IT) is as essential today as treatment given the complexities of the health care system and the necessity of balancing clinical and business functions. However, relatively few clinicians are equipped with the education or experience to design, select, and/or apply IT systems. This chapter was drafted with great trepidation given the frenetic pace at which technology is developed and becomes obsolete. The morass of emerging technologies, maelstrom of jargon, and diversified rehabilitation settings magnifies this challenge. Basic concepts, principles, and examples of diverse IT applications that may play a potential role in disability management are provided in this chapter. However, some of these technologies have yet to be fully incorporated into physical rehabilitation settings. Last, this chapter does not endorse specific hardware, software or operating platforms, services, or products.

Moran (1998) asserts that the health care sector is in its infancy relative to other sectors that possess sophisticated IT systems (e.g., financial and insurance institutions). The average health care organization's IT budget represents a mere 2% of the entire budget compared with 7% to 10% for data-intensive sectors. In 1997, health care IT investment approached $15 billion per year (Gallo & Lee, 1998). This investment is expected to nearly double early in the new millennium. The health care sector, however, has plenty of data; "Imbedded in a health care system is archaic and inadequate" (Horn & Hopkins, 1994). Ironically, those sectors with which health care providers must negotiate (e.g., insurance, managed care, employers, third-party administrators) have more advanced forms of data repositories, mining, and applications processes. Providers are at a distinct disadvantage when negotiating with payers. Kleinke (1998) remains optimistic about the health care sector's pursuit of IT:

"Every clinical situation, no matter how unique, can be digitized into a set of inputs, quantitative predictors, optimized medical decision making, and maximized results, be they lower costs, improved quality, or some combination of the two"

Information Technology Semantics

Those who provide health care services are often criticized for their use of medical jargon, abbreviations, and acronyms. IT experts are equally adept at speaking in their specialized terminology. IT is cloaked in many names including medical informatics, paperless enterprises, document management, health care informatics, and health IT (Chin, 1999a; Cross, 1991; Kleinke, 1998). Understanding the IT jargon is the first step to identifying applications that are relevant to physical rehabilitation delivery.

Purposes and Drivers of Health Data

Van Brunt (1998) identifies a number of drivers for IT development by describing a triad of influences that have collectively spawned Internet-based patient information systems. These include health care reform, emerging technologies, and consumer demand (Figure 12–1). For example, the Internet and interactive television together have created a new mode of information delivery. This combination facilitates decision support for the provider while targeting useful information to the consumer. Van Brunt asserts that the recent development of technology that stores, manipulates, and blends different types of media (e.g., text, sound, graphics, animation, video) provides opportunity to improve the learning experience.

Table 12–1 lists an array of health care data applications. Every organization must identify its own unique data collection, management, and application needs. For instance, a hospital may wish to track infection rates among various departments. These data, however, may not be as useful to an outpatient rehabilitation company. Data uses are collectively determined through the interaction of providers, payers, patients, employers, utilization review organizations, and societal needs. Data applications are rarely developed exclusively for internal use. For example, provider profiling data may assist a health care organization to understand provider performance, but these data are also useful when contracting with managed care firms. In this latter application, data that identify the most efficient providers can be invaluable when assigning staff to service a capitated population.

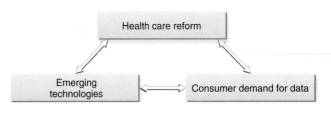

Figure 12–1. Triad of IT applications.

Table 12-1 Purposes of Health Data

- Assess public health and unmet needs (e.g., identify patterns of illness or injury within specific populations)
- Identify cost-effective providers for selective at-risk (e.g., capitation) contracting
- Provide data concerning quality of care indicators
- Create serial patient medical records that reflect the chronology of care
- Develop risk management practices and programs
- Maximization of reimbursement and accounts receivables collection
- Tracking of clinical outcomes across patient populations, treatment settings, interventions, and providers
- Satisfy requirements of accreditation and certification bodies
- Enhance delivery efficiency through process and structural alterations
- Facilitate more interactive care between patient-provider

Data collection is essential to the articulation of "quality" care. This is increasingly important as payers, patients, and other consumers look beyond cost and begin to desire outcomes measures. The management of serial patient records is another purpose of IT as it applies to rehabilitation. Physical rehabilitation providers face unique challenges in medical record keeping because of the relatively high treatment frequency and episode duration. Rehabilitation often requires protracted care versus the infrequency associated with visits to one's primary care physician, diagnostic laboratory, durable medical equipment supplier, or surgeon.

Along similar lines, the ability to identify cost-effective providers may offer rewards when the time arrives to contract with managed care organizations. Managers may be surprised to find out that their "best" or most popular clinicians may not be the most cost-efficient. Patterns of

expenditure allow the clinician to determine whether his or her staff-to-patient ratio is commensurate with profit, which is extremely critical in today's health care arena.

The Internet has permeated society swiftly and extensively. More than 22 million Americans now use the Internet to search for health care, according to research conducted by Cyber Dialogue of New York (Anonymous, 2000). Reimbursement pressures and organizational shifts represent additional drivers for IT development. The recent trend toward clinics without walls or virtual corporations demands that information be easily transportable across providers, treatment settings, and patient populations.

Figure 12-2 depicts three different IT pathways. Pathway A represents a direct provider to central database data exchange. In this model, separate databases housed within an organization (i.e., financial, clinical, legal, and regulatory) are fully integrated. Model B illustrates a common scenario in which a provider must access separate databases within his or her own organization. This is accomplished with an Intranet function: specifically, an interface engine or server. Model C portrays the flow of information between a provider and several databases via a browser that accesses a web application server. Browsers interface with web application servers to allow providers to access disparate databases housed on the World Wide Web (www).

IT plays a vital role in risk-management programs and medicolegal issues that commonly arise in today's health care environment. The need to ensure both safety and efficiency fuels IT applications. In worst-case scenarios, providers may need to defend their actions and the subsequent outcomes if adverse consequences result from disability management. An entire chapter of this book is devoted to risk management principles and practices.

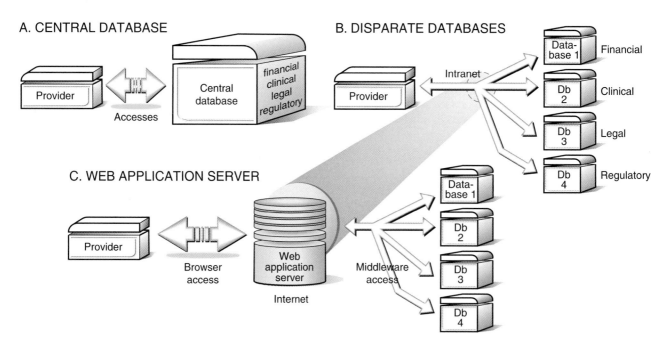

Figure 12-2. Three integrated database models.

Compound Integration

Today's health care data require what McCormack (1999) describes as "compound integration." Health data must satisfy business, clinical, and legal and regulatory needs. Data management involves multiple disciplines, divergent data elements, vendor diversity, absence of universally accepted definitions, and different operating platforms (e.g., DOS, Windows).

Figure 12–3 depicts the complexities associated with IT directed at compound integration. Compound integration involves the union of health care business applications and clinical support systems. Clinical support systems are the computerized elements of a delivery system that assist the rehabilitation provider in the development and application of clinical interventions. Examples include clinical treatment guidelines, pathways or protocols, treatment precertification data, case definitions, and clinical outcomes measures. Business applications include contract management, scheduling, insurance verification, treatment coding, cost reporting, compliance programs, confidentiality protocols, marketing program, accounts receivables, and disbursements.

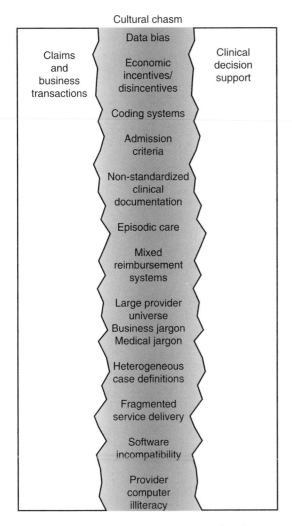

Figure 12–3. The disconnect between business and clinical IT applications.

The episodic nature of rehabilitation interventions, i.e., fragmented delivery (multiple providers, settings, patient irritability stages), medical-business language barriers, software incompatibility, and various coding systems can stifle integration efforts. The compound integration challenge begins the moment a patient contacts or is referred to a rehabilitation center. New patients must be scheduled with consideration to business hours of operation and appropriate provider availability. A non-integrated system may pair a patient with an inappropriate provider, appoint an inappropriate time for service, or wrong treatment setting.

Preauthorization of care (requirements vary between payer sources) then takes place. This further requires melding the clinician's plan of care with insurance coverage provisions and preauthorization requirements. If the treating provider is not provided this information, insurance verification and/or treatment cannot ensue. Front and back office staff must collaborate with providers within integrated delivery models. Upon arrival, the patient completes a morass of paperwork that includes medical history, insurance forms, and Health Insurance Portability and Accountability Act (HIPAA) acknowledgements. The interface between provider and patient then begins the clinical support system process as initial evaluations are performed, case definitions are formulated, interventions are selected, and a plan of care is constructed. Ongoing treatment requires further linkage of patient progress reports (clinical) with billing documents (business) for reimbursement purposes.

Information Technology Goals Differ by Stakeholder

The purpose of health data management shifts according to the stakeholders involved. For instance, although it may be an oversimplification to say insurers and health plans are fundamentally interested in financial data, cost is high on their priority scale (Milbank Memorial Fund, 2000). Payers are very concerned about loss ratios, premium dollars collected versus medical expenditures. Similarly, it is an oversimplification to assume that providers are only interested in clinical measures and not financial ones. Patients may be principally driven by a want or need to select the so-called "best" providers for their problems at no personal cost. The purpose of data management is as diverse as the universe of stakeholders. Stakeholders may include employers, indemnity insurers, HMOs, PPOs, attorneys, regulatory agencies, accrediting bodies, patients and their families, providers, utilization review organizations, insurance brokers, and others. Refer to Table 12–2 for a comparison of IT purposes by stakeholder type. On a societal level, health data are critical in gauging public health. Vaccination programs and other preventive-health programs, such as breast cancer screening, are good examples of this application of data. Data can be useful in the identification of injury and illness patterns. This allows for intelligent allocation of human and capital resources. For the clinician, these data can assist in the development and marketing of programs that are consistent with demographics or patient populations. Diversification of services into areas or conditions that

Table 12-2 IT Incentives by Stakeholder

Stakeholder	Incentive
Health plans/insurers	1. Selection and profiling of preferred providers
	2. Low medical cost vs. premium price
Employers/business coalitions	1. Value purchasing: cost vs. benefit
	2. Early and safe return-to-work
	3. Productivity
Provider organizations	1. Efficiency in care delivery/ standardize care/reduce variations
	2. Competitive contracting
	3. Maximum reimbursement
	4. Optimize clinical outcomes measures
	5. Promise of a paperless office
Patient/consumer	1. Access to providers
	2. Informed selection of different treatment options
	3. Minimum financial outlay
	4. Optimal outlays

are underserved can be profitable if injury or illness incidence is high.

INTEGRATION OF INFORMATION SYSTEMS

The Healthcare Financial Management Association (HFMA) conducted a study of 17 delivery systems considered by many to be the leaders in the application of IT (Van Brunt, 1998). This study clearly illustrates that most health care delivery systems have disproportionately addressed the business versus the clinical side of IT.

Eighty-seven percent of health care delivery systems have applied IT to business functions such as payroll and accounting, whereas only 20% reported implementation of provider profiling, outcomes management, demand forecasting, or patient tracking systems through a delivery network. There are many reasons for the disconnect between business-driven and clinical-driven IT applications.

Integration Caveats

There is a plethora of variables that inhibit a harmonious melding of clinical and business transactions. A wholly integrated IT system may be implausible for health care because of the "human element." Health care has many qualitative features, unlike banking and finance, which are highly quantitative in nature. Medicine has been

called an art, not a science. This observation raises a number of questions:

1. Can art and science truly be integrated from an IT standpoint?
2. Will artificial intelligence augment or supplant human intelligence in some facets of health care delivery?
3. What role will IT experts have in the delivery of health care?
4. Will future health care providers also need to be IT experts?
5. Will tomorrow's providers be programmers or practitioners?

Interface Engines

Interface engines are software packages that permit the flow of information from one application to another without the need for point-to-point interfaces.

This technology makes it possible for large multi-site health care systems to communicate between sites. For instance, a rehabilitation organization may have inpatient, outpatient, and homecare divisions. Each of these divisions has its own unique IT requirements. However, the parent organization requires that certain data be accessible across sites. Common examples include patient demographics, referral sources, insurance data, and tax data. An interface engine may allow each division to access these data while preserving clinically specific databases. Data can be managed in real time or stored in a repository for later use.

Figure 12-4 illustrates a variety of IT applications that are available to rehabilitation providers. A number of these require compound integration between clinical and business elements. These applications present a confounding array of technology choices. It is not surprising that clinicians who are trained to "treat" may have an aversion to technology. Some may even view it as "high tech [technology] over high touch [treatment]." In an ever-complex world wherein tomorrow's entry-level providers will undoubtedly be better equipped with IT knowledge.

Before the 1990s, many large health care organizations owned all of their facilities, which made data-system integration relatively easy. In today's strategic partnering era, data integration has become a greater challenge, which is especially true of the rehabilitation sector, which shrank.

BALANCING DATA ACCESS AND CONFIDENTIALITY

Health Insurance Portability and Accountability Act of 1996

The enactment and subsequent promulgation of patient confidentiality statutes under the 1996 Health Insurance Portability and Accountability Act (HIPAA) has profoundly altered how patient-specific data are acquired, stored, and accessed (Figure 12-5). Informal patient discussions in the hallways between providers and patient sign-in sheets placed in public view have been replaced by

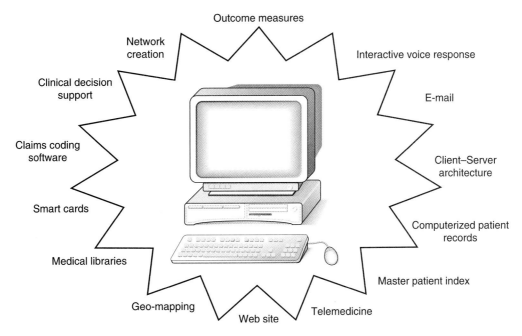

Figure 12–4. Computer-based IT applications.

security passwords, written authorizations, and sterilized data. HIPAA is not strictly an IT issue because it has fundamentally changed how many health care organizations conduct business, from patient scheduling to discharge planning. Some have called HIPAA "the full employment act for chief security officers" (Goedert, 2000).

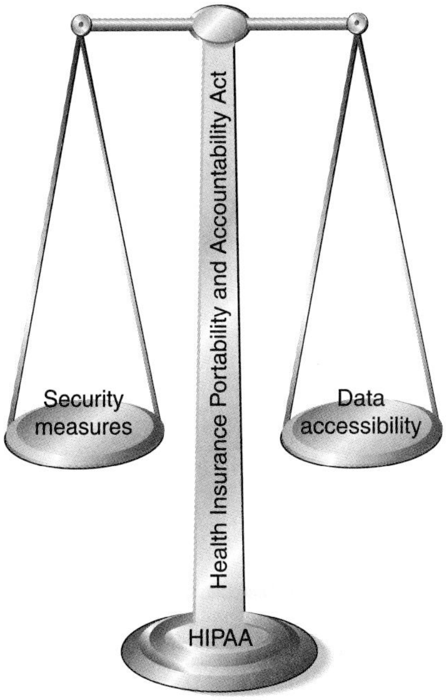

It is essential that rehabilitation providers fully understand the impact of HIPAA on health care delivery. Information is available to providers at the United States Health and Human Services Department. Specifically, a Fact Sheet entitled "Protecting the Privacy of Patients' Health Information" is available at http://www.hhs.gov/ocr/hipaa.

HIPAA permits patients access to their medical records within a 30-day period from time of request. Providers may charge for copying and mailing fees; however, providers must post a notice of HIPAA compliance and request a patient sign-off, acknowledging that they have been notified of their rights. Patients may restrict access of their records from certain entities not directly involved in their treatment or care. Data that identify specific patients may not be used for marketing purposes without written permission.

Tips for Selecting an Information Technology Vendor

Providers can place their IT needs out for bid but must understand that high cost does not necessarily assure high quality in IT development, nor does low cost condemn an organization to poor quality. The better defined an organization's needs are the more likely a compatible vendor can be identified. Seek references from similar health care providers before choosing a vendor for IT applications. A good reference from a hospital administrator may not guarantee performance when solutions are applied to an outpatient rehabilitation facility.

Determine what level of commitment your organization is prepared to make in order to become IT literate. *Are you prepared for business interruption while systems are being installed or the staff is getting trained?* It might be wise

Figure 12–5. Balancing patient confidentiality with record accessibility.

to purchase business interruption insurance under such circumstances. As previously cited, the average health care organization only allocates 2% of their annual budget toward IT. Ask yourself, "Is this a reasonable amount for my organization?"

Currently, there is no public policy posture to guide us in the development of IT capabilities that meet the needs of all health care providers, especially in rehabilitation. Therefore, when in doubt about how to approach an IT investment, rely on common sense, not the sales pitch of various vendors.

OVERVIEW OF INTERNET APPLICATIONS

Educated Consumers

The Internet promises to change the ways in which health care is delivered in the future. There may be unprecedented collaboration between patients and providers, particularly in the management of chronic disease and injury. By 1999, over 24 million Americans searched for health information using the Internet (Bickert, 1999). Baby boomers account for the greatest use of the Internet for health purposes. This medium will surely lead to more educated consumers who will have access to information through "net surfing." However, this information can be good or bad, as anyone who has surfed the net has observed. Therefore, patient education requirements may actually increase because of the Internet. Consumers will need to be educated about how to identify and avoid corrupt or inaccurate data. Consumers must learn to differentiate "informational web pages" from "advocacy web pages," which tend to be less accurate (Alexander & Tate, 1999). Refer to Chapter 15 for an expanded discussion of Web pages and other sources of data.

Breadth of Internet Applications

Rehabilitation providers will capitalize on Internet applications that span program development, billing and reimbursement, clinical care, patient education, provider continued education, patient-provider communication, peer-to-peer communication, telemedicine, and others. Table 12-3 provides a listing of Internet applications that span research, clinical, communications, reimbursement, and marketing purposes. Additional applications are certain to evolve as health care organizations explore means to enhance their competitiveness.

Internet Applications

Clinical Use of Electronic Mail

Electronic mail (e-mail) provides a valuable avenue for clinician-patient interaction. This information transmission mode can prevent telephone tag between the patient and the provider's office. E-mail represents a hybrid between letter writing and verbal communication. It is a low-cost option that is expeditious and leaves a written record that can be attached to the patient's chart. E-mail is not without its limitations, especially in regard to the issue of confidentiality. Also, e-mail is not routinely reimbursed by health plans. Time spent on e-mail usually does

 Table 12–3   Internet Applications Available to Providers

Research
- Access to research databases
- Ability to collect, store, and analyze data generated at disparate sites
- Access to government sources of research grant monies

Clinical
- Telemedicine/telerehab—access to diagnostic results
- Access to treatment guidelines, protocols, and pathways
- Provider credentialing and facility benchmarking
- Clinical documentation management
- Durable medical equipment procurement

Communications
- Patient education
- Provider continued education
- Insurance–health plan specifically claims adjuster or case manager education
- Employer education
- Regulatory, legislative, and compliance updates

Reimbursement
- Coding applications
- Electronic billing
- Electronic payment
- Health plan eligibility–benefits authorization

Marketing and Sales Support
- Website access for patient referral, education, advertisement, and branding

not result in revenue. Additionally, many providers do not wish to be accessible to patients, especially on a 24-hour basis. Productivity may be perceived to diminish when providers must pull away from "live" patients to transact with remote or "electronic" patients. Lastly, some providers prefer face-to-face encounters to the depersonalized electronic data exchange pathway. Rehabilitation providers have much to gain from utilizing e-mail. For instance, a home exercise or pain amelioration program can be periodically adjusted without the need to schedule an office visit. Attachments can be forwarded along with the provider's principal message. A recent survey revealed Internet access by age group: 77% of 18- to 29-year-olds, 75% of 30- to 49-years-olds, 58% of 50- to 64-year-olds, and 22% of persons 65 years or older currently go online (Fox, 2004). E-mail represents an opportunity to improve communication efficiency between the patient and clinician as well as between professional peers. It actively engages the patient in his or her own care, enhances patient accountability and compliance through accurate instruction, and is far less cumbersome than other forms of communication. E-mail is very advantageous for those providers who treat patients over a protracted period such as those in mental health, disease state management, and physical rehabilitation.

The start-up needs for e-mail are relatively simple and include access to a computer, telephone modem, e-mail software, and payment of a monthly access fee to an Internet Service Provider (ISP). In fact, some ISPs are actually free! The American Medical Informatics Association

(AMIA) has promulgated *Guidelines for the Clinical Use of Electronic Mail with Patients* (McCormack, 1998). This document provides some outstanding recommendations for the effective interaction between clinician and patient and the observance of medicolegal prudence. The AMIA acknowledges the paucity of published research regarding electronic exchange and cautions that a universal guideline is non-existent. E-mail is very useful for information that a patient would typically have to copy or receive orally. Examples include test results, exercise prescriptions, medication instructions, dressing changes, and discharge or postoperative instructions. E-mail messages can be embedded into educational resource universal resource locator (URL) links.

Rehabilitation providers can supply patients with a directory of sites that specifically address the diseases, injuries, and conditions of their respective patient populations. For instance, national associations or educational institutions that deal with diabetes, heart disease, musculoskeletal problems, pulmonary conditions, and neurological diseases can be readily located on the World Wide Web. Providers can direct their patients or clients to the search engines that specialize in certain areas.

E-mail Security

E-mail communication can never supplant face-to-face communication between patient and provider. If used discretely, however, it can be an asset to today's busy providers who do not have the time to engage in telephone tag. The liability stakes have never been higher with the enforcement of HIPAA confidentiality rules. E-mail transmissions are an especially risky form from at least two different perspectives: (1) the sender must be confident that the recipient is the intended recipient; (2) the recipient must be secure knowing who the sender is; and (3) both parties must be confident that the message was not altered by a third party while in transit.

E-mail is paradoxically both insecure and permanent by design. E-mail messages are actually more durable than paper communications, especially when broadcast to numerous recipients. This poses challenges when using a provider-patient e-mail system to communicate clinically-relevant and personal data. Some patients have expressed concerns that their employers may be privy to e-mail communication between providers and patients (Fridsma et al, 1994).

Providers are well-advised to consult with third-party IT experts and perhaps an attorney before commencing a patient-based e-mail system. These experts should ensure that effective communications combine efficiency with medicolegal prudence. Professional trade associations specializing in IT applications are additional sources of security guidelines.

The AMIA has developed valuable communication guidelines for rehabilitation providers (see Table 12–4).

The AMIA also recommends the use of headers on e-mail messages such as "CONFIDENTIAL medical communication." Providers are cautioned not to use their personal e-mail accounts for any patient transmissions. All transmissions should be relegated to business computers within the office itself. Recognize that e-mail does

Table 12–4 Medicolegal Administrative Guidelines

The following guidelines do not constitute legal advice. These guides have been adapted from the American Medical Informatics Association (AMIA). Readers are encouraged to consult with qualified legal counsel regarding their own specific needs.

- Obtain the patient's informed consent for e-mail participation.
- Provide operational definitions in terms of e-transmissions. Establish the types of transactions (i.e., appointment scheduling, testing-evaluation, education-training, home exercises).
- Inform patients about privacy issues in writing, consistent with HIPAA requirements. Draft an agreement with signature execution of both the provider and patient. Consider inclusion of an indemnification clause that limits liability in the event of network infractions beyond one's organization's control (e.g., system crashes, hacking, power outages at the Internet Server Provider [ISP] level).
- Provide patients with precise instructions on when and how to use e-mail. Instruct them to identify the category of transmission in a designated subject line (e.g., "test result," "medication question").
- Use patient identification numbers and protected screen savers for all desk workstations.
- Never transmit e-mail from home-based computers that include confidential data.
- Never use a patient's e-mail address for any sales-marketing purpose.
- At a minimum, perform weekly backups of e-mail onto long-term storage.
- Waive an encryption requirement, if any, at the patient's request. Do not use unencrypted wireless communication with patient-identifiable data.
- When sending an e-mail, be sure to double click the "To" section to ensure the right recipient is listed.
- Configure an automatic reply acknowledgement.
- Print all messages and place them in the patient's chart contemporaneously with office-based treatment notes.
- Train all staff in proper e-mail use; never assume that they already have the knowledge.
- Generate a list of permissible and non-permissible transmissions.
- Avoid use of a patient's full name, social security number, or other identity markers.
- Avoid leaving unopened e-mail messages on computer screens. Establish turnaround times for e-mail messages.
- Establish a written triage system for filtering e-transmissions to the appropriate party.

From American Medical Informatics Association (AMIA): Guidelines for Clinical Use of Electronic Mail with Patients, http://www.amia.org/pubs/pospaper, accessed December 13, 1999. Reprinted with permission from the Journal of the American Medical Informatics Association.

not supplant the need for office visits or face-to-face discussions. Something is always lost in e-mail translation, especially patient responses about their signs and symptoms. E-mail cannot reflect voice intonation, body language, facial grimacing, or other indicators of health status. Also, there is no guarantee that the patient has transmitted or received a clinician's message himself or herself. The AMIA provides a set of recommendations designed to secure e-mail transmissions. Again, rehabilitation providers are advised to consult with their legal counsel before implementing any risk management policies and procedures. The aforementioned suggestions neither represent nor replace qualified legal opinions.

Rehabilitation Providers as Mentors

The Internet will spawn a new breed of patients (McCormack, 1999; Kane & Sands, 1998). Currently, 22 million adults in the United States use the Internet to search for health care information according to research conducted by Cyber Dialogue. With the Internet, no man or woman will be an island, including providers. There will be unprecedented collaboration in health care and disability management. The Internet will facilitate more expeditious and efficient integration of health care products, services, and communication. Electronic exchanges are sure to eventually lead to patient selection of providers, treatment approach, and ownership of their own medical records. For some providers this represents a threat, to others, an opportunity to engage in a truly cooperative approach to health care. This should be a welcome change for physical rehabilitation providers who have already selected a profession because of the hands-on approach, degree of patient education, quality and quantity of patient-provider exchanges, and the cornerstone of patient involvement through exercise, home modality use, and behavioral modifications. Unlike the traditional passive role of "doctor heal me," tomorrow's patient will be expected to participate in "healing thyself." This may lead to a completely new paradigm shift for providers because they may no longer be as actively engaged in "giving treatment," instead serving as both architect and teacher. Actual treatment plans may be rendered by the patient, his or her family, or other supportive personnel. In any event, it will behoove rehabilitation providers to become as literate of Internet capabilities as possible to ensure their participation in new delivery paradigms.

Internet Applications: Provider Decision Support

Clinical or treatment protocols, also known as clinical pathways or clinical guidelines, have been promulgated by variety of organizations including industry associations, government agencies, specialty societies, medical or professional trade associations, and for-profit companies. Guidelines or protocols are generally evidence-based or based on best practices per se. The quality of the data utilized in the development of these protocols is generally uneven and may potentially include the good, the bad, and the ugly.

When applied, guidelines can assist in individual cases or dictate health care policy. Gillespie (2000) and McCormack (1999) reported two cases that involved an analysis of aggregate data from two developers of guidelines. MedStat Group of Ann Arbor, Michigan, reviewed 15,893 diabetic cases and discovered that only 29% had received an annual eye exam and only 46% had taken their annual cholesterol test (Gillespie, 2000). Both tests were underutilized despite clear guidelines developed by the American Diabetes Association. Similarly, an analysis of 6404 asthma cases revealed that only 27% of sufferers received anti-inflammatory medication to control their asthma (McCormack, 1999). In this case, the National Heart, Lung, and Blood Institute had developed the clinical guideline. These two cases provide convincing evidence regarding the value of clinical protocols when they are appropriately developed, disseminated, and applied by providers. So far, rehabilitation providers have not produced universally accepted databases or protocols. Despite the benefits of these data, some providers may resent the imposition of treatment protocols, especially when developed by payers or health plans.

The Evolution of Practice Guidelines

The early generation of clinical guidelines was mainly used to determine medically necessary care or to reduce cost. Quality improvement and interest in underutilization were only given lip service for much of the 1990s. There has been a surge of interest in using clinical guidelines as a component of total quality management (TQM) or continuous quality improvement (CQI) programs. This interest has spiked partly due to the growth of accrediting bodies (e.g., HEDIS/NCQA) and the legal and legislative backlash against managed care organizations. Provider organizations have also begun to realize that they must standardize their procedures in order to offer consistent value to payers.

One major initiative undertaken by the American Medical Association is the formation a not-for-profit entity, Medem Inc. (www.medem.com), which pools data from 6 professional associations and 45 medical societies. These include the American Academy of Ophthalmology, American Academy of Pediatrics, American College of Obstetrics and Gynecologists, American Psychological Association, American Society of Plastic Surgeons, and the American College of Allergy, Asthma & Immunology. Medem's partnering societies represent more than two-thirds of physicians currently practicing in the United States. Both physicians and consumers can access their databases. There does not appear to be similar collaborative efforts representing the physical rehabilitation sector. There are, however, efforts under way by individual professional organizations that pool data. The American Physical Therapy Association's "Hooked on Evidence" is one example (www.apta.org).

However, skeptical or cynical providers continue to equate treatment protocols to "cookbook medicine," when in reality, they can be adjunctive to clinical judgment. This, of course, assumes that treatment protocols are well-designed; involve provider input; are grounded in the clinical literature, research, peer consensus, and curriculum; and are not designed purely as a cost-containment measure. Decision support systems (DSS) also known as Clinical Decision Support (CDS) enable the provider, who may be sequestered from his or her peers, to benefit from the collective wisdom of many. They may do so by tapping into databases that are generated through the downloading of treatment information across practice settings, patient populations, insurance lines, and geographic regions. CDS systems apply rules to clinical and demographic data. In well-designed systems, these rules are written by clinicians that are well versed in the literature, prevailing practice patterns, clinical research, peer consensus documents, and other accepted sources of data.

DSS can supply providers with valuable information about intervention selection, length of stay or treatment duration, episodic care cost, and expected or anticipated outcomes measures. Gillespie (2000) describes the evolution of CDS through several generations. The first generation of CDS entailed employing assisted diagnostic work-ups designed to augment or corroborate the provider's clinical findings. These tools have limited utility in the physical rehabilitation field where a "functional diagnosis" is of principal concern versus a "medical diagnosis."

Second generation CDS provides the clinician with guidelines for treatment decisions. Treatment guidelines are most useful when a high degree of standardization exists. Standardization of medical nomenclature, physical assessment criteria, and case definitions and outcomes measures allow the application of treatment rules to similar cases. Again, these rules are designed with peer input after meticulous analysis of clinical literature, research, and prevailing practice patterns.

Advanced, or third generation, CDS systems provide decision support across all caregiver levels. For instance, in disease state management of diabetes, treatment is rendered by a host of caregivers ranging between nutritionists, nurses, physical therapists, physicians, and others.

The chief goal of CDS is to reduce treatment and outcome variation, which is of concern to virtually all stakeholders, but most notably providers and payers. A reduction in treatment variation hypothetically results in lower cost and improved care. Computerized patient records (CPR) are pivotal to the success of clinical decision support because it is from these records that data are secured about diagnosis, treatment intervention, and outcomes (Gillespie, 2000; Gillespie, 1999). Ideally, treatment protocols should be housed on the same computer in which the electronic patient records reside.

Sophisticated CDS systems involve artificial intelligence that allows computers to analyze patient data via complex algorithms. A customized care plan is then generated by the computer (artificial intelligence) to augment the clinician's clinical judgment. Minimally, it provides the boundaries of care, and under ideal circumstances, it prescribes or prohibits specific interventions based upon data from thousands, if not millions, of similar cases. To date, there are no systems that analyze rehabilitation cases and prescribe universally accepted customized treatment.

Some CDS systems attempt to address fiscal concerns. If costs will be impacted, then financial and billing information must be linked to clinical information in a meaningful manner. Gillespie (2000) asserts that, "The lack of a standardized medical nomenclature, for example, can hamper the deployment of computer-based patient records or decision support systems." Some national medical organizations have, or are developing, generic databases for treatment protocols. For example, the National

Guideline Clearinghouse is a publicly available repository for clinical guidelines developed by following the abstract review of thousands of clinical protocols. Clinical guidelines can be compared with different sources and selected by the user based upon his or her particular need. This network is cosponsored by the Agency for Health Care Research and Quality (formerly the Agency for Health Care Policy and Research/AHCPR), the American Association of Health Plans, and the American Medical Association. The Web site (www.guideline.gov) was launched in January of 1999 and, to date, it includes over 600 different clinical guidelines.

Internet Applications: Provider Credentialing Service

Provider credentialing is a cornerstone of managed care. Heretofore, credentialing and recredentialing have been performed through a paper process or via site visits. Managed care organizations (MCOs) use standardized forms for credentialing providers. This form is completed either by the provider or with input from a site auditor. Provider organizations and networks also perform credentialing of their members. Information that is collected during the credentialing process may include, but is not restricted to the following:

- Facility location
- Hours of business
- Provider's educational background
- Provider's licensure or board certifications
- Professional liability coverage levels (aggregate and per incident)
- History of malpractice claims
- Criminal history
- History of licensure revocation or judicial or ethics committee actions
- Fee schedule
- Available services
- Financial interest in other facilities to which one refers (e.g., laboratories, PT, SNFs)

The credentialing process for some providers is now handled through the Internet. Providers are assigned an identity code that only they and the MCO can decipher.

Provider Accreditation

Provider organizations can refer to the National Committee on Quality Assurance (NCQA) or the Joint Commission for the Accreditation of Health Organizations (JCAHO) for further guidelines associated with Internet use. Please refer to Appendix for additional information on the organizations. NCQA reviews health plans' consumer protection and quality improvement programs, whereas JCAHO reviews and conducts audits of health care organizations' quality assurance programs, including management information system processes. JCAHO accreditation requires that provider organizations develop and maintain a written plan for IT management. Both organizations determine whether an entity has standardized operating procedures; common messaging protocols; data verification processes; security and confidentiality provisions; and clearly defined policies and procedures, including enforcement.

There is concern about the potential for hacking or computer virus infiltration. Organizations must produce evidence that security measures address both of these potentialities. The profusion of Internet transmissions has generated a proportional concern for privacy and confidentiality. For more information, readers are advised to review the Department of Health and Human Services' privacy rules provisions published November 3, 1999. This 149-page draft is available in portable document format (PDF) or via HTML format in more than 630 pages at www.dhhs.gov.html.

Internet Applications: Telemedicine and "Telerehab"

Telemedicine is a technology that enables providers to render their professional opinions regarding diagnostic tests or treatment options via telecommunication lines. Currently, the preponderance of telemedicine involves the provision of second or consultative opinions regarding medical tests. For instance, it is a common practice in rural-area facilities to forward diagnostic tests to satellite locations where specialists can interpret the findings. For example, telemetry results in a cardiac case may be reviewed by a physician at a heart institute. Emerging technologies and patient demographics are certain to fuel advances in telemedicine and "telerehab" (Hersh et al, 2003; Brown, 2003; Hatzakis et al, 2003; Russell et al, 2003). Some key rehabilitation areas that are compatible with telemedicine applications include functional capacity evaluation or assessment, functional job analyses, EMG/NCV studies, disability evaluations, therapeutic exercises, sports medicine, and specialized treatment for catastrophic injury. Catastrophic injury, for the sake of this discussion, involves either expensive treatments or conditions that require intensive service. Spinal cord injury, traumatic brain injury, serious hand injury, amputation, and neurological conditions (e.g., amyotrophic lateral sclerosis, multiple sclerosis, and muscular dystrophy) are examples of potentially catastrophic injuries or illnesses. IT may foster the growth of "telerehab," especially in the management of chronic conditions (Temkin et al, 1996).

Telemedicine is not without its controversy or risk (McCrossin, 2003). One of the most hotly debated issues is that of practicing medicine out of state without proper licensure. Because telemedicine crosses state lines, some question whether it equates to practice without a license. It raises a larger debate concerning the issue of global versus local medicine. Since the health care system evolved long before the advent of telecommunications and the Internet, most people view it as a local phenomenon. Although most practitioners are licensed to practice their profession in the state in which patients reside, many now offer their expertise beyond the local area. Most states interpret medical treatment as being rendered where the patient is located. Siwicki (1999) reports that a number of states have passed or are considering legislation akin to a "mini-license" to practice telemedicine. Again, providers will need to conduct their own legal and ethical benefit-risk analysis before embracing

telemedicine and telerehab (Silverman, 2003). This new paradigm appears imminent, considering the combination of reimbursement pressures and the explosion in IT applications.

Internet Applications: Strategic Planning

Strategic planning is one of the business (versus clinical or regulatory) functions that is well served by the Internet. E-mail allows for the broadcasting of simultaneous information to staff members or clients. Virtual companies that are electronically linked can engage in instantaneous communication and reverse directions quickly when market trends shift. Additionally, the sheer volume of information that is readily available through the Internet dramatically reduces learning curves, market-research delays, and product rollout cycles. Demographic information garnered through the linkage of clinical, business, and regulatory databases enables an organization to reposition itself relative to the competition or under-served patient populations.

Internet Applications: Interactive Voice Response Technology

Interactive voice response (IVR) technology has been around for years but has only recently been applied to health care. IVR is not typically considered to be an Internet application, although it may be linked to Internet-based resources. IVR is usually thought of as a separate delivery mechanism for IT services. Many of us have called a large company, typically a bank, financial, retail, or insurance company, only to find ourselves talking to a computer. Insurance companies employ IVR across different insurance lines to ascertain and explain varying benefit structures or to preauthorize care. Data are entered through a voice recognition mode or by keying it in from a touchtone telephone. IVR has been used to access performance data, determine salary and benefit levels, determine disability benefits, or to access job postings. Some health care providers have experienced IVR when calling an HMO to precertify or preauthorize treatment. This is especially common under group health or general accident insurance plans, as opposed to automobile liability or workers' compensation cases.

Figure 12–6 depicts an IVR schematic involving precertification or preauthorization of care.

Typically, a provider or its representative contacts a health plan via telephone and provides case-specific data. These data involve demographic and condition-specific information. Treatment interventions are required for the plan's computer to precertify or authorize a specific level of care. When care frequency, cost, or duration pierces pre-established thresholds, either a live person takes the call or data are routed to a computer manned by a utilization review or benefits specialist. Savvy health care organizations are using IVR to voluntarily and internally precertify their care to avoid retrospective review and denial of services after the expenditure of capital and human resources. This is an extremely valuable technology for those companies who have risk sharing contracts with managed care organizations.

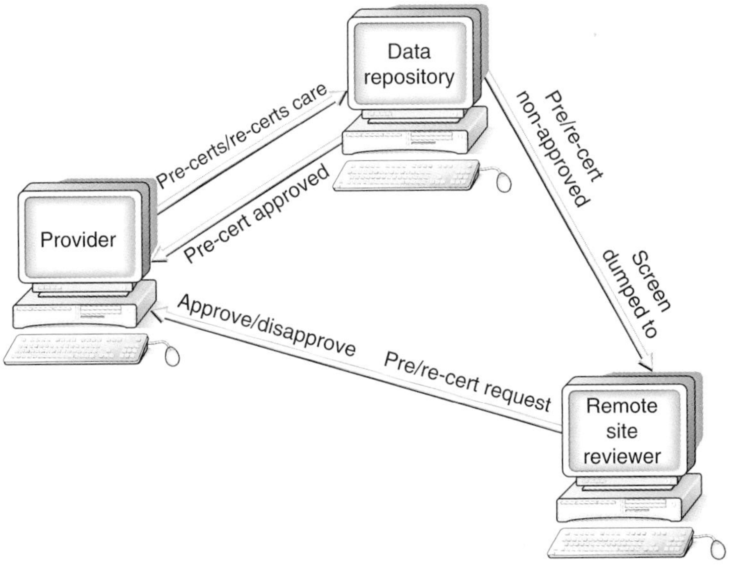

Figure 12–6. Interactive voice response (IVR) schematic.

Bar Code Technology

Bar codes or universal product codes (UPC) appear in virtually every area of commerce, including health care. Rehabilitation providers have been somewhat slow to embrace this technology with the exception of those employed in large institutions. Each product or service carries a unique bar code or magnetic strip, which is recognized by computer software. Bar code labels also identify individual patients so that appropriate records can be paired with them. Codes from a patient's chart, test result, or durable medical equipment prescription are scanned by a device linked to a personal computer. Some of these devices are wireless to accommodate clinically based transactions. Rehabilitation services present several unique obstacles to the use of bar codes. The frequent encounters that patients have in rehabilitation require that each episode has its own code. Diverse providers often provide rehabilitation, therefore provider identifiers are essential. Rehabilitation is often billed under CPT-4 codes shared by physical therapists, occupational therapists, physicians, nurse practitioners, physician assistants, and many others.

Applications in rehabilitation for bar code or magnetic strip technology include the following:

- Medication management
- Durable medical equipment, wound dressings, therapeutic exercise equipment
- Coupling modality or therapeutic exercise parameters to a patient's condition
- Pairing patient test or evaluation results to their rehab chart (e.g., FCEs)
- Categorization of medical records (e.g., outpatient, inpatient, home care)

The rehabilitation field can learn from the hospital-based system wherein nurses track a patient's medication use via bar codes. This technology can be transferred to enable clinicians to track therapeutic exercise compliance, home modality use, ambulatory assistive device histories, DME usage, and any other function that is repetitive or serial in nature. The author has applied bar code technology in an occupational health surveillance program for carpal tunnel syndrome risk assessment in order to ensure that a tested employee's nerve conduction velocity result is paired with the patient's medical history and functional job analysis or ergonomic assessment. Incumbent employee populations were assessed for their risk of developing and/or exposure to carpal tunnel stressors. Each employee underwent a medical-personal health history. These data were entered into a questionnaire that had an accompanying bar code identifying the employee. In addition, each employee's job was analyzed from an ergonomic standpoint to determine widely acknowledged risk factors, such as cold ambient temperatures, repetitive motion, non-physiological positions, and other documented stressors.

This form also included the unique bar code feature. Lastly, each employee received a sensory nerve conduction velocity (NCV) test to determine the neural transmission speed across the carpal tunnel. Each NCV trial incorporated the unique bar code for a given employee. Data from the three assessment tools was downloaded onto a smart card and ultimately into a personal computer. The PC integrated the three data elements. The computer analyzed one's risk of developing carpal tunnel syndrome. Then, through an artificial intelligence process, recommendations were generated for each employee. Computer software then assigned a different weighting factor to each stressor, whether it was ergonomically induced (worksite) or medically induced (worker). Evidence supportive of the weighting system was generated from extensive literature searches. Worker-specific stressors included obesity, pregnancy, diabetes, and other health conditions known to be associated with cumulative trauma disorders. The computer then generated unique recommendations for each employee or worker that were driven by ergonomic and/or health stressors (the ErgoMed approach). These recommendations were then reviewed and adjusted by clinicians including an orthopedic hand surgeon, internist, nurse, and physical therapist. The bar code technology enabled evaluators to collect and aggregate data pertaining to specific employees from disparate sources. Similar applications are possible on the treatment side of disability management.

Smart Cards

Health care smart cards contain embedded computer chips that retain medical or insurance information on a patient. They are popular in Europe but have just begun to emerge in the United States. The advantages of this new technology are enormous. A provider can access the chronological medical history of his or her patient by using a card-swipe device. This eliminates problems associated with data entry errors or patients who are poor historians. Patients who have chronic conditions, who seek frequent treatment at multiple sites, or who are engaged in disease state management programs are prime candidates for smart card applications.

Smart cards can bolster a provider's risk management program through the collection and recording of accurate medical information. Additionally, when cards contain insurance benefit information, it can save providers the heartache of a retrospective denial of benefits, particularly if there are financial limits as in automobile liability of personal injury protection or PIP limits.

Geo-Mapping Software

This software enables a provider to access demographic data within defined geographic parameters. There are multiple applications available with geo-mapping. Sophisticated systems track or plot multiple variables or characteristics such as patient gender, age, regions, neighborhoods, insurance status, consumer surveys, and standard industrial classification codes (SIC). Software presents its data in the following two formats: in geographic maps or in tabular forms. Geo-mapping has been used extensively by public health agencies to determine community health care needs (e.g., child vaccinations, breast examinations, STD tracking). Geo-mapping is advantageous to health care organizations that enter at-risk contracts. It enables some degree of patient-volume prediction based upon enrollee assessments in a given region. Health care organizations can develop a profile of their patients through zip code tracking. This technology also allows tracking of other data elements, including: referral source, employer, case manager, and insurer location. Geo-mapping offers strategic planning capabilities because an organization can identify where satellite sites may be needed or where additional staffing may be required.

INTRANET APPLICATIONS: OVERVIEW

The term Intranet generally describes the use of Internet applications to facilitate the exchange of data within an organization. Intranets are only accessible to authorized users, typically employees. In today's era of "clinics without walls" or "virtual corporations," operational functions are not required in only one location. Tip O'Neill, former U.S. representative, once quipped that

"politics is local," and so it is with health care. Although health care organizations desire critical mass and size, the actual delivery of care remains at the local level. However, organizations have a craving to aggregate their clinical and business data (compound integration) so that any department or person within the corporate umbrella has access. This is especially important with national managed care contracts serviced at multiple provider sites. Essentially, Intranets enable users to access multiple databases, avoiding piecemeal retrieval. Intranets are based on Web browsers that send a transmission to a middleware server. The server connects databases for reciprocal delivery or receipt of data. This allows providers to retrieve data, thus avoiding the need for mail, fax transmissions, or express delivery of information. Intranets also enable providers to connect with medical libraries. As with most computer technologies, Intranet applications initially tend to address the business functions of an organization versus the clinical needs. This partly explains why clinically based Intranets are still in the emergent phase of development.

Intranets house a variety of databases or functions, including the following:

- Employee directories
- Organizational charts
- Company policies and procedures
- Chat or discussion rooms-forums
- Customer–client lists
- Service descriptions
- Employee benefits

Intranet Applications: Computerized Patient Records

Computerized patient records are essential if one is to engage in meaningful computer exchange of business or clinical data. Clinical patient records (CPR) are also known as electronic medical records (EMR), electronic health records (EHR), or paperless charts. CPR systems were first developed for inpatient hospitals but have become diversified with the shift towards ambulatory services and home care.

The heart and soul of CPR is a central repository or relational database that allows for the receipt, storage, and retrieval of data. CPR is essential if providers wish to engage in outcomes measures, provider credentialing, or CDS (e.g., treatment algorithms) programs. Chin (1999b) provides a list of recommendations or tips on how to get started with CPR (Table 12–5).

Rehabilitation providers should not fret if they have not entered the CPR fray. According to Bazzoli (1996), only 5% of all physicians have CPR systems in place. However, CPR has received a jump start from the Health Insurance Portability and Accountability Act of 1996, and the increasing pressure from managed care organizations for more and more data. Although some providers may resist an organization's efforts to develop computer-based records, a wide-ranging literature review reveals that the clinical, workflow, administrative, and revenue enhancements benefits of CPR outweigh barriers and challenges (Erstad, 2003).

Table 12–5 Tips for Starting a Computer-Based Patient Record

- Select a repository that is scalable or capable of expanding as your business grows.
- Select a repository that is front-end user friendly.
- Request customer referrals for the vendor staying within your company's sector or niche.
- Buy off-the-shelf software and avoid the development of self-designed programs.
- Consider a test pilot approach and incrementally phase-in the program.
- Dedicate staff (e.g., IT specialist) to train clinicians in the use of the system.
- Upgrade your network infrastructure to assure that providers can promptly access data stored in the central repository.
- Implement an enterprise master patient index that allows each site to download and upload data. This reduces costly redundant data entries.
- Develop a standard medical vocabulary through peer consensus, and distribute it to all staff members.
- Install an interface engine that links clinical systems to the central repository.
- Involve clinicians in the entire process.
- Select a vendor that is financially sound and possesses a vision of how your business works, especially the linkage between a central repository (business applications) and computer-based records (clinical applications).

Data modified from Chin TL: Gathering clinical data: A clinical data repository provides the foundation for computer-based patient records. Health Data Manage 7(5):47, 1999b.

Components of a Computer-based Patient Record

Master Patient Index (MPI)

A master patient index (MPI) involves a software database that links financial and clinical data together throughout an enterprise network (Bazzoli, 1996). Although integrated delivery systems have pioneered MPI, this concept is applicable across large multi-service organizations or to smaller single-service organizations. The core element of an MPI is its central data repository. In these systems, patients are assigned one identification number, which is used across treatment sites or service sectors. Scalability is an important element if an MPI is to be successful. Scalability means that capability can be expanded or reduced as a network grows or shrinks. It is equally important that data exchanges occur in real time and that they eliminate redundant entries.

Client-Server Architecture

Client-server architecture is a term for the ability of multiple personal computers, known as clients, to link with more powerful computers, known as servers. Internet computing is a form of client-server architecture because data are reciprocally exchanged between the client and server. Although the client may be programmed to focus on one principal function, the server can multitask, or handle many functions. Servers can consolidate disparate sources of information and merge business, clinical, and legal-regulatory into meaningful functions. These systems are commonly used by case managers, customer service representatives, benefits managers, provider relations personnel, and by credentialing agencies. McDonald (1998) describes three types of standards that are used in IT management. All of these are found within a client-server architecture.

1. Message standards define the data structures of the records sent between individual systems. An example would be an admission department's message sent to the laboratory.
2. Clinical code standards are multiaxial nomenclature systems that are designed to index entire medical records by the patient's signs, symptoms, diagnoses, procedures, and clinical outcomes.
3. Privacy standards are the rules designed to protect the confidentiality of patients and providers. They are the identification codes or encryptions designed to protect the system from hackers, those seeking unauthorized access.

Claims Coding Software

There are now a number of software programs available that assist providers in the identification of ICD-9 diagnostic and CPT-4 treatment codes; both are requirements of Medicare participation. This capability offers several advantages to rehabilitation providers. Accurate code selection is vital to expedient and optimal reimbursement. Automation reduces the dissonance that exists between staff members who select different codes for the same treatment or diagnosis. This commonly occurs between clinical and administrative staff. Automation is also useful in tracking data for clinical outcomes measurement purposes and in formulating provider report cards. In the latter instance, resource allocation, as a product of treatment code selection, can be determined among providers. Treatment efficiency measures may address the question of, *Do some providers use fewer resources in achieving the same or superior clinical outcomes?* A clinic's profitability statement can be augmented through the automation of diagnostic and treatment codes. This is most helpful when bidding for selective managed-care contracts, which require that a provider know their cost of doing business. It can also provide guidance in assigning providers to specific patient populations. For instance, a clinic's most efficient clinician, defined as the person with optimal outcome relative to resource inputs, can be apportioned a greater volume of capitated patients. To the contrary, it would be prudent to not use a therapist who utilizes substantial resources by rendering extensive treatment to a managed-care caseload. Code automation can bolster a risk management program by documenting specifically what was provided to an individual patient and for which diagnosis. Clinical documentation (inclusive of coding choices) is the first line of defense when an adverse event occurs. Some software programs provide "red flags" or advance directives to assist the provider in appropriate selection. This is also known as a "crosswalk feature" because it guides one by the hand, so to speak. There are inherent cost savings when automation is used and manually intensive searches are reduced or eliminated. Computer software also minimizes data entry errors associated with a purely manual process. The ICD-9 book has over 63,000 diagnoses from which to choose. Large health care organizations rely on claims-processing houses. The provider downloads his or her billing information through one electronic connection to the claims processor who, through a server, broadcasts claims data to scores of health plans. This eliminates the need for a provider to be online electronically with dozens of payers using countless billing formats.

SELECTING A COMPUTER OR INFORMATION TECHNOLOGY SERVICE VENDOR

It is safe to conclude that most rehabilitation providers (including the author) are not IT experts. It is equally safe to conclude that some providers do not have access to an internally based IT expert, especially those in smaller organizations such as private practices. Providers are already challenged in staying abreast of clinical technology advances. They may not have the time, aptitude, or desire to dabble in IT applications. Therefore, some may elect to contract with an external IT consultant. This too can be a challenging task. Table 12–6 provides some basic issues to consider when selecting a computer or IT vendor. Readers are also encouraged to contact various trade organizations and entities that specialize in these applications. These include the following:

- American Medical Informatics Association, www.amia.org
- Computer Security Institute, www.gocsi.com
- International Computer Security Association, www.ncsa.com
- International Information Systems Security Certification Consortium, www.isc2.org
- International Systems Security Association, Inc., www.issa-intl.org
- National Committee for Quality Assurance (NCQA), www.ncqa.org
- U. S. Department of Health & Human Services, Health Accountability Act (HIPAA) of 1996, www.hhs.gov

SUMMARY

Some may believe that health care is entering an era of the paperless clinic whereas others think not. Some may believe that automated clinical algorithms will supplant clinical judgment whereas others may not. Some may think that clinical data elements and business elements can be seamlessly merged whereas others may not. Some may believe that computer automation will lead to improved clinical outcomes whereas others may not. However, the one thing that many can agree on is best summarized by Moran (1998, p 11):

> *"It might appear that we are poised on the brink of a dramatic new era in health care, in which the power of emerging computing and telecommunications technologies synergistically combines with rapid advances in the biological sciences to produce a quantum leap in our ability both to treat disease and to promote rapid and continuous improvement in the efficiency of clinical processes."*

 Table 12–6   How to Select a Computer Service Vendor

- Compare apples to apples: Select vendors with specific experience in your business.
- Secure a reference list.
- Demand an on-site demonstration.
- Determine the ability of the vendor to modify off-the-shelf products.
- Look for an integrated package that combines clinical and financial data elements.
- Ascertain vendor's technical support capabilities and ask how long after the sale they are available.
- Ask the vendor about its participation in standardization efforts (e.g., American National Standards Institute [ANSI], National Committee for Quality Assurance [NCQA]).
- Inquire about the vendor's future plans and product rollouts especially as they relates to the Internet.
- Request a credit rating report to determine financial solvency of the vendor.
- Review the vendor's training materials to determine user-friendliness and the potential for a "train the trainers" approach.
- Ask for published articles that highlight the vendor's products and services.
- Do not purchase anything until your legal counsel, accountant, and risk manager have examined it.

REFERENCES

Alexander J, Tate MA: Web Wisdom: How to evaluate and create information quality on the Web. Mahwah, NJ, Lawrence Erlbaum Associates Publishers, 1999.

Baldwin G: Intranets are the key to new database strategies. Health Data Manage 7(11):56-64, 1999.

Bazzoli F: Providers point to index software as key element of integration plans. Health Data Manage 4(9):61-65, 1996.

Bickert M: The impact of ecommerce on legacy health-care companies, Cyber Dialogue, New York, 1999.

Brown SJ: Next generation telecare and its role in primary and community care. Health Soc Care Community 11(6):459-462, 2003.

Chin TL: Putting an end to the paper chase. Health Data Manage 7(3): 46-58, 1999a.

Chin TL: Gathering clinical data: A clinical data repository provides the foundation for computer-based patient records. Health Data Manage 7(5):47, 1999b.

Cross M: Computers that think. Health Data Manage 7(2):146-151, 1991.

Erstad TL: Analyzing computer-based patient records: A review of the literature. J Healthcare Information Management 17(4): 51-57, 2003.

Fox S: Older Americans and the Internet. Reports: Demographics, Pew Internet and American Life Project, www.pewinternet.org, accessed August 8, 2004.

Fridsma DB, Ford P, Altman R: A survey of patient access to electronic mail: Attitudes, harriers and opportunities. Procedures Annual Symposium Computer Application & Medical Care, 1994, pp 15-19.

Gallo AC, Lee VJ: Health care information technology: Keeping health care wired. Research Report. Alex Brown Company, Baltimore, May 5, 1998.

Gillespie G: A pillar of support. Health Data Manage 7(8):58-65, 1999.

Gillespie G: Online clinical guidelines help trim costs. Health Data Manage 8(1):38-45, 2000.

Goedert J: The dawn of HIPAA: Is HIPAA the full employment act for chief security officers? Health Data Manage 8(4):92, 2000.

Hatzakis M, Haselkorn J, Williams R: Telemedicine and the delivery of health services to veterans with multiple sclerosis. J Rehabil Res Dev 40(3):265-282, 2003.

Hersh D, Hersch F, Mikuletic L: A web-based approach to low-cost telemedicine. J Telemed Telecare 9(Suppl 2):224-266, 2003.

Horn SD, Hopkins DSP: Clinical practice improvement: A new technology for developing cost-effective quality health care. Faulkner & Gray Healthcare Information Center, Washington, DC, 1994, p 35.

Kane B, Sands DZ: White paper, guidelines for the use of electronic mail with patients, for the American Medical Informatics Association (AMIA), J Am Med Inform Assoc 5(1):104-111, 1998, www.amia.org/pubs/pospaper/positio2.htm, accessed May 6, 2004.

Kleinke JD: Release 0.0: Clinical information technology in the real world. Health Aff 17(6):23-38, 1998.

McCormack J: The top 10 ways the internet is changing health care I.T. Health Data Manage 7(12):34-39, 1999.

McCormack J: The missing link: Health care organizations are using data standards and integration technologies to bridge disparate information systems. But the task is far from simple. Health Data Manage 7(9):72-82, 1999

McCormack J: Improving the odds: Health care providers are using information systems to gather and analyze data that will help make entering capitated managed care contracts less of a gamble. Health Data Manage 6(11):58-67, 1998.

McCormack J: The possibilities and perils of e-mail. Group Practice Data Manage 1(2):32-38, 1998.

McCrossin R: Managing risk in telemedicine. J Telemed Telecare 9(2):36-39, 2003.

McDonald CJ: Need for standards in health information. Health Aff 17(6):44-46, 1998.

The Medem Network—Connecting Physicians and Patients, http://www.medem.com, accessed June 24, 2004.

Milbank Memorial Fund: Better information, better outcomes? The use of health technology assessment and clinical effectiveness data in health care purchasing decisions in the United Kingdom and the United States. Milbank Memorial Fund New York, 2000.

Moran DW: Health information policy: On preparing for the next war. Health Aff 17(6):9-22, 1998.

Russell TG, Jull GA, Wootton R: Can the Internet be used as a medium to evaluate knee angle? Man Ther 8(4):242-246, 2003.

Silverman RD: Current legal and ethical concerns in telemedicine and e-medicine. J Telemed Telecare 9(1):S67-S69, 2003.

Siwicki B: Telemedicine providers' progress impeded at the border. Health Data Manage 7(5):94-102, 1999.

Temkin AJ, Ulicny GR, Vesmarovich SH: A perspective of the way technology is going to change the future of patient treatment. Rehabil Manage 9(2):28-30, 1996.

US Department of Health & Human Services, http://www.hhs.gov/ocr/hipaa, accessed May 6, 2004.

Van Brunt D: Internet-based patient information systems: What are they, why are they here, how will they be used, and will they work? J Rehabil Outcomes Measures 2(5):58-63, 1998.

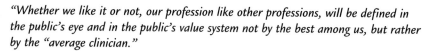

CHAPTER 13

The Quest for Quality in Health Care

David W. Clifton, Jr., PT

"Whether we like it or not, our profession like other professions, will be defined in the public's eye and in the public's value system not by the best among us, but rather by the "average clinician."

- Rothstein, 2001

KEY POINTS

- Quality is in the eye of the beholder, and there is a diversity of beholders.
- Quality assessment and improvement in health care has traditionally been associated with process and structure elements but devoid of outcome measures.
- Rehabilitation providers must consider how other stakeholders define quality.
- Quality indicators that include outcome measures, both cost-related and function-based, will resonate with other stakeholders, especially payers.
- Multiple stakeholder groups are attempting to define quality services partly because of providers' failure to do so.

Operational Definitions

Health Care Stakeholder	Any person or entity that is involved either directly or indirectly in the finance or delivery of services during an episode of care.
Quality	The extent to which health services for individuals and populations increase the likelihood of desired health outcomes and are consistent with current professional knowledge" (IOM, 1990).
"Soft" Clinical Measures	Process and structure measures that do not address functional outcomes in rehabilitation.
Value	A dimension in the disablement model that considers benefit-cost ratios in addition to clinical outcomes.

HEALTH CARE SYSTEM INPUTS VERSUS OUTPUTS

Rothstein's quote illustrates the importance of pursuing excellence and the need to define quality rehabilitation. "Quality" and "Outcomes" are distinct yet associated concepts that are treated separately in this text (two separate chapters). The traditional view of health care quality in the United States emphasizes system inputs, or process, versus outcomes (Morrison, 1996). Provider training and credentials, equipment and technology, facilities, organizational elements, and capital investment are examples of inputs. Some believe that high-quality care increases the likelihood of beneficial outcomes (Chassin et al, 1998). This model suggests a direct correlation between system inputs and outcomes. However, although the United States spends 14% of its GDP on health care, it lags behind many nations in key health measures, such as life expectancy, suggesting that health care system inputs have poor correlation with outputs or outcomes (Regnier, 2003).

A number of quality gaps exist in service organizations (O'Connor et al, 2000). These gaps are created when a chasm exists between expected service and perceived service. This gap tends to be especially broad in health care organizations that principally focus on transactions rather than consumer relationships. O'Connor et al (1991) assert that health care's most critical need is to increase awareness among providers regarding consumer expectations.

Provider Credentials

A discussion of health care quality must include provider competencies since it is providers who drive health care system inputs through diagnostic workups, treatment plan development, goal establishment, and technology selection. The current U.S. health care system is presumed to be superior to others partly because it is the world's most expensive system. The multitude of certifications and accreditations that providers and their facilities secure contributes to this perception (Sullivan, 1998; Goka & Arakaki, 1991; Neuman & Ptak, 2003; Rainwater & Romano 2003). However, these credentials predominantly focus on process and structure elements of health care delivery and not outcomes measures (Kronneger, 1999). This begs a number of questions including the following:

● Do certifications and accreditations indicate how something is done (e.g., process and structure) or how well it is done?
● Do certifications and accreditations guarantee outcomes and quality of care? Are those providers and facilities that possess selective credentials more competent than those without them?
● Do certifications and accreditations describe who should render a specific treatment?
● Do certifications and accreditations accurately identify master clinicians and "centers of excellence?"
● Do certifications correlate with outcomes? Should providers with greater credentials be held to a higher level of quality (e.g., six sigma)?

Coye and Detmer (1998) assert that purchasers have traditionally accepted facility accreditations and board certifications as "proxies for quality." Doloresco (2001) points out that accreditation can be a symbol of excellence but not a guarantee of excellence. Some illustrate the flaws in accreditation whereas others support more standards (Cross, 2003; MacDonell, 1997; Gallagher, 2003; Greenberg, 2003).

At least one study of provider credentials has correlated clinical specialty status with greater efficiency, defined by fewer visits and treatment procedures. However, this same study failed to show improved clinical effectiveness measured by change in health status (Hart & Dobrzykowski, 2000). It may be unrealistic to expect patients to define quality elements when providers themselves have failed to reach a consensus.

QUALITY BEGINS WITH EDUCATION

A provider's education begins the journey toward achieving quality in health care delivery. Currently, most professionals receive their education and training in a relatively sequestered manner; however, interdisciplinary programs are growing. The Institute of Medicine (IOM) sponsored a study in 1991 (Crossing the Quality Chasm) that resulted in the publication of *Health Professions Education: A Bridge to Quality* (Greiner & Knebel, 2003). This text outlines the following five core areas in which professionals must develop and maintain proficiency:

1. Delivering patient-centered care
2. Working in an interdisciplinary team
3. Practicing evidence-based health care
4. Focusing on quality improvement
5. Using information technology

Educators, accreditation bodies, certification entities, and licensing organizations are all encouraged to emphasize these competencies so that providers can meet the evolving needs of patients in a changing health care environment.

DEFINING QUALITY

Several visionaries largely fueled the quest for quality throughout the business world; this pursuit then trickled down into the health care sector. These change agents gave birth to terms such as "total quality management" (TQM) and "continuous quality improvement" (CQI). Juran (1988) & Gryma (1989), Deming (1986), and Ishikawa (1986) published seminal works that laid the foundation for many of today's quality improvement initiatives.

The health care sector is a relative latecomer to quality initiatives when compared to other business sectors. Franke (1990) mused that health care providers relied heavily on provider-patient rapport versus clinical outcomes. He stated, "Quality is not that the catheter is put in well, but is it put in friendly." For many, quality was taken for granted. The Japanese describe this as *atarimae hinshitsu* (acceptable or of average quality, not superior quality) (Ishikawa, 1986). Today's six sigma initiatives seek excellence in quality, which the Japanese describe as *Miryokuteki hinshitsu*, or quality that fascinates (Chassin, 1998).

The National Roundtable on Health Care Quality, sponsored by the Institute of Medicine, a component of the National Academies of Science, claims that the quality of health care can be precisely defined and measured with a degree of scientific accuracy on par with other clinical measures (Donaldson, 1998; Chassin et al, 1998). All health care stakeholders, including providers, payers, consumers, government, employers, attorneys, and others, have embarked on individual quests to define, measure, and articulate quality. It can be said that quality, like beauty, is "in the eye of the beholder." It seems that virtually everyone has their own concept of quality, and, as a result, different health care stakeholders express different interests. For instance, payers are predominantly interested in economic measures of quality (cost), whereas providers traditionally focus on clinical measures (intervention-outcome). Payers are more prone to describe cost-effective care as a good outcome, whereas a rehabilitation provider may describe desirable outcomes in terms of functionality, with little concern for cost. This may be an oversimplification, but it is not without some basis. However, both providers and purchasers of health care have become more concerned about its value, efficiency, appropriateness, and effectiveness (O'Connor & Lanning, 1991).

Although perceptions may differ between stakeholders, money is a common concern between parties because no stakeholder group wishes to be solely responsible for payment of services. The financial burden is expected to be shared among stakeholders. Risk-sharing is one of the hallmarks of managed care that is likely to survive. Although providers may yearn for the days of supplier-induced demand and fee-for-service, those days are likely gone forever. Today's providers must consider both economic (value purchasing) as well as clinical-quality indicators. Payers (e.g., employers, insurers, government) may relish the transfer of risk to providers via capitation, prospective payment, or case rate reimbursement. However, they owe at least two basic duties to taxpayers and consumers: They hold a fiduciary responsibility of supplying the best possible health care at reasonable cost, and they have an ethical obligation to ensure the quality of the health care they fund (Greenfield et al, 1996).

Although payers and providers may consider themselves adversaries, in reality, one cannot survive without the other. Providers immutably need sources of funding for their increasing costs. Payers require the services of providers to manage the risk they have assumed. Despite this interdependency, both sides tend to demand increasing control and can be relentless in seizing it. It is not a stretch to state that patients, the actual consumers of the service, demand the highest quality of care as long as someone else covers the cost. These generalizations may appear to be stereotypes of entire stakeholder groups, but again, they are not without merit.

This chapter will outline quality concerns and quality initiatives of major stakeholder groups: patients or consumers, providers or health care organizations, and payers (e.g., insurers, employers, government). The subject of outcomes measures and their contribution to quality indicators is covered in Chapter 14. Last, an attempt will be made to illustrate an alignment of quality indicators across stakeholder groups.

Institute of Medicine's Quality Initiatives

The Institute of Medicine (IOM), a component of the National Academy of Sciences, has promulgated a definition of quality that is broad enough to encompass many constituents but specific enough that it requires consideration of process (knowledge) and outcome.

> *"Quality is the extent to which health services for individuals and populations increase the likelihood of desired health outcomes and are consistent with current professional knowledge."*

(IOM, 1990)

This definition suggests that if providers demonstrate that their care is consistent with community standards, then a desired outcome may result. In turn, quality care is established.

National Roundtable of Health Care Quality

IOM has been instrumental in promoting a health care quality agenda, principally through sponsorship of the National Roundtable on Health Care Quality (Coye & Detmer, 1998). This roundtable, comprised of distinguished experts in health care policy research and development, was convened to examine the nature and scope of health care quality problems. Experts considered solutions to improve quality through a number of mechanisms including financial incentives, competition, regulation, and continuous quality improvement initiatives. Participants posed five critical questions during the course of this workshop (Coye & Detmer, 1998):

1. Why has health care lagged behind other sectors in quality improvement?

Table 13-1 Critical Features of a High-Performing Health Sector

- Defect-free processes and delivery measured through performance goals.
- Accelerated cycle time for the deployment of improvements.
- Information technology that can provide analytical reports to support patient care and organizational decision-making.
- Transfer of knowledge regarding "best practices."
- Aligned incentives for improved performance and the assignment of priority to quality objectives.
- Encouragement of innovation through the creation of "safe zones."
- Organized systems of care.
- Community-based interventions.
- Purchaser and consumer education, particularly about provider and health plan performance.
- Accountability through standardized measures and reporting, the establishment of minimally acceptable performance levels, and rewards in price or volume for those plans and providers who successfully improve quality.

From Coye MJ, Detmer DE: Quality at a crossroads. Milbank Quarterly 76(4):1-5, 1998, http://www.milbank.org/quarterly/764featcoye.html, accessed May 11, 2004.

2. Why have clinical quality improvement efforts apparently failed to move the sector as a whole?
3. How do we enlist physicians and other health professionals to work on meaningful improvements in the quality of health care?
4. How will changes in the expectations and behavior of consumers and patients affect quality?
5. What will be required to transform health care into a sector capable of delivering quality care and constantly improving care?

This last question prompted participants to elaborate on the components of a "high-performing health sector." These can be found in Table 13-1. This group continues in its work and rehabilitation providers are encouraged to follow their progress because it may lead to major national health care policy changes. Ideally, representation from the physical rehabilitation professions could be vital to enhancement of rehabilitation's role in quality management.

Medical Errors

The IOM has also taken the lead in discourse regarding medical errors due to poor quality (Fong, 2003). IOM estimates that 98,000 Americans die each year secondary to medical errors. This figure is especially disturbing for a country that touts itself and is perceived by many to have the best health care on earth. A number of studies strongly suggest that the care delivered in the United States often fails to meet professional standards (Schuster et al, 1998; Brennan, 1998; Leape et al, 1991; Leape 1994).

The National Quality Forum

The IOM is not alone in taking an aggressive posture on quality improvement. The National Quality Forum (NQF) is a private, not-for-profit, open membership, public benefit corporation established for the purpose of developing consensus concerning standardized health care performance measures, reporting mechanisms, and a national strategy for health care quality improvement (Kizer, 2001).

IOM's report, entitled "Leadership by Example: Coordinating Government Roles in Improving Health Care Quality," challenges the federal government to improve care and standardize measures (IOM, 2002). This report addresses six government programs that are certain to involve rehabilitation providers: Medicare, Medicaid, State Children's Health Insurance Program (SCHIP), the Department of Defense (DOD), TRICARE programs, the Veterans Administration, and the Indian Health Service. IOM points out the quality gap that currently exists between federal health care programs and the need for purchasing strategies that serve as incentives for providers to adopt "best practices." However, IOM recommends that the government work in collaboration with the private sector.

Viewing Quality Through Four Lenses

Lohr (1997) asserts that quality of care should be examined through four lenses. Quality across the *range of services* is a critical factor, especially now that multidisciplinary teams treat patients within integrated systems. Continuity of care demands that providers standardize their language and measures. Second, both individuals and populations must be considered in the *study of "non-events."* It can be argued that underutilization of health care services is the most methodologically demanding quality assurance task due to the difficulty of identifying or assessing "non-events" (Lohr, 1997). Third, the *range of outcomes* must include biological, clinical, functional, and general health elements. Lastly, health care providers who engage in various aspects of primary care need to achieve consensus on *common core competencies* possessed by team members. This will require a restructuring of health education programs.

Tripartite Classification of Quality Problems

Poor quality has generally been attributed to treatment variation and medical mistakes (Shipon & Nash, 2000; Merry & Crago, 2001; Moore et al, 2003). These can be further broken down into three general categories descriptive of quality problems: overuse, underuse, and misuse (Chassin, 1991; Chassin et al, 1998). The American health care system is rife with all three manifestations of poor quality. An entire utilization review industry has grown to identify and battle at least two of these causes: overuse and misuse. This industry has traditionally been grounded in exposing overutilization. Relatively few organizations have engaged in aggressive efforts to identify underutilization. The prevailing question for many years had been, "Since high cost is the demon to be exorcised, why bother with cases involving lower utilization rates and/or costs?" However, a paradigm shift has occurred as utilization review has evolved into utilization management. Utilization management includes the application of strategies that address quality indicators, clinical outcomes measures, and cost containment (Clifton, 1995).

 Table 13–2   Potential Causes of Health Care Service Overuse

- Human greed
- Lack of adequate information management systems
- Delayed referral for rehabilitation
- Health care system fragmentation and associated redundancies
- Financial gain
- Treatment variation
- Divergent definitions of quality
- Reimbursement rules that encourage code bundling or stacking (e.g., use of multiple codes when one would be sufficient)
- Provider's role of patient advocate
- Referral process to specialists with the expectation of an intervention
- Defensive medicine—"If I do everything, something will work."
- National infatuation with technology
- American culture accustomed to high consumption of resources
- Shift from not-for-profit to for-profit entities
- Intentional manipulation of the provider by the patient
- Litigation
- Lack of a universal definition of *disability*

Service Overuse

Overuse has been defined as the provision of a health service when its risk of harm exceeds its potential therapeutic benefit (Chassin, 1998). This definition evolves when service cost is factored in. Overuse occurs when cost exceeds the payer's usual, customary, and reasonable (UCR) fees or perception of value. Table 13–2 lists potential causes of overuse.

Service Misuse

Chassin (1998) defines *misuse* as "an avoidable complication of appropriate health care." Misuse, like overuse, is rarely perpetrated for outright financial or malicious reasons. Overuse, misuse, and underuse of health care services can be indicative of health care delivery system failures as much as individual provider culpability. For instance, delays in referring patients to specialists in a timely manner (gatekeeper role) may result in misuse of the specialist's services because the window of opportunity for intervention has since passed. Although errors in health care are well-documented, they are not necessarily well understood (Leape, 1994; Gaba, 1989; Leape et al, 1991). Table 13–3 addresses potential causes of misuse of health care services.

 Table 13–3   Potential Causes for Misuse of Health Care

- Failure of the provider to recognize contraindications to care
- Provider incompetency
- Human greed
- Lag between clinical research and clinical application
- Disparity among treatment protocols or treatment standards
- Fragmentation of the health care system and associated communication breakdowns
- Inaccurate patient history due to poor historian
- Patient's intentional manipulation of the provider
- Physician-driven referrals (e.g., self-referral for physical therapy)

The sheer complexity and fragmentation of the American health care system sets the stage for adverse consequences. These and other system attributes further confound the task of defining quality.

In the midst of this complexity, consumer expectations are certain to rise as they assume an increasing financial risk through higher deductibles, co-payments, and denied services or access. Additionally, the legal tort system has fanned the flames regarding this issue. Investigation of adverse effects from health care has been an under-studied area but has recently gained much attention on a national level (Lieberman, 1998; ERIC, 1998).

Service Underuse

Underuse involves a different set of factors than overuse or misuse of services (Chassin, 1998; Lieberman, 1998). Underuse is defined as a failure to provide an effective service or services during an appropriate time with a probability of favorable outcomes. Little has been written about underuse compared to overuse (Fetterolf, 1999). However, several studies have revealed underuse, even under fee-for-service (FFS) reimbursement (Wells et al, 1989; Retchin & Preston, 1991; Udvarhelyi et al, 1991). It remains clear that the FFS system and supplier induced demand jointly invited overuse, but now the inverse is evident. Managed care entices providers to underuse services due to provider at-risk contracts. For example, a physical therapist who is paid 28 cents per member per month (PMPM) to manage an HMO's members may be more tempted to undertreat than a therapist receiving $1.28 PMPM. Of course, incidence rates ultimately determine one's profitability under capitation. For example, if the provider receiving 28 cents PMPM (10,000 plan members) treats only 10 patients a month, their costs associated with treatment are much lower than the therapist who receives $1.28 PMPM but treats 100 patients per month. Ironically, health care delivery has flip-flopped from a potential for referral for profit (under FFS) to a non-referral for profit potential (gatekeeper and capitation). Table 13–4 identifies potential causes of underuse or underutilization.

Table 13–4 Potential Causes of Underuse or Underutilization

- Capitation and non–referral-for-profit schemes
- Provider failure to embrace proven new technologies
- Underinsured
- Non-insured
- Primary care physicians and gatekeeper role
- Managed care's focus on acute problems a detriment to chronic cases
- Perplexing volume of information available to provider
- Restrictive treatment protocols imposed by MCOs
- Defensive medicine— "If I do less, I can't harm them" attitude
- Physician-driven referrals (e.g., gatekeeper or primary care physician)

MEASURING QUALITY: PROCESS-STRUCTURE-OUTCOMES

Another conceptual model for viewing quality of care involves a focus on process, structure, and outcome (Donabedian, 1988; Westaway et al, 2003). Quality under this model is derived from all three components. Process involves the methodologies employed within a given structure or stable set of resources. Structure can include the facility itself, administrative organization, staff allocation, and equipment, whereas process describes how these things are applied. Process in health care involves the professional standards of care, practice guidelines, and general policies and procedures.

Various methodologies that fall within the process and structure domains are used by health care stakeholders to qualify and quantify health care: access to care, appropriateness of care, technical proficiency of the care provided, interpersonal care, and health and functional status (Greenfied et al, 1996). Patients principally relate best to these "service" indicators because they can understand them. Consumers tend to understand and value process structure elements when describing quality (outcomes) (Coye & Detmer, 1998; Shilling et al, 2003; Rahman et al, 2002).

Patients are not attuned to clinical outcome measures, nor should they be because providers have difficulty reaching consensus on standardized measures among themselves. Timeliness of scheduling, friendliness of staff, waiting room time, cleanliness of the facility, and fresh coffee are features of a rehabilitation encounter to which patients can relate. However, process and structure demands a third dimension to intelligently discuss quality. Unless process and structural elements of care are linked to outcomes, they are inadequate measures of quality.

Outcome measures represent the third dimension when process and structure converge with a purpose. Unfortunately, until very recently (i.e., the past decade), many equated outcome as the additive sum of process and structural components. This model has been applied to physical rehabilitation (Jette, 1995).

Outcome measures are covered in great detail in Chapter 14. However, to round out this discussion, outcomes in Donabedian's (1988) model address morbidity, disability, or quality of life.

Physical rehabilitation cases require unique outcome measures with an emphasis on patient function and related quality of life issues (Rothstein, 1994; Jette, 1995).

The Three *E*s of Quality

Quality is often used interchangeably with terms like, efficiency, efficacy, and effectiveness. Efficiency and effectiveness describe the production of desired or intended results, but quality and efficiency are frequently considered antonyms. *Quality* implies that the more service one receives, the higher their quality will be. This has not been demonstrated through controlled studies. Inversely, greater efficiency or less care does not equate to lower

Table 13–5 Consumer Quality Rating Scales

- Consumer Assessment of Health Plans Survey or CAHPS (AHCPR, 1998)
- Hulka Patient Satisfaction with Medical Care Survey (Hulka, 1970)
- Picker Institute's Adult Medical Surgical Inpatient (Picker Inst.) Patient Judgments of Hospital Quality (Rubin et al, 1990)
- Outpatient Satisfaction Questionnaire or OSQ-37 (Hays, 1995)
- SERVQUAL Scale (Parasuraman et al, 1988)

quality of service. Similarly, high cost may not yield high quality nor may low cost yield low quality.

One could argue that in the majority of cases, the most efficient or effective provider delivers the highest quality of service, and if carefully used, efficiency can be a proxy for quality of care.

There is no universal quality assessment tool that satisfies the multifaceted needs of patients; addresses multi-setting care; or crosses insurance or financing schemes, patient populations, or diagnostic categories. Instead, there is a confusing array of quality assessment instruments in use today that allow consumers to gauge quality of care. Some contain common denominators whereas others may actually be contradictory in nature. Table 13–5 contains a partial listing of these.

Quality accountability initiatives are evolving across a broad spectrum of special interest groups and government (Gosfield, 1997; Silberman, 1997, Blumenthal & Kilo, 1998). Governments tend to dwell on patient or consumer issues, but providers and payers under the new delivery paradigm will encourage, if not demand, consumer empowerment. Patients in the next era of health care will accept more risk in finances and active participation to derive benefit. In some instances, self-pay and self-care will represent the principal delivery modes.

Standards of Quality

The American health care system has some serious and widespread quality problems; this was the conclusion of the IOM-sponsored roundtable meetings conducted between February 1996 and January 1998 (Chassin et al, 1998). This group of 20 representatives of the private and public sectors (The National Roundtable on Health Care Quality) concluded that a very large number of persons are harmed as a direct result of poor quality.

The following three major goals resulting from the National Roundtable on Health Care Quality are paraphrased:

1. To afford effective services to all who need them.
2. To eliminate unnecessary interventions.
3. To avoid preventable complications of care.

Accomplishment of these goals will require a concerted effort among all stakeholders, most notably consumers–patients, providers, and employers, who fund health care and insurers. These stakeholders must begin to embrace a common language; collect standardized data elements; disclose their findings; and apply quality

measures across all treatment settings, conditions, patient populations, funding sources, and provider types.

Shipon and Nash (2000) offer a more detailed six step approach to quality improvement:

1. Increased accountability at all levels of the health care sector including stakeholders.
2. Continuous quality improvement (CQI).
3. Standardized treatment guidelines.
4. Patient-consumer empowerment to make educated choices.
5. Centralized information management.
6. Incentives for both providers and patients to make appropriate treatment selections.

Field and Lohr (1992) propose three levels for standards of quality: (1) minimum levels of acceptable performance or results, (2) excellent levels of performance or results, or (3) the range of acceptable performance or results. Providers and their organizations must agree upon which level best describes their goal before embarking on any cogent discussion of quality.

For some organizations, minimum levels of acceptable performance and results (outcomes) are sufficient. So-called "Centers for Excellence" strive for excellent levels of performance or results, or in the absence of hard data, they seek the perception of excellence. These organizations may strive for six-sigma level of quality. *Six sigma* is a term coined by Motorola Corporation during the 1980s to describe near-perfect quality. Six sigma is a measurement standard that tolerates only 3.4 errors for every one million encounters. This translates to a quality measure of 99.99966% accuracy. A defect or mistake can range from a faulty part to laxity in scheduling patients for treatment. Metrics are at the heart of six sigma, which requires extremely rigorous data collection and analysis. Centralized data collection and a high degree of standardization is required to execute at the six sigma level. This has been one of the most daunting challenges of a relatively fragmented health care industry. Some question whether health care is ready for six sigma (Chassin, 1998). Chassin cites health care quality frequency rates between 2% and 50%, or 200,000 to 500,000 per million. Rand Corporation studies indicate poor quality that fails to meet professional standards of care (Schuster et al, 1998).

CONSUMERS' ROLE IN QUALITY IMPROVEMENT

Consumers are playing an increasingly larger role in quality improvement initiatives, particularly as they are placed at more financial risk, suffer benefit restrictions, and must private pay (O'Connor et al, 2000). Health care quality improvement efforts no longer ignore the needs of the patient or consumer, which was a tendency underFFS. The American health care system is currently in an era of consumerism that values patient input and strives to meet patients' expectations (Kizer, 2001). Consumer service expectations have many of the following points of origin:

- External communication
- Word-of-mouth

- Past experiences
- Direct product inspection
- Provider image and reputation
- Provider marketing

Patient and Provider Expectations

A number of quality gaps have been identified between the patient's expectation of service and the provider's perception of these expectations (O'Connor et al, 2000). For instance, consumers and patients often blindly assume that one provider is as good as the next or that standards of care are universal. This could not be further from the truth as there is significant evidence of wide quality variations in the delivery of health care services (Chassin et al, 1986; Lewis, 1969; Roos & Roos, 1982; Wennberg & Gittleson, 1982; Gomick, 1977).

In fact, practice variation is perhaps the most important reason for managed care's existence. Practice variation is synonymous with unpredictable costs—the very antithesis of managed care. The United States has an employer-based health care finance system. Employers, in their race to curb spiraling health costs, have traditionally placed a disproportionate emphasis on cost-reduction versus quality assurance. They initially attacked cost because of its tangible nature while, to a large extent, they ignored quality until consumer, employer, and regulatory pressures mounted resulting in the current anti–managed care backlash. This cost-based approach is understandable when one considers that many managed care executives are generally not clinicians. Cost indicators are easier to quantify than quality is. A failure of providers to define *quality* further invites a focus on cost instead.

Although process and structure elements are important to patients, some believe these do not necessarily have a direct correlation with quality (Lieberman. 1998). Outcomes measures alone are not necessarily indicative of quality care. There are multiple variables that impact quality of care, some of which have little or nothing to do with treatment.

Table 13–6 provides a listing of process and structure elements that are important to patients but may or may not equate to quality of care.

Although access, patient choice, and a claims denial appeal process are important components of any patients' bill of rights, they are not necessarily descriptors of high quality services (Darby & Dervin, 1997). Access and choice simply guarantee the right to treatment by a particular provider but do not address quality.

The federal government sponsors a consumer Web page (http://www.talkingquality.gov) via the Agency for Healthcare Research & Quality (AHRQ), the Centers for Medicare & Medicaid (CMM), and the Office of Personnel Management. This Web page provides information about different government agency quality initiatives, various health plan structures, and a host of other educational resources.

The Foundation for Accountability (FACCT), www.facct.org, is a national consumer advocacy organization dedicated to helping Americans make better health care decisions. It is a collaboration of consumers and purchasers representing 80 million persons. Organized as a forum where parties work towards a quality-focused health care system, FACCT was formed in 1995 and established

Table 13–6 Common Examples of Process & Structure Elements

The following items are commonly addressed in quality assessment and improvement initiatives. Unfortunately, these elements alone fail to address functional outcomes. Yet, some of these are routinely found in patient satisfaction surveys generated by provider organizations or health plans.

- State-of-the-art equipment
- Certified specialists
- Facility accessibility
- Ample parking
- Minimal waiting room time
- Prompt scheduling of visits
- Current treatment protocols-practice guidelines
- Clean environment-facility
- Friendly-cordial staff
- Consumer educational materials available
- Cost of care
- Convenient location

offices in 1996. FACCT publishes an "Accountability Resource Series," "Prototype Guidebook for Performance Measurement," and "Consumer Satisfaction Sets." FACCT conducts seminars-symposiums on quality-related topics. The following lists summarize FACCT's objective for each health care stakeholder:

Consumers

1. Appreciate the value of quality in health care
2. Make decisions based on clear, reliable quality data
3. Provide direction to the health care system about important consumer needs and expectations
4. Balance personal and societal needs in health care decision making

Purchasers

1. Hold the health care system accountable for quality and value
2. Provide data and support for quality-based decisions
3. Provide real choices for employees and beneficiaries
4. Create health-focused partnerships with beneficiaries, providers and the community at large

Providers and Plans

1. Understand what consumers want
2. Monitor and improve performance in the areas that matter the most to consumers
3. Mobilize consumers as partners in their health care
4. Compete on quality as well as price

Patient Satisfaction Surveys: Do They Really Describe Quality?

Quality can be described as the strong link between service providers and users of a service (Rahman et al, 2002). The patient-provider relationship represents the heart of patient–satisfaction instrument use. However, some have raised issue with this approach because patients frequently do not distinguish between the art and technical aspects of care (Like & Zyzanski, 1987). Patients are not inherently equipped with the ability to gauge the clinical aspects of quality, so system inputs (process and structure) are what they tend to focus on instead of system outputs (clinical outcomes) (Monnin & Perneger, 2002; Ware et al, 1983).

Rothstein (1994) provides an interesting observation about providers' reliance on patient reports. On one hand, therapists may accept a patient's complaint as justification for treatment initiation. They recognize, however, that more than the patient's word is required to justify discharge or to prove effectiveness. This observation acknowledges the limitations of patient reports. Although patient satisfaction surveys enjoy a high degree of use among providers and health plans, there is no universal instrument. Patient satisfaction instruments can be highly variable and confusing (Abramovwitz et al, 1987; Aharony & Strasser, 1993; Allen, 1998).

Is Patient Satisfaction a Validation of Treatment Quality?

Patient satisfaction is clearly a multidimensional challenge that includes the following (Keith, 1998):

- Interpersonal manner
- Technology quality
- Accessibility-convenience
- Financial issues
- Physical environment
- Availability of providers and services-products
- Continuity of care between providers and facilities
- Efficacy or clinical outcomes

Hudak and Wright (2000) assert that "patient satisfaction" has two distinct meanings and caution its use in outcome measures. Patients frequently have a very difficult time differentiating patient satisfaction from outcome or care itself (Ware et al, 1983). These two separate constructs require different measurement instruments.

Patient satisfaction is often viewed as an administrative issue. Keith (1998) opines that patient satisfaction in the rehabilitation setting should serve two vital purposes:

1. To measure progress
2. To return a person to independent living

Patient satisfaction surveys, when used as administrative tools, have correlated decreased patient satisfaction with cost-cutting, high–patient volume, and the use of care extenders (Beattie et al, 2002).

Providers cannot discount the effect that patient satisfaction (or lack thereof) has on clinical outcomes. Satisfied patients have been shown to exercise greater compliance in their therapeutic regimens, resulting in better outcomes, whereas dissatisfied patients demonstrate less compliance, resulting in worse outcomes (Hudak & Wright, 2000).

Cheng et al (2003) found that interpersonal skills were more positively correlated to patient satisfaction than clinical competence in the management of stroke, diabetes, cesarean section, and appendectomy cases. These researchers concluded that facilities with a high percentage of patient satisfaction do not necessarily receive high levels of recommendation by their consumers. Recommendations were more likely to be correlated with the patient's perception of technical competence. In this study, although patients rated facilities high, they would not necessarily recommend them to others. This finding may have some applicability to physical rehabilitation. Rehabilitation providers, perhaps more than any other discipline, spend more quality time with their patients, engage in more direct communication, provide a hands-on approach to care, and treat-manage patients for longer periods of time or length of stay. However, rehabilitation directors would be well-advised not to assume that the therapist with the highest patient satisfaction survey ratings is the most effective or competent. Process and structural components of care may more fully reflect patient satisfaction. Waiting room time was negatively correlated with quality as measured via patient satisfaction (Rahman et al, 2002; Shilling et al, 2003). However, it is absolutely critical that providers deprogram consumers relative to process and structure addiction. Consumers need to be refocused toward meaningful measures of outcome such as functionally based lifestyle inventories. This will remain a daunting task until providers reach consensus on appropriate quality measures among themselves. Providers are cautioned to avoid lengthy survey instruments that require a multivariate analysis of data. Rehabilitation providers may wish to consider four simple questions for inclusion in their patient satisfaction survey instruments, at least until consensus is reached regarding the process-structure-outcome components:

1. Would you come back to our center for treatment?
2. Would you private pay for our services if other funding sources were not available?
3. Would you send your child here for treatment?
4. Would you recommend us to others?

PURCHASERS'-PAYERS' ROLE IN QUALITY IMPROVEMENT

Capturing meaningful information on health care quality that can be used to compare HMOs has yet to achieve state-of-the-art status, although great gains have recently been made (SPRY Foundation, 1997). Payer diversity is one reason for the lack of uniform quality standards. Payers comprise a variety of entities including third party insurers, re-insurers, third party administrators (TPAs), managed care organizations (MCOs), state funds (workers' compensation), and self-funded or self-insured employers.

Many employers continue to fund health care costs for their employees through group health policies. However, some have abdicated their leadership role in managing health care dollars as well. Medical premiums are escalating at rates ranging between 8.7% to 15% in 2003, depending upon insurance line (IOMA, 2003; Strunk, 2003; Abbott, 2003).

Value Purchasing Overcomes a Fixation on Price

MCOs initially effected savings and wrung excesses from the health care system by picking the "low hanging fruit." Competitive price discounting and provider at-risk contracts (e.g., capitation, case management, and selective enrollments) removed perceived excesses from the system. However, medical costs at the time of this writing continue to escalate as consumers assume more at-risk arrangements. Examples include reduced benefit plans, higher co-payments, and rising deductibles.

The *total value* of a product or service is determined by the interaction of three variables: price, service, and quality (SPRY, 1997). Quality, without question, is the most difficult component of value to describe or measure. Few argue the need for quality indicators; they simply differ on what data to collect and how to collect them (Greenfield et al, 1996). Value purchasing is a derivative of cost versus benefit. If payers believe the outcome justifies the expense, they perceive value and by proxy, quality as well. However, if payers observe an outpouring of financial resources without a reasonable and timely result or outcome, they may view health care suspiciously, namely as overutilization. Providers must educate payers regarding the adverse impact of underutilization as well. Underutilization can ultimately lead to greater incurred cost because of chronic illness and injury. Few studies have addressed this growing trend (Fetterolf, 1999). Underutilization that delays referral to rehabilitation can result in confounding psychosocial issues, which are challenging to manage. Chapters 7 and 22 provide extensive coverage of these issues. Essentially, to delay rehabilitation is to compromise it. Evidence suggests a lack or delay of referral for rehabilitation services, especially under managed care's gatekeeper model (Ostrow & Kuntavanish, 1983).

Employer's Demand Health Plan Accountability

Employer financing is the foundation of the American health care system. Approximately 80% of all health care is financed by employers in some form. Group health, workers' compensation, short- and long-term disability and retiree health care is predominantly financed by employers. Contrary to popular belief, government or public funding constitutes a significantly smaller proportion via Medicare, Social Security, Medicaid, and other assistance programs (e.g., Centers for Medicare and Medicaid). For some, there is a widespread fear that MCOs increase profits at the expense of quality (Armstead & Leong, 1999).

There are at least four basic mechanisms for assuring health plan accountability: the managed care industry itself, external review, the legal system, and marketplace demands (Gosfield, 1997). The focus of this section will be on the purchaser strategies to ensure that their employees are receiving medically necessary, cost-effective, and efficacious services. The managed care industry initially policed itself through voluntary accreditation programs. Voluntary self-policing yielded to mandatory controls within the managed care industry, especially as their trade groups grew in membership and scope. Since the mid 1990s, public concern over quality has led to skepticism regarding the degree to which MCOs self-police. Each new horror story published in the media concerning denied services (e.g., "drive-through deliveries" or "gag rules") raised the specter of suspicion among consumers. Many began to question metaphorically, was the fox designing *and* guarding the chicken coop? As a result, it is generally perceived to be far more credible when an MCO, or any entity for that matter, is held accountable by an independent arm's-length entity. Inversely, payers are somewhat suspicious of

peer review when conducted within a network, which partly explains why external utilization-peer review will continue to exist.

Employers are increasingly demanding quality measures from the health plans that serve their employees (Hibbard et al, 1997; Beauregard & Winston, 1997). Ironically, and perhaps justly so, managed care plans which aggressively hold providers accountable for their actions are now under pressure to demonstrate both financial performance (e.g., cost savings) while enhancing quality and outcomes. There was a time when few employers were self-insured; however, today more and more employers are gravitating towards self-insurance. Those employers who continue to pay insurance premiums to a third-party insurer or managed care plan indirectly control their costs though selection of carriers. They accomplish this by comparing managed care plan performance benchmarks and employee satisfaction surveys; renegotiating premium rates or benefit packages; and, ultimately, through selecting the highest-ranked plans. Through the mid1980s, it was common for employers to offer dozens of HMO choices to their employers. Today, most employers offer one or two HMO choice plans to avoid the cumbersome task of assessing multiple plans' performance. It should also be noted that consolidation within the managed care sector also contributed to a smaller selection of plans.

National Committee for Quality Assurance

The National Committee for Quality Assurance (NCQA) is a 501(c)(3) non-profit organization whose mission is to improve health care quality everywhere. NCQA was founded in 1993 and is perhaps best known by its "Health Plan Report Card." This report card is used by employers and government purchasers to compare and contrast the performance of various health plans. NCQA offers employers a set of standardized performance measures (Health Plan Employer Data and Information Sets [HEDIS]) designed to ensure that purchasers, as well as consumers, have reliable information with which to compare and contrast health plans. HEDIS involves 60 standardized performance measures developed and maintained by NCQA. These quality measures address process, structure, outcomes, and consumer satisfaction. NCQA also promotes other quality improvement initiatives including Disease Management Accreditation & Certification, Report Card for Managed Behavioral Healthcare Organizations, Physician Organization Certification, Credentials Verification Organization Certification, and Utilization Management Certification.

FEDERAL GOVERNMENT QUALITY ACCOUNTABILITY INITIATIVES

There are a number of external review mechanisms that augment self-policing activities. As managed care ran out of fuel for its increasingly hungry engine, it looked to the elderly population.

Medicare

In 1985, the Health Care Financing Administration (HCFA) first offered Medicare beneficiaries the option of enrollment in managed care plans. By 1997, Medicare had approved more than 330 HMOs to deliver services to beneficiaries (SPRY, 1997). One major HMO alone provided managed Medicare services in 40 states and subcontracted care to providers in 10 additional states. The majority of managed Medicare was provided in Arizona, California, Florida, Hawaii, New York, and Oregon. Managed Medicare enrollment had grown at an annual rate exceeding 25%. However, as we enter the new millennium, a growing number of HMOs are withdrawing from managed Medicare due to reported low profitability. This is likely to reverse itself as HMOs learn how to deal more effectively with the elderly population and chronic conditions; in neither of which have they had much experience. The growth of managed Medicare throughout most of the 1990s invited federal inspection of MCOs. The HCFA set forth rules for MCOs who managed Medicare beneficiaries. These rules addressed enrollment, grievance policies, provider credentialing, and reporting elements. In 1997, the physician incentive plan regulations were promulgated to define the thresholds of financial risk assumed by physicians in Medicare managed care. These rules were put in place to safeguard against underservice or non–referral for profit. These rules are mandated under several sections of the law, including the Stark amendment and the Medicare HMO qualification provisions (Gosfield, 1997).

Federal quality assurance policies typically do not directly affect the private sector, the commercial insurers, and the HMOs. However, when these payers enter the Medicare market, they fall within the jurisdiction of federal rules and regulations.

HCFA's quality of care program involves the following four instruments (SPRY Foundation, 1997):

1. HEDIS 3.0 or Health Plan Employer Data and Information performance measures.
2. The SF-36 or Short Form 36, which is an outcomes measure of functional changes in beneficiary health status over time. SF-36 is a component of HEDIS 3.0.
3. Beneficiary satisfaction surveys are derived from the Consumer Assessments of Health Plans Study (CAHPS).
4. Clinical outcome measures developed by FACCT augment the SF-36 measures.

It should be noted that although most changes in health care come from the private sector, those initiatives emanating from the federal government are ultimately absorbed by the private sector. Medicare documentation guidelines represent a good example of this phenomenon. Many commercial insurers embraced these guidelines with the assumption that if they were good enough for our senior citizens, they are good enough for others. One can see portions of Medicare documentation guidelines and definitions of medical necessity, reasonable care, and maintenance care in many insurer materials.

Agency for Healthcare Research and Quality

National Quality Measures Clearinghouse

The National Quality Measures Clearinghouse (NQMC), sponsored by the Agency for Healthcare Research and Quality (AHRQ), U.S. Department of Health and Human Services (DHHS), accepts the IOM definition of quality. NQMC provides information about different domains of measurement: access, outcome, patient experience, and process. Each of these domains offers a unique perspective on quality health care. Table 13–7 provides a description of each of these domains. Quality measures are designed for use in quality improvement, accountability, and research.

National Guideline Clearinghouse

The National Guideline Clearinghouse (NGC) is another quality initiative of AHRQ. The NGC is a comprehensive database of evidence-based clinical practice guidelines and supportive documents. NGC's mission is to provide physicians, nurses, and other health professionals, health plans, and purchasers with structured abstracts, full-text guidelines, and Palm-based downloads of guidelines housed in its database. *Guideline Syntheses* are unique guideline comparisons that enable users to compare and contrast one set of guidelines with others covering similar topics. An *annotated bibliography* enables users to search the database for citations. Weekly electronic mailings of new and updated guidelines are posted on NGC's Web site, www.guideline.gov. Users can browse by disease-condition, treatment-intervention, or via the developing organization(s).

Database inclusions must meet NGC's criteria:

1. The clinical practice guideline contains systematically developed statements that assist providers and patients in treatment choices for specific conditions.
2. The clinical practice guideline was produced under the auspices of medical specialty associations, professional societies, public or private organizations, government agencies (state-local-federal), or health plans. Unsponsored guides are unacceptable.
3. Corroborating documentation must be produced indicating that a systematic literature search and review of scientific evidence published in peer-reviewed journals was performed.

Table 13–7   The National Quality Measures Clearinghouse Domains of Measurement

Access	An access measure assesses a patient's attainment of both timely and appropriate care.
Outcome	An outcome of care represents the health state of a patient resulting from healthcare. Outcome-based measures describe the cumulative impact of multiple processes involved in care delivery. These measures can suggest areas that require quality assessment and improvement.
Patient experience	These measures involve a patient's observations about health care.
Process	A process measure identifies the degree to which treatment adhered to clinical practice based on evidence or consensus. These measures provide insight into specific areas that may require quality improvement since they represent the system inputs.

Data adapted from Agency for Healthcare Research and Quality (AHCRQ), http://www.qualitymeasures.ahrq.gov.

4. Guidelines must be in English and should have been developed, reviewed, and/or revised within the last five years.

STATE QUALITY ACCOUNTABILITY INITIATIVES

States employ a number of quality-accountability mechanisms that directly influence the behavior of providers, consumers, health plans, and employers. These initiatives may vary across workers' compensation, Medicaid, Medicare, public health, group health, and other forms of insurance coverage even though they may be regulated by the same department (e.g., insurance department or commissioner).

State Oversight of Medicare

At the state level, Peer Review Organizations (PROs), now known as quality improvement organizations (QIOs), comprise groups of clinicians who are paid by the federal government to oversee health care delivery to Medicare beneficiaries. Each state has one QIO whose reviewers compare care received by individual beneficiaries to medical standards. Under this arrangement, providers must fully cooperate as a condition of participation in the Medicare program.

Managed Care Organization Oversight

Managed care organizations (MCOs) are typically regulated at the state level through an insurance department, a health department, or both. Each state has its own unique requirements, but, generally speaking, they require quality assurance plans, grievance procedures, provider credentials, access, and reporting mechanisms.

Quality functions that are regulated the least frequently at the state level include outcomes standards, practice standards, utilization data validation, medical record standards or audits, peer review requirements or criteria, and disenrollment surveys (Riley, 1997).

Unique State Initiatives

Pennsylvania has the distinction of being the first state to collect and publish hospital-based performance data concerning specific conditions, (e.g., cardiac). The Pennsylvania Health Care Cost Containment Council is an independent state agency that compares individual hospital care to statewide or regional norms. The Council was established by the legislature (Act 89), which specifically assigned three responsibilities (Pennsylvania Health Care Cost Containment Council website, accessed July 15, 2000):

1. To collect, analyze, and make available to the public data about the cost and quality of health care in Pennsylvania.
2. To study, upon request, the issue of access to care for those Pennsylvanians who are uninsured.
3. To review and make recommendations about proposed or existing mandated health insurance benefits upon request of the legislative or executive branches of the Commonwealth.

The Council collects over 2 million inpatient hospital discharge records annually in addition to data from ambulatory surgery centers. Published comparative quality data have been heavily marketed by those who do well against norms. Those organizations that perform poorly have tended to downplay the results or criticize the process as invalid, unreliable, etc. It will only be a matter of time before councils such as this one begin to compare rehabilitation services across treatment settings.

Workers' Compensation Oversight

Workers' compensation represents a patchwork quilt of 50 state laws. Workers' compensation bureaus or departments have enacted various quality programs on a state-by-state basis. A growing number of states have published practice guidelines and treatment protocols as a condition of participation within the program. At least 30 states have regulated utilization review within workers' compensation and the composition of provider panels or networks.

Regulatory Activity

When industry self-policing and marketplace forces fail to assure quality, regulatory activity emerges as a significant force for managed care accountability for quality across an expanding spectrum of concerns (Gosfield, 1997). Legislative initiatives have exponentially grown now that the honeymoon with managed care is over (Weber, 1997; Silberman, 1997). Initiatives specific to tort laws, jury verdicts, and legislative activity are too numerous to discuss. Although most state legislative bodies lack expertise in health care quality accountability, they routinely attempt to legislate health care. States serve multiple masters because they serve as large health care purchasers while at the same time, they have a fiduciary duty as consumer-protection advocates. Legislation will continue to flourish in the absence of reliable systems for quality accountability (Riley, 1997). State-generated regulatory activity often conflicts with federal actions. For instance, a state may enforce antikickback provisions in Medicare but allow referral-for-profit within workers' compensation programs. Additionally, states may hold one health care profession to strict regulations under their practice act, at direct odds with federal rules and regulations. For example, in Pennsylvania, a physical therapy assistant (PTA) may not treat a home care patient because such treatment violates the "on-premise supervision" requirement (by a licensed physical therapist) of the state practice act, yet Medicare encourages the use of PTAs as a reasonable low-cost alternative to licensed physical therapists. Regulatory and legal inconsistencies can serve to further cloud an already vague definition of what constitutes quality care.

The Perspective of Special Interest Groups

Special interest groups, for the sake of this discussion, involve organizations that are created to serve the needs of consumers. They do not represent the viewpoint of all consumers, but they play a pivotal role in quality assurance.

These groups include labor organizations, unions, professional affiliations, and disease- and age-specific clusters of people. Only a small sampling of these groups will be covered here. Corporations and their unions or labor organizations are large consumers of health care services. As such, they have a vested interest in the quality of care issues, and they lobby both MCOs and government to effect changes. Some of the more powerful groups include the AFL-CIO, the Teamsters, the National Educational Association (NEA), the American Medical Association, and the National Trial Lawyers Association. Other organizations that take up health care causes may not be directly tied to any one group. Examples include Common Cause and the American Civil Liberties Union (ACLU).

American Association of Retired Persons

The American Association of Retired Persons (AARP) is one of the most powerful, vocal, and well-funded groups in the nation. This group has a seat at virtually every health care policy table and is certain to increase its leverage as 72 million baby boomers enter its ranks. In fact, the AARP, in acknowledgement of this group's numbers, power, and affluence, offers early membership in the association. AARP has its own Public Policy Institute, formed in 1985. This institute has published and disseminated a number of publications that address both state and national issues (McCloskey et al, 1996). AARP has annually published "State Health Profiles" since 1991. This publication presents nearly 90 indicators as the basis for individual profiles of state health care systems and reform efforts. Topics include demographics, utilization of services, administration and quality, health care coverage, and reform initiatives.

National Coalition on Health Care

The National Coalition on Health Care is one of the nation's largest and most diverse alliances striving to improve American health care. This non-profit, nonpartisan group is comprised of 94 different organizations representing over 100 million Americans (National Coalition on Health Care. This organization has the support of some highly influential persons including former presidents Jimmy Carter and George Bush. The coalition's founding principles include the following:

● Health insurance for all.
● Improved quality of care.
● Cost containment.
● Equitable financing.
● Simplified administration.

The National Quality Forum is another not-for-profit organization created to develop and implement a national strategy for health care quality measurement and reporting. This group supports consensus-based performance measures that assure safe, timely, beneficial, efficient, and patient-centered care. Examples of its work include *National Voluntary Consensus Standards for Adult Diabetes Care, Nursing Home Performance Measures, A Comprehensive Framework for Hospital Care Performance Evaluation*, and *Safe Practices for Better Healthcare*. This group continues its work

in a number of other areas including cancer, minority health care, and wellness-prevention. Resources such as these are invaluable to rehabilitation providers who desire to learn more about the expectations of consumers. This is especially true if one believes that significant change comes from the private sector (versus the public sector). Consumer advocacy groups, like those mentioned, wield great political and financial power generated by their critical mass and voting block. These groups will unequivocally contribute to shaping the future of health care.

THE PROVIDER PERSPECTIVE

"The time has come to think like purchasers, to place ourselves in their shoes, and to persuade them that what we are doing is humane, efficient, effective, productive, and in their best interest, as well as our patient's and society's."

- Reece, 1988

Beyond "Soft" Clinical Measures

This quotation challenges providers to satisfy the needs of multiple health care stakeholders: providers, purchasers, patients and society. This is a formidable challenge because stakeholders have divergent and often competing needs, expectations, and desires. Since quality is viewed through a prism unique to each stakeholder group, rehabilitation providers are cautioned not to define quality solely through clinical outcomes. Similarly, purchasers of health care services need to look beyond cost when gauging the relative value of an intervention.

Quality assessment methodologies have been available to providers for several decades, during which time they have evolved dramatically (Kessner et al, 1973; Rutstein et al, 1976; Jonas 1977). Traditional quality measures espouse process and structure with little attention paid to outcomes or actual performance measures. Many of these "soft" measures are weakly correlative with rehabilitation functional outcomes. For instance, "state-of-the-art" equipment as a structural measure does not necessarily ensure superior outcomes. Prompt scheduling of visits, a friendly receptionist, free waiting room coffee, and a pleasant environment (process and structure measures) may define quality in the eyes of patients but have little or no correlation to the efficacy of the treatment itself. Understanding the patient's perspective is a core critical task, but it should not obviate the need for "hard data" and outcomes-linked measures. It has only been recently that rehabilitation providers have begun to explore, embrace, and utilize evidence-based practice (Kane, 1994; Jette et al, 2003). However, great variation exists in the manner in which therapists chart rehabilitation activities, especially as they pertain to gauging functional improvement (Kane, 1994; Steffen & Meyer, 1985). Therapists are not solely culpable for these charting deficiencies. Regulatory and reimbursement pressures can influence what is recorded.

Another obstacle to quality assessment in rehabilitation is the extended course of treatment often associated with these cases. Rehabilitation providers often treat and/or manage chronic conditions. During protracted treatment courses or episodes of care that involve multiple provider types, distinguishing the contributions of one service from another is a daunting task. This is one reason for the rise in the use of global measures of function or clinical outcome.

The provision of quality care requires attention to non-medical aspects. A study involving first-year medical students exposed a lack of attention to humanistic and patient-centered needs (Ewan, 1987). This inattentiveness is attributed to tendencies toward academic and scientific pursuits. Rehabilitation providers are challenged to balance medical or scientific pursuits with patient-centered needs. A plethora of non-medical issues are discussed in Chapter 7.

Health-related quality of life (HRQL) measures were introduced to the rehabilitation community in the early 1990s (Jette, 1993). Jette cites two factors that are partly responsible for the shift to HRQL: chronic diseases and the need for cost-containment. He also observes that most physical rehabilitation services for those with chronic conditions focus on functional improvement and overall quality of life. Providers, however, often focus on improvements in impairment. Impairment measures include muscle performance, range of motion, balance, aerobic capacity, and swelling.

There is no consensus or universal definition of "quality of life" (Carr et al, 1996). Ironically, some argue that the enormous expenditures on outcomes research have yet to result in significant changes in health care practice. Anderson (1994) cites $200 million spent by the Agency for Health Care Policy & Research (now Agency for Health Care Research & Quality) as having no significant impact on practice shifts. To demonstrate the quality of their services, rehabilitation providers must find the means to link impairment measures with more global HRQL measures. Carr et al (1996) places quality of life measures in the context of the World Health Organization's model of disease impact.

Evidence-based practice is the current trend in health care at large; however, rehabilitation as a sector has been somewhat slow in fully embracing this new paradigm. The Jette et al (2003) survey of physical therapists suggested that quality of patient care is better when evidence is used in treatment. However, this survey also indicated a relative absence of evidence-based treatment. Seventeen percent of survey respondents stated that they read fewer than two articles per month, whereas only 25% stated they used literature in their clinical decision-making less than twice per month. This survey suggests that the use of evidence-based practice should increase in daily practice. To accomplish this objective, a common language of functional assessment may be required (Fisher et al, 1995; Granger & Gresham, 1993; Menard & Hoens, 1994).

Rehabilitation's Value Proposition

Assessment and accountability are the hallmarks of a new revolution in medical care according to Arnold Relman (1988), former editor of the *New England Journal of Medicine*. In this third revolution, which continues today, providers must justify their interventions through both evidence-based practice and outcomes. A rehabilitation value proposition must satisfy the demands of several customers and numerous stakeholders. Value represents an economic litmus test, especially for payers who demand fiscal accountability. Optimal functional gains may not represent quality to a payer if the cost to produce these gains is perceived as exorbitant. In this scenario, the clinical outcome does not justify high costs. Purchasers may, however, consider optimal outcomes a great value if the costs to produce them are comparatively low.

Providers must also be mindful of the cost-benefit ratio of their individual services relative to others. Comparisons of value routinely address provider type, treatment settings, insurance lines, stages of irritability (acute-subacute-chronic), and conventional versus unconventional interventions. It is not enough for rehabilitation providers to calculate and articulate their value proposition to other stakeholders. It is incumbent upon rehabilitation providers to have an understanding of the value propositions to which theirs will be compared and contrasted.

Wade (2003) describes *value* as an additional dimension in the disablement model, pathology-impairment-disability-handicap and value. Evidence-based practice and functional outcomes in rehabilitation represent only a portion of the quality proposition. Hart and Dombrozykowski (2000) define *value* as a unit of functional improvement per estimated cost. Value comparisons are critical in a competitive marketplace where consumers (patients) and purchasers must choose between alternative treatments, providers, and settings. A number of studies have demonstrated the value of rehabilitation relative to other interventions across a wide range of conditions and treatment settings. Korthals-de Bos et al (2003) used cost utility ratios and cost effectiveness ratios to differentiate physiotherapy from manual therapy and general practitioner services in neck pain. Evans and Hendricks (2001) compared subacute rehabilitation care with outpatient primary medical care. Hospital- versus home-based rehabilitation following hip replacement has been studied from a value proposition perspective (Goldie & Jonsson, 1992). Annual per capita "rehabilitation costs" were studied in the care of neuromuscular diseases (Koch et al, 1986). The economic benefits of secondary and tertiary cardiac rehabilitation have been demonstrated via cost-benefit analyses (Shephard, 1992). Kramer et al (1997) correlated outcomes and costs for hip fracture and stroke cases.

Function-based Payment Models

Function-based prospective payment systems are being employed both by government health care funding sources (Medicare) and private sector sources (managed care) (Sutton et al, 1996). Medicare has used functional status information (FSI) in patient assessment, provider performance assessment, and as integrants in payment systems. Wilkerson and Batavia (1992) purport that functional status and gain are among the best predictors of resource utilization. Functional status data serve five fundamental purposes (Clauser & Bierman, 2003):

1. To encourage innovative models of care delivery.
2. To encourage continuous quality improvement.
3. To gauge facility and provider performance.

4. For reimbursement.

5. To facilitate appropriate consumer choice.

The Medicare program has taken the lead in reimbursement decisions tied to FSI (Health Care Financing Review, 2003). Payment mechanisms are correlated with patient assessment tools and performance assessment. Payers need functional assessment measures that can be linked to cost savings because this is their bias. (Eazell & Maama, 1992).

Functional status information is now used to define quality for the purpose of consumer choice among different treatment alternatives or settings. The Centers for Medicare and Medicaid (CMS) is supporting a diverse range of quality improvement initiatives. These include the following:

- Medicare Managed Care Quality Improvement (QI)
- Home Health QI
- Hospital QI
- Doctor Office QI
- Medicaid QI
- Nursing Home QI

CMS (2003) publishes a *Quality Fact Sheet* and promotes two data collection systems: the Minimum Data Sets (MDS) and the Outcome & Assessment Information Set (OASIS). MDS is geared toward care provided in long-term-care (LTC) centers while OASIS is a home health-based database.

EXTERNAL ACCREDITATION AND CERTIFICATION BODIES

Providers who wish to demonstrate their value through quality services often do so by seeking external validation. There are a number of entities that offer seals of approval to provider organizations including rehabilitation.

Joint Commission on Accreditation of Health Care Organizations

The focus on process and structure was reinforced by those bodies that accredited or certified providers and their organizations. It was not until 1987 that the Joint Commission on Accreditation of Healthcare Organizations (JCAHO) announced its "Agenda for Change" initiative. (JCAHO, 2004). In fact, this organization was previously known as the Joint Commission on Accreditation of Hospitals because their focus was on hospitals, not integrated health care systems. The JCAHO accredits more than 16,000 health care organizations and is recognized nationwide as a symbol of provider organization quality. Health care organizations that desire accreditation must undergo on-site survey by JCAHO every three years. This survey now includes outcome and performance measures (for hospitals). Integration of performance data into the JCAHO accreditation program was accomplished through the ORYX initiative. This tool allows for the comparison of performance across hospitals. Performance measures, according to JCAHO, "represents what is done and how well it is done." Performance measures encourage quality improvement within organizations as well as provide a means for external parties to make value-driven decisions.

Commission on Accreditation of Rehabilitation Facilities

The Commission on Accreditation of Rehabilitation Facilities is a Tuscon, Arizona-based organization that accredits a variety of rehabilitation services and programs. CARF's mission is "to promote the quality, value, and optimal outcomes of services". The following represents CARF's core values:

- All people have the right to be treated with dignity and respect.
- All people should have access to needed services that achieve optimum outcomes.
- All people should be empowered to exercise informed consent.

CARF's approach involves peer-consultation in which an on-site surveyor of a similar background visits the facility applying field-driven standards of review. CARF offers education, training, and various publications—all designed to enhance the delivery of quality services. Clinicians routinely, and perhaps falsely, equate quality of their service with clinical or technical competency (Cleary & McNeil, 1988). Quality problems can begin with provider attitudes, education, and training processes that create so-called "master clinicians" (Chassin, 1998).

Rothstein (2000), in delivering the Thirty-second Mary McMillan Lecture, cautioned physical therapists:

"Evidence must supplant testimonials. Interventions born out of cult-like beliefs must be left by the wayside. How long can we tolerate the intellectual dishonesty of those who argue that to embrace new methods or to use what are called "alternative treatments" means that we must abandon scientific inquiry and clinical trials?"

The future of rehabilitation will partly be determined by the sector's ability to produce evidence or, better yet, to produce a value proposition that is acceptable to the stakeholders involved.

Quality is also defined by what providers do not do to their patients. Embracing evidence-based practice requires that unproven interventions be eliminated from the roster of services. Rothstein (2000) urges therapists to give up those areas of practice that do not make use of one's clinical expertise:

"It is however, the height of irresponsibility, and totally at odds with our [physical therapists] humanistic traditions, to proceed with interventions in the face of evidence that suggests better methods are available or that shows the chosen intervention to be ineffective."

Rothstein (2000) cites the use of thermal modalities during the acute stage of low back pain as one example of an intervention that should be voluntarily avoided by providers if they are to preserve the respect of other stakeholders. He opines that it should not require refutation by a government agency or payer to alert a profession about quality issues. Health care professionals owe a duty to the public to define what constitutes quality services and to eliminate those that do not meet standards. To otherwise would be to abdicate the responsibility to those who are not the content experts in the rehabilitation arena. Although consumer choice is a growing trend, providers, not consumers, have the responsibility to articulate their value proposition.

In their zealous pursuit of quality, some providers actually achieve "believer status" in that they believe they are doing something good for patients, despite substantial evidence to the contrary (Chassin, 1998).These persons may actually be greater harbingers of poor quality than those who underserve or undertreat. Providers who undertreat may actually be doing a favor to patients by returning responsibility to them for self-care. Of course, this assumes that the patient possesses the faculties, resources, and desire to self-manage their problem. The overtreating provider may insidiously create a co-dependency relationship and enhance neediness, the antithesis of independence.

Do Rehabilitation Providers Create Co-Dependency?

In the movie *What About Bob?*, Richard Dreyfus plays the role of a psychiatrist to whom an extremely phobic patient, played by Bill Murray, is referred. A co-dependency relationship ensues. Dreyfus goes to great extremes to break-off the relationship but fails miserably. Rehabilitation providers may be among the best at creating the *What About Bob* patients who simply won't go away. Overutilization of rehabilitation services may be correlative to the quantity and quality of time spent with patients, during which a strong rapport often results. When payers view this as overutilization, the rehabilitation value proposition suffers.

Again, consumers are not generally interested in highly technical or clinically based quality measures, which may partly explain the disconnect or gap between patient expectations and provider perceptions of these expectations (Darby & Dervin, 1997). Health care providers must share culpability for consumer ignorance and disinterest because of an inadequate job of educating patients about clinically relevant and self-responsibility issues. Most continuous quality improvement (CQI) initiatives focus on improvement of the delivery of non-clinical services to patients (Entoven & Vorhaus, 1997).

ALIGNMENT OF QUALITY INDICATORS ACROSS DIVERSE STAKEHOLDERS

Quality will continue to be defined from each stakeholder's unique perspective. However, rehabilitation providers may wish to consider embracing the following principles as they strive to define quality and satisfy the diverse needs of diverse stakeholder groups:

1. All humans have value and are entitled to optimal care.
2. All stakeholders in health care both owe a duty to others and are owed a duty by others.
3. Accept that health care is a business, but balance humanitarian concern with economic rationality. Serve as a patient's ombudsperson.
4. Restore the *care* in health *care* and managed *care* by recognizing and legitimizing psycho-social-economic needs of consumers.
5. Appreciate that one must first measure it (disability) to manage it. Data (evidence-based practice) should bolster, *not* replace, clinical judgment.
6. Communication is the adhesive of all human interactions.
7. Quality measurement should involve both processes and outcomes of care since a focus on one area is insufficient (Lohr, 1997).
8. Appreciate that involved and empowered consumers enhance the quality of care (Entoven & Vorhaus, 1997; Lorig et al, 1993; Greenfield et al, 1985).
9. Accept that scientific measures of quality may not be feasible, and common sense must prevail.
10. Understand that quality of care assessments require attention to the importance of non-events as well as events occurring among individuals and populations.

Kane (1994) provides sage advice concerning the key to quality assurance and improvement by stating the importance of "humanizing quality information and explaining its importance in simple terms, rather than in health policy verbiage."

Greenfield et al (1996) provide a lesson for rehabilitation providers as they attempt to define quality services: "Ultimately, quality of care will be measured in terms of whether the patient got the care he or she needed, whether the patient's condition stabilized, or improved, how long it took to reach that point, and what it cost to get there."

REFERENCES

Abbott RK: High-performance health plans beat the average. J Compensation 19(3):46-50, 2003.

Abramovwitz S, Cote AA, Berry E: Analyzing patient satisfaction: A multianalytic approach. Qual Rev Bull 13:122-130, 1987.

Agency for Health Care Policy and Research (AHCPR): Consumer assessment of health plans (CAHPS) 2.0 questionnaires. Rockville, MD, December 1998, http://www.ahcpr.gov/qual/cahps/cahpques.htm, accessed May 10, 2004.

Aharony L, Strasser S: Patient satisfaction: What we know about and what we still need to explore. Med Care Rev 50:49-79, 1993.

Allen H: Anticipating market demand: Tracking enrollee satisfaction and health over time. International J Quality Health Care 10:531-530, 1998.

Anderson C: Measuring what works in health care. Science 263: 1080-1082, 1994.

Armstead R, Leong D: Outcomes improvement: The true mark of quality in managed care. Am J Med Qual 14(5):202-210, 1999.

Beattie PF, Pinto MB, Nelson MK et al: Patient satisfaction with outpatient physical therapy: Instrument validation. Phys Ther 82(6):557-564, 2002.

Beauregard TR, Winston KR: Employers shift to quality to evaluate and manage their health plans. Managed Care Q 5(1):51-56, 1997.

Blumenthal D, Kilo CM: A report card on continuous quality improvement. Milbank Q 76(4):625-648, 1998.

Brennan TA: The role of regulation in quality improvement. Milbank Q 76(4):, 1998.

Carr AJ, Thompson PW, Kirwan JR: Quality of life measures. Rheumatol 35(3):275-281, 1996.

Centers for Medicare and Medicaid Services (CMS): Quality fact sheet. July 2003, Publication No. CMS-11043, http://www.cms.hhs.gov/quality/QualityFactSheet.pdf, accessed May 10, 2004.

Chassin MR: Is health care ready for six sigma quality? Milbank Q 76(4), 1998, http://www.milbank.org/quarterly/764featchas.html, accessed May 10, 2004.

Chassin MR: Quality of care. Time to act. JAMA 266:3472-3473, 1991.

Chassin MR, Galvin RW, National Roundtable on Health Care Quality: The urgent need to improve health care quality. JAMA 280:1000-1005, 1998.

Chassin MR et al: Variations in the use of medical and surgical services by the Medicare population. New Engl J Med 314(5):285-290, 1986.

Cheng SH, Yang MC, Chiang TL: Patient satisfaction with and recommendation of a hospital: Effects of interpersonal and technical aspects of hospital care. Int. J Qual. Health Care 15(4):345-355, 2003.

Clauser SB, Bierman AS: Significance of functional status data for payment and quality. Health Care Finance Rev 24(3):1-12, 2003.

Cleary PD, McNeil BJ: Patient satisfaction as an indicator of quality care. Inquiry 25:25-36, 1988.

Clifton DW: A shift toward utilization management. PT Magazine 3(7):32-34, 1995.

Commission for Accreditation of Rehabilitation Facilities (CARF), www.carf.org, accessed August 8, 2004.

Coye MJ, Detmer DE: Quality at a crossroads. Milbank Quarterly 76(4):1-5, 1998, www.milbank.org, accessed September 30, 2003.

Cross M: Money pit: Is accreditation always worth the cost? Managed Care 12(7): 26-30, 2003.

Darby C, Dervin K: Measuring consumer satisfaction under workers' compensation managed care. A presentation at Workers' Compensation and Managed Care: Challenges and opportunities in a changing health care system. Agency for Health care Policy and Research, Chicago, July 30 1997–Aug 1,1997, http://www.ahcpr.gov/research/ulpwrkrs.htm,

Deming WE: Out of crisis. Cambridge, MA, MIT Press, 1986.

Doloresco L: CARF: Symbol of rehabilitation excellence. Sci Nurs 18(3):165,172, 2001.

Donabedian A: Quality assessment and assurance: Unity of purpose, diversity of means. Inquiry 25:173-192, 1988.

Donaldson MS (ed): Statement on quality of care. Washington, DC, National Roundtable on Health Care Quality, Institute of Medicine, 1998, http://books.nap.edu/books/statement/JAMA/pdf, accessed August 8, 2004.

Eazell DE, Maama F: Demonstrating cost savings through functional gains: Payors need a functional assessment measure that clearly translates to increased savings. Rehabil Manage Aug/Sept:137-139, 1992.

Entoven AC, Vorhaus CB: A vision of quality in health care delivery. Health Aff 16(3):44-57, 1997.

ERISA Industry Committee: Policy statement on health care quality and consumer protection. Washington, DC, ERISA Industry Committee, April1998, http://www.eric.org, accessed August 8, 2004.

Evans RL, Hendricks RD: Comparison of subacute rehabilitation care with outpatient primary medical care. Disabil Rehabil 23(12):531-538, 2001.

Ewan CE: Attitudes to social issues in medicine: A comparison of first-year medical students with first-year students in non-medical facilities. Med Ed 21(1):25-31, 1987.

Fetterolf DE: A framework for evaluating underutilization of health care services. Am J Med Qual 14(2):89-97, 1999.

Field MJ, Lohr KN: Guidelines for clinical practice: From development to use. Institute of Medicine, Washington National Academy Press, 1990.

Fisher W et al: Rehabits: A common language of functional assessment. Arch Phys Med Rehabil 76:113-122, 1995.

Fong T: Things aren't getting better. Modern Healthcare 33(9):6-16, 2003.

Franke RJ: Restoring the health care paradox. 1990 Robert D. Eilers Memorial Lecture. Chicago, John Nuveen and Company, 1990.

Gaba DM: Human error in anesthetic mishaps. Intl Anesthesiol Clinics 23(3):137-147, 1989.

Gallagher RM: Physician variability in pain management: Are the JCAHO standards enough? Pain Med 4(1):1-3, 2003.

Goka RS, Arakaki AH: Centers of excellence: Choosing the appropriate rehabilitation center. J Insur Med 23(1):66-69, 1991.

Goldie MG, Jonsson E: Hospital care versus home care for rehabilitation after hip replacement. Int J Technol Assess Health Care 8(1):93-101, 1992.

Gomick M: Medicare patients: Geographic differences in hospital discharge rates and multiple stays. Soc Sec Bull 40:22-41, 1977.

Gosfield AG: Who is holding whom accountable for quality? Health Aff 16(3):26-40, 1997.

Granger CV, Gresham GE: Functional assessment in rehabilitation medicine. Phys Med Rehabil Clin North Am 4(3):417-423, 1993.

Greenberg L: Accreditation strengthens the disease management bridge over the quality chasm. Dis Manage (6)1:3-8, 2003.

Greenfield L, Cohen BD, Cleary PD et al: Evaluating the quality of health care: What research offers decision makers. New York, Milbank Memorial Fund, 1996.

Greenfield S, Kaplan S, Ware J: Expanding patient involvement in care. Ann Int Med 102(4):520-528, 1985.

Greiner AC, Knebel E (eds): Health Professions Education: A Bridge to Quality, Committee on the Health Professions Education Summit, The Institutes of Medicine, Washington, DC, The National Academy Press, 2003.

Hart DL, Dobrzykowski EA: Influence of orthopaedic clinical specialist certification on clinical outcomes. J Orthop Sports Phys Ther 30(4):183-193, 2000.

Hays RD: The outpatient satisfaction (OSQ-37): Executive summary. Santa Monica, CA, RAND Corp, 1995.

Health Care Financing Review: 24(3):1-12, 2003.

Hibbard JH, Jewitt JJ, Legnin MW et al: Choosing a health plan: Do large employers use the data? Health Aff 16(6):172-180, 1997.

Hudak PL, Wright JG: The characteristics of patient satisfaction measures. Spine J 25:3167-3177, 2000.

Hulka BS, Zyzanski SJ, Cassel JC et al: Scale for the measurement of satisfaction with medical care: Modification in content, format, and scoring. Med Care 12:611, 1970.

Institute of Management and Administration (IOMA): Report on managed care plans. Health care cost benchmarks compare HMO, PPO, & POS plans. IOM 3(3):3-5, 2003.

Institute of Medicine (IOM): Medicare: A strategy for quality assurance, vol 1. Washington, DC, National Academy Press, 1990.

Institute of Medicine (IOM): Leadership by example: Coordinating government roles in improving health care quality. Washington, DC, National Academy Press, 2002.

Ishikawa K (ed): Guide to Quality Control. White Plains, NY, Krahs International, 1986.

Jette AM: Outcomes research: Shifting the dominant research paradigm in physical therapy. Phys Ther 75(11):965-970, 1995.

Jette AM: Using health-related quality of life measures in physical therapy outcomes research. Phys Ther 73(8):528-537, 1993.

Jette DU, Bacon K, Batty C et al: Evidence-based practice: Beliefs, attitudes, knowledge, and behaviors of physical therapists. Phys Ther 83(9):786-805, 2003.

Joint Commission for the Accreditation of Healthcare Organizations, www.jcaho.org, accessed August 8, 2004.

Jonas S: Healthcare delivery in the United States. New York, Springer, 1977.

Juran JM: Juran on planning for quality. New York, The Free Press, 1989.

Juran JM, Gryma FM (eds): Juran's quality control handbook, 4th ed, New York, McGraw-Hill, 1988.

Kane RL: Looking for physical therapy outcomes. Phys Ther 74(5):425-429, 1994.

Keith RA: Patient satisfaction and rehabilitation services. Arch Phys Med Rehabil 79:1122-1128, 1998.

Kessner DM et al: Assessing health quality—The case for tracers. New Engl J Med 288(4):189-194, 1973.

Kizer KW: Establishing health care performance standards in an era of consumerism. JAMA 286(10):1213-1217, 2001.

Koch SJ, Arego DE, Bowser B: Outpatient rehabilitation for chronic neuromuscular diseases. Am J Phys Med 65(5):245-257, 1986.

Korthals-de Bos IB, Hoving JL, van Tulder MW et al: Cost effectiveness of physiotherapy, manual therapy, and general practitioner care for neck pain: Economic evaluation alongside a randomized controlled trial. BMJ 326(7395):911, 2003.

Kramer AM, Steiner JF, Schenkler RE et al: Outcomes and costs after hip fracture and stroke: A comparison of rehabilitation settings. JAMA 277(5):396-404, 1997.

Kronneger B: Perspectives: Rehab accreditors looking for more than just outcomes data. Med Health 53(34):S1-S4, 1999.

Leape LL: Error in medicine. JAMA 272:1351-1357, 1994.

Leape LL, Brennan TA, Laird N et al: The nature of adverse-events in hospitalized patients. The results of the Harvard Medical Practice Study II. New Engl J Med 324:377-384, 1991.

Lewis CE: Variations in the incidence of surgery. New Engl J Med 281:880-884, 1969.

Lieberman T: In search of quality healthcare. Consumer Rep 63(10):35-40, 1998.

Like R, Zyzanski SJ: Patient satisfaction with the clinical encounter: Social and psychological determinants. Soc Sci Med 24(4):351-357, 1987.

Lohr KN: How do we measure quality? Health Aff 16(3):22-25, 1997.

Lorig K, Mazonson P, Holman H: Evidence suggesting that health education for self-management in patients with chronic arthritis has sustained health benefits while reducing health care costs. Arthritis Rheumatol 36(4):439-446, 1993.

MacDonell C: The many benefits of facilities accreditation. J Long Term Care Adm 24(4):12-13, 1997.

McClosky AH et al: Reforming the health care system: State profiles 1996. Washington, DC, American Association of Retired Persons (AARP), 1996.

Menard MR, Hoens AM: Objective functional capacity: Medical, occupational and legal settings. J Orthop Sports Phys Ther 19(5):249-260, 1994.

Merry MD, Crago MG: The past, present and future of health care quality, urgent need for innovative, external review processes to protect patients. Physician Executive 27(5):30-35, 2001

Monnin D, Pernegar TV: Scale to measure patient satisfaction with physical therapy. Phys Ther 82(7):682-691, 2002.

Moore C, Wisnivesky J, Williams S, et al: Medical errors related to discontinuity of care from an inpatient to an outpatient setting. J Gen Intern Med 18(8):646-645, 2003.

Morrison I: The second curve: Managing the velocity of change. New York, Ballantine Books, 1996.

National Academy of Science, www.nas.edu, accessed August 8, 2004.

National Coalition on Health Care (NCHC) webpage, http://www.nchc.org, accessed June 29, 2004.

National Committee for Quality Assurance (NCQA), 2000 L Street NW, Washington, DC, http://www.ncqa.org.

Neuman KM, Ptak M: Managing managed care through accreditation standards. Soc Work 48(3):384-391, 2003.

O'Connor SJ, Trinh HQ, Shewchuk RM: Perceptual gaps in understanding patient expectations for health care service. Quality Health Care Manage Rev 25(2):7-23, 2000.

O'Connor SJ, Lanning JA: The new health-care quality: Value, outcomes, and continuous improvement. Clin Lab Manage Rev 5(4):221-223, 226-229, 232-233, 1991.

Ostrow PC, Kuntavanish AA: Improving the utilization of occupational therapy: A quality assurance study. Am J Occup Ther 37(6):388-391, 1983.

Parasuraman A, Zeithaml VA, Berry LL: SERVQUAL: A multiple-item scale for measuring consumers perceptions of service quality. J Retailing 64:12-40, 1988.

Pennsylvania Health Care Cost Containment Council website, http://www.phc4.org/glance.htm, accessed June 15, 2000.

Picker Institute, Picker Adult Medical Surgical Inpatient, http://www.pickerinstitute.org, accessed August 8, 2004.

Rahman NM, Shahidullah M, Rashid HA: Quality of health care from patient perspectives. Bangledesh Med Res Counc Bull 28(3):87-96, 2002.

Rainwater JA, Romano PS: What data do California HMOs use to select hospitals for contracting? Am J Managed Care (8):553-561, 2003.

Reece RL: And who shall care for the sick? Minneapolis, MN, Media Medicus, 1988.

Relman A: Assessment and accountability: The third revolution in medical care. New Engl J Med 319:1220-1222, 1988.

Retchin SM, Preston J: Effects of cost containment on the care of elderly diabetics. Arch Intern Med 151:2244-2248, 1991.

Riley T: The role of states in accountability for quality. Health Aff 16(3):41-43, 1997.

Roos NP, Roos LL: Surgical variations: Do they reflect the health or socioeconomic characteristics of the population? Med Care 20: 945-958, 1982.

Rothstein JM: Thirty-second Mary McMillan lecture: Journeys beyond the horizon. Phys Ther 81(11):1817-1828, 2001.

Rothstein JM: Editor's note: Disability and our identity. Phys Ther 74: 375-378, 1994.

Rubin HR, Ware JE, Nelson EC et al: The patient judgments of hospital quality (PJHQ): Questionnaire. Med Care 28(9):517-518, 1990.

Rutstein DD et al: Measuring the quality of medical care: A clinical method. New Engl J Med 294:582, 1976.

Schuster MA, McGlynn EA, Brook RH: How good is the quality of health care in the United States. Milbank Q 76(4):517-563, 509, 1998.

Shephard RJ: Economic benefits of secondary and tertiary cardiac rehabilitation: A critical study. Ann Acad Med Singapore 21(1):57-62, 1992.

Shilling V, Jenkins V, Fallowfield L: Factors affecting patient and clinician satisfaction with the clinical consultation: Can communication skills training for clinicians improve satisfaction? Psychooncology 12(6):599-611, 2003.

Shipon DM, Nash DB: Quality in health care: What are the problems and what are the solutions? Tex Med J 96(10):61-65, 2000.

Silberman P: Ensuring quality and access in managed care: How well are we doing? Quality Management in Health Care 5(2):44-54, 1997.

SPRY Foundation: Quality of care in HMOs for mature adults: An overview of current measurement & evaluation initiatives. Washington, DC, March 14, 1997.

Steffen TM, Meyer AD: Physical therapists' note and outcomes of physical therapy. A case of insufficient evidence. Phys Ther 65(2):213-217, 1985.

Strunk BC, Ginsburg PB: Tracking health care costs: Trends stabilize but remain high in 2002. Health Aff 22(4):W-3-266-W-3-277 supplement, 2003.

Sullivan B: Program accreditation. Phys Ther 78(12):1339, 1998.

Sutton JP, De Jong G, Wilkerson D: Function-based pament-model for inpatient medical rehabilitation: An evaluation. Arch Phys Med Rehabil 77(7):893-701, 1996.

Udvarhelyi IS, Jennsion RS, Phillips RS et al: Comparison of the quality of ambulatory care for fee-for-service and prepaid patients. Ann Intern Med 115(5):394-400, 1991.

Wade DT: Outcome measures for clinical rehabilitation trials, impairment, function, quality of life or value? Am J Phys Rehabil Med 82(10 supplement):S26-S31, 2003.

Ware JE Jr et al: Defining and measuring patient satisfaction with medical care. Eval Program Plan 6(3-4):247-263, 1983.

Weber DO: Second thoughts: Can managed care be ethical? Healthcare Forum J July/Aug:17-26, 1997.

Wells KB, Hays RD, Burnam MA et al: Detection of depressive disorder for patients receiving prepaid or fee-for-service care. JAMA 258:2568, 1989.

Wennberg J, Gittleson A:Variations in medical care among small areas. Sci Am 246(4):120-135, 1982.

Westaway MS, Rheeder P, Van Zyl DG et al: Interpersonal and organizational dimensions of patient satisfaction: The moderating effects of health status. Int J Qual Health Care 15(4):337-344, 2003.

Wilkerson DL, Batavia AI, DeJong G: Use of functional status measures for payment of medical rehabilitation services. Arch Phys Med Rehabil 73(2):111-120, 1992.

Ziegenfuss JT: Systems thinking and quality management. Am J Med Quality 18(4):139, 2003.

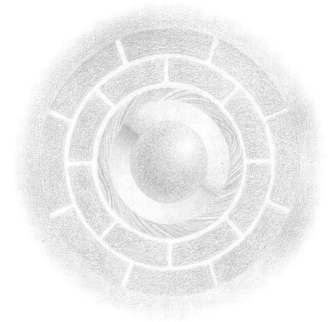

## CHAPTER 14

Outcomes Management

David W. Clifton, Jr., PT

"We were inundated by instruments that almost always measured impairments. We eschewed the 'soft' behavioral measures that reflected disabilities in favor of the seemingly more scientific measurements of impairments. We forgot to balance the elements to find the middle ground."

- Rothstein, 1994

KEY POINTS

- Health care has entered into a new era of accountability with outcomes measures playing a vital, yet evolving, role.
- Outcomes measures, in order to satisfy the needs of multiple health care stakeholders, must address clinical, cost, and patient satisfaction concerns.
- Physical rehabilitation professionals must abandon the traditional impairment-based paradigm and adopt more meaningful measures of disability status.
- Use of meta-analysis summaries can provide a relatively quick but reliable means for clinicians to ascertain which treatment interventions are efficacious, cost-effective, and efficient
- There is no universal outcomes management system that adequately satisfies all patient populations, treatment settings, provider organizations, or payer needs.

Operational Definitions*

Reliability	The consistency of information collected during assessment.
Intertester Reliability	Consistency between different evaluators.
Intratester Reliability	Consistency with same evaluator over repeated tests or trials.
Sensitivity	The ability of a test or test battery to detect true outcomes.
Specificity	The ability of a test or test battery to obtain normal results or true negatives.
Validity	The ability to accurately measure a specific test variable.
Construct Validity	Designing a measure secondary to a hypothesis or theory.
Content Validity	The measurement instrument that measures samples from knowledge contained within the variable being measured.
Concurrent Validity	Design of an alternate measure that is typically more user-friendly.
Predictive Validity	The ability of a measure to distinguish and separate variables that do or do not share attributes.
Evaluation	A judgment that is derived from a measurement.
End-Result Outcome	A change in the patient's status between two or more points in time (e.g., pretreatment and posttreatment).
Process Evaluation	Evaluation of the degree to which services meet professional standards of quality care (e.g., practice guidelines or protocols).
Structural Outcome	The stable resources required to deliver care (e.g., providers' qualifications, administrative organization, facilities, equipment).
Utilization Outcome	A type of health care outcome that demonstrates a change in the patient's status over time; status is typically described as the patient moving from one treatment setting to another.

*Sources: Data modified from Jette (1995), Rothstein & Echternach (1993); Center for Health Service and Policy Research (2004).

AN INTROSPECTIVE VIEW OF PHYSICAL REHABILITATION

Jules Rothstein's quotation was embedded in an editorial entitled "Disability and Our Identity." In this critical but constructive editorial, Rothstein contends that physical rehabilitation providers have been fixated on other matters while the central focus should be on remediation of disability. He contends that impairment measures have been an obsession with providers, who are seduced into their use in an attempt to justify treatment interventions and to establish professional credibility. Rothstein contends that clinical outcomes measures must transcend impairment measures through meaningful functional indicators.

All outcome measures attempt to compare a patient's progress or lack thereof between two points in time, typically an initial evaluation to re-evaluation comparison. The design of an outcomes management (OM) tool is what distinguishes one approach from another. Some tools use pathology or disease comparisons (the biomedical approach). Others use impairments such as muscle performance, endurance, balance, edema, or range of motion (the impairment approach). Function-based OM represents a third approach (the disability model). Physical rehabilitation providers have only in the past decade or so applied disablement models that link disease or pathology to functional consequences. However, conceptual models of disablement have been in existence for decades (Nagi, 1965).

Functionally based disability management requires objective, not anecdotal, evidence. Wilkerson et al (1992) assert that the primary goal of medical rehabilitation is to enhance patient function and independence. However, some contend that developments in clinical practice have not kept pace with the increase in evidence availability (Maher, Sherrington, Eljkins et al, 2004). This suggests that rehabilitation practice has not significantly changed because of the prevalence of non-evidence–based practice (Haynes & Haines, 1998; Metcalfe, Lewis, Wisher et al, 2001).

Rothstein (1994) asserts that goals are often expressed in terms of changing impairments or goals that do not necessarily represent meaningful changes in a person's life. He concludes that clinical goals should address the function of the person seeking treatment. Physical rehabilitation OM must therefore have function as a cornerstone.

Physical rehabilitation has some unique features that distinguish it from traditional medical care. First, rehabilitation is often considered a discretionary or elective intervention. For this reason, rehabilitation referrals are often delayed until after other services or interventions have been rendered, such as medication, surgery, chiropractic care, specialist care (e.g., orthopedics, neurology), and hospitalization. This reduces the rehabilitation provider's ability to confirm that indeed it was his or her service that affected functional outcomes, especially in chronic cases in which the original insult, trauma, or injury has less relevance and psychosocial issues have emerged. Chronicity is extensively covered in Chapter 22.

A BRIEF HISTORY OF THE REHABILITATION OUTCOMES MOVEMENT

This chapter strives to familiarize providers with the general principles surrounding the development and implementation of OM systems.

Paul Ellwood (1988), a psysiatrist, coined the term "outcomes management" during a seminal Shattuck Lecture of 1988. During this same year, Arnold Relman, the editor of the *New England Journal of Medicine* authored an editorial titled "Assessment and Accountability: The Third Revolution in Medical Care" (Relman, 1988). Both of these medical leaders envisioned the emerging importance of outcomes measures.

OM is a technology of patient experience that is designed to assist multiple health care stakeholders, including patients, payers, and providers, in making rational medical care-related choices based on the effect on the patient's life. OM incorporates clinical, financial, and health outcomes that strive to link medical interventions with health outcomes (Albrecht & Harasymiw, 1979).

Ellwood describes the centerpiece and unifying ingredient of OM as the tracking and measurement of function and well-being or quality of life (Ellwood, 1988).

Physical rehabilitation providers are uniquely qualified experts on function and as such play a vital role in both the development and implementation of OM systems. A number of rehabilitation professionals have been OM change agents, shifting the dominant treatment paradigm toward a focus on function. Jette (1995) articulated a paradigm shift from an impairment-based model toward a disability and quality of life approach. Impairment outcomes focus on anatomical or physiological measures such as edema, range of motion, or muscle performance. Disability-related outcomes measures describe the level of a patient's functioning in physical, social, cognitive, and behavioral terms. Table 14–1 contrasts impairment and disability outcomes measures.

Guccione (1991) introduced Nagi's disablement model to the rehabilitation sector. Rothstein (1985) pioneered efforts to standardize measures in physical therapy. Swanson (1995) identified six technical outcomes that satisfy the requirements of Medicare beneficiaries: prevention, cure, symptom control, elimination of impairment,

 Table 14–1 Outcomes Measures Paradigm Shift

The Old Paradigm	The New Paradigm
Defined by impairment measures	Defined by health-related and disability measures
Pain	Function/dysfunction
	Instrumental activities of daily living (IADLs)
Range of motion	Work status
Muscle performance	Cost outcomes
	Medical
	Indemnity/wage replacement
	Legal
	Administrative
Edema/swelling	Health-related quality of life (HRQOL)
Sensation	Social functioning
Balance	General well-being

Table 14–2 Integrants of an Outcomes Measures Program

- Client characteristics or needs
- Diagnostic composition of case load
- Volume of clients treated, by provider type or facility
- Average length of stay (LOS), by diagnosis compared to norms
- Average rehabilitation cost per case or episode by diagnosis
- Client age, gender, and other demographics
- Time from injury/illness to treatment
- Recidivism or reinjury data
- Return-to-work data
- Use of community services
- Referral patterns by referrer (e.g., physician)
- Program interruptions or patient compliance issues

Data modified from Forer S: Outcome analysis for program service management. In Fuhrer MJ (ed): Rehabilitation Outcomes: Analysis and Measurement. Baltimore, Brooks, 1987, pp 115-136.

elimination of disability, and elimination of handicap or disadvantage. Kane (1994) acknowledged a paucity of patient-focused outcomes measures despite a near consensus among providers regarding their patient advocacy role. Forer (1987) outlined elements for consideration in the development and implementation of an outcomes measures system. Forer's outcomes measure integrants are listed in Table 14–2. Donabedian (1988) described four broad categories of outcome determination: death, morbidity, disability, and quality of life. Granger's contribution via the Functional Inventory Measures or FIM represented a pioneering effort to describe meaningful functional measures in elderly or long-term–care populations (Granger, 1998). Ware et al's (1981). Short-form 36 or SF-36 provided impetus to define outcomes from a lifestyle or activity of daily living perspective.

Both Granger's and Ware's models transcend the traditional impairment-based approach to outcomes measures and have become universally accepted standards of disability assessment.

The urgency of OM research accelerated in the 1980s when researchers discovered that "geography is destiny" (Agency for Healthcare Policy and Research, 2000). Studies demonstrated regional practice variation in terms of health care costs and utilization rates (Wennberg, 1984; Chassin, 1980). Providers, payers, and policymakers became increasingly aware through much of the 1980s and 1990s of the need for standardized functional measures (Fratelli, 1993; Granger, 1997; Jackson & Burwell, 1989; Patrick & Deyo, 1989). This period of enlightenment led to a vortex of activity centered around the development of functionally based measures.

Historically, health care providers have relied on biomedical measures such as laboratory test results to determine treatment efficacy (Agency for Healthcare Policy and Research, 2000). Rehabilitation providers specifically relied on impairment-based measures (Jette, 1995; Badley, 1993). These paradigms persisted in the face of research indicating that patients valued non-biomedical outcomes measures (Hall & Dornan, 1988).

Biomedical measures are displaced and/or augmented under a new paradigm by measures of symptom status, functional status, disability health perceptions, and quality of life measures (Williams & Myers, 1998). Jette (1995, p 970) described this paradigm shift:

Research needs to include both impairments and disabilities when appropriate, and most importantly, it needs to explicitly investigate the nature of the relationship assumed to exist between impairments and disability-level outcomes across various target groups.

The impairment-to-function-or-disability paradigm shift has resulted in an explosion in the use of functional capacity evaluations, especially under workers' compensation and disability insurance programs (American Occupational Therapy Association, 2001; Matheson et al, 1998; Owens & Buchholz, 1995). Functional capacity evaluations, or FCEs, enjoy widespread acceptance, exemplifying a new function-based paradigm (Abdel-Moty et al, 1996).

Multidisciplinary rehabilitation programs emphasizing functional assessment and restoration have achieved return-to-work outcomes ranging from 50% to 80% (Bendix et al, 1995; Cleary et al, 1995; Niemeyer et al, 1994). These outcomes link impairments to disability status.

Worker-task relationships have been examined by rehabilitation and disability professionals (Bullock, 1990; Rodgers, 1988). Disability evaluation measures functional abilities or limitations in terms of a specific role(s) and worker-task relationships. However, a person's functional impairment represents only one-half of the picture. Worksite elements such as critical job demands represent the other half of the puzzle. A worker⇔worksite match or mismatch depends on the relationship of a person's physical and cognitive abilities to the critical functional demands of the job or task. Figure 14–1 depicts the relationship between environmental and human attributes. The left side of this diagram describes the physical or critical functional demands of the environment and identifies reasonable accommodations based upon the worker's minimal functional abilities. Reasonable accommodations, including engineering modifications or administrative changes that facilitate re-entry into the workforce, are required under the 1990 Americans With Disabilities Act. The right side of the schematic depicts a worker's physical and cognitive abilities, which are quantified in functional terms. Physical restrictions are identified that may require reasonable accommodations. A worker's true functional capacity remains enigmatic even with the application of reasonable accommodations. A worker's abilities (versus capacities) represent either a worker-worksite match or mismatch. Demonstrable functional ability is gauged through functional testing protocols; however, tests of an individual's current function do not necessarily predict his or her actual functional capacity (Matheson, 1996). In fact, the term "functional capacity evaluation" may actually be a misnomer because outcomes quantify a person's functional abilities, not capacity, which implies a theoretical construct or untestable prediction.

PURPOSES OF OUTCOMES MEASURES OR MANAGEMENT

Outcomes measures serve a variety of purposes across the following broad categories: scientific, regulatory,

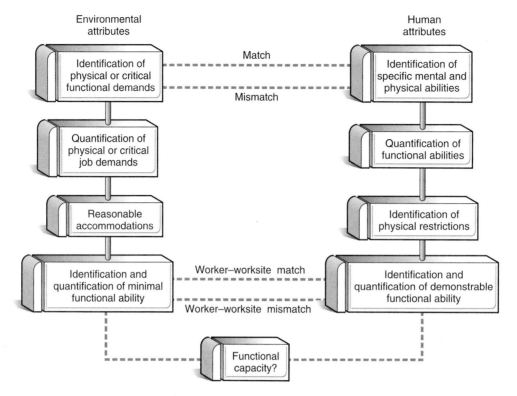

Figure 14–1. Worker-worksite interface.

reimbursement, legal and risk management, quality assurance, cost containment, and value purchasing.

It is important to note that the OM movement has not been embraced by all stakeholders despite the traction gained by some developers and users. Kessner et al (1973) cautioned that OM alone is inadequate and can be misleading if patients receive unnecessary diagnostic tests or inappropriate treatment. Anderson (1994) argued that the millions of dollars spent on outcome research have not resulted in changes in general medical practice. Others assert that rehabilitation records are commonly insufficient in documenting functional improvement (Clifton, 1995; Steffen & Meyer, 1985).

Scientific

OM facilitates scientific advances and clinically efficacious interventions. Refinements to treatment protocols and guidelines are more meaningful when they directly result from outcomes measures rather than solely from a clinician's anecdotal observations. OM enables providers to eliminate non-efficacious interventions in favor of proven strategies. This benefits a multitude of health care stakeholders, including patients, providers, and payers (Table 14–3). Evidence-based approaches bridge the chasm between healing art and science-based health care.

Regulatory

The role of outcomes measures intensifies as health care policymakers become more involved in health care finance and delivery oversight. Government programs such as Medicare, Social Security, Medicaid, Civilian Health and Medical Plan for Uniformed Services (CHAMPUS), and federal workers' compensation programs increasingly demand accountability (SSA, 1997). Health plans and providers can demonstrate their accountability via outcomes measures, especially when they include cost reports. Federal agencies such as the Agency for Healthcare Quality and Research (AHCQR) have taken a lead role in encouraging OM. In fact, this focus is exemplified by the name change of this agency: It was formerly known as the Agency for Healthcare Policy and Research, or AHCPR. This agency has promulgated a number of treatment guidelines that have had an enormous effect on both governmental and private sector payers with regard to reimbursement for rehabilitation services.

Reimbursement

Reimbursement decisions both influence and are highly influenced by OM data. Outcomes measures are routinely considered when establishing the medical necessity, appropriateness, and reasonableness of care. Those rehabilitation modalities, techniques, and interventions not found to be efficacious and or cost-effective are potentially judged as non-reimbursable. Rehabilitation services that are covered may be only those that are designed to achieve a clear functional goal and for which the need for skilled professional services can be clearly demonstrated through clinical documentation (Clifton, 1995; Moorhead & Clifford, 1992; Steffen & Meyer, 1985).

Table 14–3 Benefits of an OM System

1. Improved community acceptance of an organization
2. Informed decision making for organizational planning
3. Generation of marketing data (e.g., comparisons to industry standards)
4. Cost-effectiveness data for selective contracting or preferred provider negotiations with managed care organizations (MCOs)
5. Identification of problematic areas or triggers for process analysis and/or improvement (e.g., continuous quality improvement [CQI])
6. Alignment of provider goals with client needs or expectations
7. Reduction in practice variation/standardization of care through the identification of best practices
8. Establishment of treatment efficacy from a scientific perspective
9. Definition of quality across stakeholder groups
10. Maximization of provider reimbursement
11. Function as a risk management tool
12. Clarification of choices for informed consent
13. Provider profiling
14. Facility benchmarking
15. Linkage of process and structure elements of care to outcomes

Data modified from Forer S: Outcome analysis for program service management. In Fuhrer MJ (ed): Rehabilitation Outcomes: Analysis and Measurement. Baltimore, Brooks, 1987, pp 115-136; Eazell DE, Maama F: Demonstrating cost savings through functional gains. Payors need a functional assessment measure that clearly translates to increased savings. Rehabil Manage: Interdisciplinary J Rehabil Aug/Sept:137-139, 1992.

Legal and Risk Management

The litmus test in legal cases involving professional liability is the concept of a legal or community standard of care (Scott 1990). Standards of care can be local, regional, or national, depending on the strength of consensus and universal application associated with them.

Outcomes measures can directly lead to the development of treatment standards, which are used as evidence in medicolegal cases. Providers who render a service that results in an adverse impact may find their treatment standards to be either a shield or a sword. If their standards are found to be consistent with the community standard of care, they serve as a shield. If they breach the community standard of care, they may serve as a sword. Standardized OM tools help define the community standard of care.

Quality Assurance

Outcomes measures allow for both qualitative and quantitative comparisons of clinical performance. Data can be used to compare one clinician to another or one facility to a second facility (Ahmen et al, 1988; Melin et al, 1993; Ottenbacher et al, 1994). Quality assurance and continuous quality improvement programs are enhanced through the use of outcomes measures (Spector & Mukamel, 1998). Figure 14–2, Three Generations of Care, illustrates three distinct generations of managed health care. Each generation is defined by its principal focus or foci. For example, the first generation is defined by an exclusive focus on reducing cost without any consideration given to quality or outcomes measures. A second-generation health plan shifts to a value focus expressed as the relationship between service costs, quality, and outcome. In this scenario, the focus remains on impairment management, such as reduced pain and swelling, or increased range of motion and strength. This second generation represents the old rehabilitation paradigm described by Jette (1993). The third generation places a premium on both cost restraint and healthy lifestyles and behaviors. This approach goes beyond simply measuring anatomical or physiological impairments and is more representative of the current disability assessment paradigm. For a more detailed discussion, readers are encouraged to refer to Chapter 13.

Cost Containment

In the era of managed care, treatment cost and duration or utilization rate often dictate the profitability of a given

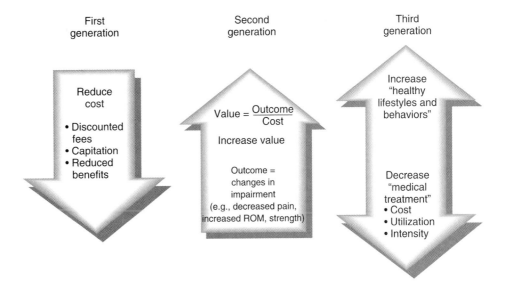

Figure 14–2. Three generations of managed care.

treatment center. Therefore, financial models that include treatment cost should be incorporated into an OM system. Providers are challenged by the problem of balancing quality with costs in a health care system that severely restricts or allocates resources (Schenke et al, 2000, 2001). This presents many ethical dilemmas, which are summed up well by Russell (1998):

> *"The ethical basis of clinical outcomes measurement is a desire to improve care in a way which will increase both clinical effectiveness and value for money—beneficence as well as comptetence."*

A Sample Cost Model

Figure 14–3 presents a sample two-dimensional model of profiling both individual providers of care (POCs) and individual facilities (FACs). The two dimensions involve rehabilitation cost and utilization expressed as visits per diagnosis. Quadrant "A" represents those providers and facilities that incur the greatest cost per episode but that are responsible for lower utilization expressed in visit count. These services render higher intensity of service, which can involve more modalities, techniques, longer visits, more highly specialized providers, or the use of expensive technology, or these providers and facilities may simply price their services higher, without a plausible explanation. Providers and facilities in quadrant "B" are responsible for lower rehabilitation costs as well as lower utilization rates. These providers may be an organization's preferred provider under managed care capitated contracts. Of course, this rubric presupposes that functional outcomes between groups do not substantially vary. Functional outcomes would represent a third dimension in this example. Quadrant "C" providers and facilities are perhaps the least desirable since both costs and utilization are the highest among groupings. Lastly, quadrant "D" houses POCs and FACs that, although low in costs, are among the highest in terms of utilization rates.

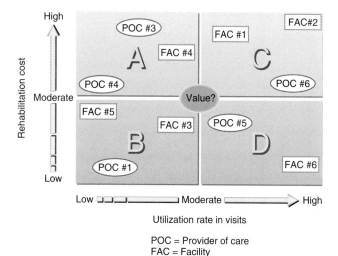

Figure 14–3. Provider and facility profiling.

GENERAL GUIDELINES FOR OUTCOMES MANAGEMENT SYSTEM SELECTION OR CONSTRUCTION

Functional Assessment and Outcomes Management

Rehabilitation providers must make a fundamental choice concerning OM system design. Will the OM system be designed with the provider's needs as the central focus or with the needs of patients, payers, policymakers, and other stakeholders as the central focus? Can one system satisfy all stakeholders' needs?

Barriers to Outcomes Management Design

There are a number of barriers to the development and implementation of outcomes indicators (Batterham et al, 1996). One obstacle involves the short-term clinical focus of rehabilitation providers and a lack of consensus among providers regarding which outcomes should be targeted. A second barrier is the lack of theory about how rehabilitation achieves its outcomes specific to disability. This is especially a problem when rehabilitation services have been rendered across the entire disability spectrum, from acute to subacute and chronic stages of illness or injury. The diversity of providers involved in rehabilitation further compounds this problem. Disability assessment also requires a great deal of subjectivity (Lamon & Lankhorst, 1994).

The Three *Es* of Outcomes Management

OM is a technology designed to assist patients, payers, and providers in making rational medical care–related choices based on the effect of those choices on the patient's life (Jette, 1995). Valuable rehabilitation is reflected by outcomes defined as the restoration and/or maintenance of appropriate personal functioning in performance and behaviors (Granger, 1998).

OM principally uses objective measures to determine the *effectiveness, efficiency,* and/or *efficacy* of treatment interventions. Effectiveness relates to the appropriateness or reasonableness of care when compared to community or professional standards of care. "Effectiveness" is a term that describes the clinical processes that produce the desired effect when applied in the real world (Helewa & Walker, 2000). Efficiency generally refers to the administrative elements associated with an episode of care. Efficiency describes structural and care process attributes, or the "how to" aspects of care. These attributes include but are not limited to the following:

- Provider credentials
- Technology
- Administrative policies and procedures
- Resource allocation
- Facilities
- Treatment protocols and standards

Efficacy measures, by contrast, address the actual clinical outcomes that result in a controlled or ideal environment (Helewa & Walker, 2000). In rehabilitation these are preferably function-based measures. "Efficacy" and "effectiveness" are not synonymous terms.

General Guidelines for Selecting an OM System

The task of selecting an appropriate OM system can be confusing at best and terrifying at worst. However, some guidance is available to clinicians (Law et al, 2003; McGlynn, 1998).

Forer (1987) provides some useful considerations when selecting or developing an OM system. The first step is to define the scope of the patient or impairment group that will be serviced. Next, consider the clinical and non-clinical outcomes that are of value to stakeholders. When selecting assessment tools, consider their accuracy and precision while avoiding poorly tested systems designed in house. The application time for an OM system is another critical consideration. In other words, is it user-friendly? Providers should ask themselves: Is there continuity of measures, or can they be applied across treatment settings? Forer suggests that providers should consider the various instruments that are currently available and that comport with the organization's existing documentation requirements.

Providers must make a difficult and potentially expensive choice between whether to embrace a commercially available OM system or to design one's own system. There are advantages and disadvantages to both approaches, described in Tables 14–4 and 14–5. Selection of an OM system demands an analysis of a multitude of issues, including the following:

- Capital investment
- Human investment
- Scientific soundness, such as reliability and validity of measures
- Standardization versus adaptability
- Reimbursement potential
- Legal and risk management considerations
- Time to rollout
- Review and modification schedule
- Receptivity to the greatest number and variety of stakeholders

- Staff acceptance
- Specificity: Does it serve the needs of current or future patient populations?

Field and Lohr (1992) provide insightful tips on practice guidelines that have direct application to the selection and/or design of OM systems. Providers should determine if an OM system has research relevancy or support. Supportive studies should be examined from a design standpoint. Specifically, do the data represent evidence-based health care? Evidence-based health care is defined as the use of current best evidence flowing from clinical care research that is explicit, judicious, and conscientious (Sackett et al, 1996).

Specific Guidelines for Selecting an Outcomes Management System

Rehabilitation providers are confronted with a daunting task when selecting an OM system because of the diversity of physical rehabilitation providers, settings, treatment interventions, patient populations, and clinical conditions. The following questions and tips may have utility in this endeavor.

1. What patient population(s) or subset(s) represents the target group?
   Tip: Caution should be exercised when adapting systems designed for one target group while applying them to another.
2. Has the OM system's reliability and validity been established via refereed journals or published controlled clinical trials?
   Tip: Be cautious of research that is funded by those persons or groups that have a financial or vested interest in a given system.
3. Is the OM system widely embraced by others in the rehabilitation community?
   Tip: Follow the lead of professionally recognized Centers of Excellence or professional associations that do not benefit from direct advertisement revenue from OM system suppliers.

 Table 14–4 Self-Constructed Outcomes Management Systems

Pros	Cons
1. Specific to center's patient	Relatively small database or client population
2. Staff easily trained	Absence of comparative databases
3. Can be quickly adapted	Potentially biased data
4. No one knows your patients better than you	May be incongruent with widely accepted OM systems (e.g., FIM, MOS)
5. Consensus building is easier in one's own practice than across settings and/or providers	Limitations of OM expertise within one's practice
6. Can be rolled out relatively quickly	Expensive, especially in human capital terms
	May tend to be used more for marketing than quality assurance purposes
	May appear to others to be self-serving

 Table 14–5 Commercially Available Outcomes Measures Systems

Pros	Cons
1. Diversity of data	May lack patient, condition, or treatment intervention specificity
2. Larger database correlates with statistical validity	Staff training may be cumbersome
3. Offers comparative databases	Provider or licensee has relatively little input in OM design methodology; one's fate is in the hands of others
4. May already be accepted by one's peer group and payers	May be slow to adapt to market shifts because of bureaucratic inertia
5. May have access to true OM experts	May be available to one's competitors
6. May assist in marketing efforts	Your data may be enriching the owners of the database, who do not share your practice risks (financial and otherwise)

4. What are the strengths and weaknesses of the OM systems under consideration?

   Tip: On a sheet of paper, draft two columns labeled "strengths" and "weaknesses." Perform an analysis of all pertinent OM systems before making a decision. Beware if the weaknesses significantly outweigh the strengths.

5. How adaptable is the OM system for different treatment settings, conditions, or provider types?

   Tip: Avoid any OM vendors who promote a one-size-fits-all system: It's probably too good to be true.

6. What are the documentation requirements, and do they conform with your current documentation system?

   Tip: Attempt to select a system that meets clinical, reimbursement, and risk management goals of documentation. Be especially aware of the reimbursement implications and educate your top ten payers before making a selection. Payers who understand your OM system are less likely to deny payment because of poor documentation. You may also wish to consult with your corporate counsel before making a selection.

7. Is the OM system impairment-based, disability-based, and/or quality-of-life–based?

   Tip: Secure your staff's consensus concerning what represents an optimal outcome emphasis for your center. Ask the OM vendor for sample outcome printouts as well as for professional references from similar practices.

8. How practical and cost-effective is it to install a given OM system?

   Tip: Track the number of man-hours required to implement the system. Assign a dollar amount per hour and determine aggregate cost to the derived benefit of having the system in place. Ask the vendor to estimate rollout time frames, and negotiate a penalty clause in the contract if time exceeds the vendor's estimate.

9. Can a commercially available system meet your needs, or should an in-house system be constructed?

   Tip: Understand that internally developed systems are potentially subject to a payer's suspicion that the fox is not only guarding but also designing the chicken coop. Externally validated systems may overcome the appearance of being self-serving or of having conflicts of interest.

10. Does the OM system incorporate financial as well as clinical outcomes measures?

Tip: Since health care is widely accepted today as being a business, providers should only consider OM systems that can provide formulas for calculating cost savings and comparisons between your data and those of other providers. Although clinical data are nice to have, they alone may not get you paid.

When treatment interventions span the broad disability continuum and involve different interventions at different levels of acuity (acute, subacute, chronic), it becomes exponentially more difficult to distinguish the contribution of a given service via outcomes measures.

An OM system must be applicable to the irritability stage or acuity level of a given patient.

Diversity of physical rehabilitation across the disability continuum magnifies the difficulty in selecting and designing an adequate OM system (Kane, 1994). Others point to poor clinical documentation as a detriment to sound OM systems (Sager et al, 1992). Even when documentation possesses clarity and uniformity, performance measures alone may not describe how well a person functions in daily living.

The presence of co-morbidities and secondary diagnoses, both common scenarios in physical rehabilitation, severely challenges standardization of an OM system. The paucity of case definitions across the rehabilitation sector further restricts OM development.

Rehabilitation operates from a completely different paradigm than does medicine. Medicine's primary goal is to cure, whereas rehabilitation's goal is to restore or maintain function and to habilitate patients to their own unique environment, whether it be work, home, sports participation, or avocational pursuits. This distinct goal demands equally distinctive outcomes measures. Physical therapy or occupational therapy diagnoses that are based on function may or may not be congruent with a medical diagnosis. All these caveats add enormous difficulty to finding an appropriate OM system.

CLASSIFICATION OF OUTCOMES MANAGEMENT SYSTEMS

OM systems can be divided into categories based on their design elements and purpose (Bakheit et al, 1995; Heald et al, 1997; Kopec et al, 1995; Leek et al, 1986; Weinberger et al, 1992). They may be based on interventions, diagnoses

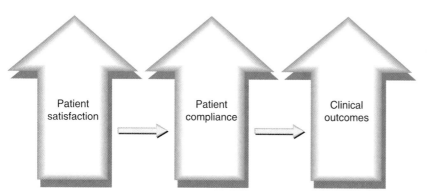

Figure 14–4. A disablement model. (Data adapted from Jette AM: Using health-related quality of life measures in physical therapy outcomes research. Phys Ther 73[8]:528-537, 1993.)

Patient satisfaction → Patient compliance → Clinical outcomes or conditions, treatment settings, providers, patient populations, payers, and others.

Patient Satisfaction Surveys: Meaningful or Meaningless Indicators of Outcomes?

There are essentially two sources of expectations that factor into all OM systems: the patient's expectations and the provider's expectations. Both can contribute data toward gauging the success or failure of a given treatment intervention. One is the seller of services, whereas the other is the consumer of those services. In simplistic terms, the patient communicates in subjective terms, whereas the provider attempts to insert objectivity. One party offers perceptions concerning quality (the patient), whereas the other (the provider), a trained observer and assessment specialist, strives to identify measurable indicators of quality. A third party, the payer, is often the actual purchaser of the service, which exponentially compounds the difficulty of achieving consensus.

Many rehabilitation providers have incorporated patient satisfaction surveys into their OM program. Patient satisfaction surveys provide an appropriate vehicle for inclusion of subjective data (Cohen & Hoffman, 2003; Mancuso et al, 2003) (Figure 14–4).

However, some assert that clinicians who equate patient satisfaction with outcomes measures are misguided because these terms require different measurement instruments (Keith 1998; Pascoe, 1983).

Patient satisfaction as a component of an OM system may logically grow in importance as patients shoulder increasing financial burdens via higher co-payments and deductibles coupled with reduced health care benefit packages.

Hall and Dornan (1988) identified 221 studies addressing patient satisfaction during a literature meta-analysis. Most patient satisfaction systems primarily focus on the perceived quality of services, which in and of itself may weaken the veracity of these instruments (Keith, 1998). Figure 14–5 illustrates the positive correlation commonly found between patient satisfaction, patient compliance, and clinical outcomes. This may be an oversimplification, but it is a pattern that is often observed by rehabilitation professionals. Patients frequently do not distinguish between the art and technical aspects of care (Like & Zyzanski, 1987). Stated another way, patients may overvalue "soft" data and undervalue "hard" clinical data relative to quality perception. Soft data include elements that reside principally in process and structure and not true quality or outcome indicators. Examples of "soft" data include the timeliness of appointments, waiting room time, clerical staff friendliness, office ambience, and a clinician's personality. Hard data reflect actual clinical outcomes in objective measurable terms, and, in rehabilitation, function reigns supreme in terms of clinical outcomes.

Clinicians routinely, and perhaps falsely, equate quality with clinical or technical competence (Cleary & McNeil, 1988). Interpersonal and communication skills are highly valued by patients and are positively associated with patient satisfaction. Despite the "softness" of these elements, providers should be cognizant of their influence in disability management. Patient expectations are a critical element of any OM program (Cole et al, 2002; Fuhrer, 1994, 2000).

Patient satisfaction surveys are generally collected near or at the time of discharge from services. This fact alone suggests that surveys may be skewed by a biased sampling. One could reasonably argue that patients who complete a rehabilitation program are more likely to be satisfied than those who drop out.

There are many difficulties in crafting a patient satisfaction instrument that considers both art and science, or qualitative and quantitative elements. This task becomes increasingly difficult when instruments are used across patient populations, treatment settings, and health care disciplines (Keith, 1998).

Although some OM forms have enjoyed extensive application within rehabilitation, a universally embraced system has not evolved (Kane, 1994). However, OM systems that address impairment, function, quality of life, and value will continue to evolve (Wade, 2003).

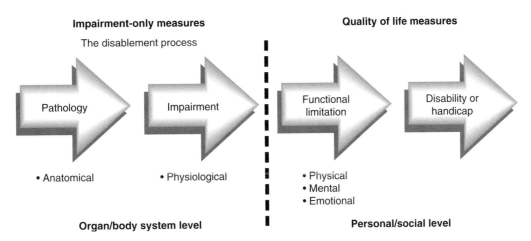

Figure 14–5. Patient satisfaction and its effect on clinical outcomes. (Data adapted from Keith RA: Patient satisfaction and rehabilitation services. Arch Phys Med Rehabil 79[9]:1122-1128, 1998.)

Outcomes Management System Based on Diagnosis or Condition

Virtually every major diagnostic category has received attention relative to outcomes measures development. However, more prevalent conditions include stroke, spinal cord injury, head trauma, and musculoskeletal conditions (Corrigan et al, 1997; DiGabio & Boissonault, 1998; Moreland & Thomson, 1994; Riddle & Straford, 1998). A number of clinicians and researchers have applied functional outcomes measures to populations of stroke survivors (Bohannon et al, 1995; Brock et al, 2002; Brosseau et al, 1995; Granger et al, 1993; Khader & Tomlin, 1994; Morgan, 1994). Outcomes measures in brain trauma cases have also received a significant degree of study (Cowan et al, 1995; Granger et al, 1995; Hall, 1992). Spinal cord trauma requires highly specific outcomes measures (Davarat et al, 1995; DiTunno, 1992; Griffin et al, 1991; Saboe et al, 1997). Musculoskeletal conditions, especially low back pain, arthritis, and soft tissue injury, have also been extensively examined (Bendtsen et al, 1995; Bigos et al, 1994; Davidson & Keating, 2002; Earhard et al, 1994; Heald et al, 1997; Kopec et al, 1995; Liang et al, 1990; Patrick et al, 1995).

Outcomes Management System Based on Population

Population-specific OM tools are directed at patient populations defined by a host of non-clinical attributes, such as age and gender (Hart, 1998; Ware et al, 1981; Washburn et al, 2002). The clinical literature is replete with studies that focus on virtually every age group; however, pediatric and geriatric conditions warrant the greatest attention. Pediatric-driven outcomes measures have been studied by numerous researchers and clinicians (Braun & Granger, 1991; Haley et al, 1989; Lewin et al, 1993; Msall et al, 1993). Clinical articles descriptive of outcomes measures targeting the elderly population run into the hundreds if not thousands (Granger, 1990; Katz & Stroud, 1989; Neuhaus & Miller, 1995; Smith, 1994). The Functional Independence Measures, or FIM scale studies, are among the most numerous. These are discussed later in this chapter.

Outcomes Management System Based on Treatment Setting

Treatment setting–specific OM is extremely prevalent in the clinical research and is sometimes, but not always, synonymous with population-based OM (Ottenbacher et al, 1994; Porell & Caro, 1998; Priebe & Rintala, 1994). For instance, not all elderly populations (population-based OM) receive treatment in the same clinical setting. Severity indices and insurance coverages (or, more accurately, limitations) often dictate where care will be rendered: the hospital (inpatient basis), the home (outpatient or home care basis), a subacute center, a skilled nursing facility, an assisted living center, or an employer site. The intensity of the rehabilitation service can vary dramatically between settings. Outcomes measures have been employed across a wide range of settings (Berg & Mor, 1995; Fischer et al, 1998; Hamilton & Granger, 1994; Hecox et al, 1994; Moore, 1993; Przybylski et al, 1996; Sutton et al, 1996; Tovin et al, 1994). Studies have compared one treatment setting to another in terms of efficacy and effect on physical functioning and health status (Evans et al, 1998; Guzman et al, 2002; Jette et al, 1994; Moller et al, 1992).

Outcomes Management System Based on Reimbursement and Cost

In today's health care system(s), providers must serve as both practitioners of the healing arts and astute business persons. Therefore, it is incumbent on rehabilitation professionals to assess OM literature from a reimbursement or provider-payer interfacement perspective. Payers over the past two decades have played an increasingly aggressive role in managing the delicate balance between cost and quality. They have done so through a newfound focus on outcomes measures (Eazell & Maama F, 1992; Mittleman et al, 1991; Murray et al, 2003; Tate et al, 1993). Specifically, the relationship between function and reimbursement has received heightened scrutiny (Batavia, 1988; Kindig, 1998; Kramer et al, 1997; Reina-Rosenbaum et al, 1997; Sutton et al, 1996; Wilkerson et al, 1992). Functional status and gains can be good predictors of resource allocation within rehabilitation facilities. Since rehabilitation is a major cost driver, payers are interested in finding cost-effective treatment interventions. Payers, like providers, have a vested interest in maximizing function at a reasonable cost. In fact, health plan performance may be gauged by how well disability is managed from a cost and functional perspective (Auerbach & Lucas, 1997). Health plans attempt to control disability duration, which in turn controls costs (Government Accounting Office, 1996). Providers themselves have become more aware of the payers' paradigm as it relates to OM (Bakker et al, 1994; DiFabio et al, 1995; Franklin et al, 1994; Freyburger, 2000; Lorig et al, 1993; Savoie et al, 1995). Friedlieb (1994) describes the effectiveness of clinical practice guidelines in physical therapy in the management of 1,796 cases of low back pain. In this study, 85% of all patients responded well to 4 to 6 weeks of conservative management including physical therapy. This study exemplifies the cost sensitivity that is evolving among providers. Friedlieb cites cost savings and ties them directly to treatment interventions, thus exemplifying the provider-payer interface, which is sure to define disability management in the foreseeable future.

USE OF META-ANALYSIS DATA IN OUTCOMES MANAGEMENT

Tabor's Cyclopedia Medical Dictionary (1993) defines a meta-analysis as "a statistical procedure for combining data from a number of studies and investigations in order to analyze the therapeutic effectiveness of specific treatment and plan future studies." Helewa and Walker (2000) opine that a systematic review of research evidence is a fundamental scientific activity, and nowhere is this more important than in OM. Although evidence-based practice, or EBP, is transforming modern health care, these authors caution clinicians about selection bias, data extraction bias, and source of support bias when considering meta-analysis. Meta-analysis can be one of the best means of summarizing the body of literature pertaining to a specific issue. (Pettit, 1994). It gives the provider a method for understanding the consistencies within otherwise inconsistent clinical literature.

Rehabilitation providers have much to gain by reading and using the data discovered during a meta-analysis. There are times in rehabilitation when support for medical necessity or reasonable care must come from external sources. Clinical documentation of a patient episode of care often fails to fully tell the story or justify services. It is helpful at times to draw upon clinical literature to support a particular rehabilitation intervention. However, external sources of data alone may not lead to authorization or reimbursement of services. When the results of a supportive meta-analysis are coupled with sound, functionally based clinical documentation, preauthorization of service is enhanced and retrospective claims denials are minimized.

Meta-analysis results can be found in several places. Professional journals routinely publish meta-analysis summaries. International collaborations offer perhaps the most expedient manner for securing these data.

The Cochrane Collaboration

The Cochrane Collaboration is an international non-profit, independent effort to publish systematic reviews of the health care literature. The Cochrane Database of systematic reviews is the principal product of the collaboration (Cochrane, 2004). The collaboration is named in honor of Archie Cochrane, a renowned epidemiologist who concluded that clinicians did not have access to reliable systematic reviews of the clinical literature (Helewa & Walker, 2000). Cochrane's 1972 text, *Effectiveness and Efficiency: Random Reflections on Health Services* (reprinted in 1999), was a seminal work on evidence-based medicine. The first results of his studies were published in 1989, and the final product was a systematic review of over 600 different interventions and treatments related to the practice of obstetrics. Cochrane Review Groups (CRGs) now focus on specific conditions that are targeted by specific countries. For instance, the United States has focused on complementary medicine, hypertensive disease, and prostatic diseases. The United Kingdom is focused on a number of fields of interest to rehabilitation providers, including musculoskeletal injuries, neuromuscular disease, pain, palliative care, and supportive care and health promotion (Helewa & Walker, 2000). The Rehabilitation and Related Therapies Field can be found on the following Internet address: http://www.epid-unimaas.nl/html/cochrane/field.htm. This field is based at the University of Masstracht in the Netherlands and coordinates a pool of international physical rehabilitation professions. The team hand-searches journals related to rehabilitation and related fields to identify and analyze randomized clinical trials pertaining to interventions. Once this task is completed, systematic reviews are published using the most reliable data available.

The Agency for Health Care Quality and Research

The Agency for Health Care Quality and Research (AHCQR), formerly known as the Agency for Health Care Policy and Research (AHCPR), was formed in 1989 as an extension of the United States Public Health Service (PHS) (AHCQR, 2000). A division of the AHCQR, "The Forum for Quality and Effectiveness in Health Care," is charged with the task of clinical practice guideline development, dissemination, review, and periodic update. The following guidelines have been published that may be of interest to rehabilitation providers:

- Acute Pain Management, Operative or Medical Procedures and Trauma: Under call # SN017-022-01180-6
- Acute Low Back Problems in Adults: Under call # SN017-026-00141-7
- Pressure Ulcers in Adults, Prediction and Prevention: Under call # SN017-026-00110-7
- Pressure Ulcer Treatment: Under call # SN017-026-00143-2
- Post-Stroke Rehabilitation: Under call # SN017-026-00147-6

Because of a change in its congressional mandate, the AHCQR no longer produces clinical practice guidelines; however, this agency is still in the business of linking clinical research to clinical practice. This is accomplished principally through the funding of evidence-based practice centers or EPCs.

Philadelphia Panel: Evidence-Based Clinical Practice Guidelines on Selected Rehabilitation Interventions

The Philadelphia Panel (2001) is an expert panel that uses a systematic approach to health care literature search, study selection, data extraction, and data synthesis. Various professional organizations nominate participants, who then develop criteria for grading the strength of clinical evidence and recommendations. Randomized controlled trials (RCTs) receive level I status, and non-randomized studies are designated level II. The panel adopts criteria developed through the Cochrane Collaboration. Consensus results for those patient-critical outcomes that are determined to be both reliable and valid. Outcome include the following:

- Pain
- Function
- Patient global assessment
- Quality of life (QOL)
- Return to work (RTW)

Philadelphia Panel methodology is used in the development of evidence-based clinical practice guidelines, or EBCPGs. For instance, for the management of shoulder pain only one positive recommendation of clinical benefit was developed: ultrasound. The efficacy of other interventions related to shoulder conditions was not established via panel consensus. Two positive recommendations of clinical benefit were developed for knee pain: (1) transcutaneous electrical nerve stimulation (TENS) and (2) therapeutic exercises. For neck pain, therapeutic exercise was the only intervention that was deemed to have a clinical positive benefit. Four recommendations were developed for low back pain management. Therapeutic exercises were found to be beneficial for postsurgical low back pain, subacute conditions, and chronic conditions, and continuation of normal activity was deemed beneficial for acute low back pain.

American Physical Therapy Association Database

Some rehabilitation organizations have embarked on grassroots efforts to identify current research evidence that supports treatment effectiveness and have incorporated this evidence into a database for member use. The American Physical Therapy Association's "Hooked on Evidence" database exemplifies such an initiative (APTA, 2004). APTA members can both download as well as extract data from the database in an effort to link clinical research with clinical practice guidelines. These guidelines, like the Cochrane and Philadelphia Panel guides, are driven by systematic reviews of the literature.

Additional Meta-Analysis Initiatives

There are a host of meta-analysis reports published in rehabilitation journals that may be of interest to providers who desire to keep abreast of current clinical practice guidelines and outcomes measures. Lokey et al. (1991) studied the effects of physical exercise on pregnancy published in eighteen studies. Flor et al (1992) examined the efficacy of multidisciplinary pain management in a meta-analysis that covered sixty-five studies. Robertson and Baker (2001) published a meta-analysis of thirty-five RCTs specific to therapeutic ultrasound. These authors concluded that RCTs provided little clinical evidence for the efficacy of therapeutic ultrasound. Beckerman et al (1992) conducted a criteria-based meta-analysis regarding laser therapy for musculoskeletal disorders and skin conditions.

However, Rothstein (2001) reminds us that "an absence of evidence is different from negative evidence." This is an especially critical distinction, considering the role of utilization review in reimbursement determinations. For example, a provider's care can be denied based on an absence of evidence instead of negative evidence or disproof. When this occurs, a clinician's documentation must rise to the challenge of proving that rehabilitation services are both medically necessary and reasonable. For example, Baker et al (2001) conducted a literature analysis of the biophysical effects of therapeutic ultrasound and concluded that they are "unlikely to be beneficial." Again, it is important to note that this conclusion is based on an absence of evidence rather than negative evidence.

PREVALENT OUTCOMES MANAGEMENT INSTRUMENTS AND METHODOLOGIES

It would be virtually impossible to cover the full breadth and depth of every outcome measure in one book, let alone a single chapter. Instead, the focus of this section will be on those instruments that are either in popular use today or have withstood the test of time and scrutiny. Inclusion does not imply endorsement. The following descriptions do not delve into an analysis of instrument reliability, specificity, validity, utility, or other attributes. Readers are encouraged to explore those OM systems that pique their interest through procurement of references and recommended readings. Refer to Table 14-6, Compendium of Functionally Based Outcomes Measures Systems, for a more comprehensive listing.

Health-Related Quality of Life

Health-related quality of life (HRQL) has emerged as a new outcome paradigm (Bergner, 1993; Bowling, 1991; Carr et al, 1996; McDowell & Newell, 1987; Ormel et al, 1997; Spector, 1990; Thompson & Kirwan, 1996).

What are health-related quality-of-life measures? A multitude of clinicians, researchers, and academics have proposed their own definitions. Jette (1993) asserts that loose definitions of "health status measure," "functional status," and "quality of life" have led to some of the ambiguity surrounding rehabilitation outcomes measurement. For the sake of this discussion, Jette's concept of HRQL is broad and incorporates functional limitations, disability, and handicap, all key components of the "disablement process." His model does not include measures of pathology, impairment, or disease. The biopsychosocial framework of HRQL includes a physical function component, a psychological component, and a social component. Refer to Figure 14-6.

Jette (1993) identified three major reasons supporting the paradigm shift to quality of life and health outcomes. The rise in chronic diseases in persons who previously were tracked via mortality or morbidity supports the use of quality-of-life (QOL) measures. An aging American population is a second driver of QOL systems. Cost containment of double-digit medical inflation also fostered QOL growth.

Jette cautions that providers must carefully select an HRQL instrument by delineating the appropriate dimensions that are likely to be impacted by one's intervention. There is no single HRQL tool that can be applied across patient populations, conditions/diagnoses, clinical interventions, or treatment settings. Of course, the selection of any HRQL technology presupposes that a provider has evaluated its psychometric properties. These include reliability, validity, specificity, utility, and practicality.

There are a number of health-related QOF measures available to rehabilitation providers.

Functional Independence Measure

In 1983 the American Academy of Physical Medicine and Rehabilitation collaborated with the American Congress of Rehabilitation Medicine in a joint task force. This collaboration resulted in the development of a national consensus known as the Uniform Data System or UDS. The Uniform Data System is designed to measure disability and rehabilitation outcomes. This initiative received

Table 14–6 Compendium of Functionally Based Outcomes Measures Systems

System	References
Barthel Index	Wade & Collin (1988)
	Mahoney & Barthel (1965)
	Mahoney & Wood (1958)
Colorado Client Assessment Record	McGinnis et al (1986)
Community Integration Questionnaire	Sander et al (1999)
COOP Charts	Nelson et al (1987)
Disability Interview Schedule	Bennett & Garrad (1970)
Disability Rating Scale	Rappaport et al (1982)
DUKE-UNC Health Profile	Parkerson et al (1981)
ESCROW	Granger et al (1979)
Fairview Self Help Scale	King et al (1980)
Functional Activities Questionnaire	Harvey & Jellinek (1981)
Functional Assessment Inventory	Crewe & Athelston (1981)
Functional Assessment of Communication Skills for Adults (FACS)	American Speech-Language-Hearing Association
Functional Life Scale	Sarno et al (1973)
Functional Limitation Scale	Williamson (1971)
Functional Status Index	Jette (1978, 1980)
Geriatric Resident Goals Scales	Cornbleth (1978)
Health Assessment Questionnaire	Fries et al (1980)
Hospital Utilization Project	Hospital of University Pennsylvania (1974)
Katz Index of Independence or Index of ADL	Katz et al (1959, 1976)
Kenney Self-Care Evaluation	Iverson et al (1973)
Lambeth Disability Screening Questionnaire	Patrick et al (1981)
Level of Rehabilitation Scale	Carey & Posavac (1978)
London Handicapped Scale	Sturm et al (2002)
McMaster Health Index Questionnaire	Chambers et al (1982)
Medical Outcomes Study (MOS) Short-form 36	Tarlov et al (1989)
Notttingham Health Profile (NHP)	McEwen (1988)
OASIS (Outcome & Assessment Information Set)	Center for Health Services and Policy Research, University of Colorado
One Hundred Point Scale	Miller & Johnston (1985)
Patient Evaluation Conference System	Harvey & Jellinek (1981, 1983)
Physical Self-Maintenance Scale	Powell & Brody (1969)
Psychosocial Functioning Inventory	Feragne et al (1983)
PULSES	Granger et al (1979)
Quality of Well being Scale	Kaplan et al (1989)
RAND 36-Item Health Survey 1.0	Hays et al (1993)
Rapid Disability Rating Scale	Linn et al (1977)
Rehabilitation Indicators	Brown et al (1984)
REHABIS	Harasymiw & Stahl (1979)
Revised Functional Status Rating Instrument	Forer (1982)
Roland-Morris Disability Index	Roland & Morris (1983)
Scaled Outcome Criteria in an Extended Care Facility	Howe et al (1980)
Self Assessment of Disability Outcomes	Susset et al (1979)
Sickness Impact profile (SIP)	Bruin et al (1992)
Social Functioning Examination	Robinson et al (1985)
Telephone Structured Interview	Alexander & Halstead (1979)
Total Outcomes & Prediction Program	Cohen et al (1997)
Uniform National Data System	Granger et al (1985)

Data modified from Forer S: Outcome analysis for program service management. In Fuhrer MJ (ed): Rehabilitation Outcomes: Analysis and Measurement. Baltimore, Brooks, 1987, pp 115-136; Jette AM: Using health-related quality of life measures in physical therapy outcomes research. Phys Ther 73(8):528-537, 1999; McDowell I, Newell C: Measuring Health: A Guide to Rating Scales and Questionnaires. Oxford, Oxford University Press, 1987.

support in the form of a federal grant and endorsement by eleven national associations:

- American Hospital Association
- American Occupational Therapy Association
- American Physical Therapy Association
- American Speech, Language and Hearing Association
- American Spinal Injury Association
- Association of Rehabilitation Nurses
- Commission for the Accreditation of Rehabilitation Facilities
- National Association of Rehabilitation Facilities
- National Association of Rehabilitation Research and Training Centers
- National Easter Seals
- National Head Injury Foundation

The UDS is housed at the Center for Functional Assessment and Research in the Department of Rehabilitation Medicine at State University of New York in Buffalo. Objectives are contained in the UDS mission to enable providers and facilities to document the severity of patients' disabilities. This facilitated the measurement of outcomes of medical rehabilitation in a uniform manner. It also resulted in a common language that allows for transdisciplinary communication and comparisons of rehabilitation data.

By 1987, the Functional Independence Measure, or FIM, was developed under the leadership of Carl Granger, MD, and Byron Hamilton, PhD (Granger, 1998). A national task force reviewed 36 published and unpublished functional assessment scales in the development of the FIM scale. The FIM consists of 13 motor and 5 cognitive measures that are rated on a 7-point scale. This scale describes stages of disability ranging from complete dependence on others (1/7) to complete independence (7/7) in the performance of essential activities of daily living. Components of the FIM scale can be found in Table 14–7. FIM was one of the first scales to assess disability and not simply impairment. It does, however, link impairment to disability (Stineman et al, 1997).

Functional Related Groups

Functional Related Groups (FRGs) were developed with length of stay or LOS as the dependent variable (Harada et al, 1993). FRGs require classification of patients into one of the nine following diagnostic groups:

1. Stroke
2. Arthritis
3. Hip fracture
4. Brain injury
5. Back injury
6. Cardiopulmonary impairment
7. Spinal cord injury
8. Neurological impairment
9. Amputation

The functional status of patients is determined upon admission and described through five activities-of-daily-living or ADL tasks: transfers, toileting, grooming, drinking/eating, and bladder management. These items are scored on a 3-level ordinal scale with a higher score indicative of a higher degree of functioning or ADL independence.

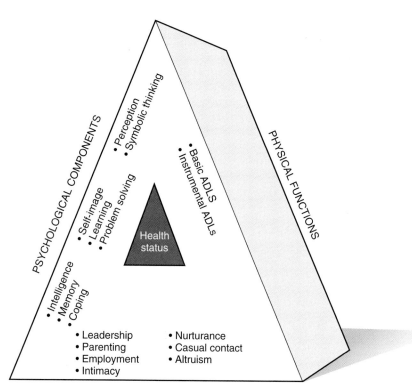

Figure 14–6. Biopsychosocial Model of Health-Related Quality of Life (Data from Engle G: The biopsychosocial model and medical education. New Engl J Med 306:802-806, 1982.)

Table 14–7   FIM Components

Self-care	Eating
	Grooming
	Bathing
	Dressing, upper extremities
	Dressing, lower extremities,
	Toileting
Sphincter control	Bladder management
	Bowel management
Transfers	Bed
	Chair
	Wheelchair
	Toilet
	Tub
	Shower
Locomotion	Walk
	Stairs
	Wheelchair
Communication	Comprehension
	Auditory
	Expression: verbal/non-verbal
	Visual
Social cognition	Social interaction
	Problem solving
	Memory

From Uniform Data System for Medical Rehabilitation, a division of UB Foundation Activities, Inc., Buffalo, New York.

FIM-FRGs

This system was designed by Stineman et al (1995) as a case-mix classification scheme for medical rehabilitation cases. Data are derived from the Uniform Data System for Medical Rehabilitation (UDS). There are 17 different impairment categories that focus on a primary rehabilitation diagnosis. The developers created an 18th category to capture those diagnoses or conditions that do not fit into one of the 17 standard categories. Patients are classified into 53 FIM-FRGs according to functional status at admission via the FIM system. The FIM-FRG system is rehabilitation-specific, but it is one of the few that incorporate medical, functional, and psychosocial elements of care. This is a critical concept given that current trends in rehabilitation delivery promote evidence-based care, transdisciplinary coordination, linkage of impairment to disability, and a shift from the medical model (biopathology) to a rehabilitation model (biopsychosocial or functionally based model). FIM-FRGs allow the rehabilitation team (inpatient) to predict treatment costs, length of stay or LOS, and patient functional status at discharge (Stineman, 1998).

Sickness Impact Profile

The SIP 68 is a generic outcomes measures system developed in 1976 with 100 self-report items (Pollard et al, 1976). It was revised in 1981 and reduced to 68 items (Bergner et al, 1981). The SIP 68 has six subscales: somatic autonomy, mobility control, psychic autonomy and communication, social behavior, mobility range, and emotional stability.

Barthel Index

The Barthel Index was originally designed for long-term care populations and measures the degree of one's functional independence (Mahoney & Barthel, 1965; Wade & Collin, 1988). This generic scale is completed by the provider and involves a 15-item ADL list addressing transfers, wheelchair propulsion, dressing, continence, and other ADL issues.

Short-Form (SF) 36 Health Survey

The SF-36 is a health survey designed for use in the general population (Ware & Sherbourne, 1992; Ware et al, 1981). It is a generic outcome measure targeting large populations, not specific patient groups. The 8 health concepts included in the scale were reduced from an original roster of 40 items contained in the Medical Outcomes Study, or MOS, sponsored by the Robert Wood Johnson Foundation, the Pew Charitable Trusts, the Agency for Healthcare Policy and Research, and the National Institute of Mental Health. The SF-36 is constructed to measure the relationship between two dimensions of self-reported health care: mental and physical health. The instrument can be self-administered by the patient or provider. The SF-12 is an even more condensed version that some think has more utility and that takes less time for completion (Ware et al, 1996). Table 14-8 lists the eight health concepts of the MOS SF-36 instrument.

Oswestry Low Back Pain Disability Questionnaire

The Oswestry Low Back Pain Disability Questionnaire is an example of a disease- or condition-specific device designed to measure a patient's disability status (Fairbank et al, 1980). This popular instrument assesses 10 areas as self-reported by the client:

- Pain intensity
- Change in pain status
- Personal hygiene
- Lifting
- Walking
- Sitting
- Standing
- Sleeping
- Social activity
- Travel

The Oswestry is scored on a 5-point scale from 0 or no limitation to 5 or maximum limitation, for a maximum of 50 points. There is a positive correlation between higher scores and greater disability level. This tool is typically used in an outpatient orthopedic setting and is especially helpful in workers' compensation cases.

Outcome and Assessment Information Set

The OASIS-B set was developed as a means of standardizing outcomes measures within the home care setting (Table 14-9). This product is the result of a 5-year national research program funded by the Health Care Financing Administration or HCFA in conjunction with the Robert Wood Johnson Foundation (RWJ). OASIS was developed via the Center for Health Services and Policy Research. This instrument comprises 79 items in a data set obtained at admission, during interim reassessments, and at discharge. The system is computerized through identifiers for each data element collected. OASIS is a mandated outcomes measurement tool for those providers or home care agencies that wish to participate in the Medicare program. This provides HCFA with a means for judging the performance of home care agencies. It is not coincidental that OASIS comes on the heels of one of the nation's most aggressive antifraud initiatives, Operation Restore Trust, and assorted fraud alerts. The methodology applied in the OASIS development and implementation process has been dubbed outcomes-based quality improvement, or OBQI. Readers are encouraged to read the Utilization Review and Long-Term Care chapters for a more in-depth discussion of quality initiatives.

OASIS has a number of objectives:

- To minimize the burden of data collection
- To increase the specificity and precision of information collected
- To maximize the consistency among different individuals collecting the same or similar information
- To make items as discipline-neutral as possible

A Convergence of Stakeholder Outcomes Measures

Figure 14-7 depicts the convergence of stakeholder outcomes measures. There must be inputs from the patient, provider, and payer, among others, for appropriate health-related quality of life outcomes (HRQOL) to result.

Table 14-8 MOS SF-36 Eight Health Concepts

1. Limitations in physical activities due to health problems
2. Limitations in social activity
3. Limitations in usual role due to health problems
4. Bodily pain
5. General mental health
6. Limitations in usual role activity secondary to emotional problems
7. Vitality (energy/fatigue)
8. General health perceptions

Table 14-9 OASIS Data Set Items

- Demographics and patient history
- Sensory status
- Respiratory status
- Integumentary status
- Elimination status
- Neurological/emotional/behavioral status
- Activities of daily living (ADLs)
- Instrumental activities of daily living (IADLs)
- Supportive assistance
- Medication use
- Equipment (assistive/adaptive)
- Emergent care
- Discharge information

From Center for Health Services and Policy Research, University of Colorado.

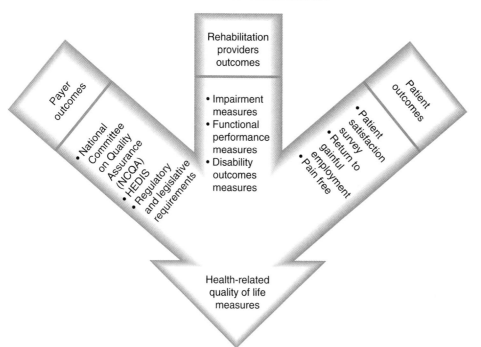

Figure 14–7. Convergence of stakeholder outcomes measures.

These inputs must contribute to vital elements of a rehabilitation program. Patients, providers, and payers in an ideal world share treatment goals and understand the value proposition of rehabilitation services. Regrettably, this is not always the case, because each stakeholder may have his or her own treatment or management goals and expectations (O'Malley et al, 2004). For instance, it is not unusual for an employer to expect an injured worker to return early or at 100% functional levels. Payers cannot expect that all treatment programs will be both expeditious and inexpensive. Conversely, providers cannot expect unlimited resources, protracted care, and full reimbursement.

Generally speaking, health plans that participate in quality assurance initiatives, such as the National Committee for Quality Assurance, are better positioned to contribute to a successful rehabilitation outcome. Patient participation is even more critical because patients are the direct recipients of services, or the primary customers. Satisfied patients are generally more compliant and more highly motivated than unsatisfied patients. However, patients or clients are satisfied by different treatment elements. One physical therapy patient may be satisfied with hot packs and massage three times a week for 12 weeks whereas another patient may desire more aggressive therapy, such as work hardening.

The Outcomes Pyramid

Figure 14–8 illustrates a hierarchy with appropriate outcomes at its pinnacle. Clinical documentation serves as the foundation that supports the medical necessity of care. "Medical necessity" can be an ambiguous term, but for the sake of this discussion it is defined as a patient's condition that warrants skilled physical rehabilitation services.

Once medical necessity has been established, reasonable and appropriate interventions follow. There is an enhanced likelihood that appropriate outcomes will result when interventions are designed and executed properly or according to an established standard of care. Rehabilitation programs geared toward disability management address all three attributes of all interventions: process, structure, and outcomes. These attributes are the underpinnings of the pyramid, from clinical documentation to appropriate outcomes. Jette (1995) defines "process" evaluation as the degree to which services meet professional standards of quality. Practice guidelines, critical pathways of care, and treatment protocols exemplify process elements. Process is essentially the how-to behind treatment interventions. "Structural" evaluation refers to the stable resources that are employed during a rehabilitation program. These are equally necessary for the delivery of services and include provider credentials, equipment, facilities, and technology. Outcomes are divided into end-result or clinically based outcomes and utilization-based outcomes. The former describe a patient's status between two or more points in time. Pretreatment and posttreatment measures are the most common example of end-result or clinically based outcomes. "Utilization outcomes" refer to the transition of a patient from one treatment setting to another or from one level of intensity of service to another.

INPUTS REQUIRED OF AN OUTCOMES MANAGEMENT SYSTEM

Designing and implementing an appropriate OM system is easier said than done. This incredibly complex endeavor is portrayed in Figure 14–9. The inner ring reveals the complexity of developing and implementing an OM program.

Figure 14-8. The outcomes pyramid.

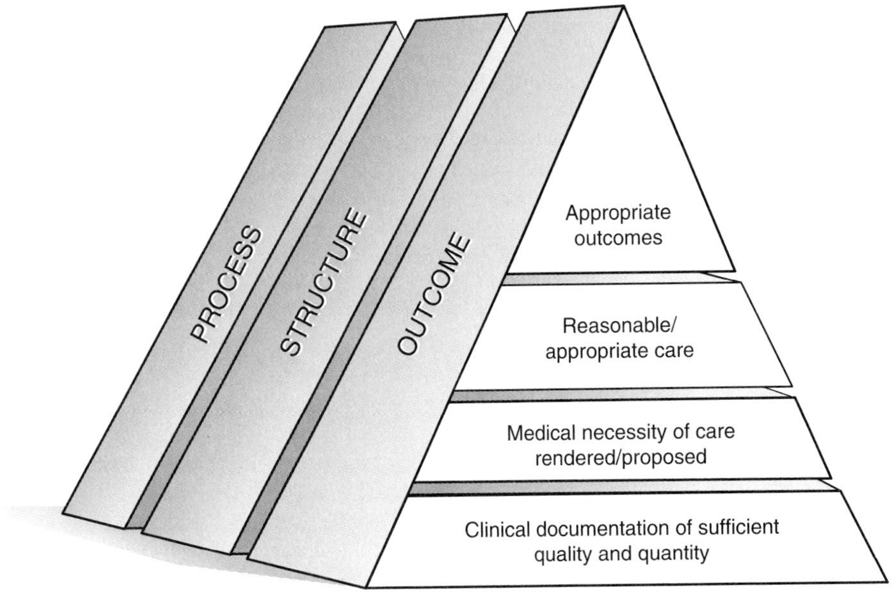
PROCESS
STRUCTURE
OUTCOME
Appropriate outcomes
Reasonable/ appropriate care
Medical necessity of care rendered/proposed
Clinical documentation of sufficient quality and quantity

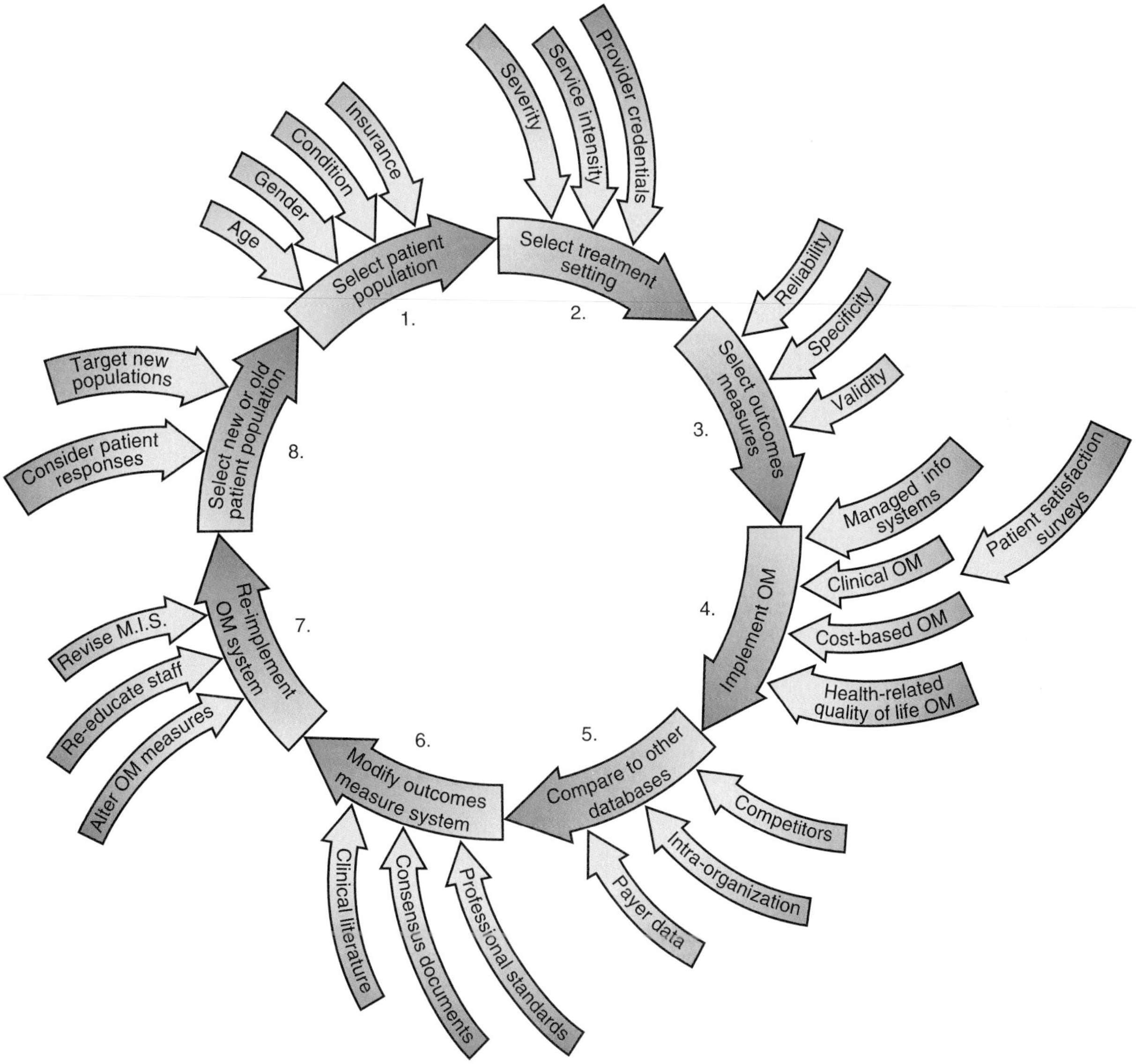
Age
Gender
Condition
Insurance
Select patient population
1.
Severity
Service intensity
Provider credentials
Select treatment setting
2.
Reliability
Specificity
Validity
Select outcomes measures
3.
Managed info systems
Clinical OM
Cost-based OM
Health-related quality of life OM
Patient satisfaction surveys
Implement OM
4.
Competitors
Intra-organization
Payer data
Compare to other databases
5.
Professional standards
Consensus documents
Clinical literature
Modify outcomes measure system
6.
Revise M.I.S.
Re-educate staff
Alter OM measures
Re-implement OM system
7.
Target new populations
Consider patient responses
Select new or old patient population
8.

Figure 14-9. Inputs of an outcomes management system.

This ring begins with the selection of a patient population. Again, there is no universal OM system that conforms to all patient populations. Patient populations dictate treatment settings and intensity of services. Treatment settings are determined by patient attributes such as age, co-morbidities, gender, insurance coverage/limitations, and availability of rehabilitation professionals. Injury severity strongly influences where a patient will be treated. Outcome measures that are most meaningful possess reliability, specificity, and validity.

Implementation of a credible OM system requires a sound managed information system (MIS) that collects, analyzes, and employs clinically based measures of function, cost-based data, health-related quality-of-life measures, and patient satisfaction data. These data can then be compared to databases managed by payers, professional organizations, government entities, quality assurance groups, and other providers. Comparison of one's data to external databases can lead to treatment modifications and best practices as employed by so-called Centers of Excellence. Professional standards of practice that flow from these databases facilitate the dynamic nature of OM. Reimplementation of an

OM system demands MIS revisions, a reeducation of staff, and alteration in clinical and cost measures. New patient populations may be targeted while others may be deselected as a result of data collection and analysis.

Hagen's (1999) "Managed Outcome Rehabilitation System" incorporates three vital management tools:

- Quality management
- Clinical management
- Cost management

In this model, potential rehabilitation goals vary by treatment setting and address one or more of these management tools. Rehabilitation goals span the entire disablement process described by Jette (1995) (refer to Figure 14–5). The ultimate outcome of Hagen's model is to optimize effectiveness and efficiency, which together create value for multiple stakeholders.

Outcomes measures both partly define and are defined by professional standards of care. For example, as more clinicians adopt the FIM outcomes measures system, this may become the standard of care. Our health care system is a long way from ameliorating practice variation driven

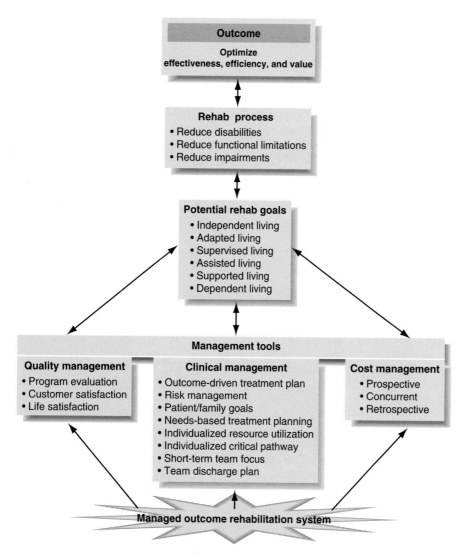

Figure 14–10. Hagen's managed outcome rehabilitation system (Data adapted from Hagen C: Rehabilitation in Managed Care: Controlling Cost, Ensuring Quality. Gaithersburg, MD, Aspen, 1999.)

by inappropriate, medically unnecessary, non-efficacious, and wasteful services. A Rand analysis of the literature concluded that some persons are receiving more care than they need, while others are receiving less (Schuster et al, 1998). This study indicated the following:

- 50% of people received recommended preventive care
- 70% received recommended acute care
- 30% received contraindicated acute care
- 60% received recommended chronic care
- 20% received contraindicated chronic care

These data represent averages across multiple studies, but they suggest poor-quality health care. The development and implementation of sound OM systems that consider multiple stakeholders can only improve the status of health care (Figure 14–10).

REFERENCES

Abdel-Moty E, Compton R, Steele-Rosomoff R et al: Process analysis of functional capacity assessment. J Back Musculoskel Rehabil 6: 223-236, 1996.

Agency for Healthcare Policy and Research (AHCPR): The outcome of outcomes research at AHCPR: Final report. Summary, Agency for Healthcare Policy and Research, Rockville, MD, www.ahrg.gov/clinic/outcosum.htm, accessed September 23, 2003.

Agency for Healthcare Research and Quality (AHCRQ): Outcomes Research Fact Sheet, AHRQ Pub. No. 00-P011, Rockville, MD, www.ahcpr.gov/clinic/outfact.htm, accessed October 5, 2000.

Ahmen M, Sullivan M, Bjelle A: Team versus non-team outpatient care in rheumatoid arthritis. Arthritis Rheum 31:471-479, 1988.

Albrecht GL, Harasymiw SJ: Evaluating rehabilitation outcome by cost function indicators. J Chron Dis 32:525-533, 1979.

American Occupational Therapy Association: Functional capacity evaluation, www.aota.org, accessed July 10, 2001.

American Physical Therapy Association (APTA): "Hooked on Evidence" website, APTA, Alexandria, VA, www.apta.org/hookedonevidence/indx.cfm, accessed August 10, 2004.

Anderson C: Measuring what works in health care. Science 263:1080-1092, 1994.

Auerbach R, Lucas B: Linking health plan performance with disability outcomes. Benefits Quarterly 13(4):46-56, 1997.

Badley EL: An introduction to the concepts and classification of the international classification of impairments. Disabil Rehabil 15: 161-178, 1993.

Baker KG, Robertson VJ, Duck FA: A review of therapeutic ultrasound: Biophysical effects. Phys Ther 81(7):1351-1358, 2001.

Bakheit AMO, Haines SR, Hull RG: Validity of a self-administered version of the Barthel Index in patients with rheumatoid arthritis. Clin Rehabil 9(3):234-237, 1995.

Bakker C, Hidding A, van der Linden S et al: Cost-effectiveness of group physical therapy compared to individualized therapy for anklylosing spondylitis: A randomized controlled trial. J Rheum 21(2):264-268, 1994.

Batavia AL: The Payment of Medical rehabilitation Services: Current Mechanisms and Potential Models. Chicago, American Hospital Association, 1988.

Batterham RW, Dunt DR, Disler PB: Can we achieve accountability for long-term outcomes? Arch Phys Med Rehabil 77:1219-1225, 1996.

Beckerman H, diBie RA, Bouter LM et al: The efficacy of laser therapy for musculoskeletal and skin disorders: A criteria-based meta-analysis of randomized clinical trials. Phys Ther 72:483-491, 1992.

Bendix AE, Bendix T, Ostenfeld S et al: Active treatment programs for patients with chronic low back pain: A prospective randomized observer-blinded study. Eur Spine J 4:148-152, 1995.

Bendtsen P et al: Cross-sectional assessment and subgroup comparison of functional disability in patients with rheumatoid arthritis in a Swedish health care district. Disabil Rehabil 17(2):94-99, 1995.

Berg K, Mor V: Medicare nursing home residents with stroke. J Aging Health 7(3):384-401, 1995.

Bergner M: Development, testing and use of the sickness impact profile. In Walker SR, Rosser RM (eds): Quality of Life Assessment. Dordrecht, Kluwer, 1993.

Bigos S, Bowyer O, Braen G et al: Acute Low Back Problems in Adults: Assessment and Treatment. Clinical Practice Guideline, Quick Reference Guide No. 14. Rockville, MD, US Department of Health & Human Services, Public Health Service, Agency for Healthcare Policy & Research (AHCPR), AHCPR Pub. No. 95-0643.

Bohannon RW, Learey KM, Cooper J: Independence in floor-to-stand transfers soon after stroke. Top Geriatr Rehabil 11(1):6-9, 1995.

Bowling A: Measuring Quality: A Review of Quality of Life Measurement Scales. Philadelphia, Open University Press, 1991.

Braun SL, Granger CV: A practical approach to functional assessment in pediatrics. Occup Ther Practice 2(2):46-51, 1991.

Brock KA, Goldie PA, Greenwood KM: Evaluating the effectiveness of stroke rehabilitation: Choosing a discrimination measure. Arch Phys Med Rehabil 83(1):92-99, 2002.

Brosseau L, Philippe P, Boulanger YL: The functional independence measure: Validity of selected assessment methods applied to stroke survivors. Top Geriatr Rehabil 11(1):75-86, 1995.

Bruin AF, Witte LP, Stevens F et al: Sickness impact profile: The state of the art of generic functional status measure. Soc Sci Med 35: 1003-1014, 1992.

Bullock M: The development of optimum worker-task relationship. In Bullock M (ed): Ergonomics: The Physiotherapist in the Workplace. London, Churchill Livingstone, 1990, pp 13-50.

Carr AJ, Thompson PW, Kirwan JR: Quality of life measures. Br J Rheum 35(3):275-281, 1996.

Center for Health Services and Policy Research: Outcomes and Outcome Measures Information, Aurora, CO, University of Colorado Health Sciences Center, www.oasis-obqi.org/computin.htm, accessed June 30, 2004.

Chambers LW, MacDonald LA, Tugwell P et al: The McMaster Health Index Questionnaire as a measure of quality of life for patients with rheumatoid disease. J Rheum 9:780-784, 1982.

Cleary PD, McNeil BJ: Patient satisfaction as an Indicator of quality care. Inquiry 25:25-36, 1988.

Cleary L, Thombs DL, Daniel EL et al: Occupational low back disability: Effective strategies for reducing lost work time. Am Occup Health Nurs J 43:87-94, 1995.

Clifton DW: Tolerated treatment well, may no longer be tolerated. PT Magazine of Physical Therapy 3(10):24, 26-27, 1995.

Cochrane A: Effectiveness and Efficiency: Random Reflections on Health Services, London: reprinted for Nuffield Trust by the Royal Medicine Press, 1999.

Cochrane Collaboration webpage: www.Cochrane.org, accessed January 22, 2004.

Cohen D, Hoffman P: When putting patients first fits the bill. Healthcare Financial Management 57(9):90-96, 2003.

Cole DC, Modndloch MV, Hogg-Johnson S: Listening to injured workers: How recovery expectations predict outcomes—A prospective study. Can Med Assn J 166(6):749-754, 2002.

Corrigan JD, Smith-Knapp K, Granger C: Validity of the functional independence measure for persons with traumatic brain injury. Arch Phys Med Rehabil 78(6):828-834, 1997.

Cowan TD et al: Influence of early variables in traumatic brain injury on functional independence measure scores and rehabilitation length of stay and charges. Arch Phys Med Rehabil 76(9):797-803, 1995.

Davarat P et al: The long-term outcome in 149 patients with spinal cord injury. Paraplegia 33(11):665-668, 1995.

Davidson M, Keating JL: A comparison of five low back disability questionnaires: Reliability and responsiveness. Phys Ther 82(1):8-24, 2002.

DiFabio RP, Mackey G, Holte JB: Disability and functional status in patients with low back pain receiving workers' compensation: A descriptive study with implications for the efficacy of physical therapy. Phys Ther 75(3):180-192, 1995.

DiGabio RP, Boissonault W: Physical therapy and health-related outcomes for patients with common orthopedic diagnoses. J Sports Phys Ther 27:219-230, 1998.

DiTunno JF: Functional assessment measures in CNS trauma [Review]. J Neurotrauma 9(Suppl):S301-305, 1992.

Donabedian A: Quality assessment and assurance: Unity of purpose, diversity of means. Inquiry 25:173-192, 1988.

Earhard RE, Delitto A, Cibulka MY: Relative effectiveness of an extension program and a combined program of manipulation and flexion and extension exercises in patients with acute low back syndrome. Phys Ther 74:1093-1100, 1994.

Eazell DE, Maama F: Demonstrating cost savings through functional gains: Payors need a functional assessment measure that clearly translates to increased savings. Rehabil Manage: Interdisciplinary J Rehabil Aug/Sept:137-139, 1992.

Ellwood P: Shattuck lecture—Outcomes management: A technology of patient experience. New Engl J Med 318(23):1549-1556, 1988.

Evans RL, Connis RT, Haselkorn JK: Hospital-based rehabilitative status. Disabil Rehabil 20(8):298-307, 1998.

Fairbank JCT, Couper J, Davies JB: The Oswestry Low Back Pain Disability Questionnaire. Physiotherapy 66:271-273, 1980.

Field M, Lohr K (eds): Guidelines for Clinical Practice: From Development to Use. Washington, DC, National Academy Press, 1992.

Fischer DA, Tewes DP, Boyd JL et al: Home-based rehabilitation for anterior cruciate ligament reconstruction. Clin Orthop 347:194-199, 1998.

Flor H, Fydrich T, Turk DC: Efficacy of multidisciplinary pain treatment centers: A meta-analytic review. Pain 49:221-230, 1992.

Forer S: Outcome analysis for program service management. In Fuhrer MJ (ed): Rehabilitation Outcomes: Analysis and Measurement. Baltimore, Brookes, 1987, pp 115-136.

Franklin GM, Haug J, Heyer NJ et al: Outcome of lumbar fusion in Washington State workers' compensation. Spine J 19(17):1897-1904, 1994.

Fratelli CM: Perspectives on functional assessment: Its use for policy making [Review]. Disabil Rehabil 15(1):1-9, 1993.

Freyburger JK: An analysis of the relationship between the utilization of physical therapy services and outcomes of care for patients after total hip arthroplasty. Phys Ther 80(5):448-458, 2000.

Friedlieb OP: The impact of managed care on the diagnosis and treatment of low back pain: A preliminary report. Am J Med Quality 9(1):24-29, 1994.

Fuhrer MJ: Subjective well-being: Implications for medical rehabilitation outcomes and models of disablement. Am J Phys Med Rehabil 73(5):358-364, 1994.

Fuhrer MJ (ed): Rehabilitation Outcomes: Analysis and Measurement. Baltimore, Brookes, 1987, pp 115-136.

Government Accounting Office (GAO): Practice Guidelines: Managed Care Plans Customize Guidelines to Meet Local Interests. Washington, DC, GAO/HEHS 96-95, 1996.

Granger CV: Health accounting: Functional assessment of the long-term patient. In Krusen (ed): Handbook of Physical Medicine and Rehabilitation. Philadelphia, WB Saunders, 1990, pp 270-282.

Granger CV: [Foreword]. In Dittmar SS, Gresham GE (eds): Functional Assessment and Outcome Measures for the rehabilitation Professional. Gaithersburg, MD, Aspen, 1997.

Granger CV: The Walter J. Zeiter lecture: The emerging science of functional assessment: Our tool for outcomes analysis. Arch Phys Med Rehabil 79:235-240, 1998.

Granger CV, Divan N, Fiedler RC: Functional assessment scales: A study of persons after traumatic brain injury. Am J Phys Med Rehabil 74(2):107-113, 1995.

Granger CV et al: Functional assessment scales: A study of persons after stroke. Arch Phys Med Rehabil 74(2):133-138, 1993.

Griffin JW, Toomis RE, Mendius RA: Efficacy of high voltage pulsed current for healing of pressure ulcers in patients with spinal cord injury. Phys Ther 71:433-444, 1991.

Guccione AA: Physical therapy diagnosis and the relationship between impairments and function. Phys Ther 71(7):499-504, 1991.

Guzman J, Esmail R, Karjalainen K: Multidisciplinary bio-psycho-social rehabilitation for chronic low back pain [Cochrane Review]. Cochrane Database Systematic Reviews 2002(1):CD 000963, www.newfirstsearch.oclc.org, accessed October 15, 2003.

Hagen C: Rehabilitation in Managed Care: Controlling Cost, Ensuring Quality. Gaithersburg, MD, Aspen, 1999.

Haley SM, Hallenborg SC, Gans BM: Functional assessment in young children with neurological impairments. Topics in Early Childhood Special Education 9(1):106-126, 1989.

Hall JA, Dornan M: Meta-analysis of satisfaction with medical care: Description of research domain and analysis of overall satisfaction levels. Soc Sci Med 27:637-644, 1988.

Hall KM: Overview of functional assessment scales in brain injury rehabilitation. Neurorehabilitation 2(4):98-113, 1992.

Hamilton BB, Granger CV: Disability outcomes following inpatient rehabilitation for stroke. Phys Ther 74:494-505, 1994.

Harada N, Kominski G, Sofaer S: Development of resource-based classification scheme for rehabilitation. Inquiry 30:54-63, 1993.

Hart DL: Relation between three measures of functionation in patients with chronic work-related syndromes. J Rehabil Outcomes Measures 2(1):1-14, 1998.

Haynes B, Haines A: Barriers and bridges to evidence based clinical practice. Br Med J 317:273-276, 1998.

Heald SL, Riddle DL, Lamb RL: The Shoulder Pain and Disability Index: The construct validity and responsiveness of a region-specific disability measure. Phys Ther 77(10):1079-1089, 1997.

Hecox R et al: Functional independence measurement (FIM) of patients receiving easy street: A retrospective study. Phys Occup Ther Geriatr 12(3):17-31, 1994.

Helewa A, Walker JM: Critical Evaluation of Research in Physical Rehabilitation: Towards Evidence-Based Practice. Philadelphia, WB Saunders, 2000.

Jette AM: Using health-related quality of life measures in physical therapy outcomes research. Phys Ther 73(8):528-537, 1993.

Jette AM: Outcomes research: Shifting the dominant research paradigm in physical therapy. Phys Ther 75(11):965-970, 1995.

Jette AM et al: Physical therapy episodes of care for patients with low back pain. Phys Ther 74(2):101-110, 1994.

Joint Commission on Accreditation of Healthcare Organizations: Glossary of Terms, Primer on Indicator Development and Application. Oakbrook Terrace, Il, Joint Commission on Accreditation of Healthcare Organizations, 1990.

Kane RL: Looking for physical therapy outcomes. Phys Ther 74(5):425-429, 1994.

Kaplan RM, Anderson JP, Wu AW et al: The Quality of Well-Being Scale. Med Care 27 (Suppl): S27-S43, 1989.

Katz S, Stroud MW III: Functional assessment in geriatrics. J Am Geriatr Soc 37:267-271, 1989.

Keith RA: Patient satisfaction and rehabilitation services. Arch Phys Med Rehabil 79(9):1122-1128, 1998.

Kessner DM et al: Assessing health quality: The case for tracers. New Engl J Med 288:189, 1973.

Khader MS, Tomlin GS: Change in wheelchair transfer performance during rehabilitation of men with cerebrovascular accidents. Am J Occup Ther 48(10):899-905, 1994.

Kindig DA: Purchasing population health: Aligning financial incentives to improve health outcomes [Review]. Health Serv Res 33(2 Part 1):223-242, 1998.

Kopec JA, Esdaile JM, Abramhamawicz M et al: The Quebec Back Pain Disability Scale: Measurement properties. Spine 20:341-352, 1995.

Kramer AM, Steiner JF, Schlenker RE: Outcomes and costs after hip fracture and stroke. A comparison of rehabilitation settings. JAMA 277(5):396-404, 1997.

Lamon H, Lankhorst GJ: Subjective weighting of disability: An approach to quality of life assessment in rehabilitation. Disabil Rehabil 16:198-204, 1994.

Law M, Hurley P, Hurley D et al: Selecting outcomes measures in children's rehabilitation: Comparison of methods. Arch Phys Med Rehabil 84(4):496-499, 2003.

Leek L, Pryor DB, Harell FE et al: Predicting outcome in coronary artery disease: Statistical models versus expert clinicians. Am J Med 80:553-560, 1986.

Lewin JE, Mic CM, Gaebler-Spira D: Self-help and upper extremity changes in 36 children with cerebral palsy subsequent to selective posterior rhizotomy and intensive occupational and physical therapy. Phys Occup Ther Pediatr 13(3):25-42, 1993.

Liang MH, Fossel AH, Larson MG: Comparison of five health status instruments for orthopedic evaluation. Med Care 28:632-642, 1990.

Like R, Zyzanski SJ: Patient satisfaction with the clinical encounter, social psychology determinants. Soc Sci Med 24(4):351-357, 1987.

Lokey EA, Tran ZW, Wells CL et al: Effects of physical exercise on pregnancy outcomes: A meta-analytic review. Med Sci Sports 23:1234-1239, 1991.

Lorig KR, Mazonson PD, Holman HR et al: Evidence suggesting that health education for self-management in patients with chronic arthritis has sustained health benefits while reducing health care costs. Arthritis Rheum 36(4):439-446, 1993.

Maher CG, Sherrington C, Elkins M et al: Challenges for evidence-based physical therapy: Accessing and interpreting high-quality evidence on therapy. Phys Ther 84(7):644-654, 2004.

Mahoney FI, Barthel DW: Functional evaluation: The Barthel Index. Maryland State Med J 14:62, 1965.

Mancuso M, Smith P, Illig S: Satisfaction with medical rehabilitation in patients with orthopedic impairment. Arch Phys Med Rehabil 84(9):1343-1349, 2003.

Matheowetz V: Role of physical performance component evaluations in occupational therapy functional assessment [Review]. Am J Occup Ther 47(3):225-230, 1993.

Matheson LN: Functional capacity evaluation. In Demeter SL, Andersson GBJ, Smith GM (eds): Disability Evaluation. St Louis, Mosby, copyright American Medical Association, Chicago, 1996, pp 168-188.

Matheson LN, Isernhagen SJ, Hart DL: Functional capacity evaluation as a facilitator of social security disability reform. WORK J 10:77-84, 1998.

McDowell I, Newell C: Measuring Health: A Guide to Rating Scales and Questionnaires. Oxford, UK, Oxford University Press, 1987.

McGlynn EA: Choosing and evaluating clinical performance measures. J Comm J Qual Improv 24(9):470-479, 1998.

Melin AL et al: The cost-effectiveness of rehabilitation in the home: A study of Swedish elderly. Am J Pub Health 83(3):356-362, 1993.

Metcalfe C, Lewin R, Wisher S et al: Barriers to implementing the evidence base in four NHS therapies: dieticians, occupational therapists, physiotherapists, speech and language therapists. Physiotherapy 87:433-441, 2001.

Mittleman M, Urso J, Baldwin B et al: Workers' compensation cases with traumatic brain injury: An insurance carrier's analysis of care, costs, and outcomes. J Insur Med 23(1):55-63, 1991.

Moore A: Functional outcomes of patients with hip fracture in the home health setting. J Home Health Care Practice 5(4):49-58, 1993.

Moorhead JF, Clifford J: Determining the medical necessity of outpatient physical therapy services. Am J Med Quality 7(3):81-84, 1992.

Moreland J, Thomson MA: Efficacy of electromyographic biofeedback compared with conventional physical therapy for upper extremity function in patients following stroke: A research overview and meta-analysis. Phys Ther 74:534-547, 1994.

Morgan P: The relationship between sitting balance and mobility outcome in stroke. Aust J Physiother 40(2):91-96, 1994.

Msall ME, DiGaudio KM, Duffy LC: Use of functional assessment in children with developmental disabilities. Phys Med Rehabil Clin North Am 4(3):517-527, 1993.

Murray PK, Singer M, Dawson NV: Outcomes of rehabilitation services for nursing home residents. Arch Phys Med Rehabil 84(8):1129-1136, 2003.

Nagi SZ: Some conceptual issues in disability and rehabilitation. In Sussman MB (ed): Sociology and Rehabilitation, Washington, DC, American Sociological Association; 1965, pp 100-113.

Niemeyer LO, Jacobs K, Reynolds-Lynch K et al: Work hardening: Past, present and future—the Work Programs Special Interest Section National Work Hardening Outcome Study. Am J Occup Ther 48:327-339, 1994.

Neuhaus BE, Miller PA: Status of functional assessment in occupational therapy with the elderly [Review]. J Allied Health 24(1):29-40, 1995.

O'Malley KJ, Roddey TS, Gartsman GM et al: Outcome expectancies, functional outcomes and expectancy fulfillment for patients with shoulder problems. Med Care 42(2):139-146, 2004.

Ormel J, Lindenberg S, Steverinh N et al: Quality of life and social production functions: A framework for understanding health effects. Soc Sci Med 45(7):1051-1063, 1997.

Owens LA, Buchholz RL: Functional capacity assessment, worker evaluation strategies, and the disability management process. In Shrey DE, LaCerte M (eds): Principles and Practices of Disability Management in Industry. Winter Park, FL, GR Press, 1995, pp 269-301.

Pascoe GC: Patient satisfaction in primary health care: A literature review and analysis. Eval Prog Plan 6:185-210, 1983.

Patrick DL, Deyo RA: Generic and disease-specific measures in assessing health status and quality of life. Med Care 27(Suppl):S217-S232, 1989.

Patrick DL, Deyo RA, Atlas SJ et al: Assessing health-related quality of life in patients with sciatic. Spine 20:1899-1909, 1995.

Pettit DB: Meta-Analysis, Decision Analysis and Cost-Effectiveness Analysis. New York, Oxford University Press, 1994.

Philadelphia Panel: Philadelphia Panel evidence-based clinical practice guidelines on selected rehabilitation interventions for low-back pain, knee pain, neck pain and shoulder pain. Phys Ther 81(10):1629-1730, 2001.

Pollard WE, Bobbit RA, Bergner M et al: The Sickness Impact Profile: Reliability of a health status measure. Med Care 14:146-155, 1976.

Porell F, Caro FG: Facility-level outcome performance measures for nursing homes. Gerontologist 38(6):665-683, 1998.

Priebe EM, Rintala DH: Functional assessment in a community setting. Top Stroke Rehabil 1(3):16-29, 1994.

Przybylski BR, Dumont ED, Watkins ME et al: Outcomes of enhanced physical and occupational therapy service in a nursing home setting. Arch Phys Med Rehabil 77(6):554-561, 1996.

Reina-Rosenbaum R, Bach JR, Penek J: The cost/benefits of outpatient-based pulmonary rehabilitation. Arch Phys Med Rehabil 78(3):240-244, 1997.

Relman A: Assessment and accountability: The third revolution in medical care. New Engl J Med 319:18, 1988.

Riddle DL, Straford PW: Use of generic versus region-specific functional status measures on patients with cervical spine disorders. Phys Ther 78:951-963, 1998.

Robertson VJ, Baker KG: A review of therapeutic ultrasound: Effectiveness studies. Phys Ther 81(7):1339-1350, 2001.

Rodgers S: Job evaluation in worker fitness determination. In Himmelstein J, Pransky B (eds): Worker Fitness and Risk Evaluation. Philadelphia, Hanley & Belfus, 1988, pp 219-240 .

Rothstein J: [Editor's page]. Phys Ther 74(5):375-377, 1994.

Rothstein JM: [Editor's notes]. Autonomous practice or Autonomous ignorance? Phys Ther 81(10):1620-1621, 2001.

Rothstein JM (ed): Measurement in Physical Therapy. New York, Churchill Livingstone, 1985.

Rothstein JM, Echternach JL: Primer on Measurement: An Introductory Guide to Measurement Issues. Alexandria, VA, American Physical Therapy Association, 1993.

Russell E: The ethics of attribution: The case of health care outcome indicators. Soc Sci Med 47(9):1161-1169, 1998.

Saboe LA, Darrah JM, Pain KS, Guthrie J: Early predictors of functional independence 2 years after spinal cord injury. Arch Phys Med Rehabil 78(6):644-650, 1997.

Sackett DL, Rosenberg WMC, Gray JAM et al: Evidence-based medicine: What it is and what it isn't. Br Med J 12:71-72, 1996.

Sager MA, Dunham NC, Schwantes A et al: Measurement of activities of daily living in hospitalized elderly: A comparison of self-report and performance-based methods. J Am Geriatr Soc 40:457-462, 1992.

Savoie FH III, Field LD, Jenkins RN: Costs analysis of successful rotator cuff repair surgery: An outcome study. Comparison of gatekeeper systems in surgical patients. Arthroscopy 11(6):672-676, 1995.

Schenke R, Berkowitz E, Ludden JM et al: Leading beyond the bottom line: Organizational assets of the new economy. Physician Executive 26(6):6-9, 2000.

Schenke R, Berkowitz E, Ludden JM et al: Leading beyond the bottom line, Part 4: The questions it has raised. Physician Executive 26(6):6-9, 2001.

Schuster MA, McGlynn EA, Brook RH: How good is the quality of health care in the United States? Milbank Q 76(4):517-563, 1998.

Scott RW: Health Care Malpractice: A Primer on Legal Issues for Professionals. Thorofare, NJ, Slack, 1990.

Sharpe VA, Faden AIU: Appropriateness in patient care: A new conceptual framework. Milbank Q 74(1):115-136, 1996.

Smith R: Validation and reliability of the elderly mobility scale. Physiotherapy 80(11):744-747, 1994.

Social Security Administration (SSA): Progress report on development of a redesigned method of evaluating disability in social security claims. Social Security Administration, June 17, www.ssa.gov/DFRT/research2.htm, accessed March 9, 1999.

Spector W: Functional disability scales. In Spiker B (ed): Quality of Life Assessments in Clinical Trials. New York, Raven, 1990, pp 115-129.

Spector WD, Mukamel DB: Using outcomes to make inferences about nursing home quality [Review]. Eval Health Porf 21(3):291-315, 1998.

Steffen TM, Meyer AD: Physical therapists' notes and outcomes of physical therapy. A case of insufficient evidence. Phys Ther 65(2):213-217, 1985.

Stineman MG: Charting outcomes. Advance for Directors of Rehabilitation 7(10):33-35, 1998.

Stineman M, Escarse J, Goin J et al: A case-mix classification system for medical rehabilitation. Med Care 32:366-379, 1995.

Stineman MG, Jette A, Fieldler R, Granger C: Impairment specific dimensions within the functional independence measure. Arch Phys Med Rehabil 78(6):636-643, 1997.

Sutton JP, DeJong G, Wilkerson D: Function-based payment model for inpatient medical rehabilitation: An evaluation. Arch Phys Med Rehabil 77:693-701, 1996.

Swanson GH: Use of outcome reports: Justifying the need for physical therapy services. Orthop Phys Ther Clin N Am 4(2):253-268, 1995.

Taber's Cyclopedic Medical Dictionary: Philadelphia, FA Davis, 1993, p 1203.

Tate DG, Forchheimer M, Daugherty J: Insurance benefits coverage: Does it affect rehabilitation outcomes? J Rehabil 59(4):6-10, 1993.

Thompson CAJ, Kirwan JR: Quality of life measures. Br J Rheum 35(3):275-281, 1996.

Tovin BJ, Wolf SL, Greenfield BH et al: Comparison of the effects of exercise in water and on land on the rehabilitation of patients with intra-articular anterior cruciate ligament reconstructions. Phys Ther 74:710-719, 1994.

van Herk IEH, Arendzen JH: Measures to assess functional capacities of stroke patients living at home: A review of literature. J Rehabil Sci 8(3):66-71, 1995.

Wade DT: Outcome measures for clinical rehabilitation trails: Impairment, function, quality of life or value? Am J Phys Med Rehabil 82(10 Suppl):S26-31, 2003.

Wade DT, Collin C: The Barthel ADL Index: A standard measure of physical disability? Int Disabil Stud 10:64-67, 1988.

Ware JE, Brook RH, Davies AR et al: Choosing measures of health status for individuals in general populations. Am J Public Health 71:620-625, 1981.

Ware JE, Phillips J, Yody BB et al: Assessment tools: Functional health status and patient satisfaction. Am J Med Quality 11(1):550-553, 1996.

Ware JE, Sherbourne CD: The MOS 36-Item Short-Form Health Survey (SF-36): I. Conceptual framework and item selection. Med Care 30:473-483, 1992.

Washburn RA, Zhu W, McAuley E: The physical activity scale for individuals with physical disabilities: Development and evaluation. Arch Phys Med Rehabil 83(2):193-200, 2002.

Weinberger M, Samsa GP, Tierney WM et al: Generic versus disease-specific health status measures: Comparing the Sickness Impact Profile and the Arthritis Impact Measurement Scale. J Rheum 19:543-546, 1992.

Wennberg JE: Dealing with medical practice variations: A proposal for action. Health Affairs (Millwood) 3(2):6-32, 1984.

Wilkerson DL, Batavia AI, DeJong G: Use of functional status measure for payment of medical rehabilitation services. Arch Phys Med Rehabil 73:111-120, 1992.

Williams RM, Myers AM: A new approach to measuring recovery in injured workers with acute low back pain: Resumption of activities of daily living scale. Phys Ther 78:613-623, 1998.

SUGGESTED READINGS

American Physical Therapy Association: Outcomes Effectiveness of Physical Therapy: An Annotated Bibliography. Fairfax, VA, American Physical Therapy Association, 1994.

Gray JA: Evidence-Based Healthcare. New York, Churchill Livingstone, 1997.

Sackett DL, Richardson WS, Rosenberg WM, Haynes RB et al (eds): Evidence-Based Medicine: How to Practice and Teach EBM. New York, Churchill Livingstone, 1997.

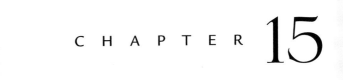

C H A P T E R 15

How to Locate Sources of Disability-Related Data

David W. Clifton, Jr., PT

"We are drowning in information and starved for knowledge."

- Naisbitt & Aburdene, 1990

KEY POINTS

- "Data" is not synonymous with "information"; "information" is not synonymous with "knowledge"; and "knowledge" is not synonymous with "wisdom."
- Clinicians must look beyond their own industrial sector for non-traditional sources of data that can be applied to practice.
- More information is not necessarily better information, and information that is not linked to clinical and/or business practices is of limited value.
- The Internet can play a vital role in securing information; however, users must learn to discriminate between useful and useless information.

Operational Definitions*

Facts	Truth, reality, circumstance.
Information	Intelligence communicated or gathered.
Data	Facts or information, facts from which conclusions can be drawn; plural form of datum.
Knowledge	Information or clear perception, facts, sum of what is known.
Judgment	Good sense, discernment, estimate, opinion, ascertaining the relationship between ideas.
Skill	Ability, knowledge united with dexterity, aptitude, expertise borne of practice, art, or craft.
Wisdom	Sound judgment and knowledge, prudence, being wise, scholarly knowledge.

*From The Random House American Dictionary, 1990; and The New International Webster's Collegiate Dictionary, Trident Press, 2002.

INTRODUCTION

A provider's knowledge, judgment, and skill are among the most important determinants of quality health care (Entoven & Vorhaus, 1997). However, a great deal of knowledge critical to success resides beyond the immediate clinical environment. Never in history has out-of-the-box knowledge been more vital or available. Today's clinicians must function in an increasingly complex health care system that interfaces with other domains. Health care is no longer autonomously delivered but is profoundly influenced by a constellation of external factors and forces. Health care has evolved from a cottage industry into sophisticated business enterprises that are publicly traded. As a result, clinicians are now expected to be savvy business persons as well as artful practitioners. To achieve success, rehabilitation professionals may need to covet knowledge in the following areas: personnel management, business administration, finance, regulatory and legislative issues, risk management, health care economics, and medicolegal expertise. In fact, success under and beyond managed care may depend more on non-clinical competencies than on clinical acumen. The term "master clinician" may actually be a misnomer because it conveys a relatively narrow band of knowledge and competency in clinical treatment. A master clinician may be one who has a command of both clinical and non-clinical knowledge. Clinicians, both entry level and advanced, may not be equipped with the necessary knowledge, wisdom, and skills to ensure successful integration with a variety of patients, clinical settings, health care funding sources, and delivery models. Perhaps a more appropriate goal is to train master disability managers, not clinicians. This implies a broader band of knowledge and competency that extends beyond the clinical box. Generally speaking, a master disability manager needs an expanded vision regarding physical rehabilitation's role within this maelstrom we call health care.

Clinicians, on entry into the health care system, may be ill prepared to serve as disability managers. Some assert that professional schools and related professional associations fail to prepare clinicians regarding the extra-clinical issues that transcend treatment per se (Huebler, 1995). There is no intended derision directed toward those who perform valuable clinical services.

This chapter strives to introduce rehabilitation professionals to alternative sources of information that may not be readily communicated during their didactic and theoretical training. A good starting point is to review operational definitions, from which discussion can flow. Operational definitions are essential to understanding the hierarchy of identification, assemblage, and application of data into practice.

Providers must be selective in their pursuit of wisdom and skill because "we now mass produce information the way we make cars" (Naisbett & Aburdene, 1990). More information is not necessarily better or accurate and, unless applied, is of little value. Wurman (1989, p 89)

contends that the great information age in which we currently reside is really an explosion of "non-information." Wisdom beyond the clinical realm implies possession and exercise of sound judgment, which allow clinicians to achieve clinical success within the matrix of a much larger and more complex system. For instance, occupational or physical therapists may be sound clinicians but still fail miserably in the delivery of services if they do not understand long-term care financing, especially Medicare rules and regulations. This knowledge and understanding may or may not be secured through formal education and clinical affiliations, yet it is vital to success.

Figure 15–1 depicts a hypothetical model of how facts evolve into clinical (in-the-box) and non-clinical (out-of-the-box) skills and competence. Facts establish truth, reality, and circumstances, which offer little utility to clinicians. Facts establish the base that supports information. Information results from facts that inform or are found to be useful. Information that is formatted for a specific application becomes data. Applied data in turn become knowledge. As a clinician secures more knowledge and connects ideas, judgment results. Judgment that leads to good decision making is considered wisdom. Wisdom is what ultimately allows clinicians to exercise their skills in disability management.

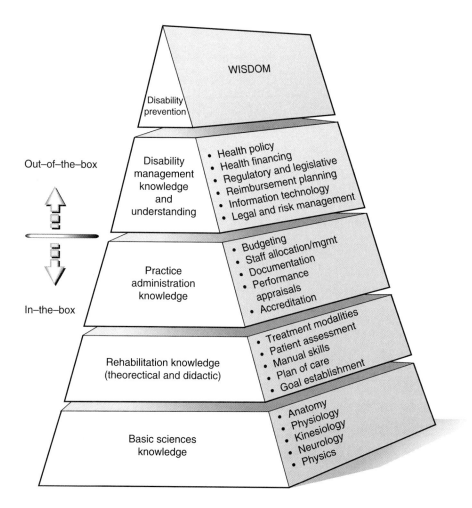

Figure 15–1. The wisdom pyramid.

This chapter will examine sources of data that hopefully clinicians can convert into knowledge, skill, and wisdom. Readers are encouraged to peruse the Appendix of this book for additional sources of data.

INTERNET SEARCHES

There are essentially five different mechanisms for accessing information on the Internet (University of Alabama Libraries, 1998):

1. E-mail discussion groups
2. Direct site access via a universal resource locator or URL
3. Browsing
4. Exploration of subject directories
5. Search engine use

Each of these mechanisms has its advantages and disadvantages. However, this chapter will focus on subject directory and search engine applications.

Corruption or inaccuracy of data remains a problem associated with Internet use. Alexander and Tate (2001) provide a concise yet comprehensive methodology for differentiating "informational web pages" from "advocacy web pages." Webpages are designed according to the user needs. Informational Webpages are generally, but not always, associated with educational institutions (edu.com) or government entities (gov.com). These sites tend to have accurate data devoid of sales and marketing messages. Advocacy Webpages are sponsored by an organization that is attempting to influence public opinion. These pages generally place spin on a topic, although it may be grounded in fact. Websites can be public or proprietary in nature. Public sites typically involve no access fee and are composed of unfiltered data presented in raw format. Private Websites routinely involve a fee and publish filtered and edited data screened by "fact checkers" (Alexander & Tate, 2001).

An examination of five criteria may assist providers in establishing the credibility of sources (Alexander & Tate, 2001).

How to Recognize an Informational Webpage*

Criterion No. 1: Authority

1. Is it clear who is responsible for the contents of the page?
2. Is there a link to a page describing the purpose of the sponsoring organization?
3. Is there a way of verifying the legitimacy of the page's sponsor (e.g., telephone number, postal address, or other contact information)?
   Note: an e-mail address is insufficient for this purpose.
4. Is it clear who wrote the material, and are the author's qualifications for writing on this topic clearly stated?

5. If the material is protected by copyright, is the name of the copyright holder given?

Criterion No. 2: Accuracy

1. Are the sources for any factual information clearly listed so they can be verified in another source?
2. Is the information free of grammatical, spelling, and typographical errors?
3. Is it clear who has the ultimate responsibility for the accuracy of the content of the material?
4. If there are charts and/or graphs containing statistical data, are the charts and/or graphs clearly labeled and easy to read?

Criterion No. 3: Objectivity

1. Is the information provided as a public service?
2. Is the information free of advertising?
3. If there is any advertising on the page, is it clearly differentiated from the informational content?

Criterion No. 4: Currency

1. Are there dates on the page to indicate:
   a. When the page was written?
   b. When the page was first placed on the Web?
   c. When the page was last revised?
2. Are there any other indications that the material is kept current?
3. If the material is presented in graphs and/or charts, is it clearly stated when the data were gathered?
4. If the information is published in different editions, is it clearly labeled what edition the page is from?

Criterion No. 5: Coverage

1. Is there an indication that the page has been completed and is not still under construction?
2. If there is print equivalent to the Webpage, is there clear indication of whether the entire work is available on the Web, or only parts of it?
3. If the material is from a work that is out of copyright (as is often the case with a dictionary or thesaurus), has there been an effort to update the material to make it more current?

How to Recognize an Advocacy Webpage†

Criterion No. 1: Authority

1. Is it clear what organization is responsible for the contents of the page?
2. Is there a link to a page describing the goals of the organization?
3. Is there a way of verifying the legitimacy of this organization?
4. Is there a statement that the content of the page has the official approval of the organization?
5. Is it clear whether this is a page from the national or local chapter of the organization?

---

*The greater number of questions answered "Yes" to the criteria in this section (Alexander & Tate, 1996), the more likely it is that the Webpage is a quality source of information.

†The greater number of questions answered "Yes" to the criteria in this section (Alexander & Tate, 1996), the more likely it is that the Webpage is an advocacy page.

6. Is there a statement giving the organization's name as copyright holder?

Criterion No. 2: Accuracy

1. Are the sources for any factual information clearly listed so they can be verified in another source?
2. Is the information free of grammatical, spelling, and typographical errors?

Criterion No. 3: Objectivity

1. Are the organization's biases clearly stated?
2. If there is any advertising on the page, is it clearly differentiated from the informational content?

Criterion No. 4: Currency

1. Are there dates on the page to indicate:
   a. When the page was written?
   b. When the page was first placed on the Web?
   c. When the page was last revisited?
2. Are there any other indications that the material is current?

Criterion No. 5: Coverage

1. Is there an indication that the page has been completed, and is not still under construction?
2. Is it clear what topics the page intends to address?
3. Does the page succeed in addressing these topics, or has something significant been left out?
4. Is the point of view of the organization presented in a clear manner with its arguments well supported?

Search Engines

A search engine is a database of Internet (IN) files that have been collected by a computer program known as a wanderer, crawler, robot, worm, or spider (University of Alabama Libraries, 1998).

Search engines consist of the following three elements:

1. A spider that traverses the Web, going from link to link until it has identified matching data.
2. An index, which is a database that includes every Webpage identified by the spider according to search parameters or syntax.
3. The actual search engine mechanism, which allows a user to query the index based upon relevancy ratings. Relevancy ratings are expressed as a percentage of how closely the retrieved data match the search parameters. One hundred percent (100%) indicates the highest relevancy rating.

Search engines are both numerous and diverse in their data assemblage (Table 15–1). Engines display a number of unique characteristics. For instance, some display both directory listings and search results. Many cluster documents by topic and provide ratings or relevance rankings. These ratings are probability-based estimates of whether a search result correlates with the keyed-in search words or parameters. Some directories are human compiled and reviewed, whereas others are not. Human-compiled directories involve the use of content experts who have read, analyzed, and rated data. Yahoo is an example of a

Table 15–1   Prominent Search Engines

Engine	Website
Alta Vista	http://www.altavista.digital.com
Excite	http://www.excite.com
HotBot	http://www.hotbot.com
InferenceFind	http://www.inference.com/infind
Infoseek	http://www.infoseek.com
The Internet Sleuth	http://www.isleuth.com

human-compiled search engine. Those engines that are non-human-compiled automatically categorize data via search results. Data are categorized strictly according to parameters that computers follow, without expert analysis.

Metacrawlers are those engines that also search other search engines to secure additional results (Table 15–2). Dogpile and Inference Find are examples of metacrawlers. Many search engines make heavy use of links as a means of ranking Websites, such as Google. A link connects two related subject directories or Websites. Search speed varies dramatically between engines. Search engines may require encrypted language or can be accessed through natural language entries. Ask Jeeves is an example of the latter.

It is important at each search engine site to read the directions about formulating a search for that particular engine. Individual engines will instruct users about appropriate syntax use. Each search engine has a form that must be completed with the user's search terms. Specific language understood by an engine ensures a successful search. Specific syntaxes, such as Boolean logic, employ terms such as "AND" or "+" to ensure that all of the search terms are included during the database search. The content and subject matter of each search will

Table 15–2   Sample Meta Search Engine Listing

- All4One
- Ask Jeeves
- ByteSearch
- Cyber411
- Debriefing
- Dogpile
- Highway61
- Inference Find
- Mamma
- Metabug
- Metacrawler
- Metafind
- MetaGopher
- MP3Meta
- PrimeSearch
- Profusion
- SavvySearch
- Seeko
- SETI-Search
- SherlockHound
- SuperSearch
- Super-seek
- The Ultimates

dictate the choices among the hundreds of search engines. The methodology employed by various search engines will also continue to evolve with consumer demands. Search engines are being refined at an impressive rate, and data are being formatted in more meaningful ways than in earlier generations.

Subject Directories

Subject directories provide an alternative to search engines because subjects are organized into categories. Subjects are organized by humans, rather than by the computer automation commonly associated with search engines. Some subject directories provide an adequate description of selection criteria, but many do not. Rarely does a subject directory reveal its reviewers' credentials. When it does, a reviewer's description is generally better than a simple list of links or related sites. The searcher must exercise caution because some directories do not omit poor-quality sites in attempts to be all-inclusive. Well-reviewed sites can suffer from serious time lapses between updates. Unfortunately, there is no universally applied rating system that standardizes content across all search engines or subject directories. This means that the user must discriminate between those data that represent high quality and those that do not.

MEDLINE is an example of a subject directory database. It is the National Library of Medicine's database, which comprises over 11 million indexed journal citations and abstracts relating to biomedicine and health. Journal inclusion is determined by a Literature Selection Committee, or LSTRC. This group is chartered by the National Institutes of Health (NIH) and is similar in function to NIH grant review committees. MEDLINE covers approximately 4500 journals published in more than seventy countries. It includes references for articles dating from 1966 to the present. Citations that predate the 1960s are found on OLDMEDLINE.

HEALTHSTAR is an online bibliographic database produced by the National Library of Medicine. HEALTHSTAR was formerly available though the Internet's GratefulMed, which is no longer in service. It focuses on the evaluation of patient outcomes and service effectiveness. Between 1978 and 1999, the American Hospital Association (AHA) co-produced HEALTHSTAR with the National Library of Medicine (NLM).

Index Medicus represents a third database that assembles literature from the biomedical domain; it is indexed by author and subject. This database is very user-friendly and allows relatively simple retrieval of information.

Government Sources of Data

Government sources of disability-related data offer providers several distinct advantages over private sources. First, data are often free because they are subsidized by taxpayers. Second, data accuracy is generally sound because government agencies recruit content experts from the private sector who commonly serve on consensus panels or peer review committees. Lastly, the private sector often follows the lead of government entities in disability prevention and management initiatives.

Brief vignettes of various government entities are presented here. These entities may have data invaluable to rehabilitation providers. This listing is by no means all-inclusive, and readers are encouraged to review the Appendix for additional sources of data.

U.S. Department of Health and Human Services

This agency is one of the nation's principal means of protecting the health of Americans. It sets the agenda for prevention programs in both the public and private sectors http://www.os.dhhs.gov Health and Human Services matches resources to targeted human needs. For instance, its "Healthy People 2000" initiative's objectives are to reduce workplace deaths, reduce cumulative trauma disorders (CTDs), and promote employer safety, health, and rehabilitation programs.

DHHS has the following strategic goals:

- Reduce the major threats to the health and productivity of Americans
- Improve the economic and social well-being of individuals, families, and communities
- Improve access to health services and ensure the integrity of the nation's health entitlement and safety net program
- Improve the quality of health care and human services
- Strengthen the nation's health sciences research enterprise and enhance its production

Centers for Disease Control and Prevention

The Centers for Disease Control just recently added "Prevention" to its name (http://www.cdc.gov). CDC's Disability and Health Branch fosters the development of knowledge and specific interventions designed to reduce and/or prevent secondary conditions that stem from congenital or acquired physical, cognitive, or sensory impairments.

The CDC has established a number of broad strategies:

- Science: ensure a strong science base for public health action
- Assessment: detect and assess threats to public health
- Policy: provide leadership for the nation in prevention, policy, and practice
- Assurance: ensure the public's health through the translation of research into effective community-based action

Occupational Safety and Health Administration

Over 100 million workers rely on OSHA to ensure safe and productive work environments (http://www.osha.gov). OSHA was created secondary to the Occupational Safety and Health Act of 1970. It employs over 2,100 inspectors who are experts in medicine, engineering, education, ergonomics, safety, and industrial hygiene. This staff establishes protective standards, enforces those standards, and encourages employers and employees to use its technical assistance and consultation programs.

During the past decade OSHA has been extremely involved in the prevention of cumulative trauma disorders (CTDs) through the encouragement of ergonomics standards and interventions. OSHA has failed to date to secure national standards for CTD prevention through rule making.

National Institute for Occupational Safety and Health

The National Institute for Occupational Safety and Health (NIOSH) is part of the Centers for Disease Control and Prevention (CDC). This agency is responsible for conducting research and providing recommendations for the prevention of workplace injury and disease (http://www.cdc.gov/niosh). NIOSH uses a three-pronged approach to accomplish its mission:

- Investigate potentially hazardous working conditions and environments at the request of employers or employees
- Provide recommendations and distribute information designed to prevent or obviate workplace disease, injury, and disability
- Provide training to occupational safety and health professionals

NIOSH complements the efforts of DHHS and CDC and participated with 500 organizations in the nation's first national research agenda to identify 21 research priorities. This initiative is known as NORA, or National Occupational Research Agenda.

NIOSH operates programs in all 50 states and has regional offices in Ohio, West Virginia, Pennsylvania, and Washington State. Like OSHA, it was created in response to the Occupational Safety and Health Act of 1970. NIOSH, however, is part of the Department of Health and Human Services, whereas OSHA is embedded in the Federal Department of Labor, or DOL. NIOSH efforts have contributed to a reduction in workplace fatalities by 78% between 1970 and 1995, and to a 25% decline in occupational injury and illness between 1973 and 1994.

Institute of Medicine

The mission of IOM is to advance and disseminate scientific knowledge to improve human health. The institute "provides objective timely authoritative information and advice concerning health and science policy" (http://www.iom.edu). IOM functions as an independent entity and uses unpaid volunteer experts in the drafting of most reports. IOM falls within the National Academy of Science (NAS), which was created by the federal government. The academy functions as a non-governmental organization but is included here because it is funded by appropriations made available to federal agencies. IOM findings and recommendations are evidence-based whenever possible and reflect the consensus of various content expert panels.

Rehabilitation Services Administration

The Rehabilitation Services Administration was established by Congress as the principal authority to enforce provisions of the Rehabilitation Act of 1973. The Rehabilitation Services Administration is one of three components of the Office of Education and Rehabilitation Services, or OCERS. Figure 15–2 illustrates RSA's relationship to other government entities. Specifically, RSA is responsible for the formulation, development, and implementation of regulations, policies, and guidelines addressing vocational rehabilitation programs, independent living, training, research, and workplace integration for those individuals with disabilities (http://www.ed.gov/offices/OSERS/RSA/rsa.htn). RSA in its advocacy role serves as a resource and clearinghouse of information for service providers at all levels: local, state, regional, and national. Removal of employment barriers is a specific goal that requires cooperation among various federal agencies, including the Social Security Administration or SSA, the Department of Labor or DOL, the National Institute of Mental Health, the President's Committee on the Employment of Persons with Disabilities, the Office of Special Education Programs, the Office of Adult and Vocational Education, and the

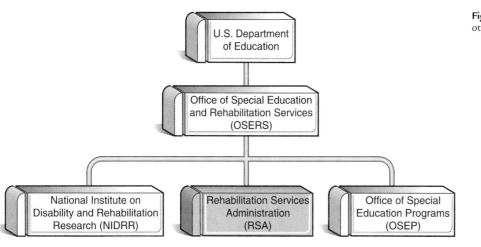

Figure 15–2. RSA's relationship to other government functions.

National Institute on Disability and Rehabilitation Research.

The National Clearinghouse of Rehabilitation Training Materials (NCRTM) is funded by the Rehabilitation Services Administration. NCRTM provides a variety of training materials that may be of interest to providers, employers, and patients. These include training manuals, forms, monographs, electronic documents, articles, audio- and videotapes, and CD-ROMs. The *NCRTM Quarterly* is published and distributed free of charge. A general catalog descriptive of available resources is also available to providers. Lastly, NCRTM provides a free reference and research service via its Webpage, http://www.nchrtm.okstate.edu.

National Institute on Disability and Rehabilitation Research

The National Institute on Disability and Rehabilitation Research conducts research under the auspices of the federal Department of Education's Office of Special Education and Rehabilitation Services (OSERS). NIDRR funds more than 300 disability and rehabilitation research projects ranging from product development to clinical research (http://www.ed.gov/offices/OSERS/NIDRR). It was created in 1978 as one of three components falling under OSERS: NIDRR, the Rehabilitation Services Administration, and the Office of Special Education Programs (OSEP). NIDRR's mission is to maximize full inclusion, social integration, employment, and independent living for persons with disabilities of all ages. NIDRR precariously balances its scientific role with that of consumer advocate.

The National Rehabilitation Information Clearinghouse (NARIC) collects, publishes, and disseminates information from NIDRR's research projects through two principal documents: *NIDRR Program Directory* and *Compendium of Products by NIDRR Grantees and Contractors*. Both volumes are available on NARIC's Website, http://www.naric.com/search.htm. NARIC's Webpage houses an "Instant Disability Information Center" database known as "REHABDATA." This database contains over 70,000 resources located in two subdirectories: from 1956 to 1994 and from 1995 to the present. Informational referral sheets, directories, statistical reports, and guides are available covering the latest disability and rehabilitation research. Informational topics include but are not limited to the following:

- Developmental disabilities
- Neurological/neuromuscular disorders
- Advocacy/self-help
- Assistive technology/devices
- Case administration/management/counseling
- Employment/transition to work
- Evaluation/needs/assessment/tests
- Home modifications
- Independent living/community integration
- Information sources
- Medical or rehabilitation facilities
- Mobility issues
- Rehabilitation success/outcomes

- Self-care/daily living
- Service delivery/rehabilitation services
- Statistics/demographics/epidemiology

National Center of Medical Rehabilitation Research

The National Center for Medical Rehabilitation Research (http://www.nichd.nih.gov) was established within the National Institutes of Health in 1990. The center is a component of the National Institute of Child Health and Human Development. A primary goal of NCMRR is to match biological, behavioral, and engineering advances to people with disabilities. Through its "Research Plan," it has established seven priority areas:

1. Improvement of functional mobility
2. Promotion of behavioral adaptation to functional losses
3. Assessment of the efficacy and outcomes to medical rehabilitation therapies
4. Development of improved assistive technologies
5. Promotion of an understanding of whole body system responses to physical impairments and functional changes
6. Development of more precise measurement methods for impairments, disabilities, and functional and societal limitations
7. Training of research scientists in the field of rehabilitation

NCMRR has funded four regional Medical Rehabilitation Research Networks located in the West, Midwest, South, and Northeast.

The National Council on Disability

The National Council on Disability is an independent federal agency that makes recommendations to the president and Congress pertaining to issues affecting 54 million Americans with disabilities (http://www.ncd.gov). NCD's 15 members are appointed by the president and confirmed by the United States Senate. Its most notable achievement to date is the 1986 "Toward Independence" report, which proposed that Congress enact a civil rights law for people with disabilities. As a result, in 1990 the Americans With Disabilities Act, or ADA, was signed into law. NCD's mission is to do the following:

1. Promote policies, programs, practices, and procedures that guarantee equal opportunity for all persons with disabilities
2. Empower individuals with disabilities to achieve economic self-sufficiency, independent living, and full inclusion into all aspects of society

NCD is currently overseeing a multiyear study addressing the implementation and enforcement of the ADA.

The Interagency Committee on Disability Research

The Interagency Committee on Disability Research is charged with facilitating interdepartmental cooperation, coordination, and consultation among all federal program activities. The ICDR derives its authority from

Section 203 of the Rehabilitation Act of 1973. Its primary focus is research related to rehabilitation of individuals with disabilities (http://www.ncddr.org/icdr.htm). ICDR compiles information about the status of rehabilitation research sponsored by all federal agencies. It also attempts to facilitate cost sharing and coordinated client/patient information exchanges between agencies. ICDR provides policy recommendations and establishes objectives and research priorities, reporting directly to the president and/or Congress. Lastly, ICDR maintains ongoing coordination and communication with the National Council on Disability, or NCD.

Agency for Healthcare Quality and Research

The Agency for Healthcare Quality and Research (AHCQR) was formerly known as the Agency for Healthcare Policy and Research (AHCPR). After AHCPR's policy charter was reexamined, policymaking was omitted, for which it was not commissioned. Reauthorization was implemented with the signing of the 1999 Healthcare Research and Quality Act. The new name reaffirms AHCQR as a scientific research agency, not a policy maker. AHCQR is the anointed lead federal agency responsible for quality-of-care research and coordination (http://www.ahcpr.gov/about/ahrqfact.htm). The agency supports 12 "evidence-based practice centers" and disseminates its findings through the "National Guideline Clearinghouse." AHCQR's philosophy and mission are to develop an extensive evidence-based database that enables providers, health policymakers, and health decision makers to make appropriate decisions. Its goals are to do the following:

- Support quality health care enhancement
- Strengthen quality measurement and improvement
- Identify strategies designed to improve access to services and ensure appropriate utilization while reducing medically unnecessary expenditures

AHRQ is also directed by Congress to promote patient safety and eliminate or reduce medical errors associated with care.

National Library of Medicine

The NLM serves as another mechanism or central command center for those interested in rehabilitation and disability management (http://www.nlm.nih.gov/pubs.htm). NLM boasts over 800,000 catalog records for books, audiovisuals, journals, computer files, and extraneous information. NLM's "Locatorplus" service is available on the World Wide Web at http://www.Locatorplus.gov.htm. Locatorplus allows for keyword, author, title, journal, and call number searches. NLM's database is diverse and includes MEDLINE and TOXNET.

NLM offers a "Health Service Technology Assessment Text," or HSTAT. HSTAT enables users to search for evidence-based reports in subdirectories entitled *technical reports, evidence report summaries,* and *evidence report/technology assessments.* AHCPR-supported guidelines and technology assessment reviews are also available through HSTAT.

Office of Women's Health

The Office of Women's Health is housed within the Department of Health and Human Services, where it champions women's health issues through research, health care services, and education. OWH coordinates women's health efforts in HHS to eliminate disparities in health status, support culturally sensitive educational programs, and encourage women to take personal responsibility for their health and wellness (http://www.4woman.gov.htm). These goals are accomplished through a variety of mechanisms, including brochures, fact sheets, reports, education and outreach initiatives, National Centers of Excellence, expert health panels, and various working groups on selected issues.

Office of Public Health and Science

The OPHS reports to the United States secretary of health, who in turn serves as a senior advisor on public health and science to the secretary of Health and Human Services (http://www.surgeongeneral.gov.htm). OPHS coordinates a number of services and offices:

- National Vaccine Program
- Office of Disease Prevention/Health Promotion
- Office of Emergency Preparedness
- Office of HIV/AIDS Policy
- Office of Global Health Affairs
- Office of Military Liaison and Veterans Affairs
- Office of Minority Health
- Office of the Surgeon General
- Office on Women's Health
- President's Council on Physical Fitness and Sports

ABLEDATA

ABLEDATA is a federally funded project whose principal mission is to provide assistive technology and rehabilitation equipment information (http://www.abledata.com). The ABLEDATA databases contain data on more than 29,000 assistive technology products ranging from computer voice-activated programs to mobility devices. The database is formatted with detailed product descriptions, prices, and supplier information. It serves as a treasure trove for rehabilitation providers who need to match technology to a patient's or client's needs.

ABLEDATA is sponsored by the National Institute on Disability and Rehabilitation Research, or NIDRR. ABLEDATA is not a government entity per se because it operates under contract. Database searches are free of charge and conducted through different mechanisms: keyword or phrase, type/function of product, brand name, supplier/manufacturer/distributor, and Boolean searches.

ABLEDATA also provides training workshops on how to access its databases. "Fact Sheets" provide detailed descriptions of different classes of devices or products. These are accompanied by supplier lists and related readings or bibliographies.

ABLEDATA supplies consumers with "Informed Consumer Guides" pertinent to products and devices. Its Webpage contains links to national and international rehabilitation- and disability-related sites.

Lastly, ABLEDATA operates "Resource Centers" that provide executive summaries of all Internet resources pertaining to selected disability-related issues. These briefings give users a quick scan of relevant issues and may preclude the need for a more exhaustive and time-consuming Internet search.

National Clearinghouse of Rehabilitation Training Materials

The National Clearinghouse of Rehabilitation Training Materials is funded through a Rehabilitation Services Administration (RSA) grant. This database locates, collects, and distributes an array of training materials, including participant training manuals, trainer training manuals, videos, and course syllabi. NCRTM supplies references and research services in either paper or electronic form (http://www.nchrtm.okstate.edu). Users who wish to be placed on NCRTM's mailing list can do so and receive a quarterly publication that provides up-to-the-minute rehabilitation training materials. NCRTM's Webpage has links to national, state, and regional rehabilitation associations, along with various commissions and accreditation organizations.

Job Accommodation Network

The Job Accommodation Network engages consultants who provide advice or recommendations regarding employment of persons with disabilities (http://www.jan.wvu.edu.htm). JAN evolved from a collaborative effort of the U.S. Department of Labor's Office of Disability Employment, the International Center for Disability Information, West Virginia University, and various private industries and persons. JAN's goals are outlined by stakeholder group on its Webpage:

Employers

- Hire, retain, and promote qualified employees with disabilities
- Provide information on accommodation options and practical solutions
- Become educated about their own responsibilities under the Americans With Disabilities Act and the Rehabilitation Act
- Address issues pertaining to accessibility

Persons with Disabilities

- Become educated about consumer rights under ADA and the Rehabilitation Act
- Acquire accommodation options
- Become aware of government resources, especially those associated with job placement

Rehabilitation Professionals

- Facilitate placement of clients
- Locate resources for workplace assessment, device fabrication, and job modification

Vocational Rehabilitation & Employment

The Vocational Rehabilitation & Employment program is housed within the Veteran's Administration, where it assists veterans who wish to reintegrate with the worksite and/or community (http://www.vba.va.gov.htm). In order to qualify, persons must have documented service-connected disabilities. Services include the following:

- Assistance in finding an appropriate employer
- On-the-job training
- Vocational counseling/assessment/placement
- Formal two- or four-year academic programs
- Supportive rehabilitation services
- Independent living support services
- Training in activities of daily living
- Evaluation of a client's skills, knowledge, and aptitude

Government Accounting Office

GAO reports examine federal health-related programs, policies, and agencies (http://www.gao.gov.htm). All unclassified reports are made available to the public. Reports dating from 1994 to the present are found in a database entitled "Blue Book." This database is updated daily, and reports are made available within two business days following public release. Titles of sample reports include the following:

- Traumatic Brain Injury: Programs Supporting Long-Term Services in Selected States
- Long-Term Care: Consumer Protection and Quality of Care Issues in Assisted Living
- Medicare Home Health Agencies: Certification Process is Ineffective in Excluding Problem Agencies
- Medicaid Managed Care: Challenge of Holding Plans Accountable Requires Greater State Effort

Government Printing Office

The Government Printing Office is a source of voluminous amounts of information for providers, consumers, and employers (http://www.access.gpo.gov.htm). GPO's Webpage contains major search categories, including the following:

- Catalog of Government Laws, Regulations, Decisions and Guidelines
- Health Care Financing Administration (HCFA) Laws, Regulations and Manuals
- Disability-Related Publications
- Health Care Resources Catalog
- National Health Interview Surveys on Disability
- Various Subject Directories arranged alphabetically

The GPO publishes virtually every unclassified federal document. Its Health Care Subject Directory houses a host of interesting documents, including the following sampler:

- Acute Pain Management: Clinical Practice Guidelines
- Acupuncture Jan 1970–Oct 1997
- Acute Low Back Problems in Adults: Clinical Practice Guidelines
- Acute and Chronic Incontinence: Clinical Practice Guidelines
- ABC's of Safe and Healthy Child Care: A Handbook for Child Care Providers

- Alternative Medicine: Expanding Medical Horizons, A Report to the National Institutes of Health on Alternative Medical Systems and Practice in the United States
- Cardiac Rehabilitation as Secondary Prevention
- Management of Functional Impairment
- Chronic Disease Prevention
- National Ambulatory Medical Care Survey

United States Code Office of the Law Revision Council, U.S. House of Representatives

The United States Code is the codification of the general and permanent laws of the United States (http://www.access.gpo.gov.htm). The code is updated in print format every six years. It is broken down by title and section, thus enabling the user to conduct a methodical search. The database is provided in ASCII text, and graphics are supplied as TIFF files. The code also comes with useful instructions: "Helpful Hints for Searching the US Code." Any and all of the aforementioned legislative initiatives, such as the Americans With Disabilities Act of 1990, can be located.

Federal Register

The *Federal Register* publishes all notices, rules, proposed rules, and presidential documents on a daily basis (http://www.access.gpo.gov.htm). Documents can be accessed through the Government Printing Office Website.

Congressional Budget Office

The CBO publishes online studies and reports pertinent to health care (http://www.cbo.gov.htm). Sample reports include the following:

- Trends in Health Care Spending by the Private Sector (April 1997)
- Expanding Health Insurance Coverage for Children Under Title XXI of the Social Security Act (February 1998)
- Projections of Expenditures for Long-Term Care Services for the Elderly (March 1999)
- Predicting How Change in Medicare's Payment Rules Would Affect Risk-Sector Enrollment and Costs (March 1999)

National Committee on Vital and Health Statistics

The National Committee on Vital and Health Statistics serves as a public advisory body reporting to the secretary of Health and Human Services (http://www.ncvhs.hhs.gov.htm). Subject areas covered by this body have included computer-based patient records systems, electronic data interchange or EDI, and patient confidentiality. NCVHS reports and publications can be found on the Government Printing Office Webpage (http://www.gpo.gov.htm).

SUMMARY

To remain competitive in a vigorous health care marketplace, rehabilitation providers must secure accurate and timely information. Many sources of these data fall outside of the usual clinical conduit. Professional schools and associations, although extremely vital, cannot possibly equip providers with the requisite knowledge to thrive in an increasingly complex health care system. It is therefore incumbent on providers to explore alternative sources of information. This chapter has provided some guidance in this regard; however, readers are encouraged to peruse the Appendix for additional data sources.

REFERENCES

Alexander J, Tate MA: July 1996, Wolfgram Memorial Library, Widener University, Chester, PA, www.2.widener.edu/Wolgram-Memorial-Library/webevaluation/inform.htm, accessed November 2, 2001.

Alexander J, Tate M: July 21 2001, Wolgram Memorial Library, Widener University, One University Place, Chester, PA, www.widener.edu/Wolfgram-Memorial-Library/webevaluation/inform.htm, accessed August 8, 2004.

Entoven A, Vorhaus C: A vision of quality in health care delivery. Health Affairs 16(3):44-57, 1997.

Huebler D: Education for allied health professionals, graduates lack clinical skills as well as knowledge of managed care. Interdisciplinary J Rehabil 7:62-65, 1995.

MEDLINE, www.ncbi.nlm.nih.gov/PUBMED/.

Naisbitt J, Aburdene P: Megatrends. New York, Avon, 1990, p 416.

The Random House American Dictionary. New York, Random House, 1990.

University of Alabama Libraries: Searching the Internet: Recommended sites and search techniques, 1998, www.albany.edu/library/internet/search.htm, accessed March 12, 2001.

Wurman R: Information Anxiety. New York, Bantam Books, 1989, p 358.

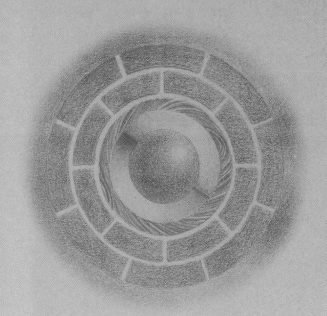

Ethical-Legal Regulatory Compliance Issues

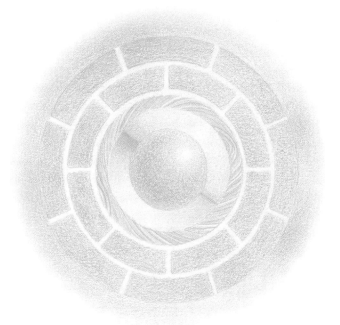

CHAPTER 16

Risk Management*

Ron Scott, LLM, EdD

"If we could only ignore risk—act as if it didn't exist, we could have much more fun in this world. But that option doesn't exist. Risk isn't going to let you forget it. And it has many voices—static and dynamic, private and public, personal and corporate—that keep calling for your consideration."

- Grose, 1987

> ### KEY POINTS
>
> - All businesses involve a degree of risk taking that may or may not be commensurate with potential benefits.
> - Rehabilitation providers must determine the degree of risk relative to their own comfort level.
> - Risk must be measured or assessed before it can be managed.
> - Risk management strategies incorporate a combination of risk acceptance, avoidance, transference, and sharing.
> - Health care providers and their patients have two basic relationships: (1) a professional (health care) relationship and (2) a business relationship.
> - Liability risk management is as integral to fostering optimal quality patient care as are peer review; credentialing, privileging, and competency assessment; equipment maintenance; and other more obvious quality management processes.

Operational Definitions

Breach of Duty	Non-compliance with minimally acceptable practice standards in a health care malpractice civil lawsuit.
Claims-Made Policy	A policy that insulates providers from professional liability for conduct *during* the policy's term.
Informed Consent	The legal right of a patient to receive adequate information to make intelligent, voluntary, and unequivocal decisions regarding acceptance or rejection of professional services.
Liability	Culpability in a civil proceeding.
Occurrence-Based Policy	A policy that covers professional liability for claims reported after the policy's term has expired.
Professional Negligence	Substandard clinical care delivery without malicious intent.
Risk Management	Use of a systematic business strategy to reduce, minimize, or, whenever feasible, avoid liability claims.
Vicarious Liability	The legal and financial responsibility for the conduct of another person.

INTRODUCTION

Rehabilitation professionals bear a particularly onerous (yet fulfilling) set of obligations to participants within the health care delivery system: to patients and clients under their care; to the families and significant others of patients and clients; to their employers; to professional colleagues; to complementary disciplines; to business associates, to product and equipment vendors; to publication professionals; to third-party payers; to governmental officials and representatives; and to themselves as professionals and human beings.

Health professional licensure and certification impose special solemn responsibilities upon conferees, including the duty to act as fiduciaries toward patients and clients. Licensed and certified health care professionals must place patients' and clients' best interests above those of all other persons, including their employer and themselves.

---

*DISCLAIMER: The material contained in this chapter is intended as legal information only, and not as legal advice for any individual or health care organization. Such advice must be obtained from personal and/or institutional legal counsel, with whom a legally privileged confidential relationship may be formed. Legal advice is highly dependent on state and federal law, which is subject to change as new case law precedents are established.

This lofty duty is strictly enforced by courts of law. Subordinate to the special fiduciary duty owed by health professionals toward patients are other important duties, including the duty of loyalty and trustworthiness to employing entities. This duty is most often a common law duty, fashioned and refined through court case opinions, but it exists in strong force nonetheless. It is this duty that requires health professionals to safeguard employer confidential information, including patient and client lists, and not to expropriate their names for personal use after leaving the employer's employ. The fidelity owed by an employee to an employer similarly permits an employer to require a health professional contractually to refrain from disparaging the employer before third parties, including patients (the "anti-disparagement" clause in many employment contracts for health professionals?).

The professional relationship between health professionals and patients or clients is always an implied or express contractual business relationship. In an express agreement (i.e., a typical business contract), the terms of the agreement are relatively clearly defined. The names of the parties, the nature and duration of the agreement, the amount of compensation paid by the patient or client and reciprocal consideration from the provider, and other tailored terms are spelled out, orally or (preferably) in writing. It is always a prudent liability risk management strategy to reduce all business contracts to writing and to employ attorneys to draft and review them.

In the event that a provider-patient/client contract is not in writing, certain legally binding obligations are incumbent upon the contracting health care professional. Among these are the duty to carry out care competently (i.e., within the legal standard of care) and to comply with the fiduciary legal and professional ethical duties of fidelity, truthfulness, and confidentiality to patients and clients. Additional implied-in-law duties may attach, dependent upon applicable state or federal law.

Whenever possible, providers should have patients and clients contractually agree to cooperate with prescribed examinations and interventions. In this way, patients and clients, even those under otherwise implied (non-specific) contracts, are contractually bound to perform under the care agreement.

Course of Action: Ethical Versus Legal Consideration

A clinician's specific course of action regarding the avoidance, transfer, acceptance, or sharing of risk requires an examination of whether or not the particular action is considered ethical and/or legal. These terms ("ethical"/"legal") are not necessarily synonymous, since what is ethical may not be legal and vice versa. The upper left quadrant of Figure 16–1 depicts a course of action that may be perceived as legal but may not be considered ethical. The upper right quadrant inversely illustrates a perceived ethical yet potentially illegal action. The lower right quadrant displays an action that is considered neither legal nor ethical.

This four-quadrant figure may have utility when prioritizing responses to specific risks.

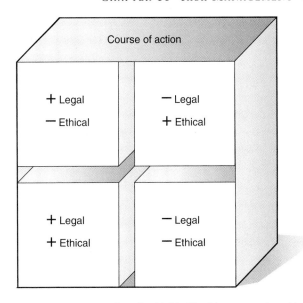

Figure 16–1. Four-quadrant legal/ethical health care practice grid. (From Scott RW: Professional Ethics: A Guide for Rehabilitation Professionals. St Louis, Mosby, 1998.)

PROFESSIONAL LIABILITY ISSUES

Rehabilitation clinical professionals are exposed to considerable risk because of their interaction with patients and clients. From a single allegation of substandard care, a provider may face adverse legal and administrative proceedings in multiple venues: criminal court (*People v. Doe*), civil court (*Patient v. Doe*), administrative licensing agencies (*State v. Doe*), and professional association judicial committees for ethical infractions. The consequences of a finding or findings of culpability include possible monetary damage awards, incarceration, loss of licensure, loss of professional association affiliation, and loss of certification(s), among other possible adverse events.

Because of the serious nature and consequences of a finding of liability, the best risk management measure is to take all reasonable prudent preventive steps to avoid allegations of substandard care and patient/client-related misconduct. This truism applies to planning, implementation, dissemination, and ongoing revisions of clinical liability risk management policies and procedures designed to protect patients and clients, health care organizations, and individual providers from harm.

The best risk management measure that can be undertaken in health care clinical practice is to take all reasonable prudent preventive steps to avoid allegations of harm to patients and clients.

Civil liability for patient or client physical and/or psychological injury incident to health care malpractice may be based on one or more of five recognized legal bases for liability imposition:

1. Professional negligence, or objectively determined substandard care delivery
2. Intentional care-related misconduct
3. Breach of an express therapeutic promise made to a patient or client

4. Patient or client injury from dangerous defectively designed or manufactured care-related products or equipment
5. Patient or client injury from abnormally dangerous clinical care activities

Professional negligence, or objectively substandard clinical care delivery, involves patient or client care that fails to comport with expected standards of practice for the health care provider's professional discipline. The classic elements of proof in a professional negligence patient-initiated lawsuit include the following:

● Proof that the defendant-provider (and/or health care organization) owed a special **duty** toward the plaintiff-patient or client to carry out care competently and within acceptable legal practice standards
● Proof that the defendant negligently failed to carry out care within such standards (**breach of duty**)
● Proof of resultant patient or client **injury**
● Proof of resultant losses (lost income, consequential medical and related expenses, pain and suffering, etc., called "**money damages**")

In order to prevail in a health care malpractice civil case, the plaintiff must prove these four elements of proof by a preponderance, or greater weight, of evidence (i.e., more credible than the defendant's evidence). This same standard of proof normally applies to administrative agency and professional association adverse proceedings. The standard of proof in criminal cases, however, is much higher: guilt beyond a (i.e., any) reasonable doubt. This higher proof standard in criminal cases applies because the consequences of a finding of criminal culpability are much more severe than with civil or administrative proceedings: loss of freedom and the lifelong stigma of a criminal conviction on a defendant's record.

Breach of legal duty, or non-compliance with minimally acceptable practice standards in a health care malpractice civil lawsuit, is normally established through expert witness testimony on the standard of care, which focuses on whether minimally acceptable practice standards were met or not met. Often, expert witness testimony is in conflict in pretrial discovery (depositions) and at trial, and must be weighed by a judge or jury in determining the issue of breach of duty. The standard of care may also be established or supported through the introduction of relevant authoritative reference texts and peer-reviewed journals (i.e., evidence-based practice) and discipline-specific and/or institutional/system clinical practice protocols and guidelines.

Although every legally competent person bears legal responsibility for his or her conduct (especially rehabilitation professionals for their conduct toward patients), certain persons and entities also bear legal and financial responsibility for the conduct of others. This concept is called vicarious liability.

Employing health care organizations normally bear legal responsibility for the official conduct of their employees when they are acting within the scope of their employment. Thus, it is a health care organization, and not its supervisory licensed health care professionals, that is vicariously liable for the official conduct of employee assistants and extender personnel.

Employing entities normally escape vicarious liability under two sets of circumstances. First, when an employee engages in unforeseeable conduct or blatantly impermissible misconduct, an employer might not be vicariously or indirectly liable for that conduct. For example, when an employee brings a knife to the clinic and stabs a patient, the employer might not be vicariously liable for that employee's misconduct (assuming that there was no known or reasonably discoverable propensity to violence on the part of the offending employee). Second, the employer is not normally vicariously liable for the conduct of contract professionals and their staffs. An exception occurs when the employer fails to undertake reasonable measures to distinguish contract from employed staff and a court imposes vicarious liability for contract staff under apparent or ostensible agency principles.

Irrespective of whether patient injury results from employee, contract staff, consultant, or volunteer official conduct, the legal concept of corporate liability holds health care organizations liable for injuries to patients and others incident to non-delegable duties such as quality management, appropriate hiring and retention, and facility safety, among other possible parameters.

Ordinary negligence is not health care malpractice. It involves injury to anyone (including patients) on premises from non-care-related physical hazards, such as unsecured electrical cords, wet surfaces, or sharp objects. Ordinary premises liability is insured against under general and not professional liability insurance policies. A payment or settlement to an injured person in an ordinary negligence claim or lawsuit is not normally reportable as health care malpractice pursuant to the National Practitioner Data Bank (NPDB), which otherwise requires reporting of malpractice payments and judgments involving licensed health care providers irrespective of whether a case is litigated in court or settled. Additionally, there is no minimum threshold for jury awards or settlements triggering reports to the NPDB.

Professional Liability Insurance

In consultation with their legal counsel, all health care professionals should consider obtaining and maintaining individual professional liability insurance to transfer the risk of monetary loss incident to health care malpractice to their insurers. Although an employer always carries professional liability insurance on its health professional employees, the primary purpose of that insurance coverage is to protect employer interests. Supplemental (and often relatively inexpensive) individual professional liability insurance coverage adds an additional layer of liability risk transfer potential to a health professional's insurance portfolio.

There are two principal types of health professional liability insurance. They are claims-made and occurrence policies. *Claims-made policies* generally insulate health professionals from liability for covered conduct only while a policy remains in force, that is, during a period of employment when premium payments are being made. *Occurrence policies*, on the other hand, provide longer-term coverage, so that even if employment is ended and a policy terminated, conduct that occurred during the term of the policy is protected from liability exposure.

In many or most cases, health care malpractice claims and lawsuits are filed months or years after alleged patient injury. For that reason, occurrence coverage may be more advantageous for health professionals, albeit more costly. To achieve similar protection under claims-made policies, insured professionals must normally purchase relatively expensive tail or prior acts (post-policy period) insurance coverage.

In any event, a health professional should discuss his or her individual situation and needs with state-licensed legal counsel before purchasing a professional liability insurance policy. Keep in mind, too, that professional liability insurance normally does not (and cannot by law as a matter of social policy) insure against malicious intentional misconduct, such as sexual assault or battery committed by a health care professional upon a patient or client.

Principles of Liability Risk Management

Risk management means "liability risk management," that is, self-protection from personal exposure to monetary losses incident to a settlement or court judgment in a civil legal action. In this sense, risk management equates to prophylaxis, or prevention.

Risk management is an integral component of an overall quality management program in a health care organization. However, unlike competency assessment, process and outcomes analyses, documentation and information management, and resource utilization management, liability risk management seemingly serves health professional and organizational interests directly, and not those of patients and clients. The deliberate processes of risk appraisal and avoidance (and fear of malpractice consequences), though, probably help lessen the incidence of patient and client injury incident to care, and thus do co-directly serve their interests.

Risk management strategies and tactics span a continuum from mundane through sophisticated processes, and all are potentially invaluable as liability avoidance tools. At the simplest form, vigilance on the part of all health care workers toward area safety and security is critically important. In every health care setting, every worker should be a safety manager.

More sophisticated measures, like systematic and ad hoc equipment calibration and maintenance, fire and other evacuation drills, universal staff CPR certification, interpersonal communication training (with input from human resource management specialists), control of hazardous substances, and other devices, are important as well.

Figure 16-2 depicts a hypothetical model for gauging relative risk in a rehabilitation facility. A similar model can be constructed through consensus building among a facility's staff. Since each facility is unique, each facility's relative risk will vary because of differences in staff credentials, patient populations, technology applications, and a host of other variables. The bull's-eye illustrates "no-risk" at its center with increasing levels of risk moving outward toward the perimeter. Risk is inherent in all businesses, and a true "no-risk" zone probably does not exist. It is included here as an optimal goal. Risk in this model is defined via two dimensions: (1) prevalence or incidence

of risk and (2) severity of risk. An issue can be located in an outer ring if (a) it occurs frequently or (b) when it occurs (irrespective of frequency), its severity warrants "high-risk" designation. "High-risk" can imply financial cost, human suffering, business interruption, loss of licensure, and decertification, among other considerations.

In this example, the bull's-eye is divided into four quadrants: treatment, administration, external, and physical. However, each center can select its own areas of demarcation. For instance, provider credentials, clinical treatment, clinical documentation, and facility safety could constitute individual quadrants.

Since many persons are visual learners, this model can be an effective means of illustrating the potential for risk and communicating it throughout an organization. Priority actions can then be taken as incremental steps toward risk avoidance or minimization.

One critically important aspect of liability risk management programs is the systematic involvement of legal counsel in in-service education processes. Whether institutional legal counsel or consulting legal advisors, attorneys' input into proposed liability risk management strategies and tactics may spell the difference between liability and non-liability for providers and organizations. Attorneys should also be called upon to review important salient legal cases and pronouncements, especially those including sexual harassment and misconduct issues.

In every health care setting, every worker should be a safety manager.

Informed Consent

Strict and universal adherence to a formal patient informed consent clinical policy is an important risk and quality management strategy. All patients with legal and mental capacity must be given disclosure information by their health care providers to enable them to weigh their options and choose to accept or reject proposed health-related physical examinations and care interventions. To obtain patient informed consent to examination and intervention is to evidence strong respect for patient autonomy and dignity.

Informed consent typically involves disclosure of the following information (to patients or to their surrogate decision makers):

- Examination and evaluative findings
- Diagnosis
- Recommended interventions, with explanation of potential benefits and risks of harm or complication
- Reasonable alternatives to proposed interventions, and their relative benefits and risks (It has been argued that former managed care "gag rules" interfered with providers' ability to comply with this mandate.)

After disclosure of this information, at the level and in a language that a patient (or surrogate) understands, a provider must additionally actively solicit, and satisfactorily answer, patient (or surrogate) questions and formally ask for consent to proceed before doing so.

In many health care organizations, patient informed consent is routinely memorialized in patient care documentation; however, the law typically only requires such

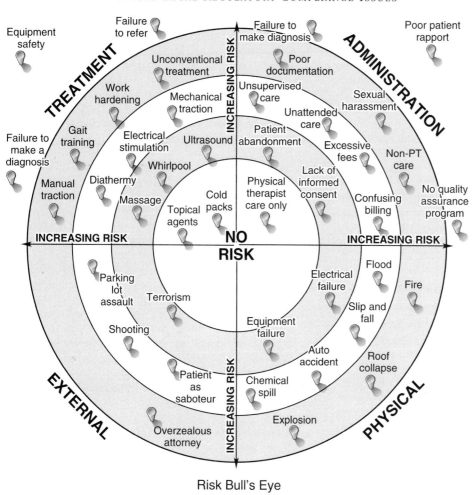

Figure 16–2. Hypothetical model for gauging relative risk in a rehabilitation facility. (From Clifton DW: Risk management in work therapy, orthopaedic physical clinics. Industr Phys Ther 1[1]:171, 1992.)

Risk Bull's Eye

documentation for surgery or anesthesia procedures. Universal documentation of patient informed consent for other procedures may be counterproductive, in that it may create an inference in patients that their relationship with their health care professionals is unduly business-like, perhaps increasing their propensity to file claims or to sue in the event of injury or serious dissatisfaction with care. A better option for memorializing patient informed consent may be through a mandatory policy documented in a facility's policies and procedures manual and displayed in patient intake and care areas.

To universally obtain patient informed consent to examination and intervention is to evidence strong respect for patient autonomy and dignity.

Information, Communications, and Documentation Management

The primary purpose for creating and maintaining patient care documentation is to expeditiously communicate important patient information to other health care providers who have a legitimate need to know the information. All other purposes for documenting patient care activities—from creating a record for reimbursement to creating a legal record to creating a historical record for peer review, quality oversight, or research—are of secondary importance. It is a form of professional

negligence (which is legally actionable if a patient suffers resultant injury) to fail to document patient care-related findings and activities in a timely manner and in a form that is accurate, clear, comprehensive, concise, and objective. Risk management security processes involving computerized patient care documentation effectively protect against breaches of patient confidentiality and spoliation (impermissible alteration or destruction of patient care records to hide their meaning) by limiting access to authorized system users and by disallowing the substitution of altered record entries for original ones.

The primary purpose for creating and maintaining patient care documentation is to expeditiously communicate important patient information to other health-care providers who have a legitimate need to know the information.

Appropriate and effective adverse incident reporting is a critically important liability risk management tool. Incident reports should be properly generated anytime a patient, staff member, visitor, or other person (or animal) is injured; when a patient expresses serious dissatisfaction with care delivery or care personnel; and when a crime or breach of security occurs on the premises.

Normally, incident reports are deemed privileged documents under law, meaning that they are exempt from release to any third parties without the health care organization's consent. Incident reports then are proprietary documents.

On advice of legal counsel, incident reports should be prominently labeled as quality assurance/management or institutional attorney work-product documents, or both, in order to be protected from release. Incident reports must contain factual information that is accurate and objective and that is written, whenever possible, by percipient witnesses to adverse events. Never speculate as to the cause of an adverse incident, nor assign blame to anyone for an adverse event. Leave that to investigators who carry on once the incident report is expeditiously hand-carried to the facility risk manager for processing. If a health care professional is involved as a potential defendant in an adverse incident, then report that fact immediately to the institutional risk manager and to the provider's own attorney and professional liability insurance carrier.

Influences That Contribute to One's Professional Conduct

One's professional conduct is shaped by many variables that rarely operate in splendid isolation. Some of these are depicted in Figure 16–3. Influences can be positive or negative and are rarely neutral in nature. Tort law can affect how rehabilitation providers render treatment. For instance, so-called "defensive medicine" may lead to overutilization of services because of the notion that more treatment is better. However, shorter length of stays (LOS) are also feasible if providers believe that less exposure to patients results in a reduced likelihood of professional liability/malpractice lawsuits.

Payer expectations, especially those directed at less costly and less frequent care, can influence how providers treat or do not treat their patients. Underutilization is often the assumption in this case. Financial considerations may lead to increased use of care extenders, decreased use of technology, and expenditure of fewer resources. In addition, legislative initiatives can adversely affect entire business sectors, especially when related to reimbursement shifts. Corporate risk management policies may determine conduct at the individual level. For instance, a rehabilitation company may mandate the use of a Hoyer lift or other assistive device rather than the manual transfer of patients. Patient expectations can also exert enormous pressure on provider behavior. This pressure is certain to grow as patients/clients assume an increasing financial burden in the form of co-payments, deductibles, and reduced benefit offerings.

Staff expectations, especially peer pressure, may encourage rehabilitation providers to adopt clinical treatment guidelines, protocols, or pathways of care. An organization's corporate culture can be reflected in or driven by its mission or vision statement. For instance, not-for-profits have traditionally been expected to be more sensitive to the needs of indigent populations than for-profit organizations. This oversimplification may not be in evidence in today's health care system. Conformity to organizational policies and procedures (or lack thereof) can directly influence behavior at the individual level. Professional organizations often codify conduct and ethics for acceptance by their voluntary members. A health care organization's sales and marketing department can also package its messages to produce behavioral changes among providers. For instance, if an organization's brochure or Webpage promises 24-hour scheduling from time of referral to first visit, providers may be obligated to

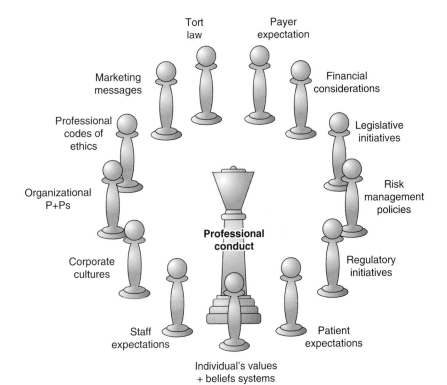

Figure 16–3. Influences that contribute to one's professional conduct.

fulfill this pledge even if it means paying less attention to other patients or responsibilities. Lastly, each and every individual's own value or belief system dictates professional conduct. Individual value and belief systems are rarely static and evolve over time as the result of a combination of variables.

CONCLUSIONS AND FUTURE DIRECTIONS

Liability risk management is as integral to fostering optimal quality patient care as are peer review; credentialing, privileging, and competency assessment; equipment maintenance; and other more obvious quality management processes. Although risk management seems exclusively self-centered and self-protective, in fact, it optimizes the quality of patient care by focusing attention on ambient safety and security.

Attorneys and risk managers are systematic risk management consultants to health care providers and clinical managers and should be consulted regularly, as well as utilized in in-service education processes on a regular basis. Through effective risk management, optimal quality patient care and liability minimization become mutually inclusive goals of providers and health care organizations.

Ultimately one's professional conduct will be influenced both positively and negatively by a myriad influences, ranging from an organization's policies and procedures to regulatory initiatives. How one balances these elements will determine relative risk and the individual's response (professional conduct).

REFERENCES AND SUGGESTED READINGS

Furrow BR, Greaney TL, Johnson SH, Jost TS, Schwartz RL: Health Law, 2nd ed. St Paul, MN, West Group, 2000.

Grose VL: Managing Risk: Systematic Loss Prevention for Executives. Englewood Cliffs, NJ, Prentice Hall, 1987, p 10.

Hall MA, Ellman IM. Health Care Law and Ethics. St Paul, MN, West Group, 1990.

Scott RW. Health Care Malpractice, 2nd ed. New York, McGraw-Hill, 2000.

Scott RW. Legal Aspects of Documenting Patient Care, 2nd ed. Gaithersburg, MD, Aspen, 2000.

Scott RW. Professional Ethics: A Guide for Rehabilitation Professionals. St Louis, Mosby, 1998.

American Health Lawyers Association, www.healthlawyers.org, accessed August 10, 2004.

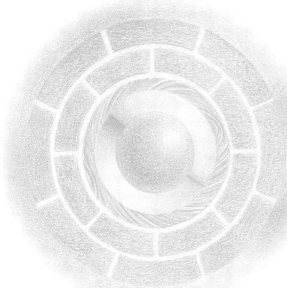

## chapter 17

Ethical Considerations in Disability Management

David W. Clifton, Jr., PT

"Rehabilitation practitioners will face important moral challenges in the coming years. Certainly, they must strive to ensure excellent patient care undergirded by scientific study, but they also must examine whether patients are treated with compassion and respect in an era dominated by financial competition and technological development."

- J. F. Haas, 1993

 KEY POINTS

- Medical/clinical ethics may not be congruent with acceptable business ethics.
- Ethical practice conforms to established professional standards and codes of conduct, at least on a theoretical basis.
- Professional conduct is the resultant action that flows from one's core values and beliefs influenced by external forces.
- A clinician's ethical conduct may be challenged by the need to balance economic accountability with humanitarian concern.
- Ethical dilemmas tend to escalate when a provider must serve in a dual moral agency role, wherein he or she must balance what is good for the patient with what is good for the health care organization.

Operational Definitions

The following definitions have been adapted from cited sources and are included here for the convenience of the reader.

Autonomy — The concept of patient self-governance or control over clinical decision making, autonomy is the opposite of the "doctor knows best" attitude (Scott, 1998).

Beneficence — The clinician's duty to help those in need and to consider their best interests or benefit when making decisions on their behalf. The principle that a provider holds a fiduciary responsibility to the patient (see fiduciary) (Scott, 1998).

Competence — The concept that providers will provide only those services and use those techniques or interventions for which they are qualified by education, training, experience, and expertise (Andre & Velasquez, 2000).

Dual Moral Agency — The concept that providers are confronted with responsibilities that are in conflict and require reconciliation. These responsibilities may be owed to different persons or health care stakeholders (Golenski & Cloutier, 1994).

Ethics — Theories or systems that guide an individual's personal actions, relations, and decisions (Guthrie, 1994).

Justice — A sense of fairness when a provider makes decisions on a patient's behalf.

Morals — The belief and conformity of acts involving right versus wrong, morality is a subcomponent of ethical theory (Guthrie, 1994).

Nonmaleficence — The dictate to do no harm (Scott, 1997).

Paternalism — This concept describes a provider who serves in the role of patient advocate, guardian, or steward and makes decisions on the patient's behalf.

| | Paternalism is a synonym for beneficence (Scott, 1998). |
| **Utilitarianism** | The moral principle that everyone is obligated by duty to do whatever will achieve the greatest good for the greatest number of persons (Andre & Velasquez, 2000). |

The nature of health care has changed dramatically during the past several decades. During this period, a large body of literature evolved that addressed medical ethics, or bioethics. Acute care services and hospital-based ethics received a disproportionate focus in this literature. By contrast, a relative paucity of ethics data exists specific to physical rehabilitation and the management of chronic conditions (Blackmer 2000; Haas, 1993; Kirschner et al, 2001).

Health care developments in the 1980s, namely, the prowess of managed care, fostered an increase in literature specific to rehabilitation ethics that continues today (Bonder, 1985; Caplan, 1988; Cottone, 1983; Coy, 1989; Haas, 1993; Haddad, 1988; Meier, 1994; Kyler-Hutchison, 1988; Purtilo, 1978, 1979).

Some authors have succeeded in systematically linking medical ethics to the circumstances that are routinely confronted by physical rehabilitation professionals (Guccione 1980; Purtilo, 1976; Ramsden, 1975). This chapter is dedicated to these early pioneers.

This chapter provides an overview of fundamental ethics principles and an attempt to relate them to rehabilitative services administration. Specific ethics issues are briefly discussed along with case scenarios. The magnitude of the field of ethics does not permit an extensive examination, and readers are highly encouraged to explore reference citations and the recommended reading list, in particular the works of professional ethicists (Table 17–1).

MEDICAL AND PHYSICAL REHABILITATION ETHICS: A COMPARISON

Ethics are theories or systems that guide personal actions, decisions, and relations, while *morality* refers to the dichotomous belief that something is either right or wrong (Guthrie, 1994). A number of distinctions exist between medical ethics and physical rehabilitation ethical dilemmas. Medical ethics predominantly address the acute care hospital-based environment, an environment that under managed care has become less relevant to rehabilitation. Rehabilitation rarely involves the life and death circumstances that give rise to many of today's ethical dilemmas such as advance directives, gene therapy, human cloning, embryonic research, euthanasia, and abortion. This distinction has great import relative to autonomy and paternalism. These and other ethics principles are addressed later in the chapter.

Unlike many medical services, rehabilitation is often considered a discretionary service, especially in the management of persons with chronic conditions. With few exceptions, rehabilitation services are non-invasive and devoid of the medical complexity that to date has sparked much of the bioethical debate. Bioethicists have essentially overlooked the less obtrusive issues such as those common to rehabilitation (Caplan et al, 1987).

 Table 17–1 Sources of Ethics Information

- American Journal of Law & Medicine
- Bioethics
- Cambridge Quarterly of Health Care Ethics
- Hastings Center Report
- Healthcare Analysis: Journal of Philosophy & Policy
- Healthcare Ethics Committee Forum (HEC)
- International Journal of Bioethics
- Issues in Law & Medicine
- Journal of Clinical Ethics
- Journal of Contemporary Health Law & Policy
- Journal of Law, Medicine & Ethics
- Journal of Medical Humanities
- Journal of Medicine & Philosophy
- Kennedy Institute of Ethics Journal
- Linacre Quarterly
- Philosophy & Public Affairs
- Second Opinion
- Social Science & Medicine
- Theoretical Medicine

The predominance of the medical model of health care delivery in the United States partly explains the focus on medical ethics or bioethics. Within this model, providers tend to perceive disability from a patient-centric or treatment-focused approach (Imrie, 1997).

The individual patient's medical condition has principally determined the intervention, while the provider has traditionally ignored the broader context in which a condition is embedded. This broader context, which rehabilitation providers tend to appreciate relatively more than other medical providers, involves professional psychological, social, vocational, environmental, and other non-medical variables that often dictate the degree of rehabilitation success. A detailed analysis of these and other variables is contained in Chapter 7.

Rehabilitation tends to be more multidisciplinary than the medical model of acute care delivery (Haas, 1993). New and complex ethical dilemmas can arise when physical therapists, occupational therapists, primary care physicians, specialty physicians, social workers, case managers, vocational counselors, psychologists, and others who may subscribe to divergent codes of ethics must work together in a collaborative model.

Rehabilitation is often the lead service in disability management of persons with chronic conditions. Chronic conditions are typically more complex than acute conditions as a result of multiple diagnoses, comorbidities, psychosocial issues, reimbursement challenges, and environmental barriers (Table 17–2).

Disability management of persons with chronic conditions generally warrants more patient education, family involvement, and self-care than do acute conditions. These cases are generally preselected and referred to physical therapists (PTs) and occupational therapists (OTs) by other medical professionals. The expectations of others follow these patients into rehabilitation. For instance, the goals of the rehabilitation professional may be at odds with the goals of the referral source. It is important to note that the medical model works to find a

Table 17-2 Medical Versus Rehabilitation Attributes That Influence Ethics

Medical Attributes	Rehabilitation Attributes
Focus on the person's anatomy, physiology, pathology	Focus on function or quality of life
Patient-centric approach	Focuses on patient, his or her environment, psychosocial issues and other non-medical issues
Acute care focus	High prevalence of chronic care
Single discipline focus	Multiple disciplines
Well-established reimbursement mechanisms	Poorly established reimbursement mechanisms
"Patient" tends to be passive recipient of treatment	"Client" actively participates in self-care, education
Provider treats	Patient self-care
Institutionally-based	Service-based
Lower degree of family involvement	High degree of family involvement
Shorter durations of care	Longer durations of care
Goal is to "cure"	Goal is to "habilitate," prevent disability
Physician operates in paternalistic manner	Provider-client partnership

Adapted from Caplan AL, Callahan D, Haas J: Ethical and policy issues in rehabilitation medicine. Hastings Cent Rep 17(Suppl):S1-S19, 1987.

cure for many conditions, whereas rehabilitation operates to maximize function and habilitation of the client to her or his environment, be it home, school, work, or the sports arena. Each setting presents unique ethical dilemmas. For instance, providers treating long-term-care patients may confront the challenge of physical restraint use (Hunt, 1990; Knapp, 1992, Sturmpf & Evans, 1991).

The semantics that surround the referrer-rehabilitation professional relationship can create conflict between parties. For example, basic confusion often exists involving the difference between a "prescription" for and a "referral" to rehabilitation (Clifton, 1995). These terms are often used interchangeably even by therapists themselves. Yet the distinction between these terms has great bearing on how others may perceive the role of rehabilitation. "Prescription" implies that allied health professionals must adhere to whatever order the referring physician recorded on the so-called "prescription" form.

In other words, no room exists for a substitution permissible option because rehabilitation is subjugated to a technician role. This perception alone can lead to ethical dilemmas when the therapist wishes to embark on a different and, perhaps, more appropriate treatment path than that outlined by the referring physician. In reality, some rehabilitation providers such as physical therapists practice on referral not on prescription. Historically, a significant number of physical therapy state practice acts included the term "prescription." Furthermore, a majority of the states allow for direct access or the ability to evaluate and/or treat without referral, which at least hypothetically renders the need for a referral or prescription null and void.

A similar dilemma presents itself when medical versus physical therapy diagnoses are discussed. This

dilemma relates to the earlier discussion in this chapter about the medical model of delivery, which focuses on finding a cure for an anatomical or physiological problem.

What Ethical Issues Are of Interest to Rehabilitation Providers?

Relatively few studies have cited data concerning which ethical issues are of greatest interest to rehabilitation providers (Guccione, 1980; Kirschner et al, 2001; Triezenberg ,1996). Guccione's landmark (1980) study was one of the earliest assessments of provider attitudes conducted. His study had the two-fold purpose of identifying which ethical problems were perceived by physical therapists to be the most frequently encountered. This survey also addressed those ethical challenges most difficult to solve during daily professional practice. This pioneering effort surveyed 450 physical therapists and presented them with 30 situations involving an ethical dimension. Forty-one percent responded ($N = 187$) with usable results. Respondents collectively identified seven primary and eleven secondary ethical issues. The following four categories comprise these issues: (1) decisions regarding the choice to treat, (2) obligations derived from the patient-provider relationship, (3) moral obligation relative to economic issues, and (4) a physical therapist's relationship with other health professionals. Guccione (1980) defined ethical dilemmas in his survey as two or more ethical principles or values in conflict in a given situation.

Survey results are summarized in Table 17-3. Survey respondents were sensitive to the role that other stakeholders played in the management of disability. Specifically, therapists expressed concern about how to resolve conflict when a patient's goals are inconsistent with those of their family. A second concern involved other health care professionals aside from therapists. Patient and family confidence in other health care practitioners was of concern. Providers also raised issues specific to medical economics and third party payer limitations. Patient-specific issues of concern included non-compliance, postrehabilitation psychological support, and the

 Table 17-3 Seven Ethical Concerns of Physical Therapists

1. Establishment of priorities for patient treatment when time or resources are constrained.
2. Discontinuance of treatment when patients are non-compliant
3. Continuation of treatment in terminally ill persons
4. Continuation of treatment through the provision of psychological support after physical therapy goals have been achieved
5. Determination of professional responsibilities when a patient's needs or goals conflict with those of his or her family
6. Deciding whether to represent patient services in a manner that meets third party payer limitations
7. Maintenance of patient and family confidence in other health care professionals regardless of personal opinions

Adapted from Guccione AA: Ethical issues in physical therapy: A survey of physical therapists in New England. Phys Ther 60:1264-1272, 1980.

management of terminally ill patients. It is important to keep in mind that this survey predated the zenith of managed care.

Respondents to a more recent survey of one acute rehabilitation facility were asked to identify three conflicts or ethical dilemmas that confronted them in practice (Kirschner, 2001). Respondents included treatment staff as well as administrative staff. The various response rates by profession are interesting. Eighty percent of admitting nurses responded, compared with just 52% for PTs and 68% for OTs.

Psychologists responded at an astounding 91% rate, leading all professions. The survey authors do not discuss the reasons behind such disparate response rates especially as they pertain to the relatively low response rate of physical rehabilitation practitioners. Twenty-four percent of respondents identified pressures resulting from health care reimbursement changes as a major ethical dilemma (Kirschner, 2001). Health care reimbursement issues were composed of a number of sub-issues, including the following:

- A lack of insurance benefits or coverage for conditions treated.
- Rationing and allocation of limited hospital resources.
- Medicare's 3-hour rule for inpatient rehabilitation.
- Unsafe discharge plans as the result of coverage issued for community-based support services.
- Documentation of the medical necessity for rehabilitation services.
- Restructure of health care delivery resources, namely, in the increased use of extenders of care as the result of fiscal concerns.

Relationship conflicts between patients, family, and team members specific to *goal setting* was the second most prevalent issue. At 7%, assessment of clinical decision making capacity was the third most prevalent response. The authors concluded that a team-based approach to rehabilitation was laden with ethical dilemmas, and that rehabilitation providers were generally troubled by issues of justice and the potential harm that may result from reimbursement decisions. Table 17–3 summarizes respondent interests relative to what they would like to see as topics for future education designed to equip them for dealing with ethical challenges. Triezenberg's survey of ethical dilemmas sixteen years after Guccione's landmark survey provides additional insight into how providers view ethical dilemmas. His survey had the luxury of hindsight relative to managed care strategies and influence on service delivery. Sixteen priority issues were identified spanning a variety of topics. Key issues derived through consensus addressed business versus medical or health care ethics.

A growing body of literature examines aspects of cost versus utilization. (Emanuel, 1995; Hildred and Watkins, 1996; Radel et al, 2001) Providers expressed concern about over-utilization of physical therapy services, which may come as a surprise given that capitation is the dominant reimbursement model under managed care. Involvement of therapists in business relationships that have a potential for patient exploitation also received substantial focus. It is important to point out that Mitchell's study correlating physician ownership of physical therapy centers and over-utilization was contemporaneous to Triezenberg's (1996) survey and, as such, may have influenced respondents (Mitchell, 1995). Physical therapist use of extenders of care such as physical therapy assistants (PTAs) and aides commanded significant interest. Fraudulent billing practices were also identified as a priority concern. Again, this issue was extensively covered by the media, especially as it pertained to Medicare fraud, abuse, and compliance. It thus comes as little surprise that it too was high on provider radar screens.

Kornblau and Starling (2000) provide a comprehensive array of ethical dilemmas potentially confronting physical rehabilitation providers. Readers are encouraged to refer to their "Ethical Dilemma Worksheets" for samples of issues that cover the entire gamut including the aforementioned ethical dilemmas. These may be useful tools for the training and education of practitioners.

ETHICS: KEY PRINCIPLES AND CONCEPTS

A discussion of disability management is incomplete without a fundamental examination of principles and concepts associated with ethical decision making. Some contend that ethics or decisions of a moral nature may be influenced, but are not necessarily dictated by issues associated with law, religion, technology, politics, or social issues (Haas 1993; Kornblau & Starling, 2000).

Ethical practice theoretically conforms to discrete established professional standards and codes of conduct (Guccione, 1980). Because professional associations are voluntary in nature, however, the application of ethical guideposts is likewise of a volitional nature and can actually conflict with the individual provider's moral and value belief systems. Professional ethos or ideology may therefore be of limited use in dealing with day-to-day ethical dilemmas that depend on individual judgments.

Although professional associations commonly formulate codes of ethics, some authors have noted that relatively few practitioners receive formal training to enhance their sensitivity to moral challenges (Haas, JF, 1993). Consequently, ethical decisions are often based on cultural and personal experience and not professional standards per se. Cultural beliefs impact on how providers view ethical issues such as social justice (Banja, 1996). Others claim that ethics have long been incorporated into professional rehabilitation educational programs (Callahan et al, 1961; Purtilo, 1979).

Personal values and beliefs are ultimately at the very core of provider decisions related to patient care. Professional conduct is the resultant action that flows from a combination of core values and the influence of external forces that serve to shape and reshape these values and beliefs. (Bailey and Schwartzberg, 1995; Rousseau, 2001; Caplan, 1988; Tepper, 2000; Gunderson, 1997; Gray, 1991). Figure 17–1 illustrates a modified Maslow hierarchy beginning with the individual's value system. Individual values evolve into principles, rules, and standards. Organizational policies and procedures, regulatory and legislative initiatives, and the expectations of other stakeholders in health care both individually and collectively influence provider ethical decision making. Provider decision making regarding ethics does not take

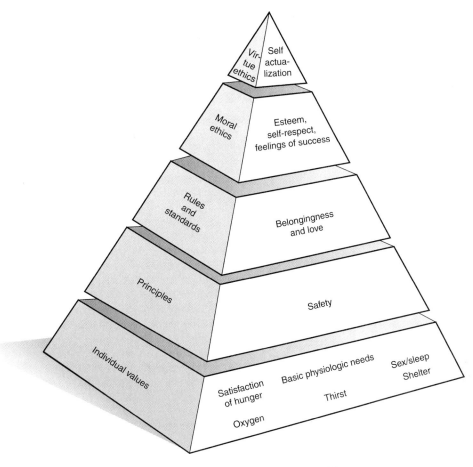

Figure 17–1. Ethic pyramid: A modified Maslow model.

place in a vacuum and is highly interdependent on these and other extrinsic variables.

Beneficence

Beneficence is a term used to describe the notion that health care professionals assume a moral obligation to help others in a charitable and kind manner. However, beneficence is not the same as the provider making decisions for the patient. A provider's duty to make health care decisions on behalf of his or her patients is not the inalienable right that some may believe or expect it to be. Instead, providers are endowed by the patient with the right to make decisions that are of benefit to the patient (Scott, 1997). The concept of beneficence stems from the Hippocratic Oath in that providers shall strive to help and certainly do no harm to their patients.

Providers in today's increasingly complex and frenetically paced health care sector must balance benefit with risk or potential for harm. For example, the discharge of a patient from an outpatient setting to a home exercise program may be viewed by the patient and his or her family as an abdication of the provider's responsibility to provide care and the patient's right to receive medically necessary and reasonable care. In this example, the clinician views a home exercise program of pain abatement combined with therapeutic exercise to be of benefit to the patient as well as the most judicious use of limited economic resources. The clinician may perceive this to be a balance between economic rationality and humanitarian concern, especially when dealing with chronic conditions or disease state management.

Clinical experience suggests that quality of care and outcome is not negatively impacted and may actually be heightened through the patient's acceptance of self-responsibility and active participation in her or his disability management program. However, other stakeholders may not share this view and demand more institutionally based service. Now imagine if this patient had a workers' compensation or automobile liability claim for which they had retained an attorney. The attorney's goals may be to highlight the degree of disability, encourage protracted treatment, and demonstrate the dependency or sick role of their patient to achieve a more financially appealing settlement or award. The strength of the legal argument may rest on the patient's dependence, the very antithesis of the rehabilitation provider's goal for this patient. This is not an uncommon example of an ethical dilemma that is routinely seen by those who manage workers' compensation, disability insurance, or automobile liability cases.

Beneficence must be considered unique to each and every case that is managed by a rehabilitation provider. Assessment of risk versus benefit may vary from patient to patient.

Autonomy and Informed Consent

Autonomy provides a patient with an inherent right to self-determination or self-governance. Autonomy is grounded in respect for the value and belief systems of patients. Autonomy is the underpinning of informed consent according to some experts (Haas, 1993). Informed consent remains, however, a controversial concept in health care relationships (Caplan, 1988; Sadan, 2000).

Under some state laws, informed consent is only required when an invasive procedure such as surgery is performed. However, Scott (1998) argues that informed consent is a fundamental obligation of all providers including rehabilitation providers irrespective of whether the patient is referred or not by a physician (Scott, 1998). The rehabilitation provider's obligation to secure informed consent is not obviated by or transferred to the referring physician. Scott contends that informed consent is the most important mixed legal-ethical clinical issue that affects a provider's practice.

Sadan (2000) purports that informed consent takes on greater significance for providers with diminished independence and practice autonomy in the milieu of managed care, especially when patient-unfriendly agendas exist (Sadan, 2000). Autonomy recognizes patients as integrated beings whose physical, emotional, and spiritual welfare are intertwined (Cohen et al, 2000). In their fulfillment of beneficence, a provider must recognize these realities.

Autonomy can be viewed as the opposite of beneficence, but this need not be the case. Patient self-determination can harmoniously co-exist with provider decision making on the patient's behalf. This situation occurs when a provider explains a treatment option (informed consent) and outlines both the benefit and risk. The patient then selects to accept or reject the treatment regime. Both autonomy and beneficence have been preserved in this example. When health care providers behave in a paternalistic manner, however, wherein the health care provider makes all treatment decisions, autonomy is stifled. This situation commonly occurs in acute care settings (e.g., emergency care) in which the patient is a passive recipient of services and does not traditionally participate in clinical decision making (Caplan, 1988). In general, the patient-provider interaction represents a contractual relationship. Informed consent serves as the cement between two consenting persons.

Emergency medicine perhaps best typifies the paternalistic approach. Provider paternalism reduces autonomy in other situations such as pediatric care and in the case of services rendered to those declared mentally incompetent. In these examples, someone other than the patient has engaged in the informed consent process, serving in a guardianship role.

When a patient and his or her provider disagree on what is best for the patient, beneficence can clash with autonomy (Maier, 1993). Several ethical dilemmas are conceivable in this situation. First, the provider may elect to perform two separate and distinct services, both the patient's and provider's preferred treatment. This decision may raise the issue of overutilization or medically unnecessary care, particularly in the eyes of a utilization reviewer or claims adjuster. If the provider succumbs to the patient's preference (even if she/he disagrees with it), this then raises the issue of the provider's abdication of fiduciary or professional responsibility. A fiduciary is one in a special position of trust (Scott, 1997).

Finally, if the provider disregards the patient's preference and fails to secure informed consent, then autonomy may be quashed. Informed consent, if it is to be useful in rehabilitation, requires serious examination, especially when unexpected trauma or an extended course of treatment alters relationship dynamics. For instance, posttraumatic catastrophic cases such as spinal cord injury or traumatic brain injury may necessitate that the provider engage in more of an educational model of intervention than a contractual treatment model. Once this person is medically stable, habilitation of him or her to the environment or instruction in the use of assistive or adaptive equipment represents the educational approach.

Likewise, persons with chronic conditions may require instruction in self-help strategies and the use of assistive or adaptive devices. In these cases, informed consent loses some of its utility because there is minimal laying on of hands, and the relationship is one of teacher-patient rather than provider-patient.

A review of the medical literature supports the concept that patients prefer to have decisional control over outcomes but prefer to delegate technical decisions about how to achieve expected outcomes (Bruhn, 2001). These patient preferences may have great significance to rehabilitation providers, who must be assured that their clinical goals are commensurate with the outcome goals of their patients. For instance, if the therapist is focused on functional goals but the patient is most interested in quality of life, a reconciliation of goals is required. Providers acknowledge that not all functional gains directly lead to enhanced quality of life. Resolution of impairments does not necessarily reduce the degree of one's disability or handicap. Shared crafting of goals between the patient and provider may be necessary in order to avoid ethical conflict.

Nonmaleficence

Nonmaleficence is the equivalent of the "do no harm" covenant. Because of the "do" in do no harm, some may equate this concept with the act of *doing something to a patient*, otherwise known as an act of commission. Scott (1997) defines an "act" as "an affirmative, volitional, intended conduct in furtherance of a specific result" (Scott, 1997, p 88). Providers should be aware that omissions or a failure to take action may also potentially violate the "do no harm" covenant from both a legal and ethical perspective. Omissions describe an intentional and wrongful failure to act when under a legal duty of care for a patient (Scott, 1997).

Logically, examples of omissions are more likely to occur when providers receive incentives to perform fewer services (e.g., managed care) than when they receive more for doing more (e.g., fee-for-service). Issues such as health care rationing, denial of care, patient abandonment, refusal to treat, unsupervised care, and underutilization of services are frequently cited by critics of managed care

(Banja, 1999; Haas, JF, 1993; Rosenblatt & Harwitz, 1999; Rodwin 1993).

Justice

Justice as an ethical (versus legal) principle refers to fairness consistently applied at various levels including the individual patient, group, societal, and global levels (Brody, 1988; Scott, 1997). Purtilo (1981, 1982) analyzed the perception of justice in the distribution of health care resources. She found marked differences of justice interpretations among three different professions: physical therapists, nurses, and physiatrists. Physical therapists were found to use a "needs-based" approach when making clinical decisions about distribution of services, whereas rehabilitation nurses and physiatrists were divided between utilitarian and needs-based distribution. Utilitarian-based decisions tend to be more responsive to external factors such as resource allocation, health care benefit schemes, staffing availability, reimbursement schemes, and political concerns.

Confidentiality

Confidentiality is a core tenet of health care practice and research. Providers must respect the patient's fundamental right to privacy by restricting access of non-authorized persons to personnel information. Confidentiality is legislatively and legally protected by a number of federal initiatives including but not restricted to the 1974 Federal Privacy Act, the 1990 Americans with Disability Act, the 1973 Rehabilitation Act, and the Health Insurance Portability and Accountability Act of 1996 (HIPAA).

Patient or client confidentiality issues have become more complicated and increase in complexity as more providers and non-provider stakeholders enter into a case. For instance, a long-term disability case involving a person with chronic illness or injury may involve a panoply of participants including an attending physician, specialist physicians, PTs, OTs, vocational counselors, case managers, claims managers, psychologists, human resource staff, social service professionals, risk managers, utilization review agents, and attorneys. Imagine the potential for ethical conflict within this assemblage of people, each possessing her or his own unique view of treatment goals, outcomes, quality, confidentiality, and other ethics issues. The ethical preservation of and disclosure of patient-specific information is severely challenged by the sheer number and diversity of participants.

Computerized record keeping, the use of electronic mail, and the Internet pose new and relatively unexplored challenges to providers. Chapter 12 explores these issues in greater detail.

Release of medical records is governed by a combination of business and clinical communications, ethical codes, practice standards, and statutory and federal laws. A team-based episode of care is unequivocally more complex than when physical or occupational therapy are the only active services.

Disclosure of confidential patient-specific information typically requires the written consent of the care recipient and identification of the entity requesting the data.

Table 17–4 Sample Confidentiality Covenant

1.2 Confidential Information

A. Information related to the physical therapist/patient relationship is confidential and may not be communicated to a third party not involved in that patient's care without the prior written consent of the patient, subject to applicable law.

D. Information may be disclosed to appropriate authorities when it is necessary to protect the welfare of an individual or the community. Such disclosure shall be in accordance with applicable law.

From American Physical Therapy Association: Code of Ethics and Guide for Professional Conduct. Alexandria, VA, APTA, 1990.

This person(s) has a moral obligation for the protection of the patient's welfare. Refer to Table 17–4 for a sample confidentiality clause.

Confidentiality does not restrict providers from disclosing information that is vital to the best interests of a patient. Defining the best interests of patients becomes the challenge. One example involves situations wherein the harm of preserving confidentiality is greater than that brought on through actual disclosure (University of Washington Medical School, 2002). Several legal circumstances warrant a breach in confidentiality even when it may be against the wishes of the patient.

For instance, clinicians have a duty to protect identifiable persons from serious threat of harm if they can potentially prevent harm through disclosure of otherwise confidential information. A patient who is diagnosed with an extremely contagious and threatening disease such as hepatitis C or AIDS may forfeit under certain circumstances their right to privacy and confidentiality. In this example, legal action may be more pertinent than ethical decision making. State law may in fact require that providers report certain communicable or infectious diseases to authorities in order to protect the public. Public health, safety, and welfare may be placed ahead of the individual's right to confidentiality in these cases.

Rehabilitation providers who work with school-age children may find themselves in the position of reporting potential child abuse to authorities without the consent of their parent or guardian. Disclosure of information to a patient's family member generally requires explicit permission (Scott, 1997). When a family member is at risk as the result of a unique condition, however, disclosure may be permissible from both a legal and ethical perspective.

APPLICATION OF ETHICS THEORIES

Virtue Ethics

Virtue ethics has its roots in ancient Greece, most notably in the philosophers Aristotle and Plato (Bivins, 2000). Aristotle described the concept of the golden mean to describe the mean between two extremes. Moral virtue occupies one pole and deficiency represents the opposite pole. Those who subscribe to the Aristotelian method identify extremes in their pursuit of moderation. Proponents of virtue ethics contend that attributes like personal courage, integrity, honesty, compassion, fidelity, fairness, self-discipline and control are more important than strict adherence to specific rules of conduct (Andre & Velasquez, 2000; Hall & Berenson, 1998). These character traits are manifested in habitual action not simply through occasional use.

Application of these virtues or character traits to actual situations represents one major criticism of virtue ethics (Bivins, 2000; Tiel, 1999). For instance, if one accepts that rehabilitation professionals as a group universally possess traits such as kindness, compassion, and fairness; how does this translate into clinical actions? How are these traits to be codified? How can they be standardized in repeatable models of conduct? Bivins illustrates both the strengths and weaknesses in virtue ethics (Bivins, 2000). Strengths include proper moral motivation that builds character and can lead to but does not guarantee ethical actions. Virtue ethics and the ideal of the golden mean assume that persons are willing to compromise, which is unrealistic in some circumstances.

Rule-Based Ethics

Rule-based or action-imperative systems for ethical decision making generally provide a formula or calculus for the determination of specific action in a given situation (Tiel, 1999). Kant's categorical imperative is an example of a rule-based ethics system that considers an act to be good in itself, unconditional, and independent of any things, circumstances, goals, desires, merits, or rewards (Guthrie, 1994). A categorical imperative can be considered a universal and binding law, that is, a moral law that is applied to all rational beings at all times. Simply put, a categorical imperative is a non-negotiable theory. Kant's theory and Mill's utilitarian principle are two examples of rule-based ethics theories.

Situational Ethics

Scott (1997) offers rehabilitation providers with some guidance through "situational ethics." Situational ethics facilitates selective compliance or non-compliance with rules of conduct depending on the mitigating and extenuating circumstances of a given ethical dilemma. Situational ethics represents an opposite approach to Kant's categorical imperative, which demands consistent conduct in specific circumstances. Situational ethics are malleable and do not represent absolutes in terms of one's professional conduct. As such, they may appear to be hypocritical or ambiguous at times, especially if the observer is accustomed to a rule-based or imperative-based approach.

Situational ethics are well positioned for today's rapidly evolving health care sector with its exponential complexity. Flexible times may very well demand flexible ethical decision making. Situational ethics appear to be well suited to those who subscribe to virtue ethics or character-based ethics.

MANAGED CARE: ETHICAL CHALLENGES

According to some, managed care strategies do not mix easily with traditional modes of ethical analysis (Hall & Berenson, 1998; Hofmann, 1995; Khushf, 1999).

Managed care has challenged medical ethics, the underpinning of health care for centuries (Friedman, 1993; Higgins, 2000; Newman & Dunbar, 2000). Medical practitioners traditionally have placed the needs of their patients ahead of all others. Providers strove to treat anyone in need of services and whom they believed could be helped. The provider-patient relationship was sacred and immune to the intrusiveness of those peripheral to this relationship. For better or worse, managed care has essentially resulted in the selective rationing of services through a variety of mechanisms. These are not discussed here. Readers are encouraged to refer to Chapter 23.

Rationing creates many conflicts of interest and quality questions (Gostin, 2000). When rationing interferes with the provider-patient relationship, considered by some to be at the heart of health care, ethical dilemmas are both common and complicated (Degnin, 1999; Kaplan, 1997; Shapiro et al, 2000).

FINANCIAL ISSUES IN ETHICAL DECISION MAKING
Dual Moral Agency

Ethical dilemmas escalate when providers serve in a dual "moral agency" role wherein they must balance that which is good for the patient with that which is good for the health care organization (Golenski & Cloutier, 1994). Providers can also be trapped between two frequently opposing paradigms: business ethics and health care ethics (Hofmann, 1995). Conflict can arise when a provider is deemed a "preferred provider" by a managed care organization. The provider executes a provider contract that incorporates a variety of fiscal issues that may or may not be conducive to the delivery of adequate care (Howard, 1991; Smoak, 1999). Capitation as a prepaid per member per month (PMPM) fee hypothetically rewards a provider for performing fewer services. If a provider's resource allocation (both human and capital resources) exceeds the rate of reimbursement, temptation may exist to reduce the intensity and duration of service. This may be viewed as unethical from a clinical perspective but prudent from a business standpoint.

This pressure is compounded by the gatekeeper's reimbursement, which is designed to influence more judicious use of discretionary services. The traditional reimbursement scheme for primary care physicians is via withhold funds. These funds essentially reward PCPs for cost savings. Cost savings result when services are restricted. Restrictions in the use of discretionary services is quite common. Physical rehabilitation is often considered a discretionary service by managed care organizations (MCOs) (Figure 17–2).

Wennberg (1992) asserts that when there is more than one reasonable option for treatment, patient preferences, a shared decision-making model, and patient empowerment should be considered.

Preferred providers are thus potentially torn between contractual or legal requirements, fiscal considerations, and ethical decision making. Balancing these interests is extremely difficult. Technology use, resource allocation, care rationing, and managed care can be vexing challenges

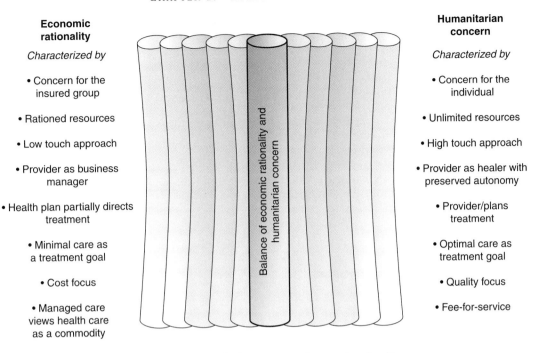

Figure 17–2. Humanitarian concern and economic rationality.

(Andre, 1999; Callahan, 195; Daniels, 1991, Evans, 1983, Evert, 1993; Weber, 1997).

Weber identified four key values that must be considered when balancing managerial and clinical ethics (Weber, 1999). Balance is achieved when the individual's or patient's rights harmonize with provider self-interest, the organization's best interest, and the public good. Thompson asserts that this daunting task can be accomplished through what he calls "ethical reasoning" (Thompson, 2000). Ethical reasoning describes a balance between business and health care goals achieved by the search for reasonable profit through the provision of dependable yet accessible health care services. Ethical reasoning accepts a certain degree of provider and organizational self-interest, provided that treatment efficiencies, economic growth, and clinical outcomes are ensured. This idea is a dramatic departure from the traditionally held belief that health care decision making should be altruistic.

Ethical reasoning hypothetically represents a classic win-win scenario; however, it cannot be achieved without some degree of compromise. Such compromise is seldom seen in today's managed care setting, in which patient selection, provider credentialing, treatment limits (cost and duration), and precertification of care are preordained by the managed care organization. In fact, the literature is replete with allegations that managed care, in particular the gatekeeper or primary care physician (PCP) model, has diminished access to care, intensity of service, and quality of service (Newman & Dunbar, 2000).

Health Care: A Commodity?

Some argue that health care in the era of managed care is a traded commodity (Zoloth & Dorfman, 1995). One study

of HMO financial incentive contracts revealed that gatekeeper physicians earned an average of 10¢ in personal profit for every $1 reduction in medical utilization expenditures (Gaynor et al, 2001).

During the past 10 years, an anti-managed care backlash has grown steadily. By 1996, more than 1000 different pieces of legislation had been introduced designed to wrest control from MCOs and return it to providers and consumers (Bodenheimer, 1996).

The impact of financial issues on ethical decision making has been widely discussed in the health care literature including rehabilitation (Banja, 1999; Burke & Cassidy, 1991; AOTA, 1990, Waldman, 1996, Gray, 1991; Kane & Kane, 1990; Mitchell, 1995; Hillman et al, 1989; PPRC, 1995). The health care sector's dramatic and rapid shift from the fee-for-service reimbursement model to the at-risk model of capitation, episodic, or case rates has fueled many ethical dilemmas. Financial impacts can involve overutilization and underutilization of services. Disclosure of financial incentives serves as one example of ethical debate (Kaplan, 1997).

Although MCOs may not always be legally bound to disclose to patients data about provider remuneration, some contend that MCOs have an ethical responsibility to do so (Figa & Figa, 1990; Levinson, 1987; Morreim, 1997). Providers too may assume a fiduciary responsibility of disclosure. The issue of financial incentive disclosure has served to align ethical and legal principles (Gunderson, 1997; Miller & Sage, 1999).

Some ethicists recommend incentive neutrality as a means of alleviating conflict and moral crisis (Hall & Berenson, 1998). No model for incentive neutrality, however, has yet been created that will satisfy the needs of diverse health care stakeholders. Some have argued against any disclosure of financial incentives and consider health care and business principles to be separate (Noone & Ubel, 1997).

MCOs share culpability with others for a number of ethical dilemmas that confront today's providers. Long-term care funding sources (Medicare) and referring physicians must shoulder some responsibility for the cost and degree of service (Friedman, 1996). Medicare intermediaries are legendary for their inconsistent application of supposedly standardized rules for the establishment of what constitutes medically necessary and reasonable rehabilitation service. Medicare rules and regulations frequently place rehabilitation providers in the position of choosing the lesser of two evils, especially as they pertain to which services are covered on a treatment setting basis. For more details about long-term care please refer to Chapter 4.

Referral for Profit and Ethical Dilemmas

Referral for profit has been associated with increased cost, duration, and intensity of service (AOTA, 1990; Mitchell & Sass, 1995; Rodwin, 1993; Waldman, 1996). Referral for profit is not likely to be an issue in managed care scenarios because under capitation models, providers reap more profits from providing less, not more, treatment. Data suggest that when referring physicians have a financial interest or stake in a rehabilitation facility, utilization rates and costs rise above those in similar cases treated in non-physician affiliated centers (Mitchell & Sass, 1995). Conversely, when referring physicians are reimbursed in a gatekeeper or PCP role for non-referral, as in the case of withholding payment, rehabilitation utilization declines. Rehabilitation professionals must share responsibility for appropriate utilization of their services and must confront the ethical dilemmas that are presented by both referral-for-profit and non-referral-for-profit.

The American Physical Therapy *Code of Ethics and Guide for Professional Conduct* addresses this very issue under Principle 7 (Table 17–5).

> *"Physical therapists accept the responsibility to protect the public and the profession from unethical, incompetent, or illegal acts.*
> *B. Physical therapists may not participate in any arrangements in which patients are exploited due to the referring sources enhancing their personal incomes as a result of referring for, prescribing or recommending physical therapy."*
>
> - APTA, 1996

Providers as Advocates

Providers must assume a patient advocate responsibility when services are restricted by reimbursement or regulatory policies when a provider believes them to not be in the best interests of the patient. The patient remains the provider's primary customer even when others are funding the care. The provider enters into the two following contracts with their patients: a professional, or clinical, contract and a business contract. Both must be honored, and reimbursement pressures are often the wedge that is driven between these two obligations. For instance, Banja (1999) describes the following five impediments to reimbursement:

Table 17–5 American Physical Therapy Association "Code of Ethics" Preamble

This *Code of Ethics* of the American Physical Therapy Association sets forth principles for the ethical practice of physical therapy. All physical therapists are responsible for maintaining and promoting ethical practice. To this end, the physical therapist shall act in the best interest of the patient/client. This *Code of Ethics* shall be binding on all physical therapists.

Principle 1:	A physical therapist shall respect the rights and dignity of all individuals and shall provide compassionate care.
Principle 2:	A physical therapist shall act in a trustworthy manner toward patients/clients and in all other aspects of physical therapy practice.
Principle 3:	A physical therapist shall comply with laws and regulations governing physical therapy and shall strive to effect changes that benefit patients/clients.
Principle 4:	A physical therapist shall exercise sound professional judgment.
Principle 5:	A physical therapist shall achieve and maintain professional competence.
Principle 6:	A physical therapist shall maintain and promote high standards for physical therapy practice, education, and research.
Principle 7:	A physical therapist shall seek only such remuneration as is deserved and reasonable for physical therapy services.
Principle 8:	A physical therapist shall provide and make available accurate and relevant information to patients/clients about their care and to public about physical therapy services.
Principle 9:	A physical therapist shall protect the public and the profession from unethical, incompetent, and illegal acts.
Principle 10:	A physical therapist shall endeavor to address the health needs of society.

From American Physical Therapy Association, House of Delegates, June 2000.

1. Erosion of private insurance.
2. Insurers' refusal to reimburse for services.
3. Lack of empirical data to justify the medical necessity of rehabilitation.
4. Financial incentives to reduce care.
5. Employers' Retirement Income Security Act (ERISA).

Rehabilitation providers are in the position to influence three of these impediments. Providers have an ethical responsibility to demonstrate the medical necessity of their services. Medical necessity is a term used by payers to justify payment of health care services (Howard, 1991; Oberg et al, 1997; Rosenblatt & Harwitz, 1999; Smoak, 1999). Medical necessity determinations can be part of a preadmission or precertification process through concurrent telephonic case management or retrospectively through a clinical record review.

Medical Necessity Determination

Medical necessity is an ambiguous term with no universal definition embraced by payers or providers (Jacobson et al, 1997). Ethical dilemmas are created for rehabilitation providers who may desire to treat or manage persons with similar conditions in a fair and consistent manner. Health plans use varying reimbursement criteria, however, to describe medical necessity. This practice means that patients may receive varying levels, duration, and intensity of service. This variance is dictated more by coverage limitations than by a patient needs-based approach. Rehabilitation providers, therefore, must understand how the various payers with whom they engage define and execute policy. This understanding may avoid and/or ameliorate ethical challenges. Establishment of the medical necessity of care can overcome an insurer's refusal to pay and partly fulfill the fiduciary responsibility (business obligation) owed to the patient. A failure to do so can potentially place the patient in the position of paying for services to which the patient believed she or he was entitled.

Providers can support research efforts that assist in demonstrating the value of rehabilitation services. Lastly, financial incentives to deliver fewer or inferior services present ethical dilemmas that must be addressed by providers. Resolving these issues may require an introspective examination of therapist attitudes and practices as they relate to the principles of beneficence, autonomy, justice, non-maleficence, and paternalism. Clearly, few hard and fast rules exist that apply to all situations, however, providers are encouraged to consult with their profession's practice standards and code of ethics. These core documents can be invaluable guideposts that can assist providers in the development of consistent responses to moral dilemmas. Rehabilitation providers are challenged to address disparities between a reimbursement-driven practice and a patient needs-based practice (Burke & Cassidy, 1991).

Those in a position to question and modify provider treatment selection, duration, and intensity (e.g., utilization reviewers) have been historically immune to legal liabilities because they do not have a legal contract with the patient. Gray (1991) recommends that if utilization reviewers are entitled to make or influence clinical decisions, then regulators should proclaim utilization review as the practice of medicine. This situation would ensure that only providers would determine the medical necessity (Gray, 1991).

Patient Selection and Admission

Clinicians must consider both clinical and non-clinical issues when determining who is a candidate for their service. This determination is multifaceted and involves several layers of decision making. Clinicians face ethical dilemmas when a patient qualifies for service on one level but not another. For instance, a person's medical condition may warrant rehabilitation services and be well aligned with the professional capabilities of the provider and the facility. If the patient's health benefit plan does not cover rehabilitation intervention, however, then a policy issue interferes with an ethical obligation to treat those in need.

This situation raises several issues for the provider. One, he or she must serve in an advocacy role and attempt to justify treatment to a third-party payer. If this attempt is unsuccessful, the provider may need to consider whether or not to extend pro bono services, which some consider to be a hallmark of professionalism (Scott, 1997). Realistically, a provider may not be able to offer pro bono or free services to all those whose benefit plans fail to cover necessary interventions. So how does one determine who receives free care and who does not? What criteria for patient selection do the provider use? These perplexing questions require that each and every case be judged on its own merits. Individual cases may require that the provider reconcile his or her own beliefs with those of the health care organization for whom the provider works, a need that raises another important question: *Should an individual provider's moral beliefs and ethical actions outweigh those of the health care facility?* No easy or universal answers to these dilemmas exist. As professionals, rehabilitation providers must consider the needs and welfare of the patient above all others. This notion is easily stated, but more difficult to honor in today's increasingly complex environment.

Patient-Provider Relationship

Many ethical issues are presented during the patient-provider relationship period, beginning with how the provider describes the person with a problem (Meier & Purtilo, 1994). Debate exists concerning whether the person in need of rehabilitation services is a "patient" or a "client" (Herzberg, 1990). This issue is more than a debate about semantics, because how the rehabilitation provider addresses the individual may indeed set the tone of the relationship. As stated earlier in this chapter, the term "patient" implies a hands-on, "provider-will-treat" approach. The "client" label implies that there is greater client participation, especially in decision-making. It also implies that the individual will engage in more self-help activities and the provider in more teaching opportunities. "Client" also implies more of a business relationship than does "patient," which is clearly a paternalistic clinical term.

According to Meier and Purtilo, the caregiver and the person with a disability develop an intermittent interdependence, with a relationship that alternates between autonomy and paternalism. This interdependence is also consistent with "situational ethics" as described by Scott (1997).

Legal Versus Ethical Dilemmas

These scenarios are examples of situations in which a provider may choose to solicit a legal opinion in addition to an ethical recommendation. Providers can experience intense conflict when their ethical principles are challenged by legal issues. Employment contracts between the provider and a health care organization are one example of this conflict. Scott's (1997) legal-ethical rubric provides clinicians with an excellent means of gauging the relationship between legal and ethical actions. This rubric illustrates that legal and ethical issues may be congruent at times and incongruent in other circumstances (Figure 17-3).

Legal and ethical issues can be mutually inclusive or mutually exclusive depending on the facts involved in a situation. For instance, rehabilitation provider employment contracts that contain treatment or revenue quotas may be legal but unethical. This example would fall in the left lower quadrant of the rubric. Billing for services not rendered would fall into the lower right quadrant as it

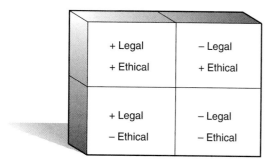

Figure 17–3. Legal and ethical rubric.

potentially could be viewed as both illegal and unethical behavior. Disclosure of a potentially harmful public health issue may be both a legal and ethical action occupying a place in the left upper quadrant. Provider forgiveness of a deductible or co-payment in the case of an indigent or impoverished patient may be a kind, charitable and ethical gesture, but highly illegal under insurance law (upper right quadrant). This discussion does not constitute a legal opinion. Providers are advised to seek qualified legal counsel when addressing perplexing ethical and legal scenarios.

Evidence-Based Practice

The long-held clinical belief of doing everything possible is challenged by evidence-based practice. Evidence-based practice strives to achieve optimal outcomes from minimal expenditures (Maynard, 1997). Evidence-based practice recognizes that there are limited resources and that efficacy alone cannot support the intensity, duration and cost of service. The three "Es" of efficacy, effectiveness and efficiency are incorporated in evidence-based practice. Evidence-based practice does not imply dispassionate care. The use of clinical research supportive of an intervention does not mean that the rehabilitation provider is any less compassionate in the delivery of services. It simply means that they are appreciative of limited resources and their dual moral agency of business and clinical administration. Evidence-based practice does not supplant the art of health care. Disability management goes well beyond simply the treatment of a clinical impairment and incorporates a holistic approach that addresses psychosocial, economic, vocational, and many other non-medical factors.

Physical rehabilitation has embraced a new paradigm regarding disability (Jette, 1995; Rothstein, 1994). Providers are seeking evidence to support their treatment interventions. There is acknowledgement that rehabilitation has not always focused on outcomes, but often dwells on process items, especially impairments (Jette, 1995). Providers are now obligated to incorporate an evidence-based approach that results in functionally-based outcomes. Compassionate care and evidence-based practice are not mutually exclusive terms. Ignoring evidence in the design and implementation of health care services could

arguably be considered unethical (Christenson & Lou, 2001).

Prayer as Therapy

Perhaps no other issue raises the degree of controversy and ethical challenges than that of prayer as therapy (Howe, 1995; Jaret, 1998; Friedman, 1996; Levin, 1994; Matthews & Larson, 1997). A discussion of ethics is incomplete without at least a cursory mention of the subject, and it is included here for several reasons. First, therapists may find themselves in clinical situations that require hospice care, particularly with today's aging population and the survivability of persons with various ailments such as AIDS, cancer, spinal cord injury, and traumatic brain injury. Second, if rehabilitation considers a holistic approach to be of value, then shouldn't prayer and spirituality be considered important components? Third, some evidence suggests that prayer is effective in healing (Friedman & Myers, 1996; Matthews & Clark, 1998).

Americans increasingly seek non-medical or non-traditional means of solving their health care problems, especially chronic illnesses or terminal conditions (Astin, 1998; Matthews et al, 1998). The use of complementary and alternative medicine and health care is a growing trend (Astin, 1998; Ernst, 2000). Some consider prayer to be a form of complementary and alternative health care (Cohen et al, 2000).

The Hastings Center, a well-known institution that studies ethics, has published an article entitled "Prayer as Therapy: A Challenge to Both Religious Belief and Professional Ethics." This seminal piece clearly outlines the ethical issues that surround prayer (Cohen et al, 2000). These authors note that religion and medicine have been historically closely linked as they share the following common human goals: compassion, comfort, and understanding. Yet, religion and health care have points of distinction as well as points of intersection. Cohen and cohorts contend that religious and spiritual beliefs are viewed by some patients as critical in coping with disease and injury. Through a logical extension, they therefore assert that providers should consider their patients' religious faith when co-designing treatment plans. Others go so far as to advocate that providers initiate bedside prayer in their treatment interventions (Dossey, 1993).

Cohen and associates believe that providers have a duty of beneficence in attending to the religious convictions of their patients. How this goal is achieved will clearly be the decision of the individual provider of service.

The ethical dilemmas presented when a provider introduces faith-based healing are obvious. Not all patients are religious or spiritual, nor do they all wish to be approached in this regard. One could reasonably argue that patients are in a position of vulnerability and that initiating spiritual counseling to them may be potentially exploitative. Training of providers raises another issue for debate. There are perhaps more questions than answers concerning the role of prayer in health care: *What happens when patient-provider religious beliefs differ? Are rehabilitation providers the best choice for this intervention? How are results measured? Should clinical documentation incorporate spiritual issues?*

Ultimately, for all ethical dilemmas each clinical situation requires assessment on its own merits. The patient's expectations and the provider's interpretation of what differentiates ethical from unethical behavior must be taken into account (Table 17–6).

The following actions may be prudent in light of the relative infancy of rehabilitation ethics in an ever-complex health care system:

- Consult with an attorney when in doubt about what constitutes legal versus ethical behavior. The National Healthcare Lawyers Association is a good starting point.
- Consult with an ethicist when facing ethical dilemmas that have no easy solutions.
- Consult with a hospital or organization's ombudsman or contact an ombudsman hotline.
- Consult with your patient concerning spiritual and religious needs.
- Refer to the Suggested Readings at the end of the chapter.
- Refer to the *Bibliography of Bioethics* by Walters and Kahn (Walters & Kahn, 1995). This bibliography strives to cite all English literature related to bioethics from multiple media sources. It uses a cross-disciplinary monitoring system that cites introduction, list of journals, subject entry, and author index. This reference is

organized by subject entries, such as "AIDS testing and screening" and "informed consent." Providers may find it useful in establishing guidelines for ethical conduct. However, providers are encouraged to refer to professional associations for guidance on these matters as well.

CHAPTER SUMMARY POINTS

- Ethical dilemmas occur when two or more ethical principles or values are in conflict.
- A provider's personal moral and belief system may or may not be congruent with a profession's code of ethics.
- Providers may need to serve in a dual moral role, and seek a balance between divergent agendas.
- Providers can adopt different ethics theories (e.g., virtue ethics, rule-based ethics, situational ethics) to solve ethical dilemmas.
- Ethical and legal issues may or may not be in conflict.
- Ethical challenges are certain to grow along with the complexity of the health care environment.
- Ethical dilemmas for rehabilitation providers will grow in both frequency and complexity as providers assume increasing levels of clinical and fiduciary responsibilities.

Kirschner (2001) outlines in Table 17–7 a set of priorities for future education of rehabilitation professionals. These priorities were identified by professionals according to their importance, with a "high" rating assigned to the issues with greatest priority, a "low" rating to the least prioritized items, and a "moderate" rating to those that fall between these extremes.

Table 17–6 Tips for Rehabilitation Providers in Avoiding and Mitigating Ethical Dilemmas

- When appropriate, co-develop goals with the patient, their family and other caregivers.
- Clarify the goals and expectations of referring physicians, especially primary care or gatekeepers.
- Clearly articulate in writing patient, family, and provider responsibilities.
- Consult with both an ethicist and attorney when crafting an informed consent document.
- Clearly articulate in writing assessment measures to be used to gauge patient functional and/or quality of life measures.
- Read and understand the limitations imposed by a patient's insurance or benefit plan before commencing treatment.
- Do not assume that the patient and his or her family comprehends benefit structures.
- Post your facility's Code of Ethics, Value Statements, Reimbursement Collection Policy, and Patient Bill of Rights in range of patient's sight.
- Design ethics education programs for new and experienced clinicians. Use case scenarios for discussion of ethical dilemmas. Refer to Kornblau & Starling (2000) under Suggested Readings in this chapter.
- Provide educational workshops to case managers, claims adjusters, and other non-medical stakeholders so that they gain a greater understanding of the principles, practices, and outcomes of physical rehabilitation.
- Attend seminars, symposia, monthly meetings of local claims associations, case management associations, employer groups, legal associations, and risk management societies so that providers gain a greater appreciation of their goals, expectations and desires as they relate to rehabilitation.
- Consult with your professional association about specific ethical dilemmas. Refer to core documents (e.g. Codes of Ethics, Practice Guidelines), review the clinical literature, and consult with known experts or ethicists.

Table 17–7 Topics of Interest for Future Education

Topics	High (%)	Moderate (%)	Low (%)
1. Decision making: patient's role	87	10	2
2. Conflict resolution: between health care team-patient	84	13	3
3. Assessment of decision-making capacity	74	23	3
4. Patient's rights	72	23	5
5. Withholding or withdrawal of care	67	27	6
6. Confidentiality issues	67	22	11
7. Decision-making: family's role	63	34	3
8. Ethical issues: goal setting	61	35	4
9. Advance directives	61	32	6
10. Informed consent	60	30	8
11. Assessing patient "potential"	53	40	6
12. Decision-making: provider's role	51	40	8
13. Allocation of limited resources	47	47	6
14. Conflict resolution: between providers	42	48	10
15. Ethical issues: outcomes scales	38	48	13
16. Research ethics	28	48	24
17. Decision making: third-party/payers	22	27	51

Key: Respondents assigned the numeral "1" to those issues of highest priority, "2" to those of "moderate" priority, and "3" to those of lowest priority.
Data from: Kirschner KL et al: Ethical issues identified by rehabilitation clinicians. Arch Phys Med Rehabil (82)(Suppl 2):S7, 2001.

REFERENCES

American Occupational Therapy Association (AOTA): Referral for profit (white paper). Am J Occup Ther 44(9):852-853, 1990.

American Physical Therapy Association (APTA): Code of Ethics and Guide for Professional Conduct. Alexandria, VA, APTA, 1990.

Andre J (1999): The alleged incompatibility of business and medical ethics. HEC Forum 11(4):288-292, 1999.

Andre J, Velasquez M: Ethics and virtue. Ethics Connection 1(3):1-3, 2000, Makula Center for Applied Ethics, www.scu.ed/SCU/Centers/Ethics/publications.html, accessed September 8, 2000.

Astin JA: Why patients use alternative medicine: Results of a national study. JAMA 279(19):1548-1553, 1998.

Bailey DM, Schwartzberg S: Ethical and Legal Dilemmas in Occupational Therapy. Philadelphia, FA Davis, 2003.

Banja JD: Ethics, values, and world culture: the impact on rehabilitation. Disabil Rehabil 18(6):279-284, 1996.

Banja JD: Patient advocacy at risk: Ethical, legal and political dimensions of adverse reimbursement practices in brain injury rehabilitation in the US Brain Inj 13(10):745-758, 1999.

Benson H: Timeless Healing: The Power and Biology of Belief. New York, Scribner, 1996.

Bivins TH: Virtue ethics, Oregon, 2000, University of Oregon, http://jcomm.uoregon.edu/~tbivins/J397/Links/VirtueEthics.html, accessed March 12, 2002.

Blackmer J: Ethical issues in rehabilitation medicine. Scand J Rehabil Med 32(2):51-55, 2000.

Bodenheimer T: The HMO backlash-Righteous or reactionary. New Engl J Med 335(21):1601-1604, 1996.

Bonder B: Standardized assessments: Ethical principles for use. Am J Occup Ther 39(7):473-474, 1985.

Brody BA: Justice in allocation of public resources to disabled citizens. Arch Phys Med Rehabil 69:333-336, 1988.

Bruhn JG: Equal partners: Doctors and patients explore the limits of autonomy. J Okla State Med Assoc 94(2):46-54, 2001.

Burke JP, Cassidy JC: Disparity between reimbursement-driven practice and humanistic values of occupational therapy. Am J Occup Ther 45(2):172-176, 1991.

Cadette WM: Regulating HMOs: An ethical framework for cost-effective medicine. Annandale-on-Hudson, NY, The Levy Economics Institute, Public Policy Brief No. 47, 1998.

Callahan D: Allocating health care resources: The vexing case of rehabilitation. Am J Phys Med Rehabil 72:101-105, 1995.

Callahan ME, Addoms EC, Schulz BF: Objectives of basic physical therapy education. Phys Ther Rev 41:795-797, 1961.

Caplan AL: Informed consent and provider-patient relationships in rehabilitation medicine. Arch Phys Med Rehabil 69(5):312-317, 1988.

Caplan AL, Callahan D, Haas J: Ethical and policy issues in rehabilitation medicine. Hastings Center Rep 17(Suppl):S1-S19, 1987.

Christenson C, Lou JQ: Ethical considerations related to evidence-based practice. Am J Occup Ther 55(3):345-349, 2001.

Clifton DW: Is the threat within? Workers compensation and physical therapy reimbursement. Phys Ther Today 18(2):10-13, 1995.

Cohen CB, Wheeler SE, Scott DA, et al: Prayer as therapy: A challenge to both religious belief and professional ethics. The Anglican Working Group in Bioethics. Hastings Center Rep 30(3):40-47, 2000.

Coy JA: Autonomy-based informed consent: Ethical implications for patient noncompliance. Phys Ther 69(10):826-833, 1989.

Daniels N: Duty to treat or right to refuse? Hastings Center Rep 21(2):36-46, 1991.

Degnin FD: Between a rock and a hard place: Ethics in managed care and the physician-patient relationship. Managed Care Q 7(2):15-22, 1999.

Dossey L: Healing Words: The Power of Prayer and the Practice of Medicine. San Francisco, Harper, 1993.

Emanuel EJ: Medical ethics in the era of managed care: The need for institutional structure instead of principles for individual cases. J Clin Ethics 6(4):335-338, 1995.

Ernst E: Prevalence of use of complementary and alternative medicine: A systematic review. Bull World Health Organ 78(2):252-257, 2000.

Evans RW: Health care technology and the inevitability of resource allocation and rationing decisions. Part I. JAMA 249(75):2047-2053, 1983.

Evert MM: Competency: Ethical issues and dilemmas. Am J Occup Ther 47(6):487-489, 1993.

Figa SF, Figa HM: Redefining full and fair disclosure of HMO benefits and limitations. Seton Hall Legislative J 14:151, 1990.

Friedman E: Managed care and managing ethics. Healthcare Forum J 36(4):13-15, 1993.

Friedman E: A matter of value, profits and losses in healthcare. Health Progress 77(3):28-34, 48, 1996.

Friedman R, Myers P: Spiritual intervention may help patients. JAMA 347:1320, 1996.

Gaynor M, Rebitzer JB, Taylor LJ: Incentives in HMOs. National Bureau of Economic Research, Inc., NBER Working Paper #w8522, 2001, www.papers.nber.org/papers/expecting/w8522, accessed January 2, 2004.

Golenski JD, Cloutier M: The ethics of managed care. Med Group Manage J 41(5):22, 24-26, 28, 1994.

Gostin LO: Managed care, conflicts of interest, and quality. Hastings Center Rep 30(5):27-28, 2000.

Gray BH: The Profit Motive and Patient Care. The Changing Accountability of Doctors and Hospitals. Cambridge, MA, Harvard University Press, 1991.

Guccione AA: Ethical issues in physical therapy: A survey of physical therapists in New England. Phys Ther 60(10):1264-1272, 1980.

Gunderson M: Eliminating conflicts of interesting managed care organizations through disclosure and consent. J Law Med Ethics 25(2-3):192-1983, 1997.

Guthrie SL: Immanuel Kant and the categorical imperative. The Examined Life-on-Line Philosophy Journal 2(7):1-9, 2001, http://guthrie.net/kant.html, accessed March 19, 2002.

Haas JH: Ethical considerations of goal setting for patient care in rehabilitation medicine. Am J Phys Med Rehabil 72:228-232, 1993.

Haas JF: Ethical issues in rehabilitation medicine. In DeLisa JA, Gans BM (eds): Rehabilitation Medicine: Principles and Practice. 2d ed. Philadelphia, JB Lippincott, 1993, pp 28-39.

Haas JH, MacKenzie CA: The role of ethics in rehabilitation medicine. Am J Phys Med Rehabil 74(1)(Suppl):S3-S6, 1995.

Haddad AM: Teaching ethical analysis in occupational therapy. Am J Occup Ther 42(5):300-304, 1988.

Hall MA, Berenson RA: Ethical practice in managed care: A dose of realism. Ann Intern Med 128:395-402, 1998.

Harris WS: Effects of remote intercession prayer on outcomes in patients admitted to coronary care unit. Arch Int Med 159:2273-2278, 1999.

Herzberg SR: Client or patient: Which term is more appropriate for use in occupational therapy? Am J Occup Ther 444(6):561-564, 1990.

Higgins W: Ethical guidance in the era of managed care: An analysis of the American College of Healthcare Executives Code of Ethics. J Healthcare Manage 45(1):32-42, discussion 43-45, 2000.

Hildred W, Watkins L: The nearly good, the bad and the ugly in cost-effectiveness analysis of health care. J Econ Issues 30:755-775, 1996.

Hillman AL, Pauly MV, Kerstein JJ: How do financial incentives affect physicians' clinical decisions and the financial performance of health maintenance organizations? New Engl J Med 321:86-92, 1989.

Hofmann PB: Caught between two paradigms...ensuring that quality of care is not affected by managed care. Healthcare Executive 10(2):39, 1995.

Howard BS: How high do we jump? The effect of reimbursement on occupational therapy. Am J Occup Ther 10:875-881, 1991.

Howe EG: Influencing a patient's religious beliefs: Mandate or no-man's land? J Clin Ethics 6(3):194-201, 1995.

Hunt AR: Legal issues involved in the use of restraints: Analyzing the risks. In Untie the Elderly: Quality Care Without Restraints, A symposium before the Special Committee on Aging, U.S. Senate, Serial No. 101—111. Washington, DC, US Government Printing Office, 1990, pp 197-202.

Imrie R: Rethinking the relationships between disability, rehabilitation, and society. Disabil Rehabil 19(7):263-271, 1997.

Jacobson D et al: Defining and implementing medical necessity in Washington state and Oregon. Inquiry 34:143-154, 1997.

Jaret P: Can prayer heal? Health March:48-54, 1998.

Jette A: Outcomes research: Shifting the dominant research paradigm in physical therapy. Phys Ther 75(11):965-970, 1995.

Kane RL, Kane RA: The impact of long-term-care financing on personal autonomy. Generations 14(Suppl):S86-S89, 1990.

Kaplan D: Managed care: Gag clause and doctor-patient communication: Sate responses. J Law Med Ethics 25(2-3):213-218, 1997.

Khushf G: The case for managed care: Reappraising medical and sociopolitical ideals. J Med Philos 24(5):415-433, 1999.

Kirschner KL, Stocking C, Wagner LB: Ethical issues identified by rehabilitation clinicians. Arch Phys Med Rehabil 82(Suppl 2):S2-S8, 2001.

Kapp MB: Nursing home restraints and industry practice. J Legal Med 13:1-32, 1992.

Kornblau BL, Starling SP: Ethics in Rehabilitation. Thorofare, NJ, Slack, 2000.

Kyler-Hutchison P: Ethical reasoning and informed consent in occupational therapy. Am J Occup Ther 42(5):283-287, 1988.

Levin JS: Religion and health: Is there an association, is it valid, and is it causal? Soc Sci Med 3:1475-1482, 1994.

Levinson DF: Toward full disclosure of referral restricting and financial incentives by prepaid health plans. New Engl J Med (317): 1729-1731, 1987.

Limentani AE: The role of ethical principles in health care ad the implications for ethical codes. J Med Ethics 25:394-398, 1999.

Maier E: Rehab and self-determination. Can Nurse 89(6):32-34, 1993.

Matthews DA, Larson DB: Faith and medicine: Reconciling the twin traditions of healing. Adv Mind Body Med 2:3-6, 1997.

Matthews DA et al: Religious commitment and health status. Arch Family Med 7:118-124, 1998.

Matthews DA, Clark C: The Faith Factor: Proof of the Healing Power of Prayer. New York, Viking, 1998.

Maynard A: Evidence-based medicine: An incomplete method for informing treatment choices. Lancet 349:126-128, 1997.

Meier RH 3rd, Purtilo RB: Ethical issues and the patient-provider relationship. Am J Phys Med Rehabil 73(5):365-366, 1994.

Miller TE, Sage WM: Disclosing physician financial incentives. JAMA 281(15):1424-1430, 1999.

Mitchell JM, Sass TR: Physician ownership of ancillary service: Indirect demand inducement or quality assurance? J Health Econ 14(3): 263-289, 1995.

Morreim EH: To tell the truth: Disclosing the incentives and limits of managed care. Am J Managed Care 3(1): 35-43, 1997.

Newman JF, Dunbar DM: Managed care and ethical conflicts. Manage Care Q 8(4):20-32, 2000.

Noone GC, Ubel PA: Managed care organizations should not disclose their physicians' financial incentives. Am J Managed Care 3(1): 159-160, 1997.

Oberg CN, Bosse LL, Moscow SR et al: Appropriate and necessary healthcare: New language for a new era. Am J Managed Care 3(3):423-428, 1997.

Physician Payment Review Commission (PPRC) (1995) Arrangements between Managed Care Plans and Physicians. Washington, DC, Health Care Financing Administration (HCFA), 1995.

Purtilo RB: Reading "physical therapy" from an ethics perspective. Phys Ther 55(4):361-364, 1976.

Purtilo RB: Protecting the "care" in managed care. Phys Ther Magazine 3(7):69-71, 1995.

Purtillo RB: Managed care: Ethical issues for the rehabilitation professions. Trends Health Care Law Ethics 10(1-2):105-108, 111, 1995.

Purtilo RB: Structure of ethics teaching in physical therapy: A survey. Phys Ther 59(9):1102-1109, 1979.

Purtilo RB: Ethics teaching in the allied health fields. Hastings Center Rep 8(2):14-16, 1978.

Purtilo RB: Justice in the distribution of health care resources. The position of physical therapists, physiatrists and rehabilitation nurses. Phys Ther 61(11):1594-1600, 1981.

Purtilo RB: Justice in the distribution of health care resources. The position of physical therapists in the United States and Sweden. Phys Ther 62(1):46-50, 1982.

Radel L, Pearso SD, Sabin JE et al: How managed care can be ethical. Health Aff (Project Hope) 20(4):43-56, 2001.

Ramsden E: Patients' right to know: Implementation for interpersonal communication processes. Phys Ther (55):133-138, 1975.

Rodwin MA: Medicine, Money and Morals: Physicians' Conflicts of Interest. New York, Oxford University Press, 1993.

Rosenblatt L, Harwitz DG: Fairness and rationing implications of medical necessity decisions. Am J Managed Care 5(12):1525-1531, 1999.

Rothstein JL: Disability and our identity. Phys Ther 74(5):375-377, 1994.

Rousseau P: Ethical and legal issues in palliative care. Primary Care 28(2):391-400, 2001.

Sadan B: Adapting informed consent to contemporary managed care. Med Law 19(3):545-547, 2000.

Scott R: Promoting Legal Awareness in Physical and Occupational Therapy. St Louis, Mosby, 1997.

Scott R: Professional Ethics: A Guide for Rehabilitation Professionals. St Louis, Mosby, 1998.

Shapiro RS, Tym KA, Gudmunson JL, et al: Managed care: Effects on the physician-patient relationship. Cambridge Q Healthcare Ethics 9(1):71-81, 2000.

Smoak RD Jr: Medical necessity: Who cares, who decides? Healthplan 40(4):19-20, 22, 1999.

Sturmpf F, Evans LK: The ethical problems of prolonged physical restraint. Geriatr Nurs 17(2):27-30.

Tepper D: The patient's bill of rights as a necessary step for now. Manage Care Interface 13(10):52, 56, 2000.

Thompson RE: Managed care's Achilles heel: Ethical immaturity. Physician Executive 26(2):33-36, 2000.

Tiel JR: Virtue ethics & core values. 1999, Ashland University, www.usafa.af.mil/jcope/JSCOPE99/Tiel99.html, accessed March 12, 2002.

Triezenberg HL: The identification of ethical issues in physical therapy. Phys Ther 76(10):1097-1107, 1996.

University of Washington School of Medicine: Ethics in medicine: Confidentiality, www.eduserv.hscer.washingto.edu/bioethics/topics/confidentialityhtml, accessed March 16, 2002.

Waldman M: Conflict of interest, physicians and physiotherapy. Can Med Assoc J 154(11):1737-1739, 1996.

Weber D: Second thoughts: Can managed care be ethical? Health Forum J 40(4):17, 20-25, 1997.

Weber LJ: The business of ethics: Hospitals need to focus on managerial ethics as much as clinical ethics. Health Progress 71(1):76-78, 1990.

Wennberg JE: A challenge to HMOs. HMO Practice/HMO Group 6(2): 5-10, 1992.

Wiener JM, Haley RJ: Winners and losers: Primary and high-tech care under health care rationing. Brookings Rev 10:46-49, 1991.

Zoloth-Dorfman L, Rubin S: The patient as commodity: Managed care and the question of ethics. J Clin Ethics 6(4):339-357, 1995.

SUGGESTED READINGS

Beauchamp TL, Childress JF (eds): Principles of biomedical ethics, 4th ed. New York, Oxford University Press, 1994.

Purtilo RB: Team challenges. Regulatory constraints and patient empowerment. Am J Phys Med Rehabil 5:327-330, 1993.

Purtilo RB: Rehabilitation and technology: Ethical considerations. Int J Technol Aging 4(2):163-170, 1991.

Purtilo RB: Thirty-first Mary McMillan lecture. A time to harvest, a time to sow: Ethics for a shifting landscape. Phys Ther 80(11):1112-1119, 2000.

CHAPTER 18

Fraud and Abuse Prevention: Legislative and Regulatory Issues of Importance for Rehabilitation Providers

Corrine Propas Parver, JD, PT

> ### KEY POINTS
>
> - The American health care system is currently undergoing dramatic and profound changes relative to fraud, abuse, and waste investigations and prosecutions. Antifraud initiatives are at an all-time high in both the private and public health care sectors.
> - To be effective under publicly funded benefits programs, rehabilitation providers must understand the legislative intent and regulatory rules/procedures.
> - Allegations of fraud and abuse can result when clinicians or health care organizations fail to understand and adhere to the rules and procedures of participation under federal and state-funded insurance programs.

This chapter provides an overview of pertinent legislative and regulatory issues that affect provider fraud and abuse in connection with federal and state health care programs, and discusses how providers can create an effective business ethics and corporate compliance program for their companies. Readers are encouraged to refer to the citations throughout the text for further guidance and more detailed elaboration.

FEDERAL ANTIKICKBACK STATUTE

The federal antikickback statute (the "Statute") (42 U.S.C. § 1320a-7b[b].) prohibits individuals and entities from knowingly and willfully offering or paying remuneration (including any kickback, bribe, or rebate), directly or indirectly, overtly or covertly, in cash or in kind to any person to induce such person to: (1) refer an individual to a person for the furnishing or arranging for the furnishing of any item or service for which payment may be made in whole or in part under a federal health care program; or (2) purchase, lease, order, or arrange for or recommend purchasing, leasing, or ordering any good, facility, service, or item for which payment may be made in whole or in part under a federal health care program.

Remuneration to induce referrals of items or services paid for by a federal health care program violates the Statute. By its terms, the Statute attributes criminal and civil liability to parties on either side of an illegal "kickback" transaction. Under the Statute, "remuneration" means the transfer of anything of value, in cash or in kind, directly or indirectly, covertly or overtly.

Violation of the Statute is considered a felony, which may result in criminal penalties and civil fines. Criminal sanctions can consist of a fine of not more than $25,000 or imprisonment for not more than 5 years, or both. Medicare law demands mandatory exclusion from all federal health care programs if one is convicted of a felony. Even without a conviction, the Department of Health and Human Services (HHS) is authorized to take administrative action to exclude a provider for an undetermined amount of time. For false or improper claims for payment, HHS may impose civil monetary penalties of as much as $10,000 and triple damages for each improper claim filed.

Although the Statute is viewed as an intent-based law—the parties must form the necessary intent to violate the law—a number of courts have interpreted the requisite level of intent differently. Some courts, for example, have held that if one of the purposes of remuneration under a given arrangement is the referral of services or the inducement of future referrals, the Statute has been violated, even if the payments made were also intended to compensate for professional services. The First Circuit upheld an instruction that the jury could find the defendant guilty if the "primary purpose" of the payment was an improper one of inducing referrals [*United States v. Bay State Ambulance and Hospital Rental Service, Inc.*, 874 F.2d 20, 29-30 (1st Cir. 1989)]. In contrast, in a subsequent decision the Ninth Circuit held that the phrase "knowingly and willfully" under the Statute means that the government must prove beyond a reasonable doubt that the defendant had a "specific intent to disobey the law." [*Hanlester Network v. Shalala*, 51 F.3d 1390, 1400 (9th Cir. 1995)]. Later cases, however, have declined to follow the reasoning of the *Hanlester* decision.

"Safe Harbors"

The Antikickback Statute includes six statutory exceptions and confers authority upon the HHS Office of Inspector General (OIG) to promulgate regulations excepting other transactions. [*See* 42 U.S.C. § 1320a-7b(b)(3).] Presently, statutory exceptions apply to the following:

1. Discounts
2. Payments to employees by employers
3. Vendor payments to particular group purchasing organizations
4. Particular waivers of patient co-payment or deductible amounts
5. Particular payment practices specified in regulations under section 14(a) of the Medicare and Medicaid Patient and Program Protection Act of 1987
6. Payments under particular risk-sharing arrangements

In addition, safe harbor regulations specifically delineate certain transactions to which civil fines and criminal penalties for the violation of the statute do not apply, provided that the transactions meet the requirements for such protection. [*See* 42 C.F.R. § 1001.952 (listing the attributes for various exceptions to the Antikickback Statute)].

Until the OIG's recent promulgation of new safe harbor regulations, safe harbors existed only for the following conditions and entities:

- Investment interests
- Space rental
- Equipment rental
- Personal services and management contracts
- Sale of practice
- Referral services
- Warranties
- Discounts
- Employees
- Group purchasing organizations
- Waiver of beneficiary coinsurance and deductible amounts

- Increased coverage, reduced cost-sharing amounts, or reduced premium amounts offered by health plans
- Price reductions offered to health care plans

The Centers for Medicare and Medicaid Services' (CMS) (formerly the Health Care Financing Administration [HCFA]) 1999 final safe harbor rule clarified many of the existing safe harbor regulations, including large and small entity investments, space and equipment rental and personal services and management contracts, and discounts. [*See* 64 Fed. Reg. 63518, 63521-63530 (November 19, 1999)]. This rulemaking was based on comments garnered in response to the 1993 proposed rule [58 Fed. Reg. 49008 (September 21, 1993)], the 1994 proposed clarifications [59 Fed. Reg. 37202 (July 21, 1994)], and the annual solicitations for suggestions for modified and new safe harbors (required under Section 205 of the Health Insurance Portability and Accountability Act of 1996 [HIPAA]).

In addition to modifying the "sale of practice" safe harbor, the OIG outlined the following seven new areas for safe harbor protection: investment interests in underserved areas, ambulatory surgical centers, group practices, practitioner recruitment, obstetrical malpractice insurance subsidies, referral agreements for specialty services, and cooperative hospital service organizations described in section 501(e) of the Internal Revenue Code.

"STARK" LAW

Section 1877 of the Social Security Act, otherwise known as the "Stark" law (named for the Congressman who introduced and sponsored the legislation, Fortney ("Pete") Stark (D-CA), prohibits a physician from referring a Medicare patient to an entity for certain designated health services if the physician has a financial relationship with the entity, unless an exception applies. (42 U.S.C. § 1395nn.)

Specifically, Section 1877(a)(1) of the Act states that:

[I]f a physician (or an immediate family member of such physician) has a financial relationship with an entity ... then (A) the physician may not make a referral to the entity for the furnishing of designated health services for which payment otherwise may be made under this title, and (B) the entity may not present or cause to be presented a claim under this title or bill to any individual, third party payor, or other entity for designated health services furnished pursuant to a referral prohibited under subparagraph (A).

Under Section 1877(g) of Stark, the statutory sanctions for violating this prohibition can include denial of payment to an entity furnishing services under a prohibited referral, refunds of billed amounts to any individual who has paid for a service furnished under a prohibited referral, assessment of civil money penalties, or exclusion from the Medicare program.

The original Stark law (Stark I) was passed in 1989 and became effective on January 1, 1992. Stark I prohibited physicians from referring Medicare patients to an entity furnishing laboratory services, where the physician has a financial relationship with that laboratory. Reimbursement claims for clinical laboratory services provided pursuant to a prohibited referral must not be presented for payment to the Medicare program. In 1993, Congress expanded Stark I by passing Stark II as part of the Omnibus Budget Reconciliation Act of 1993, and modified the Act yet again in the Social Security Act Amendments of 1994. The then HCFA promulgated regulations under Stark I, and CMS recently issued its final rules for Stark II.

Stark II expanded the self-referral restrictions in Stark I to apply to both the Medicare and Medicaid programs. The self-referral prohibition was extended beyond clinical laboratory services, and applied to ten additional designated health services (DHSs), including durable medical equipment (DME) and supplies, such as nebulizers and the drugs needed to use them, physical therapy, and orthotics and prosthetics.

Stark I and II prohibit the presentation of claims for payment for DHSs that were furnished pursuant to a prohibited referral. Such claims will be denied by Medicare and refunds sought for amounts previously paid by these programs. Stark is a civil statute that provides for civil money penalties of as much as $15,000 for each service that violates the prohibition on the presentation of such claims.

Under the Stark prohibition, a physician may not make a referral for a DHS to an entity in which he or she (or an immediate family member) has a financial interest. Health care entities may not submit or cause to be submitted a bill or claim for reimbursement to a federal health program for services provided pursuant to a prohibited referral. A referral includes any request by a physician for an item or service reimbursable under Medicare Part B (including a consultation with another physician, and any test or procedure ordered by or to be furnished by or under the supervision of another physician). The request or establishment of a plan of care by a physician that includes furnishing a DHS is also a referral.

The Stark statute defines a financial relationship as a direct or indirect relationship between a physician (or a member of a physician's immediate family) and an entity in which the physician (or family member) has the following interest:

- An ownership or investment interest through equity, debt, or other means including an interest in an entity holding an ownership or investment interest in the entity actually furnishing the services, or
- A compensation arrangement involving any remuneration to the physician or immediate family member.

An ownership or investment interest may be established through equity, debt, or other means, and includes an interest in an entity that holds an ownership or investment interest in another entity furnishing DHS. A compensation agreement is defined under Stark as any arrangement involving any remuneration, whether direct or indirect, between a physician (or an immediate family member) and an entity.

HEALTH INSURANCE PORTABILITY AND ACCOUNTABILITY ACT OF 1996

The Health Insurance Portability and Accountability Act of 1996 (HIPAA) was signed into law by President Clinton on August 21, 1996. [Pub. L. No. 104-191 (1996).] This act provided powerful new tools and a stable source of funding of more than $100 million dedicated to fighting health care fraud. HIPAA dedicates money each year for program integrity activities under the Medicare Integrity Program. For example, in fiscal year (FY) 2001, the then HCFA received $680 million for these activities.

Key fraud and abuse provisions of HIPAA include the following: theft or embezzlement, obstruction of criminal investigations into health care fraud, and making of false statements.

Fraud and Abuse Control

A new Health Care Fraud and Abuse Control Program is created, to be coordinated by HHS OIG and the Department of Justice. Funds for this program, the highlights of which are described below, are appropriated from the Medicare Hospital Insurance trust fund. The program accomplishes the following goals:

- Establishes the Medicare Integrity Program to be funded through appropriations from the HI trust fund
- Requires exclusion from Medicare and Medicaid for felony convictions related to health care fraud or controlled substances
- Creates a program encouraging Medicare beneficiaries to report fraud and abuse and offer suggestions to improve efficiency of the Medicare program, and provides for payment to beneficiaries in certain cases
- Requires issuance of OIG Advisory Opinions, additional safe harbors, and OIG Fraud Alerts regarding the Antikickback Statute
- Creates a new exception to the Antikickback Statute for certain risk-sharing organizations
- Expands conditions under which civil monetary penalties and intermediate sanctions can be imposed on health maintenance organizations participating in Medicare
- Establishes a database of final adverse actions taken against health care providers
- Makes knowing and willful transfer of assets to gain Medicaid eligibility subject to criminal penalties

BALANCED BUDGET ACT OF 1997

The Balanced Budget Act (BBA) of 1997 [Pub. L. No. 105-33 (1997)] contained sweeping payment changes to the Medicare program and provided new tools to combat fraud and abuse.

OPERATION RESTORE TRUST

In 1995, the Clinton Administration and the Department of HHS launched Operation Restore Trust (ORT), a comprehensive antifraud initiative in five key states designed to demonstrate new partnerships and new approaches in finding and stopping fraud and abuse in Medicare and Medicaid (HHS Press Release, 1995).

As part of ORT, HHS created an interdisciplinary project team of federal and state government and private sector representatives, including the HHS OIG, the then HCFA, the Administration on Aging, and the Department of Justice, to target Medicare and Medicaid abuse and misuse. Initially the project was conducted in the five states that comprised more than a third of all Medicare and Medicaid beneficiaries: California, Florida, New York, Texas, and Illinois. The ORT team focused primarily on the following three health care sectors of high spending growth: home health care; medical equipment; and nursing home care.

Special objectives for ORT included the following:

- Identify and penalize those persons and companies who willfully defraud the Medicare and Medicaid programs
- Identify systemic problems with special vulnerabilities to fraud and abuse in the Medicare and Medicaid programs
- Alter the public and health care sector to health care fraud schemes
- Demonstrate a new effort that provides especially for voluntary disclosure of evidence of fraud

During the initial 2-year demonstration, ORT identified $23 in overpayments for every $1 spent in the three targeted areas, and the OIG excluded 2700 fraudulent providers and companies from doing business with federal and state health care programs. Because of its successes, HHS expanded ORT to 24 states. Ongoing ORT activities that continue even now that the ORT demonstration has long concluded and which HHS has incorporated to prevent attempts to defraud Medicare and Medicaid include the following:

- Financial audits by OIG and CMS contractors
- Criminal investigations and referrals by OIG and other law enforcement officials
- Surveys and inspections of health care facilities by CMS and state officials
- Studies and recommendations by OIG and CMS for program adjustments to prevent fraud and reduce waste and abuse
- Issuance of Special Fraud Alerts to notify the public and the health care community about schemes in the provision of health care services, products, supplies, devices
- Fraud and Abuse "Hotline"
- Voluntary Disclosure Program
- Training of individuals within the aging network on how to identify and report suspected fraud and abuse

Today Medicare, Medicaid, and all other federal health care program contractors are trying to prevent fraud and abuse by supporting the investigation and prosecution of defrauders. Many law enforcement actions were started through contractors, such as carriers and fiscal intermediaries, and CMS regional office staff identification of problems and issues, and then through referrals by the contractors to the OIG.

RECENT FEDERAL FRAUD AND ABUSE INITIATIVES

As previously noted, HIPAA established a national Health Care Fraud and Abuse Control Program, under the joint direction of the attorney general and the HHS, acting through the HHS/OIG, which is designed to coordinate federal, state, and local law enforcement activities with respect to health care fraud and abuse. In its sixth year of operation, the program relies on a collaborative approach to identify and prosecute the most egregious instances of health care fraud, to prevent future fraud or abuse, and to protect Medicare beneficiaries and Medicaid recipients.

According to the OIG's most recently published statistics, in 2002, the federal government won or negotiated more than $1.8 billion in judgments, settlements, and administrative impositions in health care fraud cases and proceedings. As a result of these activities, as well as prior year judgments, settlements, and administrative impositions, the federal government collected more than $1.6 billion, of which approximately $1.4 billion was returned to the Medicare Trust Fund. An additional $59 million was recovered as the federal share of Medicaid restitution. This is the largest return to the government since the inception of the program.

Federal prosecutors filed 361 criminal indictments in health care fraud cases in 2002. A total of 480 defendants were convicted for health care fraud–related crimes during the year. There were also 1529 civil matters pending, and 221 civil cases filed in 2002. HHS excluded 3448 individuals and entities from participating in the Medicare and Medicaid programs or other federally sponsored health care programs, most as a result of convictions for crimes relating to Medicare or Medicaid, for patient abuse or neglect, or as a result of licensure revocations.

The following is an Internet link to the OIG's full report on the program's results:

http://oig.hhs.gov/publications/docs/hcfac/HCFAC%20Annual%20Report%20FY%202002.htm#1.

FRAUD PREVENTION AND COMPLIANCE FOR HEALTH CARE PROVIDERS

Combating health care fraud and abuse is a growing federal government enforcement priority, with 2278 civil matters pending at the end of 1999 and 371 criminal indictments in health care fraud cases in 1999 and even more in the 21st century. Significantly, the federal government imposes high standards on health care companies in an attempt to ensure that they comply with the Byzantine regulations and guidance that make up the federally funded health care programs. Many health care entities are turning to corporate compliance programs to address these concerns. Compliance plans have come to be seen as the key to staying on the right side of the fraud and abuse laws.

A compliance program has several benefits. First, an effective program can reduce the likelihood of violations by training employees as to what behavior is impermissible. Second, creating and implementing such a program can reduce certain criminal penalties for a health care provider or entity if violations do arise. Third, an effective corporate compliance plan may be helpful in settlement negotiations with the federal government on both civil and administrative matters, framing the entity as a responsible corporate citizen. Finally, when done correctly, a compliance plan also can be good business, helping to discover little problems before they develop into big ones and providing employees with an outlet to disclose perceived wrongs.

During the past several years, HHS OIG, one of the major health-related enforcement arms of the federal government, introduced several compliance guidance documents (Guidance) involving health care industry entities. Compliance guidance is the OIG's attempt to engage the private health care community in addressing and fighting fraud and abuse.

> *"While enforcement is an essential element of the government's anti-fraud and abuse campaign, so is prevention," former OIG Inspector General June Gibbs Brown stated. "And the cornerstone of our prevention efforts is the development of voluntary compliance guidance that will help the health care industry meet the high ethical and legal standards we expect of those doing business with the government."*

The foundation of the OIG's Guidance documents mirrors the compliance elements set forth in the United States Federal Sentencing Guidelines. The Guidelines articulate the following seven elements: (1) implementation of written policies, procedures, and standards of conduct; (2) designation of a high-level compliance officer and other appropriate compliance officials; (3) development of training and education programs; (4) measures for receiving complaints; (5) enforcement of standards through well-publicized disciplinary directives; (6) performance of internal audits; and (7) prompt response to detected offenses through corrective action.

Weaving compliance into the fabric of an organization is consistent with the culture and values of most health care providers and entities. Because of cost, complexity, or unfeasibility, however, some elements suggested by OIG may not be appropriate for all such entities. Nevertheless, OIG instructs health care companies to implement each of the seven elements and believes that every provider regardless of size or structure can and should strive to accomplish the objectives and principles underlying all of the compliance policies and procedures recommended within the OIG's Model Guidances.

Superficial programs that have the appearance of compliance without being wholeheartedly adopted by the health care company will be ineffective. A "paper" compliance plan that says all the right things but is not embraced by the entity is worse than no plan at all. The following examines each of the seven recommended Guidance elements in turn.

1. Written Policies and Procedures

The OIG believes it essential that all health care entities develop written, company-wide compliance policies and procedures to be followed by all employees. Every health care company can articulate in writing a commitment to comply with federally-funded health care program standards, and demonstrate an ongoing commitment to prevent and detect fraud and abuse in its operations. Policies and procedures should be related to risk areas noted by the OIG—for example, a company's compliance policy should indicate that billing for items not actually provided will not be tolerated.

2. Designation of a Compliance Officer and Compliance Committee

The OIG suggests that health care companies should designate a Chief Compliance Officer to serve as the focal point for compliance activities, who should report directly to the chief executive and governing body.

3. Conducting Effective Training and Education

Under the Guidances, companies must take steps to communicate compliance standards and procedures to all employees and other agents. The OIG expects that complex publications and training programs may not be feasible for many smaller entities. For example, OIG has suggested posttraining examinations to ensure efficacy. For a smaller provider or entity, training can be more informal and ongoing. The OIG also has suggested publishing monthly compliance newsletters.

4. Developing Effective Lines of Communication

Anonymous reporting procedures, such as a confidential hotline, are desirable where the idea of a secret reporting mechanism makes logical sense. The same is true for the OIG recommended intake form for compliance issues. An open-door policy of a personable and approachable compliance ombudsman can satisfy the same underlying concerns about having a channel for reporting potential fraud, waste, or abuse.

5. Enforcing Standards Through Well-Publicized Disciplinary Guidelines

The OIG suggests that compliance standards be enforced through appropriate disciplinary mechanisms, requiring a written policy statement setting forth the degrees of disciplinary actions that may be imposed for various infractions. In certain situations, the health care company can handle human resource problems on an ad hoc basis. A concise statement that all questionable actions will be investigated and appropriate disciplinary action will be taken is effective.

6. Auditing and Monitoring

Auditing and monitoring are important pieces of a corporate compliance plan. For example, the OIG encourages testing of billing staff by use of hypothetical scenarios or assessing awareness through validated survey instruments. A successful business operation usually has in place some type of system for periodically reviewing an employee's actual work product.

7. Responding to Detected Offenses and Developing Corrective Action Initiatives

The OIG has stated that if an entity discovers credible evidence of misconduct from any source and, after a reasonable inquiry, has reason to believe a violation may have occurred, then the entity should promptly report the misconduct to the appropriate governmental authorities within a reasonable period but not more than 60 days after determining that credible evidence exists of a violation.

Health care companies must exercise discretion when responding to detected misconduct and preventing it from reoccurring.

CONCLUSION

Adopting and implementing an effective corporate compliance program can help health care providers and entities avoid pending enforcement actions. A "canned" compliance plan will not be effective. Rather, a program that is custom-tailored to the size, culture, and pertinent risk areas of an organization is the only way for a compliance plan to be woven into the fabric of the organization and remain successful in today's aggressive and overly harsh enforcement environment.

REFERENCES

42 U.S.C. § 1320a-7b(b).

United States v. Kats, 871 F.2d 105, 108 (9th Cir. 1989); *United States v. Greber*, 760 F.2d 68, 72 (3d Cir. 1985), *cert. denied*, 474 U.S. 988 (1985).

See 42 U.S.C. § 1320a-7b(b)(3).

42 C.F.R. § 1001.952 (listing the attributes for various exceptions to the Anti-kickback Statute).

64 Fed. Reg. 63518, 63521-63530 (November 19, 1999). This rulemaking was based on comments garnered in response to the 1993 proposed rule (58 Fed. Reg. 49008 (September 21, 1993), the 1994 proposed clarifications (59 Fed. Reg. 37202 (July 21, 1994), and the annual solicitations for suggestions for modified and new safe harbors (required under HIPAA's Section 205).

42 U.S.C. § 1395nn. Pub. L. No. 104-191 (1996).

Pub. L. No. 105-33 (1997).

HHS Press Release, Secretary Schalala announces "Operation Restore Trust," May 3, 1995.

HCFA Fact Sheet, April 2000.

CHAPTER 19

Federal Reimbursement-Focused Statutes for Rehabilitation Providers

Corrine Propas Parver, JD, PT

KEY POINTS

- Success in securing reimbursement for rehabilitation services is predicated on an understanding of the rules, policies and procedures related to rehabilitation services.
- To successfully achieve payment for services, rehabilitation providers must be able to distinguish between what is medically necessary and unnecessary, and to grasp the differences between restorative service and maintenance service and skilled service versus unskilled services.
- Clear, concise, functionally based clinical documentation is a key to reimbursement success under government-sponsored insurance plans.

This chapter provides a general description of pertinent legislative issues of importance to physical rehabilitation providers and entities that provide services to beneficiaries and recipients of federal and state health care program benefits. Readers are encouraged to refer to the citations throughout the text for further guidance and more detailed elaboration.

MEDICARE

Title XVIII of the Social Security Act, "Health Insurance for the Aged and Disabled," is commonly known as Medicare. (*See* 42 U.S.C. §§ 1395 *et. seq.*)

As part of the Social Security Amendments of 1965, the Medicare legislation established a health insurance program for aged persons to complement the retirement, survivors, and disability insurance benefits that exist under other titles of the Social Security Act. When first implemented in 1966, Medicare covered most persons aged 65 years and older. Since then, legislation has added the following groups: (1) persons who are entitled to disability benefits for 24 months or more (1972), (2) persons with end-stage renal disease requiring dialysis or kidney transplant (1972), and (3) certain otherwise non-covered persons who elect to buy into the Medicare program (1973).

The Medicare program, which is administered by the Centers for Medicare and Medicaid Services (CMS) (formerly the Health Care Financing Administration or [HCFA]), consists of two parts: hospital insurance (HI), also known as Part A; and supplementary medical insurance, also known as Part B. HI (Part A) is usually provided automatically for persons aged 65 years and older and to most persons who are disabled for 24 months or more who are entitled to Social Security or Railroad Retirement benefits. Part A covers an estimated 40 million aged and disabled beneficiaries, and a slightly smaller number are covered by Part B, which requires payment of a monthly premium. A major aspect of HI is the "benefit period," defined as the measurement of time-duration for inpatient care. No limit exists on the number of benefit periods covered by HI during a beneficiary's lifetime.

The following list describes the health services for which Part A of Medicare reimburses providers, such as inpatient hospital, skilled nursing facility, home health, and hospice services that are rendered to beneficiaries enrolled in Part A.

- Inpatient hospital care coverage includes costs of meals, X-rays, drugs, intensive care, laboratory tests, a semi-private room, regular nursing services, operating and recovery room, and all other medically necessary services and supplies.
- Skilled nursing facility care is covered by Medicare HI only if it follows a hospitalization of 3 or more days and is certified as medically necessary. Covered services

are similar to inpatient hospital, plus rehabilitation services and certain medical devices and supplies. The number of Part A skilled nursing facility care days provided under Medicare is limited to 100 per benefit period. Part A does not cover nursing facility care if the patient does not require skilled nursing, or other skilled rehabilitation services that must be given on an inpatient basis.

- Home health agency care, including a home health aide, may be furnished by a home health agency in the residence of a "homebound" beneficiary if intermittent or part-time skilled nursing, physical therapy, or rehabilitation care is necessary. A plan of treatment must be in place and periodical review by a physician must occur. Home health care under Part A has no co-payment or deductible.
- Added in 1983, hospice care is a service provided to terminally ill persons with a life expectancy of 6 months or less who elect to forgo traditional medical treatment for the terminal illness and to receive only limited (hospice) care. Such care includes pain relief, nursing services, physical therapy, supportive medical and social services, and symptom management for a terminal illness.

Part B benefits are available to almost all resident citizens aged 65 years and older. Benefits are also available to certain resident aliens aged 65 years or older—even those who are not entitled (on the basis of eligibility for Social Security or Railroad Retirement benefits) to Part A Medicare services, and to disabled beneficiaries who are entitled to Medicare Part A. Part B coverage is optional, and must be paid for through a monthly premium. Almost all persons entitled to Part A choose to enroll in Part B.

Although Part B is often thought of primarily as coverage for physician services (in both hospital and non-hospital settings), it also covers certain non-physician services, including most supplies, diagnostic tests, ambulance services, clinical laboratory tests, durable medical equipment, some other therapy services, certain other health care services, blood that is not supplied under Part A, and drugs that cannot be self-administered (except certain anticancer drugs).

Expenditures for certain medically necessary services in hospital outpatient departments, ambulatory surgical centers, and certain other centers are also covered. Certain medical services and related care are subject to special payment rules, including deductibles (for blood); maximum approved amounts (for independently practicing, Medicare-approved physical or occupational therapists); or higher cost-sharing requirements (such as for outpatient mental illness treatments). Non-covered services under Medicare include long-term nursing care or custodial care and certain other health care needs such as dentures and dental care, eyeglasses and hearing aids, and most prescription drugs (except certain self-administered drugs).

The size and nature of the Medicare program make CMS unique in authority and responsibility among health care payers. Fee-for-service Medicare serves more than 35 million beneficiaries and processes a high volume of claims from hundreds of thousands of providers, such as physicians, therapists, hospitals, skilled nursing facilities,

home health agencies, and medical equipment suppliers. CMS is also responsible for paying and monitoring more than 400 managed care health plans that serve more than 5 million beneficiaries.

In Medicare's fee-for-service program—used by more than 80% of the program's beneficiaries—physicians, hospitals, and other providers submit claims and are paid for each service rendered to Medicare beneficiaries. Medicare's managed care program covers beneficiaries who have chosen to enroll in a prepaid health plan rather than purchase medical services from individual providers. The managed care program, which is funded from both the Part A and Part B trust funds, currently consists mostly of risk contract health maintenance organizations (HMOs). Medicare pays these HMOs a monthly amount, fixed in advance, for all the services provided to each beneficiary enrolled.

The Balanced Budget Act (BBA) of 1997 [Pub. L. No. 105-33 (1997)] granted HCFA substantial authority and responsibility to reform Medicare and, specifically, introduced new health plan options and major payment reforms. BBA provided for a dramatic expansion of health plan choices available to Medicare beneficiaries and made reforms to payment methods in traditional fee-for-service Medicare and managed care. Under the BBA's Medicare + Choice program, beneficiaries have new health plan options, including preferred provider organizations, provider sponsored organizations, and private fee-for-service plans.

The BBA also provided for revamping many of Medicare's payment systems to contain the growth in certain program components. Specifically, the BBA mandated prospective payment systems for services provided by approximately 1100 inpatient rehabilitation facilities, 14,000 skilled nursing facilities, 5000 hospital outpatient departments, and 8900 home health agencies. In addition, it made changes to the payment methods for hospitals, including payments for direct and indirect medical education costs. The BBA also adjusted fee schedule payments for physicians and durable medical equipment, and authorized the conversion of the remaining reasonable charge payment systems to fee schedules. Finally, the BBA granted the authority to conduct demonstrations on the cost-effectiveness of purchasing items and services through competitive bids from suppliers and providers. Congress appropriated between $20 million and $30 million for CMS's administration of BBA-related activities immediately after its enactment.

MEDICAID

Title XIX of the Social Security Act, known as Medicaid, is a federal-state matching entitlement program which provides medical assistance for certain individuals and families with low incomes and resources (See 42 U.S.C. §§ 1396 et. seq.). Medicaid became law in 1965 as a jointly funded cooperative venture between the federal and state governments to assist states in the provision of more adequate medical care to eligible needy persons. Medicaid is the largest program providing medical and health-related services to America's poorest people.

Within broad national guidelines provided by the federal government, each of the states establishes its own eligibility standards; determines the type, amount, duration, and scope of services; sets the rate of payment for services; and administers its own program. Thus Medicaid programs vary considerably from state to state, and within each state over time.

Medicaid does not provide medical assistance for all poor persons. Even under the broadest provisions of the federal statute, Medicaid does not provide health care services even for very poor persons unless they are in one of the groups designated in the list below. Low income is only one test for Medicaid eligibility for these individuals. Their resources and assets are tested against established thresholds (as determined by each state, within federal guidelines).

States generally have broad discretion in determining which groups their Medicaid programs will cover and the financial criteria for Medicaid eligibility. To be eligible for federal funds, however, states are required to provide Medicaid coverage for most individuals who receive federally assisted income-maintenance payments, as well as for related groups not receiving cash payments.

The following groups have mandatory Medicaid eligibility:

- Recipients of Aid to Families with Dependent Children (AFDC).
- Children younger than 6 years who meet the State's AFDC financial requirements or whose family income is at or below 133% of the Federal poverty level (FPL).
- Pregnant women whose family income is below 133% of the FPL (services to the woman are limited to pregnancy, delivery, complications of pregnancy, and 3 months of postpartum care).
- Supplemental Security Income (SSI) recipients (or those elderly, blind, and disabled individuals who qualify in States that apply more restrictive eligibility requirements).
- Recipients of adoption assistance and foster care who are under Title IV-E of the Social Security Act.
- All children born after September 30, 1983 in families with incomes at or below the FPL. (They must be given full Medicaid coverage until the age of 19 years. This guideline phased in coverage and by 2002, all poor children younger than 19 years should be covered.)
- Special protected groups (typically, individuals who lose their cash assistance from AFDC or SSI as a result of earnings from work or increased Social Security benefits. but who may keep Medicaid for a period of time).
- Certain Medicare beneficiaries.

States also have the option to provide Medicaid coverage for other "categorically needy" groups. These optional groups share the characteristics of the mandatory groups, but the eligibility criteria are somewhat more liberally defined. The broadest optional groups for which states will receive federal matching funds for coverage under the Medicaid program include the following:

- Infants (1 year old and younger) and pregnant women not covered under the mandatory rules whose family income is no more than 185% of the FPL (exact percentage of FPL is set by each state).

- Children younger than 21 years who meet the AFDC income and resources requirements, but who otherwise are not eligible for AFDC.
- Recipients of state supplementary income payments.
- Certain blind, elderly, or disabled adults who have incomes greater than those requiring mandatory coverage, but less than the FPL.
- Persons receiving care under home and community-based waivers.
- Persons infected with tuberculosis (TB) who would be financially eligible for Medicaid at the SSI income level (but eligibility is only for TB-related ambulatory services and for TB drugs).
- Institutionalized individuals with income and resources below specified limits.
- "Medically needy" (MN) persons.

The option to have an MN program allows states to extend Medicaid eligibility to additional qualified persons with significant health care expenses who have income in excess of the mandatory or optional categorically needy levels. The MN Medicaid program does not have to be as extensive as the "categorically needy" program in a state, but there are certain requirements. If a state has any MN program, certain services must be provided as a minimum (the state may also choose to include additional services); and in any MN program, a state is required to provide coverage to certain children younger than 18 years and pregnant women who are MN. A state may elect to provide eligibility to other MN persons who are elderly, blind, and/or disabled persons, caretaker relatives of children deprived of parental support and care, and certain other financially eligible children age 21 years and younger.

To receive federal matching funds, a state must offer the following basic services to the categorically needy populations:

- Inpatient hospital services.
- Outpatient hospital services.
- Prenatal care.
- Physician services.
- Nursing facility (NF) services for persons 21 years or older.
- Family planning services and supplies.
- Rural health clinic services.
- Home health care for persons eligible for skilled-nursing services.
- Laboratory and x-ray services.
- Pediatric and family nurse practitioner services.
- Nurse-midwife services.
- Certain federally-qualified ambulatory and health-center services.
- Early and periodic screening, diagnostic, and treatment services for children younger than 21 years.

States may also receive federal assistance for funding if they elect to provide other approved optional services. A few of the optional services under the Medicaid program include the following:

- Clinic services.
- Nursing facility services for the elderly and disabled.

- Intermediate care facilities for the mentally retarded.
- Optometrist services and eyeglasses.
- Prescribed drugs.
- Prosthetic devices.
- Dental services.
- TB-related ambulatory services and drugs for qualifying persons.

Within broad federal guidelines, states determine the amount and duration of services offered under their Medicaid programs. States may limit the number of days of hospital care or the number of physician visits covered. States are prohibited, however, from limiting the duration of coverage for medically necessary inpatient hospital services provided to Medicaid-eligible children younger than 6 years who are in "disproportionate share hospitals" and to infants in all hospitals.

With certain exceptions, a state's Medicaid Plan must allow recipients to have freedom of choice among participating providers of health care. States may provide and pay for Medicaid services through various prepayment arrangements such as HMOs.

In general, states are required to provide comparable scope, amounts, and duration of services to all categorically needy eligible persons. Two important exceptions are as follows:

- Health care services identified under the early and periodic screening, diagnostic, and treatment services program as being "medically necessary" for eligible children must be provided by Medicaid, even if those services are not included as part of the covered services in that state's plan (i.e., only these specific children might receive those specific services); and
- States may request "waivers" for home and community-based services under which they offer an alternative health care package for persons who might otherwise be institutionalized under Medicaid (i.e., only those persons so designated might receive home and community-based services). States are not limited in the scope of services they can provide under such waivers as long as they are cost effective (except that, other than as a part of respite care, they may not provide room and board for such recipients).

Medicaid operates as a vendor payment program, with states paying providers directly. Providers participating in Medicaid must accept the Medicaid reimbursement level as payment in full. With a few specific exceptions, each state has broad discretion in determining (within federally imposed upper limits and specific restrictions) the reimbursement methodology and resulting rate for services. States may impose nominal deductibles, coinsurance, or co-payments on some Medicaid recipients for certain services.

Certain Medicaid recipients must be excluded from cost sharing. These recipients include pregnant women, children younger than 18 years, categorically needy enrollees in HMOs, and hospital or nursing home patients who are expected to contribute most of their income to institutional care. In addition, emergency services and family planning services must be exempt from co-payments for all recipients.

MEDIGAP

"Medigap" refers to private insurance policies that cover various costs and provide additional medical insurance benefits not covered by the traditional Medicare fee-for-service program. Medigap is also known as "Medicare Supplemental Insurance." Medigap has been regulated by the federal government since 1980. Beneficiaries do not need Medigap and it is illegal for anyone to sell a Medigap policy to a beneficiary who is enrolled in a Medicare managed care plan, a private fee-for-service plan, a Medicare Medical Savings Account Plan, or a religious fraternal benefit plan.

Since 1990, Medigap policies provided by private insurance are required to offer specific sets of additional benefits in ten standardized plans lettered "A" through "J." (Except in Massachusetts, Minnesota and Wisconsin, which have their own standardized Medigap plans.)

All ten plans offer the following basic (core) Medigap benefits:

- Part A coinsurance for days 61 to 90 of a hospital stay in each benefit period.
- Part A coinsurance for days 91-150 of a hospital stay.
- Payment in full for as many as 365 additional days of inpatient hospital expenses.
- Part B coinsurance (20% of the Medicare –approved amount of the bill).
- Three pints of blood per calendar year.

Plans "B" through "J" also offer to pay the hospital deductible.

The following chart illustrates the benefits offered under the plans (Table 19-1).

Plans I and J, which are the most comprehensive, generally have higher deductibles before the co-payments become available. Additionally, under federal law, states

 Table 19–1 Medigap Benefits and Plans:

Benefits	Plans: A B C D E F G H I J
Core benefits	A B C D E F G H I J
Hospital deductible	B C D E F G H I J
Skilled nursing facility coinsurance[a]	C D E F G H I J
Part B annual deductible	C F A J
Foreign travel emergency care[b]	C D E F G H I J
At-home recovery[c]	D G I J
Part B excess charge[d]	F G (80%) I J
Preventive care[e] E	J
Prescription drugs[f]	H I J

[a]Skilled nursing facility insurance for days 21 through 100.
[b]After a $250 deductible, the Plans pay 80% of as much as $50,000 of lifetime expense related to emergency care received outside the United States during the first 60 days of each trip.
[c]Assistance with activities of daily living and home health care for as long as 8 weeks, not to exceed 40 visits at $40 per visit or $1600 per year.
[d]Physicians not accepting assignment may charge their patients as much as 115% of the Medicare-allowed charge for a service. This benefit pays as much as 100% of the full physician charge under plans F, I, and J. Plan G pays 80% of this full charge.
[e]Payment for up to $120 per year for routine checkups, serum cholesterol screening, hearing tests, diabetes screening and thyroid function test.
[f]After a $250 yearly deductible, payment of 50% of drug costs of as much as $1250 a year under Plans H and I and as much as $300 a year under Plan J.

are allowed to let private insurers add additional benefits to the benefits in a standard policy. Some of the items the standard Medigap plans do not cover include hearing aids, long-term care, vision or dental expenses, private-duty nursing, and unlimited prescription drugs.

Medicare SELECT is a type of Medigap insurance. Medicare SELECT policies are offered under the same A through J configuration, but they restrict the beneficiary to a specific set of preferred providers in order to obtain full benefits.

Medigap policies are best obtained during the "open enrollment period," which is 6 months after the first day of the month in which a beneficiary is 65 years or older and is enrolled in Medicare Part B. In 1997, laws were passed to protect a beneficiary's right to obtain Medigap insurance after the individual had allowed it to lapse when he or she joined a Medicare managed care plan or HMO. Other problems, such as a steady increase in premiums as beneficiaries grow older, remain to be addressed. Inquiries and complaints about the availability and marketing of Medigap polices are appropriately directed to state insurance departments. The HHS Office of Inspector General (OIG) operates a toll-free hotline (800-447-8477) for reports of Medicare fraud and abuse.

MEDICARE MODERNIZATION ACT OF 2003

Heralding the most significant expansion of the Medicare program since its creation in 1965, President Bush signed into law on December 8, 2003, H.R. 1, the "Medicare Prescription Drug, Improvement, and Modernization Act of 2003" [Pub. L. No. 108-173], which includes prescription drug coverage for millions of people with disabilities and senior citizens. (Between April 2004 and 2006, Medicare beneficiaries will be entitled to sign up for and use a transitional "prescription drug discount card." Estimated savings of this program are between 15% and 25% per prescription. Low-income beneficiaries will be eligible for up to $600 per year in prescription drug assistance, both in 2004 and 2005.) Implementation of this new Medicare "Part D" program begins January 1, 2006. Costs are estimated to reach $400 billion, at a minimum. (Federal budget experts and many Democratic members of Congress disagree with this estimate; some have projected costs to rise into the trillions of dollars, depending on the number of Medicare beneficiaries participating in the program.)

The Act also includes numerous regulatory reforms, including incentives for private health plans, an experiment in competition between private health plans and Medicare, a limited form of means testing, and provisions regarding health savings accounts. Unquestionably, however, the Act's hallmark is its voluntary prescription drug benefit. But what is missing from the new benefit is equally important, if not more significant, than what's there.

Essentially, after paying an annual deductible amount of $250, approximately 75% of enrolled Medicare beneficiaries' drug costs would be covered, up to a cap of $2500. Thereafter, eligible seniors would have *no coverage* of their drug costs, until they reach $3600 in out-of-pocket expenses—the so-called "doughnut hole" —whereupon catastrophic coverage would commence. This means that many, if not most, of our nation's elderly population will be responsible for paying all out-of-pocket expenditures between $2501 and $3599 for their prescription drugs, a fact glaringly omitted from or poorly explained in presidential Administration press releases. Beneficiaries with annual incomes below 150% of poverty will receive additional assistance.

Beneficiaries will be able to obtain drug coverage either through prescription drug plans (PDAs) or through the new Medicare Advantage program that replaces Medicare + Choice. Such entities that provide drug plans will be allowed to offer either the standard benefit or its actuarial equivalent, and will bear some of the financial risk for drug costs. A bidding process will determine monthly premium amounts for Part D.

Finally, the Act brings to bear a host of provider-related anti-fraud and payment provisions, including the following:

- Quality ratings for hospitals: 0.4% decrease in reimbursement to those hospitals that do not submit quality of care information to CMS.
- Patient referrals to "specialty" hospitals: 18-month moratorium on exception to physician self-referral prohibition, which allowed physician investors to refer their patients to specialty hospitals in which they have an ownership interest. Specialty hospitals in operation or under development as of November 18, 2003, would be exempt from this provision.
- Payment changes for durable medical equipment: imposition of a competitive bidding process for high-cost, high-utilization DME items, as well as a payment freeze for three years.
- Physician fees: 1.5% increase in the update to the physician fee schedules for 2004 and 2005.
- Numerous Medicare regulatory relief provisions and contractor corrections regarding overpayments, appeals, extrapolations, responses to providers, and retroactivity of policy applications, all of which have the potential of easing health care providers' administrative burdens if adequately implemented.

The Act took a tortured path from its initial bill introduction to enactment. Policy "wonks," legislative specialists, and attorneys alike continue to find its provisions highly complicated and controversial, notwithstanding the Act's modest benefits. In fact, liberal groups have opened a year-long campaign to seek changes in the new prescription drug law they say benefits pharmaceutical companies over senior citizens. What remains to be seen, despite the American Association of Retired Person's enthusiastic endorsement, is how our nation's senior citizens, once they begin to glean a more complete understanding of the prescription drug benefit's grants and loopholes, will react to what their increased premiums actually are purchasing.

HEALTH INSURANCE PORTABILITY AND ACCOUNTABILITY ACT OF 1996

The Health Insurance Portability and Accountability Act of 1996 (HIPAA) [Pub. L. No. 104-191 (1996)] includes important new protections for an estimated 25 million Americans (approximately 1 in 10) who move from one job to another, are self-employed, or have preexisting medical conditions. HIPAA is designed to improve the availability of health insurance to working families and their children, and also dedicates money each year for fighting health care fraud (see Chapter 18).

Key provisions of HIPAA include the following:

Insurance

Guaranteed Access for Small Business

Small businesses (50 or fewer employees) are guaranteed access to health insurance. No insurer can exclude an employee or a family member from coverage based on health status.

Guaranteed Renewal of Insurance

Once an insurer sells a policy to any individual or group, they are required to renew coverage regardless of the health status of any member of a group.

Guaranteed Access for Individuals

People who lose their group coverage (because of loss of employment or change of jobs to a firm without insurance, for example) will be guaranteed access to coverage in the individual market, or states may develop alternative programs to assure that comparable coverage is available to these people. The coverage will be available without regard to health status, and renewal will be guaranteed.

Pre-Existing Conditions

Workers covered by group insurance policies cannot be excluded from coverage for more than 12 months because of a preexisting medical condition. Such limits can only be placed on conditions treated or diagnosed within the 6 months prior to their enrollment in an insurance plan. Insurers cannot impose new preexisting condition exclusions for workers with previous coverage.

ENFORCEMENT. States have primary responsibility to enforce these protections. If states fail to act, HHS can impose civil monetary penalties on insurers. The Secretary of Labor will enforce these rules for the self-insured through Employee Retirement Income Security Act (ERISA) plans. The tax code is modified to allow the Secretary of Treasury to impose tax penalties on employers or insurance plans that are out of compliance.

Self-Employed Individuals

The tax deduction for insurance costs of self-employed individuals is gradually increased from 30% in 1996 to 80% in 2002.

Other HIPAA Issues

Long-Term Care Insurance

Minimum federal consumer protection and marketing requirements are established for tax-qualified long-term care insurance policies, including a requirement that insurers start benefit payments when a policy-holder cannot perform at least two "activities of daily living" (i.e., bathing, incontinence care, eating, toileting, transferring, dressing). Subject to certain limitations, the requirements clarify that long-term care insurance premium payments and unreimbursed long-term care services costs are tax deductible as a medical expense, and benefits received under a long-term care insurance contract are excludable from taxable income. Employer-sponsored long-term care insurance is to receive the same tax treatment as health insurance.

Medigap Insurance

Revises the notices requirement for health insurance policies that pay benefits without regard to Medicare coverage or other insurance coverage. Long-term care policies are permitted to coordinate with Medicare and other coverage and must disclose any duplication of benefits.

Administrative Simplification

All health care providers and health plans that engage in electronic administrative and financial transactions must use a single set of national standards and identifiers. Electronic health information systems must meet security standards.

Health Information Privacy

Congress did not enact privacy legislation within 3 years of HIPAA's passage and, as such, health care providers, health plans, and health care clearinghouses are required to follow privacy regulations promulgated by HHS for individually identifiable electronic health information.

Finally, HIPAA also provides CMS with explicit authority to contract with firms outside its existing claims processing contractor network to perform payment safeguard functions while avoiding conflicts of interest.

BALANCED BUDGET ACT OF 1997

The BBA of 1997 resulted from extensive negotiations between Congress and the Clinton Administration [(Pub. L. No. 105-33 (1997)]. The bill represented the most sweeping changes to the Medicare program since its establishment in 1965. At the time of its passage, the BBA was expected to save the Medicare program $112 billion during a period of 5 years, and the Medicaid program approximately $7 billion. The major changes made by the BBA include the following:

- Expanded preventive benefits for Medicare beneficiaries, including pap smear tests and colorectal cancer screenings.
- Encouraged seniors to participate in more managed care alternatives, such as preferred provider organizations, through the establishment of Medicare + Choice managed care programs.
- Created a pilot program for medical savings accounts (MSAs). As many as 390,000 seniors would be allowed to participate in the new program.

- Provided $20 billion to create a state grant program, known as the Children's Health Insurance Program, to provide health insurance to roughly 3.4 million uninsured children. This initiative was funded by a new 15¢-per-pack tax on cigarettes.
- Adjusted payments to physicians, hospitals, and other Medicare and Medicaid providers.

(See also Chapter 18 for a discussion of fraud and abuse issues.)

Not long after the passage of the BBA, physicians, hospitals, and nursing homes began to complain that the cuts in the BBA were too deep and patient care would suffer. In 1998, Congress increased payments for home health care agencies. In 1999, Congress passed the Balanced Budget Refinement Act of 1999 (BBRA) [Pub. L. No. 106-113 (1999)], which restored $16 billion to hospitals, nursing homes, Medicare + Choice plans and rural health. The BBRA also limited the outpatient hospital co-payment, increased funding for pap smears, and extended benefits for immunosuppressive drugs.

Beginning in early 2000, health care providers began lobbying Congress and the Administration to further modify the reimbursement provisions in the BBA. After a series of hearings in the House and Senate and a vigorous lobbying campaign by the provider groups, Congress passed a Medicare "give-back" bill , estimated to cost $31.5 billion during a 5-year period. The bill was part of a year-end tax package. The give-back bill included $11 billion for hospitals, $11 billion for managed care plans, $1.8 billion for home health and hospice providers, and $1.6 billion for skilled nursing homes. The Clinton Administration initially had objected to increased funding for managed care plans.

MEDICAL SAVINGS ACCOUNTS

MSAs are tax-exempt accounts that can be used for medical expenses. In Congress, MSAs are usually supported by Republicans, who see them as a way to return "purchasing power" and control over health care decision making to patients. Democrats and traditional health insurers, on the other hand, oppose MSAs, arguing that they would "siphon off" healthy beneficiaries from the universal risk pool and raise rates dramatically for the less healthy.

MSAs first surfaced as a plausible alternative to traditional health insurance in the mid-1990s. Republican Members of Congress included MSAs for senior citizens in their 1995 Medicare reform package, which was subsequently vetoed by President Clinton. During negotiations on Medicare reform two years later, Republicans secured inclusion of an MSA demonstration plan into the BBA of 1997, which established a pilot project for 390,000 seniors around the country to try MSAs.

In 1999, the House of Representatives passed a health care tax bill as a companion bill to managed care reform. Sponsored by Jim Talent (R-Missouri) and John Shadegg (R-Arizona), the bill would have allowed any taxpayer to establish an MSA. The bill passed by a 227 to 205 vote. The bill would also have allowed taxpayers who purchased their own health insurance to take a tax deduction equal to 100% of their premiums and would have allowed the self-employed to deduct 100% of premiums. The package

was expected to cost approximately $48 billion during a 10-year period. Most Democrats in Congress opposed the measure, arguing that it would primarily help the healthy and wealthy and do little to help the uninsured. The Senate's version of managed care reform legislation did not include any tax provisions.

The future of MSAs for non-Medicare beneficiaries is unclear. Managed care reform remains a contentious issue, and Democrats remain strongly opposed to including MSAs in any HMO package. Meanwhile, one of the strongest champions of MSAs, former House Ways and Means Committee Chairman Bill Archer (R-Tennessee), retired from the House of Representatives at the end of the 106th Congress.

EMPLOYEE RETIREMENT INCOME SECURITY ACT

Former President Gerald Ford signed ERISA into law on September 2, 1974, after years of intensive debate [Pub. L. No. 93-406 (1974)]. ERISA, enacted primarily to address abuses in the U.S. pension system in the 1960s and 1970s, established a uniform system of federal requirements that, generally speaking, preempted state laws but preserved state insurance regulation. The Pension and Welfare Benefits Administration administers ERISA, which is now the primary federal statute that governs employment-based health care plans. ERISA plans are provided either by employers or jointly trusted "Taft-Hartley" plans negotiated by unions with groups of employers. Roughly 50 million Americans are covered by ERISA health plans, which are exempt from state laws governing minimum hospital stays, gag clauses for physicians, and insurance discrimination, among other exemptions.

Except for the passage of the Consolidated Omnibus Reconciliation Act (COBRA) in 1986, ERISA's substantive health care requirements remained essentially unchanged from 1974 until the mid-1990s. COBRA required employers to allow certain employees and their families who lose coverage under their employer-sponsored plan to continue to buy coverage for a limited amount of time.

During the last several years, however, Congress passed several major health bills that amended ERISA, including the following:

- HIPAA
- Newborns' and Mothers' Health Protection Act
- Mental Health Parity Act
- Women's Health and Cancer Rights Act

The most significant legislation that would have affected ERISA included the managed care reform proposals passed by the House of Representatives and the Senate in the 106th Congress. Championed by Republican Charlie Norwood of Georgia and Democrat John Dingell of Michigan, the bill would have made extensive changes to the ERISA system. This bill would have preempted many state laws to guarantee comparable patient protections for all America with private health insurance, regardless of whether the plan is self-funded. The Senate bill, co-sponsored by then Senate Republican Majority Leader Trent Lott of Mississippi and then Deputy Majority Leader Don Nickles of Oklahoma, made some modifications to

ERISA but in general did not override state insurance laws. This legislation was not enacted into law.

PATIENTS' "BILL OF RIGHTS" LEGISLATION

The issue of patients' rights in health care—especially in managed care plans—has been front and center on Capitol Hill in recent years, where dozens of bills have been introduced to regulate the health insurance industry. Specific proposals that have received the most publicity and legislative attention include the following:

- A ban on "gag" clauses in provider–insurer contracts.
- A requirement for insurers to reimburse beneficiaries for emergency room trips based on a "reasonable person" standard, rather than the ultimate diagnosis.
- A ban on the practices known as "drive-through deliveries" and "drive-through mastectomies."
- A prohibition on bonuses provided by insurers to physicians for failure to refer patients to specialists.
- Provision of a uniform and expeditious appeals process for beneficiaries whose health plans have denied coverage for a treatment option recommended by the beneficiary's provider.
- Removal of the legal protections that insurers and employers currently enjoy under ERISA.

In the House of Representatives, earlier efforts to reform the managed care system were spearheaded by a pair of unlikely allies: conservative Congressman Charlie Norwood, a dentist from Georgia, and long-time Democratic Congressman John Dingell, the top-ranking Democrat on the House Commerce Committee. Their efforts culminated in the passage of a managed care reform bill in the House in the fall of 1998. The Norwood-Dingell bill (H.R. 2723), which was strongly opposed by the Republican leadership and business groups, would have allowed patients to sue their managed care plans for negligence, ensuring that all Americans with private health insurance, including those plans traditionally regulated by the states, have federally-guaranteed patient protections. Republicans argued that the Norwood-Dingell bill would have been a boon only for trial lawyers, and that it did nothing to address the ever-increasing number of uninsured Americans.

In the Senate, the Republican leadership made a conscious decision early on to respect the rights of states to regulate health insurance, and as a result their managed care proposals applied only to beneficiaries of ERISA-regulated plans. Co-sponsored by then Majority Leader Trent Lott of Mississippi and then Deputy Majority Leader Don Nickles of Oklahoma, the leadership bill (S. 1344) did not expand beneficiaries' rights to sue their managed care plans. Democrats argued that the Lott-Nickles plan paled in comparison to Dingell-Norwood, but they were able to persuade only two of their Republican colleagues to join their efforts. This bill, however, did not gain sufficient Congressional support and was not enacted into law.

AMERICANS WITH DISABILITIES ACT

After years of lobbying by concerned groups (e.g., civil rights, disability rights, public health, and AIDS support groups) and extended negotiations over several months, Congress passed the groundbreaking Americans With Disabilities Act (ADA, [Pub. L. No. 101-336 (1990)]), which provides extensive protections to approximately 43 million Americans with mental and physical disabilities, despite concerns of some business interests that compliance is costly. The ADA forbids discrimination against people with disabilities in employment, public services and public accommodations, mandates that common carriers make telecommunications relay services available to hearing- and speech-impaired individuals. Currently, the ADA applies to employers of 15 or more people, including Congress [Pub. L. No. 104-1 (1995) (Congressional Accountability Act)], and protects employees in a workplace in a foreign country [Pub. L. No. 102-166 (1991) (Civil Rights Act of 1991)].

The ADA's protections are in addition to those already afforded persons with disabilities under the 1973 Rehabilitation Act [Pub. L. No. 93-112 (1973)] and the 1988 Fair Housing Act Amendments, laws which prohibit discrimination in federally funded activities and housing, respectively. Although people with disabilities were not included as a protected class along with race, sex, religion, and national origin under the historic 1964 Civil Rights Act [Pub. L. 88-352, (1964), as amended by Pub. L. No. 102-166 (1991)], which prohibits discrimination in employment and public accommodations, the sweeping ADA is broader in scope than is the Civil Rights Act.

Under Title I, which applies to employment discrimination, the ADA requires that employers make "reasonable accommodations" for disabled employees, but does not demand changes that would constitute an "undue hardship." Title II mandates that all newly purchased or leased buses and rail cars be made accessible to the disabled, although retrofitting of existing vehicles is not necessary. Title III, involving public accommodations, covers not only the lodgings, restaurants, gasoline stations, and places of entertainment to which the Civil Rights Act applies, but also applies to dry cleaners, pharmacies, grocery stores, museums and sports stadiums, doctors' offices and hospitals, and other types of retail and service establishments. These varied businesses must make new and renovated facilities accessible to the disabled and craft "readily achievable" modifications in existing facilities to accommodate the disabled.

The ADA does not set forth particular due process procedures. Instead, persons with disabilities may use the same enforcement remedies available as under Title VII of the Civil Rights Act of 1964, as amended in 1991 [Pub. L. 88-352, as amended by Pub. L. No. 102-166].

As a result, qualified individuals who experience discrimination may file complaints with the pertinent federal agency or sue in federal court. Informal mediation and voluntary compliance are favored by enforcement agencies.

The U.S. Supreme Court has heard a number of cases regarding the rights of people with disabilities provided by the ADA and during the last few years has begun to erode several protections initially assumed to be included within the meaning of the law.

FAMILY AND MEDICAL LEAVE ACT

On February 5, 1993, Congress passed the pioneering Family and Medical Leave Act (FMLA) [Pub. L. No. 103-3 (1993)], which mandates that employers allow all but the highest-paid 10% of employees, including individuals employed by the U.S. House and Senate, as much as 12 weeks of unpaid leave annually for any of the following reasons:

- The birth of a child.
- The adoption of a child or the placement of a foster child.
- The serious illness of a child, spouse, or parent.
- The employee's own serious health condition.

Under FMLA, employers must also continue to provide employment and health care benefits that the employee accrued prior to the leave.

The Act covers employees who had worked for the employer for a minimum of 12 months and for a minimum of 1250 hours during that time period. For married employees who work for the same employer, the Act limits the total number of weeks of leave to 12. Individuals who work for a business that employs fewer than 50 persons within a 75-mile radius are excluded from FMLA.

The Act mandates that when employees return to work after taking leave under the law, employers must restore them to their original position or an equivalent one with equivalent pay, employment benefits, and other conditions. Employers may require employees who took intermittent leave for planned medical treatment to transfer on a temporary basis to an open alternative position for which the worker had the necessary qualifications, as long as the position has comparable pay and benefits and is better suited to the worker's schedule. FMLA allows employees who receive paid leave for less than 12 weeks to take without pay the additional weeks of leave, up to the 12-week maximum. Employees may also substitute any accumulated paid vacation leave, personal leave, or family leave for any portion of the unpaid 12-week leave.

Under the Act, employers may demand that the employee supply certification by a health care provider of the medical condition of the employee's child, spouse or parent (e.g., the date the serious health condition commenced; the likely duration of the condition and other germane medical information; a statement that the employee's assistance in caring for the child, spouse or parent is required; and an estimate of the amount of time needed for the leave. When the employee is ill, the certification should indicate that the employee could not perform his or her job. A certification for intermittent leave for planned medical treatment should include the expected dates and length of treatment.

When certifying the need for a leave of absence, an employer may also demand, at its own cost, that the employee secure the opinion of a second health care provider, or a third health care provider when the opinions of the first and second providers differ (the opinion of the third provider binds the employer and the employee). When the leave is foreseeable, employees must give their employers 30 days' notice of the leave (e.g., for an anticipated birth or adoption of a child). Employers may also demand that employees on leave report occasionally on their status and intent to resume employment.

INDIVIDUALS WITH DISABILITIES EDUCATION ACT

In November 1975, startling statistics provided by the Office of Education indicated that one-half of the United States' eight million disabled children were receiving an inadequate education or no education at all. Motivated by these findings, Congress passed and President Ford signed into law (albeit with some reservations) a major bill, the Education for All Handicapped Children Act [Pub. L. No. 94-142 (1975)].

The Act would assure free and adequate public school education for the country's disabled children and amend the 1967 Education of the Handicapped Act [See Section 154 of the Elementary and Secondary Education Amendments of 1967, Pub. L. No. 90-247 (1967)].

Later, as a part of the law's 1990 reauthorization, the Education of the Handicapped Act was renamed the Individuals with Disabilities Education Act (IDEA); the word "disabled" was substituted for "handicapped" throughout the law.

Initially, the Ford Administration was opposed to the 1975 bill, and threatened a veto because of its high cost and its shifting of responsibility for the education of disabled children from the local to the federal level. The U.S. House and Senate passed the bill by overwhelming margins, however, and President Ford agreed ultimately to sign the final version of the bill, which included scaled-back authorization levels.

Once in full operation, the original 1975 law was intended to provide a maximum of 20% of the additional costs of educating a child with a disability, which was then estimated by the National Educational Finance Project to be 1.9 times that of educating a non-disabled child. The major final provisions of the original bill accomplished the following goals:

- Set forth new grant formula that authorized grants equal to the number of handicapped children ages 3 through 21 years who received a special education multiplied by 40% of the national average per pupil expenditure in fiscal year 1978 (beginning in fiscal year 1982).
- Required that no state could count as disabled more than 12% of all its children aged 5 to 17 years, and mandated that only one-sixth of the children counted as disabled could have specific learning disabilities.
- Required that by September 1980, each state must provide a free and appropriate education to all its handicapped children between the ages of 3 and 21 years, except with regard to children aged 3 to 5 years and 18 to 21 years when state law or court order is contrary to federal law.
- Mandated that states give first priority to children who are not currently receiving an education and that states give second priority to those children with the most acute disability in each disability category who were receiving an inadequate education.

- Provided incentive grants to states of $300 per disabled child aged 3 to 5 years to encourage them to offer educational services for this population.
- Required that federal funds be used only to cover the additional costs of educating disabled children, rather than to supplant state or local funds (i.e., per-pupil spending by the state and local school district must be the same for disabled and non-disabled children).
- Mandated that the local school district collaborate with teachers, parents, and the disabled child (when appropriate) to develop an individualized educational program for the child, which must be written and should include annuals goals, short-term objectives, and certain services for the child. An initial meeting between interested parties when the child first enters the school system, an additional review meeting that school year, and subsequent annual reviews are required.
- Required that, when appropriate, disabled children should be educated with non-disabled children.
- Increased existing due process procedures available to ensure the rights of disabled children (placement, identification, and evaluation of the child; prohibited against testing materials that are racially or culturally discriminatory; and provided for the confidentiality of information held by the state).
- Mandated that the commissioner of education submit an annual report to Congress that includes a range of data on the education of disabled children (e.g., the number serviced, the amount of funds earmarked at the federal, state, and local levels, and the number of children in need of special services), and authorized monies for conducting evaluation studies.
- Authorized necessary appropriations for grants to state and local education agencies to remove architectural barriers that hamper the access of the disabled to certain buildings.
- Provided for the promulgation of final regulations related to the bill.

Subsequent reauthorizations of the law in 1983 and 1986 established incentive (rather than mandatory) programs directed at providing services to disabled infants and toddlers. Later, the 1990 reauthorization authorized funds for a variety of discretionary programs, such as early education for children with disabilities, postsecondary educational opportunities, training of personnel who teach the disabled, and funding for research involving new methods for educating disabled children and the advancement of new technology, materials, and educational media. In the 1990 reauthorization, Congress also clarified that it intended to allow litigants the right to sue in federal court to enforce their rights under the IDEA. Since 1990, IDEA has been reauthorized or amended numerous times.

REHABILITATION ACT OF 1973

President Nixon signed H.R. 8070, the Rehabilitation Act of 1973 [Pub. L. No. 93-112 (1973)] into law on September 26, 1973. The Act replaced the Vocational Rehabilitation Act of 1920 [Vocational Rehabilitation Act of 1920, ch. 219, 41 Stat. 735 (1920)], which President Wilson signed to establish the first system of federal aid to the states for rehabilitation services for civilians injured in industry.

The stated purposes of the 1973 Act are as follows:

- Provide a statutory basis for the Rehabilitation Services Administration.
- Authorize programs to:
  - Develop and implement comprehensive state plans to provide vocational rehabilitation services to handicapped individuals and to provide services for the benefit of such individuals.
  - Evaluate the rehabilitation potential of handicapped individuals.
  - Develop methods to provide rehabilitation services to handicapped individuals for whom a vocational goal is not possible or feasible.
  - Assist in the construction and improvement of rehabilitation facilities and assist in improving the number of rehabilitation personnel and their skills.
  - Develop methods to apply scientific and technological developments to provide rehabilitation services.
  - Initiate and expand services to groups of handicapped individuals who have been underserved in the past.
  - Promote and expand employment opportunities for handicapped individuals.
  - Establish client assistance pilot projects.
  - Evaluate approaches to architectural and transportation barriers confronting handicapped individuals and develop solutions to eliminate such barriers.

The Act also authorized appropriations of $1.55 billion in fiscal years 1974-1975.

Title III of the Act, entitled "Special Federal Responsibilities," authorizes grants and contracts to states and public or non-profit organizations to pay for part of the costs for construction of rehabilitation facilities, initial planning, and staffing assistance. Title III also authorized appropriations of $15,000,000 and $17,000,000 for fiscal years 1974 and 1975 in special project and demonstration grants.

Title III authorized the then-Secretary of Health, Education, and Welfare (now HHS), in consultation with the Secretary of Housing and Urban Development, to insure mortgages for rehabilitation facilities and specified conditions to be met before the issuance of any such mortgage. In addition, Title III created a Rehabilitation Facilities Insurance Fund to carry out the insurance provisions of the Act. The total amount of outstanding mortgages insured under the Act is not to exceed $200,000,000. Title III set forth specific grant and contract requirements for all projects approved and assisted under Title III.

DEVELOPMENTAL DISABILITIES ASSISTANCE AND BILL OF RIGHTS ACT OF 1984

The Developmental Disabilities Assistance and Bill of Rights Act of 1984 [Pub. L. No. 98-527 (1984)] permitted significant increases in spending for developmental disabilities programs. The Act amends the Mental Retardation Facilities and Community Mental Health Centers

Construction Act of 1963. The stated purposes of the Act are to:

● Assist in the provision of comprehensive services to persons with developmental disabilities, giving priority to those individuals whose needs are not met under The Rehabilitation Act of 1973 or other health, education, and welfare programs.
● Assist states in their planning activities.
● Make grants to states and to public and private nonprofit organizations to establish programs, to foster use of innovative habilitation techniques, and to train personnel to provide services to persons with developmental disabilities.
● Make grants to university-affiliated facilities to assist them in the administration and operation of services for persons with developmental disabilities and to support interdisciplinary training programs for personnel needed to provide services to persons with developmental disabilities.
● Make grants to support a system in each state to protect the legal and human rights of persons with developmental disabilities.

The Act authorizes appropriations of $75.7 million in fiscal year 1985, $80.4 million in 1986, and $85.2 million in 1987 for the development of programs for the developmentally disabled. Most of the funding is for state grants to provide and coordinate services for the developmentally disabled, emphasizing states' provision of job-related services for the disabled.

To receive funding to protect the legal and human rights of the developmentally disabled, the Act requires states to have systems in place to protect and advocate the rights of persons with developmental disabilities. States must provide assurances to HHS that the funds are being used for the appropriate purposes. The Act requires that HHS prepare a report for Congress 6 months after the Act's enactment that offers recommendations for improvements in services for the developmentally disabled and the delivery of those services.

REHABILITATION ACT AMENDMENTS OF 1986

The Rehabilitation Act Amendments of 1986 [Pub. L. No. 99-506 (1986)] extended programs created under the Rehabilitation Act of 1973 that are designed to help the handicapped become self-sufficient through employment. The Amendments authorized $1.28 billion in fiscal year 1987 for state rehabilitation grants, the principal source of job-related aid to the handicapped, and $200 million for a number of smaller programs. Congress appropriated $1.1 billion for state grants in fiscal year 1986 and $167 million for other programs authorized by the Act. These programs included research and special aid for disabled Native Americans and migrant workers.

Section 502 of the Act established an Architectural and Transportation Barriers Compliance Board to investigate problems of handicapped persons in the areas of architecture and transportation and to promote the elimination of architectural and transportation barriers for handicapped persons, especially with respect to monuments, public buildings, and residential and institutional housing. Specifically, the Board is to determine what measures are being taken to eliminate barriers, to make legislative recommendations to the President and Congress, and to ensure compliance with the standards prescribed pursuant to the Architectural Barriers Act.

Title VI of the Amendments, entitled "Architectural and Transportation Barriers Compliance Board," amends Section 502 of the Act by:

● Amending the membership and quorum requirements of the Architectural and Transportation Barriers Compliance Board ("the Board").
● Requiring that the Chair and Vice-Chair of the Board be members of the general public and federal government on an alternating basis.
● Enabling the Board to establish bylaws (including quorum requirements) and rules so as to carry out its functions.
● Adding to Section 503(g) of the Act a requirement that the Board submit two additional reports of its activities—one in the field of transportation barriers for the handicapped and the other on its activities in the field of housing needs of handicapped individuals—to be submitted no later than February 1, 1988.
● Extending the Act from October 1, 1986 through fiscal year 1987 to 1991.

QUALITY ASSURANCE REFORM INITIATIVE

Responding to a perceived need for stronger programs in the early stages of Medicaid managed care development, the then HCFA (now the Centers for Medicare and Medicaid Services or CMS) began the Quality Assurance Reform Initiative (QARI) in 1991 to provide technical assistance tools and other assistance to state Medicaid agencies. QARI produced a guide for Medicaid agencies entitled: "A Health Care Quality Improvement System for Medicaid Managed Care — a Guide for States." This publication contained the following four guidance areas for state-based Medicaid managed care programs:

● A framework for quality improvement systems.
● Internal quality assurance programs of Medicaid HMOs.
● Clinical and health services areas and use of quality indicators and clinical practice guidelines.
● Conduct of external quality reviews.

One outcome of QARI was the development of a Medicaid version of the Health Plan Employer Data and Information Set, the private sector's standardized quality performance measurement system, as modified for state Medicaid agency use. Other quality assurance tools and guidance developments stemmed from the QARI program, historically focusing on structural standards and a plan's infrastructure and capacity to improve care. In recent years, the demand from consumers of managed care services for performance measures has refocused HCFA's efforts into performance measures that hold plans accountable for actually improving the care provided. This new focus on accountability has resulted in the development of the Quality Improvement System for Managed Care.

QUALITY IMPROVEMENT SYSTEM FOR MANAGED CARE

The Quality Improvement System for Managed Care (QISMC) was the then-HCFA's initiative to create incentives for high-quality care and provide for accountability within Medicare and Medicaid. Working through the National Academy of State Health Policy in consultation with managed care plans, beneficiary groups, quality measurement experts, and state Medicaid agencies and regulators, QISMC developed objective, measurable standards to measure and hold plans accountable for improving care.

QISMC has produced the following changes to existing quality assurance standards:

- Managed care plans are required to meet minimum performance levels on standardized measures (the Health Plan Employer Data and Information Set and the Consumer Assessment of Health Plans Study).
- Plans are required to show demonstrable and measurable improvement in specified broad clinical areas (e.g., chronic care, hospital care, preventive services, and acute ambulatory care) on the basis of self-identified performance improvement projects.

By defining in advance for the plans what are acceptable, demonstrable, and measurable improvement parameters, HCFA intends to measure not whether plans have an infrastructure to improve care, but whether the care provided actually improved.

HEALTH CARE QUALITY IMPROVEMENT PROGRAM

The then-HCFA and peer review organizations (PROs) initiated the Health Care Quality Improvement Program (HCQIP) in 1992. HCQIP looks to partner with practitioners, beneficiaries, providers, plans and other purchasers to improve Medicare beneficiaries' health. Through HCQIP, the Medicare agency will:

- Develop scientific quality indicators.
- Measure care patterns and identify opportunities to improve care.
- Communicate with professional and provider communities about these patterns of care.
- Foster quality improvement through system improvements.
- Measure again to evaluate success and redirect efforts.

The Cooperative Cardiovascular Project in 1992 was the first national quality improvement project under HCQIP. On the basis of public health importance and the feasibility of measuring and improving quality, HCQIP now covers seven clinical priority areas:

- Acute myocardial infarction
- Breast cancer
- Diabetes
- Heart failure
- Pneumonia
- Stroke
- Reducing health disparities within the Medicare population

HCQIP is carried out locally by PROs, which develop and implement cooperative projects with health care providers to improve the quality of care and to assist beneficiaries to make informed health care choices. The cooperative projects are expected to result in measurable improvement in the processes and outcomes of the clinical issues involved. Additionally, PROs are required to provide quality improvement consultation to providers, including data analysis, educational materials, quality improvement consulting, custom assistance with local quality improvement activities, the dissemination of quality indicators and data collection instruments, and provider collaboration opportunities to improve care and reduce expenditures.

NATIONAL PRACTITIONER DATA BANK

HCQIA [Title IV of Pub. L. No. 99-660 (1986)] established the National Practitioner Data Bank (NPDB), which is a central clearinghouse for certain information on providers, including sanctions and malpractice actions. In enacting HCQIA, Congress intended to address, at a federal level, both an increase in medical malpractice litigation and needed improvements in the quality of medical care nationwide. These problems called for more resources than any individual state could provide.

To support the professional review of medical practitioners, the law provides immunity from private damages in civil suits to the professional review bodies of hospitals and other health care entities, and to the individuals serving on or otherwise assisting such bodies. Civil money penalties of as much as $25,000 may be assessed against any individual or entity that fails to report information on medical malpractice payments in accordance with HCQIA, and as much as $11,000 against any individual who breaches the confidentiality of information reported to the data bank.

Final regulations from HHS are codified at 45 Code of Federal Regulations Part 60. Under the regulations, hospitals must request information from the NPDB at the time a health care practitioner applies for any regular or courtesy position on its medical staff or for clinical privileges at the hospital. Also, a hospital must request information every 2 years (biennially) on all health practitioners who are on its medical staff who have clinical privileges at the hospital. Hospitals must also report to the NPDB all professional review actions, based on reasons related to professional competence or conduct that adversely affect a practitioner's clinical privileges for a period longer than 30 days, including the practitioner's voluntary surrender or restriction of clinical privileges while under, or to avoid, investigation.

HCQIA confers immunity from private damages in civil suits under federal and state laws to professional review bodies of hospitals and other health care entities and their assistants, when their activities are conducted with the reasonable belief of furthering the quality of health care and with proper regard for due process.

NPDB information addresses the professional competence and conduct of health care practitioners and is intended to augment other sources of data used to evaluate a practitioner's credentials. The data bank provides for a direct yet discreet inquiry into and scrutiny of specific areas of a practitioner's licensure, professional society memberships, medical malpractice payment history, and record of clinical privileges. The NPDB collects and disseminates the following information:

- Professional liability payments made on behalf of a health care practitioner.
- Adverse action reports based on a practitioner's professional competence or conduct that adversely affects the practitioner's privileges for more than 30 days. These actions include reducing, restricting, suspending, revoking, or denying privileges, and also include an entity's decision not to renew a practitioner's privileges if the decision was based on competence or professional misconduct. It also includes voluntary surrender or restriction of privileges either while under investigation or in lieu of an investigation.
- Disciplinary actions related to competence or professional misconduct taken against a practitioner's license, including revocation, suspension, censure, reprimand, probation, and licensure surrender.
- Professional society review actions taken for reasons related to competence or professional misconduct that adversely affect professional society membership.
- Medicare and Medicaid exclusion reports containing sanctions against a practitioner as the result of fraud and abuse.

The information in the NPDB is considered confidential and is released only to eligible entities or to physicians and other health care practitioners who wish to conduct a self-query. Practitioners may be given information about their own records, including the information a requesting entity would receive and a complete listing of those entities or individuals that have queried the file. A practitioner may dispute the reported information, whether the report should have been made, or both, but the practitioner must first attempt to resolve the dispute with the reporting entity. As an alternative to disputing the report, a practitioner may submit a statement to accompany the report to all future inquiries.

NURSING HOME REFORM

Nursing home reform refers to changes in the regulation of skilled nursing facilities (SNF) under Medicare and NFs under Medicaid as authorized under Title IV, Subtitle C of the Omnibus Budget Reconciliation Act of 1987 [Pub. L. No. 100-203 (1987)].

The nursing home reform provisions regulate the certification of long-term–care facilities under the Medicare and Medicaid programs. These provisions became effective for services rendered on or after October 2, 1990, even though final regulations implementing the reforms were not issued by the HCFA until 1994 and were not effective until July 1, 1995 [59 Fed. Reg. 56116 (Nov. 10, 1994)].

The catalyst for the nursing home reform legislation was a 1986 Institute of Medicine study which declared that the care provided in most of the nation's nursing homes was "shockingly inadequate" and "likely to hasten the deterioration of the resident's physical and emotional health." The Institute's study blamed the Medicare and Medicaid nursing home standards then in existence for placing too much emphasis on nursing homes' physical plants and capacity to provide care, and not enough emphasis on the quality of that care. The resulting nursing home reform legislation required both Medicare SNFs and Medicaid NFs to provide, directly or under arrangements, the same basic range of services that includes those nursing services and specialized rehabilitative services needed to attain or maintain each resident's highest practicable level of mental, physical, and psychosocial well-being.

Specific nursing home reform provisions, most of which were determined to be largely self-effectuating, included:

- Elimination of the previous regulatory distinctions between skilled and intermediate nursing facilities;
- Establishment of a single standard of skilled care for all Medicare and Medicaid beneficiaries.
- Maintenance of a quality assessment and assurance committee.
- Development of a written plan of care for each resident upon admission to the facility.
- Provision of needed physician, nursing and specialized rehabilitative and other service.
- Disclosure of residents' rights on admission.
- Twenty-four hour, seven-day-a-week nurse staffing requirements.
- Standards and requirements for nurse training and education and competency evaluations.
- Enhanced survey and certification requirements.
- A significantly broadened range of available penalties and sanctions to target and improve quality services delivery without displacing residents.

Because of the requirement for increased specialized services, the then-HCFA cited the law as the cause for a rapid increase in the relative demand for therapist labor in SNFs. In 1997, the BBA placed a cap on facility therapy Part B Medicare payments of $1500 for occupational therapy and a combined cap of $1500 for physical and speech therapy, but the implementation of the cap was suspended by the BBRA [Pub. L. No. 106-113 (1999)] in 1999, and the moratorium continues to this date. In the BBRA, Congress directed HHS to conduct focused medical reviews of Part B therapy in nursing homes and report back to Congress in 2001 and 2002 [See OIG Report, Monitoring Part B Therapy for SNF Patients, November, 2000 (OEI-09-99-00550)].

Other legislative efforts in the recent past have focused on repealing parts of the nursing home reform.

Finally, in a recent report titled: "Nursing Homes: Sustained Efforts Are Essential to Realize Potential of the Quality Initiatives," the General Accounting Office assessed initiatives intended to address significant weaknesses in federal and state survey and oversight activities monitoring quality assurance in nursing homes. The General Accounting Office reported that the quality initiatives require continued federal and state attention to maximize their full potential. Coordination by state and federal governments, through fine tuning the survey process and limiting survey predictability, for example, would increase detection of serious nursing home deficiencies and assure quality care for nursing home residents [*See* GAO Report, GAO/HEHS-00-197 (September 2000)].

A fundamental understanding of legislation, benefits structure, and regulatory activity is essential to rehabilitation providers engaged in disability management. Success or failure in navigating complicated, amorphous, and ever-changing health care finance and delivery systems may be influenced both positively and negatively by a provider's non-clinical knowledge. Ignorance of the law is not blissful and can directly lead to risk and legal entanglements for providers.

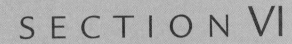

Trends and Issues in Health Care Finance and Delivery

C H A P T E R 20

Transition to Change in a Complex Health Care Sector

David W. Clifton, Jr., PT

By identifying the forces pushing the future, rather than those things that have contained the past, you possess the power to engage with your reality.

- Naisbett & Aburdene, 1990

KEY POINTS

- Change is constant, not episodic; change is external, and transitioning to it is an internal function.
- How individual and organizations transition to change, not the nature of the change itself, determines success or failure in disability management.
- Rehabilitation providers and their organizations must develop a comprehensive strategy for transition to change. This strategy preferably would be proactive and not reactive.
- Most people inherently tend to resist change, but organizations have individuals who serve as change agents.
- Transition is not an outcome but the process of bridging endings and beginnings.
- Polarization may occur between those who embrace change and those who resist it.
- Information and communication are the two vital keys to successful transition.

Operational Definitions

Change	Alteration of the status quo by an external event(s).
Transition	The response of individuals or organizations to change.
Information Anxiety	Anxiety experienced by persons/organizations because of a bombardment of data and information without instructions on application.
"The Neutral Zone"	The period of time between endings and beginnings, referred to as "limbo," or "a nowhere between two somewheres."

THE NATURE OF CHANGE

The purpose of this chapter (and of this book) is to assist rehabilitation professionals in transitioning to change in a rapidly evolving health care environment. Fundamental principles of change and transition are covered, as well as various coping strategies that can be applied at both the individual and organizational levels. Effective disability management demands that both individuals and organizations understand and adapt to change, especially change driven by factors external to one's industrial sector.

Dolphins-Carps-Sharks

Success in any business, including health care, requires an understanding of people and organizations. This is especially true when significant change affects an organization. Human resources directors use a variety of individual personality typing tools to encourage a greater appreciation of workplace diversity. These include instruments such as the Meyers-Briggs Type Indicator (MBTI), the Keirsey Temperament Sorter, the Jung-Meyers-Briggs typology, and the Gray-Wheelwright Temperament (Keirsey, 2004). These instruments are used to facilitate improved communication among employees. They are especially important during times of crisis or change. Change and transition to change can bring out the best or worst in people and their organizations. People, not products, services, or companies, determine successful transition to change.

Lynch and Kordis (1988) propose both an entertaining and instructive business theory that categorizes people and organizations as one of three creatures of the sea: carps, sharks, and dolphins. In this model, the sea can be viewed as a metaphor for the business environment. Innovations exist in a vast sea of chaos, unrest, and uncertainty. *Does this sound like the health care sector?* These innovations tend to be the product of carps and dolphins, not sharks. Carps, sharks, and dolphins share this sea, each bringing a different set of values, beliefs, traits, and action tendencies. Carps are the bait fish preyed upon by sharks. Carps, although intelligent, lack confidence as they swim in a tumultuous sea. Carps swim in large schools to create the appearance of being larger or more formidable. This is a defense tactic to fend off the predatory sharks. Carps represent moralistic persons or organizations that often have creative ideas snatched from them by fiercely aggressive "sharks." Sharks, unlike carps, are not very intelligent nor are they ethical in nature. Instead, they are remorseless and amoral creatures that ravage the carps. Little or no loyalty exists among sharks; hence, when they run out of bait fish (carp), they reveal their cannibalistic tendencies. Sharks have cold, lifeless eyes, and they lack a soul or conscience. Sharks kill indiscriminately, bloodying the waters. Sharks tend to be loners who do not swim in a school or pod. MacKay and Blanchard (1998) described business sharks in their seminal book entitled *Swim with the Sharks: Without Being Eaten Alive.*

Dolphins, to the contrary, are highly intelligent creatures with a perpetual smile. Dolphins prefer to be team players so they prefer to swim in a pod. However, they are comfortable swimming alone, especially when leading the pod. Dolphins often create waves of innovation and feed only when hungry. They will swim playfully among the carps and prefer dolphin or carp companionship to that of sharks. Dolphins are loyal and trustworthy, yet they strike fear in the heart of the shark, for they are the only sea-borne creatures that can kill the shark. Unlike the sharks, dolphins do not bloody the waters during feeding frenzies. Instead, they repeatedly batter the rib cage of the shark until it drifts lifelessly to the ocean depths. Dolphins can survive in a sea of sharks, and it is often they who prosper most from change. If a handful of dolphins are placed into a closed tank devoid of bait fish, but occupied by a hundred sharks, in due time there will be no sharks. This purging is accomplished through a combination of shark cannibalism and the coordinated battering of the sharks by dolphins, which represents business collaboration. When "dolphins" equipped with data, knowledge, and wisdom "swim in business pods" along with "carps," they are unstoppable (collaborative model of care). This chapter is devoted to the "carps" and "dolphins" of the business world and, specifically to physical rehabilitation providers!

Drivers of Change

Managed care has substantially contributed to significant paradigm shifts over the past several decades out of necessity to provide cost-effective health care services in a world of limited resources. A number of paradigm shifts have fundamentally, and perhaps irrevocably, changed how rehabilitation services are financed and delivered. Regulatory activity tends to most profoundly reshape the health care landscape (Buckley, 1999; Havighurst, 2000). See Chapter 21 for a more detailed discussion.

Americans consider the current health care system to be seriously flawed from at least three perspectives: access to care, cost of care, and quality of care (Pawlson, 1994; Greenwald, 2002; Webb, 2002). Depending on one's perspective, these three issues are responsible for or are the result of many of the changes and paradigm shifts that have occurred over the past decade. These paradigm shifts involve the provider-payer relationship (Gold, 1999). Many paradigm shifts have centered around re-structured financial arrangements between health benefit plans and providers. Capitation, discounted fees, and prospective payment systems (PPS) are notable examples. These and other financial models induce providers to modify practice to accommodate health plan demands and gain leverage during contract negotiations. These examples illustrate how external changes (e.g., regulatory, reimbursement) can lead to innovations that can revolutionize an entire sector.

Change Fuels Innovation

It has been said that necessity is the mother of all invention. The health care sector has had to re-invent itself due to a plethora of forces (Flower 1999). Some of these are discussed in Chapter 21.

Drucker (1982) asserts that innovations are incubated under certain circumstances and conditions This world-renowned business consultant outlines seven conditions from which all true innovation flows:

1. Unexpected change resulting from unexpected events leads to unexpected success or failure.
2. Incongruity between "what is" and "what ought to be."
3. Innovation based on a process need, invention, or opportunity. This innovation may involve something that exists that solves a process problem, as in technology transfer (e.g., the use of Velcro in artificial heart surgery).
4. Changes in industry structure or market structure that catch everyone off guard. Examples could include the diagnosis-related groups that ended the era of facility-based reimbursement under Medicare.
5. Shifting demographics (e.g., the graying of America).
6. Changes in perceptions, moods, and paradigms. For instance, during the past several decades, there has been a paradigm shift away from "medical" treatment and toward "health" and "wellness." The rise in use of alternative medicine exemplifies this shift (see Chapter 24.
7. The development of new knowledge, both scientific and nonscientific. Examples include genetic research, stem cell research, and human cloning.

Innovation can only result if people understand the nature of change and learn how to transition to it. This understanding is especially vital to rehabilitation professionals who have witnessed breathtaking change at a time when demand for their services has skyrocketed.

Change Is Not an Exception: It Is the Rule

The first lesson in dealing with change is to appreciate that change is constant and not periodic in nature. In today's society "perpetual unrest" displaces "contiguous progression" or incremental changes (Conner, 1998). Change is virtually a constant state. Internationally renowned business experts support this observation: "Everything is changing. This is not an overstatement. It is a fact. We are in the midst of the most profound change since the beginning of the Industrial Revolution, over two centuries ago. Perhaps, the most profound change since the Chinese more or less invented hierarchy thousands of years ago" (Peters et al, 1999).

Social historians have observed that dramatic social changes occur in cycles of approximately 30 years, or every other generation. This cycle seems to occur in health care. The first three decades of this century involved industrialization, during which employer-based insurance (e.g., workers' compensation) evolved. The next 30 years was spent in recovery from The Great Depression. The 1960s were highlighted by the advent of insurance for the disabled and elderly via Social Security, Medicare, and Medicaid. The 1990s was defined by astronomical growth in managed care as well as the appearance of chinks in its armor, namely, consumer, legislative, and regulatory backlash.

The Internet is poised to compress these 30-year cycles. It is safe to conclude that future changes and paradigm shifts will be swifter as a result of the information highway.

Change and Its Effect on Control

The human species, above all others, seeks and prizes control of its environment (Conner, 1998). Control allows an individual to balance opposing forces: threats and opportunities, fight and flight, benefit and risk, and perceptions versus reality.

Change can threaten to disrupt control over one's environment. Transition or adaptation to change must occur in order to restore a semblance of equilibrium. This demands an alignment or realignment of the expectations of individuals within organizations. Predictable responses to change occur when the expectations of individuals and organizations are in alignment. Predictable responses can restore control, which allows individuals and organizations to secure, retain, or recoup competitive advantage. Control is perennially threatened when a disconnect occurs between an individual's and organization's expectations and perceptions.

Rehabilitation providers generally do not receive formal training and education in how to respond to change, especially change driven by external forces beyond their control. Specific transition to change techniques and strategies will allow a person to make informed choices

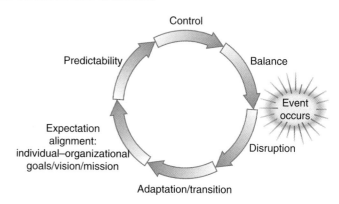

Figure 20–1. The change cycle. (Data from Conner DR: Leading at the Edge of Chaos: How to Create the Nimble Organization. New York, John Wiley and Sons, 1998.)

that preserve some degree of control over their environment. Figure 20–1 illustrates the relationships between control-balance, balance-transition/adaptation, transition-expectations, expectations-predictability and predictability-control.

Response-Ability

Health care providers today must confront and adapt to rapid and dramatic changes in how they conduct both their clinical and business practices. Clinical and business practices are frequently at odds and place the provider in a precarious position on many issues. The success of physical rehabilitation may be predicated more on how one adapts to an ever-changing environment than on one's competence or clinical skill sets. Step one is to accept that change occurs and that it most likely has its genesis in something beyond the provider's direct control.

Drucker (1982) asserts that most innovations in the public sector are imposed by outside forces or catastrophes. Although others may impose change on health care providers, an individual's response or transition to it is critical. In his seminal work, *The 7 Habits of Highly Effective People: Powerful Lessons in Personal Change,* Covey (1990) describes "response-ability." Figure 20–2 depicts the concept of "response-ability" and the freedom to choose when a stimulus demands a response. Responses require self-awareness, imagination, independent will, and conscious choices. Choices both good and bad become habits when knowledge is combined with skills and desire. Figure 20–3 portrays the overlap between knowledge, skills, and desire that leads to habit formation. Sound disability management through physical rehabilitation can only result when habits are built on a strong foundation of knowledge, wisdom, and skills. These foundational blocks begin with data, however. Distinctions exist between data and information, data and knowledge, facts and knowledge, and knowledge and wisdom.

Information Anxiety

Data have become a driving force of change. To remain relevant in today's society, health care providers must collect, analyze, assimilate and apply vast quantities of information.

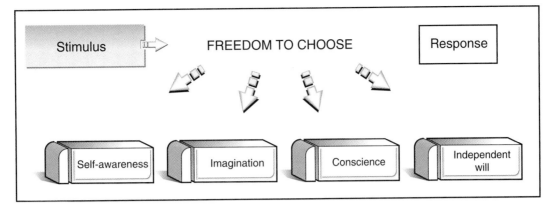

Figure 20–2. Response-ability. (From Covey S: The 7 Habits of Highly Effective People: Powerful Lessons in Personal Change. New York, Simon and Schuster, 1990.)

This information is often controlled by others and is created at a dizzying pace. Information technology is an exploding field of endeavor, and rehabilitation providers are directly affected by innovations in this sector.

Wurman (1990) coined the term "information anxiety" to describe the anxiety experienced by persons and organizations in response to an escalating deluge of information. For example, the number of books in existence doubles every 14 years. In addition, more than 9600 different periodicals are published in the United States every year.

The interpretation and ultimate use of information are often dictated by the source of the information. Information is received through various channels, as depicted by concentric rings in Figure 20–4. These sources of information have varying degrees of immediacy to one's life. In this schematic, *internal information* stems from within

an individual. This information enables individuals to function through cerebral messages, over which the individual sometimes has little or no control. For instance, anxiety and resistance may be natural sympathetic nervous system responses to change. Next in the hierarchy is *conversational information*, which is the product of human interactions on a day-to-day basis, involving both internal and external sources. The third ring in the hierarchy, *reference information*, flows from external sources that have filtered data. Health care reference information specific to

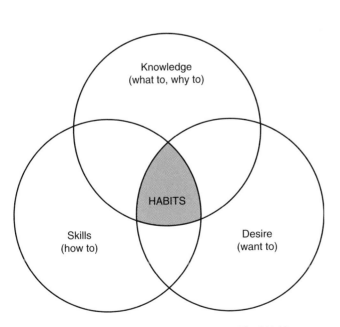

Figure 20–3. Foundation of habits. (From Covey S: The 7 Habits of Highly Effective People: Powerful Lessons in Personal Change. New York, Simon and Schuster, 1990.)

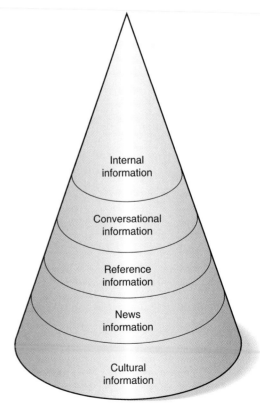

Figure 20–4. Sources and types of information. (From Wurman RS: Information Anxiety. New York, Bantam Books, 1990.)

populations or conditions falls within this ring. *News information* is broadcast over broad populations by major media. The last ring, *cultural information*, is the least quantifiable form of information dissemination. History, philosophy, and the arts that define a civilization exemplify cultural information. Information can flow between rings and influence other spheres. Rehabilitation providers assimilate information from all spheres when managing persons with physical disabilities. Understanding the sources of information can assist providers in several ways. The source of information can help distinguish trends from fads. Generally speaking, trends have at least a 10-year trajectory, whereas fads are relatively short-lived. Sources also can hint at the scope of change (e.g., societywide or cultural). Changes that affect an entire culture are most difficult to resist and can threaten to place one outside of the mainstream.

Data alone do not enlighten, however, unless they lead to knowledge and wisdom. Data consist of facts, while information is the meaning that human beings assign to these facts (Davis & McCormack, 1979). Individual data elements have little meaning or value unto themselves. Raw data cannot be valuable unless they inform or provide assistance in resolving challenges or reducing uncertainty.

What constitutes information to one person on one level may function on a different level for others. More data does not necessarily mean better data. In fact, data overload may stymie progress and true innovation. Health care providers can be so overwhelmed with data that they have difficulty relating them to the actual provider-patient encounter. For example, providers may have a disdain for excessive paperwork driven by reimbursement pressures, clinical outcome data collection, and risk management purposes. To a provider, attention spent on these issues may divert his or her attention and quality time away from the patient-provider encounter.

The pressure to balance sound business practices with quality clinical care can lead to significant provider anxiety. Anxiety has long been associated with an overstimulation by data. Table 20–1 cites the symptoms and signs associated with information anxiety. For instance, the inability to stay abreast of unfolding events or to explain a concept, resistance to new technology, and spending time on non-essential details may all suggest information anxiety.

Anxiety can only be eliminated when data lead to action. Wisdom is the product of knowledge and experience not, data and information. Wisdom is the antithesis of information anxiety. Wisdom can only be achieved through responsiveness to many mistakes made over time.

The Change Cycle

Change is not in and of itself an event but a process triggered by an event or events. Change can be planned or occur serendipitously. Change can have its genesis outside of one's sector or flow from within it. The primary purpose of transition to change is to array an organization's resources in ways that optimize its ability to manage ever-shifting external environments (Harvard Business Review, 2003). The first step in responding to changes is to identify them. This may sound overly simplistic but some physical rehabilitation providers may not perform systematic monitoring of trends and countertrends that immutably lead to changes in practice.

Conner (1998) states that "acknowledgement is the first line of defense in the struggle with constant change and hyper contingency." Transitional steps to change are depicted in Figure 20–5. In this schematic, internal or external events demand early recognition at both the individual and organizational levels. The second step involves the identification of factors that require transition. These factors include change agents, time frames, technology, capital needs, management style, and human resource needs. Action steps are next outlined that incorporate staff, timing, and financial issues. Execution of a transition plan must consider these three elements. Last, results are measured at both the individual and organizational levels. Modifications in the process may result when new changes impact an organization. Naisbett and Aburdene (1990) contend that even if one does not endorse the direction of trends, empowerment comes through the knowledge of this direction.

Stages of Change and Transition

Change is external to the individual or organization, and transition is an internal phenomenon. Transition is essentially one's response (individual or organizational) to change. Bridges (1991) describes three stages of change and transition: endings, the neutral zone, and beginnings. These stages are depicted in Figure 20–6. In this model old ways of thinking and/or acting diminish and eventually yield to new ideas and actions. When changes and transition are dramatic, paradigm shifts occur. (Please refer to Chapter 21 for comprehensive coverage of paradigm shifts that have impacted the physical rehabilitation sector.)

A transition zone known as the "neutral zone" represents the time frame during which people begin to let go of the past and begin to embrace the future. This period has been described by a number of analogies, such as an emotional wilderness, being caught between two trapezes, being lost in space, being in limbo or trapped in a nowhere between two somewheres (Bridges, 1991).

Most organizations fail to transition their staff to change because they do not provide an environment for

 Table 20–1   Signs and Symptoms of Information Anxiety

- Chronic complaints about an inability to keep up with unfolding events.
- Guilt associated with an inability to keep up with professional reading.
- An inability to explain something that an individual believed he or she understood.
- Resistance to new technology without an effort to understand and apply it.
- Spending time and resources on details that are unimportant to an individual's core business.
- Emotional responses to information without full comprehension.
- An assumption by the individual that co-workers comprehend what he or she does not and that they will cover his or her back.
- An individual's trepidation and embarrassment about his or her ignorance or poor understanding.

Data from Wurman R: Information Anxiety. New York, Bantam Books, 1989.

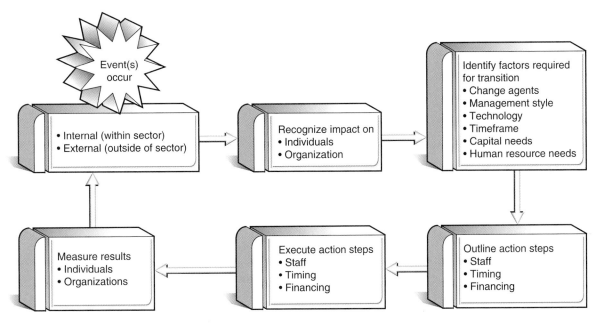

Figure 20–5. Transition to change flow diagram. (Data from Conner DR: Leading at the Edge of Chaos: How to Create the Nimble Organization. New York, John Wiley and Sons, 1998.)

employees to work through the mixed emotions often associated with the neutral zone. As a result employees tend to resist change (Page, 2002; Lawrence, 1969). Organizations and companies often expect staff to accept abrupt endings and to blindly embrace new ways of conducting business or treating patients. Mergers and acquisitions within the physical rehabilitation arena may exemplify this approach. Ownership shifts in the rehabilitation sector occurred virtually overnight with little or no transition. One large publicly traded rehabilitation company acquired nearly a billion dollars worth of their competitors' assets in 1 year alone! Literally overnight, fierce competitors became allies, without any substantive transition period.

The neutral zone is an extremely critical time frame and state of mind when employees are confused, anxious, and often without accurate and timely information or direction. Paradoxically, it is a time of both substantial threat and enormous opportunity. For some, change is

an opportunity for innovation, entrepreneurialism, and growth, yet for others change represents a threat to stability and predictability and an abandonment of traditions.

Force Field Analysis

The term *force field analysis,* coined by Stephen Covey (1990) in *The 7 Habits of Highly Effective People: Powerful Lessons in Personal Change,* describes a phenomenon that can assist providers in better understanding the genesis and depth of change.

Figure 20-7 illustrates the relationship between driving forces and restraining forces. Driving forces encourage an upward change or movement while restraining forces discourage movement. Equilibrium, the antithesis of change, is established when two equal but opposite forces exist. A perfectly balanced ball atop a hill depicts equilibration. Driving forces have distinguishing characteristics. They tend to be positive, reasonable, logical, conscious

Figure 20–6. Stages of change and transition. (From Bridges W: Managing Transition: Making the Most of Change. Reading, MA, Addison-Wesley, 1991.)

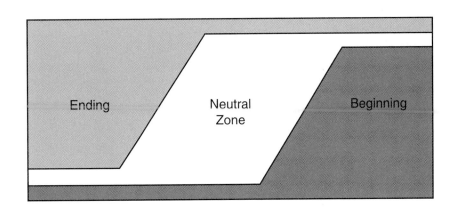

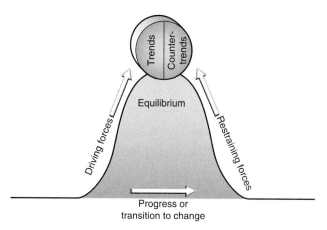

Figure 20–7. Force Field Analysis. (Modified from Covey S: The 7 Habits of Highly Effective People: Powerful Lessons in Personal Change. New York, Simon and Schuster, 1990.)

and economically driven. On the contrary, restraining forces are negative, emotional, illogical, unconscious, social, and psychological by nature. When driving forces overwhelm restraining forces, transition to change or progress results.

When of equal strength, trends and countertrends can create a static condition. In physical rehabilitation, publicly traded corporations are offset by the concurrent growth and strengthening of independently owned proprietary companies.

Economic challenges demand cost-effective rehabilitation services. As profit margins shrink, health care administrators search for less costly means of conducting business or treating patients. In fact, participation as a preferred provider under managed care may demand reduction of treatment cost. The driving force in this case is economic rationality. One means of reducing cost may be increasing the use of extenders of care such as physical or occupational therapy assistants. These assistants can manage selective aspects of care traditionally rendered by therapists, but typically at lower cost. When this occurs, staff therapists may potentially resist their administration's approach and engage in turf wars designed to protect their practice domain from less-expensive alternatives. Transition to change in these scenarios may be arrested if none of the administration's alternatives is favorably viewed by clinicians.

TRANSITION TO CHANGE

Once mere noise has been distinguished from profound change, transition can occur at the individual and/or organizational level. Flower (1998) suggests the use of three questions to gauge truly important change. Flower poses the following questions:

1. What are the changes occurring in the health care industry?
2. Is one's organization prepared for change?
3. How likely is it that one's organization can transition to this change?

Responses to these questions may hint at the degree of resistance an organization demonstrates during periods of change.

Responses both at the individual and organizational level are varied and unpredictable. Transition to change requires a comprehensive plan (McConnell, 2002; Weber & Joshi, 2000). South (2000) describes the "three D's" as a means for organizations to become more comfortable and committed to the change process. To effect successful transition to change, individuals and organizations must first feel a degree of discontent. Fear, especially fear of losses, is a remarkable motivating factor. Discontent can create a state of fear, or fear can drive discontent. Drucker (1982) states, "most innovations in public service institutions are imposed on them either by outsiders or by catastrophe." Discontent drives decision making, both good and bad. South (2000) cautions, however, that deciding to transition to change does not guarantee success unless determination exists to reposition oneself or one's organization in an ever-changing environment.

During the past decade, rehabilitation providers have experienced a decline of rehabilitation services and its resulting impact on disability benefits structures (Grahame, 2002). Trends have included declining employment opportunities, increased role of "gatekeepers," diminished referrals, shrinking reimbursement, turf infringement, the corporatism of health care, resistance to direct access, and a general loss of clinical autonomy.

Responses to change include causing change, accepting change, rejecting change, fighting change, and ignoring change (Buckley, 1999). Buckley encourages providers to become change agents; otherwise, providers may only have a chance to react to change imposed on the health care industry by external forces.

Perhaps the ultimate goal of all transition to change is to restore or retain some degree of control over one's environment. One should heed the warning, however, in this paraphrase of George Bernard Shaw (1903): The reasonable man/woman adapts himself/herself to the world: the unreasonable one persists in trying to adapt the world to himself/herself.

Figure 20-1 provides an insightful schematic for understanding the change cycle and the relationships among balance, disruption, adaptation/transition, expectations (both individual and organizational), predictability, and, ultimately, control. Virtually all change navigates this pathway, which can serve as a map for providers.

A balanced state can exist when people and their organizations command control of many variables. This balance can be disrupted when external events introduce changes in how someone conducts his or her clinical practice. Disruptions are created by events emanating from any of the following:

- Legislative activity
- Regulatory and compliance activity
- Professional standards
- Reimbursement/payer initiatives
- Corporate restructuring
- Market economics
- Public opinion

Transition to change and adaptation to new conditions and environments facilitate alignment of individual and organizational expectations, goals, vision, and mission. Alignment in turn results in a degree of predictability and, eventually, restoration and/or retention of control.

Half Empty or Half Full?

People and organizations can essentially be classified as either pessimists or optimists. Pessimists view the glass as half empty, whereas optimists view it as only half full with remaining capacity. Social scientists label pessimists as "Hobbesian" and optimists as "Lockean" (Secretan, 1998). Thomas Hobbes (1588-1679) and John Locke (1632-1704) were both English philosophers. In general, Hobbes viewed man/woman as inherently evil, greedy, selfish, and violently power seeking. Locke's view of humanity is more gentle and sees man/woman as inherently benign. In Locke's philosophy, however, antisocial behaviors are rooted in malevolent conditioning. Persons with Hobbesian traits strive to control their environments as well as their subordinates. These persons do well when external changes drive corporate changes. Transition to change is difficult for Hobbesians, who tend to reject or resist change. Behavioral and motivational theorists contend that Hobbesians thirst for power, and Lockeans strive for achievement and excellence (Secretan, 1998).

Organizational Transition to Change

At its simplest, transition involves human responses to various changes that impact the status quo (Bridges, 1991). The interaction between group and individual responses must be considered during transition. Individuals influence organizations and, reciprocally, organizations influence individuals.

Because people are the most valuable resources within an organization, individual goals, expectations, and needs must be aligned with the those of the organization for successful transition to change. Figure 20-8 depicts the overlap between individual and organizational goals, vision, and mission.

The Corporate Soul

The core culture of one's organization can determine whether change and the transition to it will be highly successful or a complete failure. The provider's ability to recognize the core culture of his or her organization may suggest to him or her whether particular changes will be properly managed (Muller-Smith, 1996). In a very insightful article, Stegall (2002) contends that individuals collectively instill a soul in their organization, and if they fail to do so, they risk losing their souls to the organization itself.

Muller-Smith (1996) cautions that the very culture of an organization may have to undergo radical change to

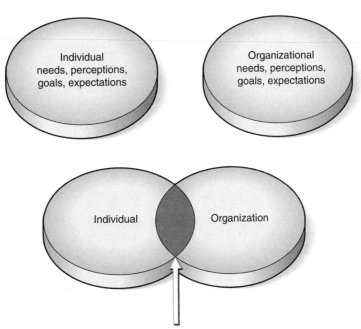

Figure 20–8. Transition to change: Alignment of individual and organizational needs, perceptions and expectations. (Modified from Lance HK, Secretan LH: Management Moxie. Rocklin, CA, Prima Publishing, 1993.)

survive paradigm shifts occurring in the health care sector. Providers must therefore understand their institution's core culture or soul if they are to transition to change without compromising their individual values, beliefs, and ethics (Izzo & Klein, 1998; Secretan, 1998). Areas of incongruence between the individual's and the organization's beliefs, values, and ethos will seriously inhibit successful transition to change. One example of this involves an overemphasis on "the bottom line" by a company's upper management (Schenke et al, 2001).

Entrepreneurial Versus Bureaucratic Management Styles

Antinomy is the contradiction or inconsistency between two apparently reasonable approaches to the same challenge (Secretan, 1993). For example, Secretan contrasts the entrepreneurial approach to the bureaucratic approach to business management. Both approaches serve a purpose and, in reality, a blending of management models most likely occurs when persons and organizations transition to change. Hospitals have traditionally employed a bureaucratic style of management with many layers between a physical or occupational therapist and the chief executive officer. This hierarchy created inertia when hospitals were required to respond to change. Hospitals over the past 20 years have become more entrepreneurial in nature as evidenced by a growing diversity of treatment settings as well as semantics (e.g., health system versus hospital). Private practice physical therapy companies, to the contrary, are devoid of hierarchal levels and thus very agile. Both models have their advantages and disadvantages. When traits are combined, provider organizations provide direction and focus while encouraging flexibility. This model is more likely to successfully adapt to environmental demands (Talbot, 1999; McConnell, 2000).

Table 20–2 compares and contrasts the entrepreneurial and administrative/bureaucratic approaches to management. Personal achievement and ego gratification fuel the entrepreneur, whereas the bureaucrat focuses on corporate image creation through achievement (Secretan, 1998). An entrepreneurial management style credits individuals for their accomplishments and not the group. By definition, entrepreneurs accept greater levels of risk than do bureaucrats. Reward systems between these styles are dramatically different as entrepreneurs tend to reward energy and effort. Bureaucrats reward individuals for conformity to standard operating procedures. Stated another way, entrepreneurialism rewards out-of-the box thinking and

 Table 20–2 Management Styles: Entrepreneurial Versus Administrative/Bureaucratic

Entrepreneur	Administrator/Bureaucrat
Seeks personal achievement and gratification	Seeks control
Gives credit to individuals	Enhancement of corporate image
Assumes moderate risk	Risk averse
Motivation derived through feedback	Motivation through merit awards
Energy and activity drive goal achievement	Conformity is preferred
Mastery of the environment	Mastery of the individual
Lateral organizational structure	Vertical organization
Encourages participation at all levels	Encourages participation only at upper levels
Authority is derived from task performance	Authority is ordained through hierarchy
Opportunity to explore hunches or to follow one's gut	Systems approach

Data from Secretan LH: Creating organizations that inspire the soul. Healthcare Des 10:3-6, 39, 1998.

risk-taking, the very antithesis of a bureaucratic management style. Entrepreneurial organizations communicate with less formality than their bureaucratic counterparts and involve workers in participatory decision making. Entrepreneurial companies are led by charismatic individuals and not by hierarchal corporate culture or image. Bureaucracies view innovation as a threat and consider adaptation to be an inconvenience instead of an opportunity for personal and corporate growth.

Kübler-Ross Model Applied to Transition to Change

When individuals face dramatic changes in their lives, they not uncommonly experience stages similar to those described in Elizabeth Kübler-Ross's (1969) seminal book, *On Death and Dying*. Figure 20–9 represents a theoretical model patterned after Kübler- Ross's theories.

Persons and organizations who wish to understand the emotions associated with change and transition may benefit from examining Kübler-Ross's theory of the five stages of loss. Because change often involves losing one thing in exchange for another, this model may have relevance in the context of organizational change. Sudden or traumatic change can often lead to feelings of denial and isolation. The mergers, acquisitions, and consolidation of the physical rehabilitation sector during the 1990s are

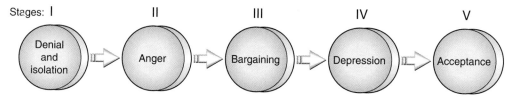

Figure 20–9. Transition to change depicted by the Kubler-Ross model. (Data from Elizabeth Kübler-Ross: On Death and Dying. New York, MacMillan, 1969.)

good examples of traumatic change. Literally overnight, thousands of physical and occupational therapists became employees of former competitors. In many cases, these new entities had different objectives, vision, mission, policies and procedures, and structure than their predecessors. It is understandable and perhaps to be expected that some persons entered into the denial or isolation stage (Stage I). Stage II is characterized by anger, a natural response especially in situations over which the affected person had little or no control. The anger stage can yield to bargaining behaviors (Stage III). During this stage, persons and organizations begin to assess changes from two poles; positive and negative. This is a stage during which one might conduct a SWOT analysis. Individual and/or organizational strengths-weaknesses and opportunities-threats are assessed during this stage. The results of the bargaining stage can dictate whether persons reach the depression stage (Stage IV) or acceptance stage (Stage V) of Kübler-Ross's model. Additional interventions may be necessary for those who enter the depression stage.

Figure 20–10 illustrates a transposition of the Bridges Model of Change-Transition that involves endings-neutral zone-beginnings with the Kübler-Ross model. This visualization may be useful in fostering a greater understanding of responses to change commonly faced by rehabilitation employees and colleagues. Rehabilitation professionals who routinely apply the Kübler-Ross model when dealing with grieving patients or families should have little difficulty in applying it to organizational change.

It is important to note that these behavioral theories are depicted as linear models of behavior. In reality, behavioral shifts may not be linear or predictable.

Although Kübler-Ross applied these stages to losses, her model may have relevancy for any change perceived by persons to significantly affect their lives. Many external events trigger changes that involve losses. Losses in physical rehabilitation may be of a financial, status, autonomy and/or control nature. Examples of such losses include:

Financial

- Reduced reimbursement
- Lower salary
- Decreased continued education allowance
- Reduced medical benefits
- Lower pension or 401K benefits

Status

- Center closings
- Demotion
- Staff terminations
- Shifts in patient populations treated
- Title changes

Autonomy and control

- Introduction of new treatment standards/protocols by others
- Increased use of extenders of care
- New supervision or reporting mechanisms
- Change implemented by home office without local input

Burnout

Although changes can occur quickly, burnout usually has an insidious trajectory. Freudenberger (1980) was among the first to define burnout: "someone in a state of fatigue or frustration brought about by devotion to a cause, way of life, or relationship that failed to produce the expected reward." Changes imposed without providers serving as stakeholders can easily change one's clinical way of life,

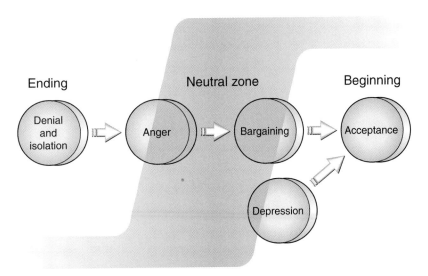

Figure 20–10. Using the Kübler-Ross stage theory to understand individuals' and organizations' response to change.

interfere with established relationships, and fail to result in expected rewards.

Rehabilitation providers need to be aware of the signs of burnout for the sake of patients/customers, their subordinates, and themselves. As previously discussed, it is important to recognize that individuals react differently to change. When incorporated into staff training and education, transition strategies can help to stem the rise of burnout conditions. Employee education is clearly the first step in preparing for change. Figure 20–11 provides a burnout scale that can be used by rehabilitation professionals to gauge their response to rapid and frequent changes in how clinical care is rendered.

Corporate Support for Change

In a watershed book, Peters and Waterman (1982) identified the following three major characteristics of well-run organizations:

1. Customers reign supreme.

2. A high level of employee dedication and enthusiasm is essential.

3. Trial and error is not only accepted, but encouraged.

These characteristics should be considered in the design of employee training and educational programs. The third characteristic, a work environment that does not condemn, but actually encourages trial and error, is particularly important for burnout prevention and transition to change.

The Role of the Change Agent

During periods of change and transition, certain individuals within every organization rise to the occasion and serve as change agents. These persons often share characteristics that allow them to develop an effective action plan for transition to change (Heifetz & Linsky, 2002). One motivating factor is to secure and/or retain a degree of personal control. Change agents attempt to develop strategies that capitalize on their unique characteristics

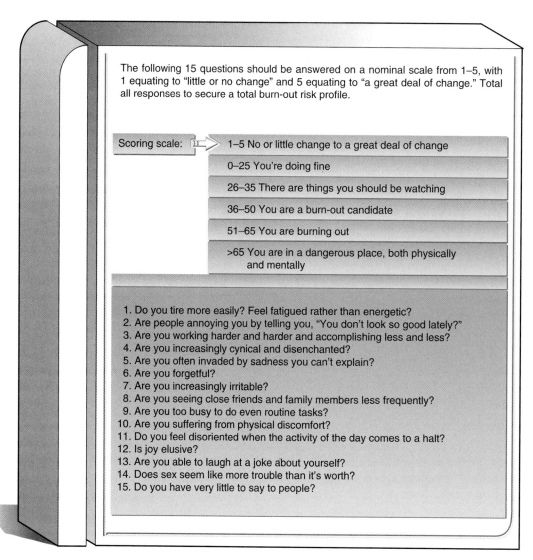

The following 15 questions should be answered on a nominal scale from 1–5, with 1 equating to "little or no change" and 5 equating to "a great deal of change." Total all responses to secure a total burn-out risk profile.

Scoring scale:
- 1–5 No or little change to a great deal of change
- 0–25 You're doing fine
- 26–35 There are things you should be watching
- 36–50 You are a burn-out candidate
- 51–65 You are burning out
- >65 You are in a dangerous place, both physically and mentally

1. Do you tire more easily? Feel fatigued rather than energetic?
2. Are people annoying you by telling you, "You don't look so good lately?"
3. Are you working harder and harder and accomplishing less and less?
4. Are you increasingly cynical and disenchanted?
5. Are you often invaded by sadness you can't explain?
6. Are you forgetful?
7. Are you increasingly irritable?
8. Are you seeing close friends and family members less frequently?
9. Are you too busy to do even routine tasks?
10. Are you suffering from physical discomfort?
11. Do you feel disoriented when the activity of the day comes to a halt?
12. Is joy elusive?
13. Are you able to laugh at a joke about yourself?
14. Does sex seem like more trouble than it's worth?
15. Do you have very little to say to people?

Figure 20–11. The burn-out scale. (Modified from Freudenberger HJ: Burn-Out: The High Cost of High Achievement. Garden City, NY, Anchor Press Doubleday and Company, 1980.)

and circumstances. For instance, a change agent may be someone who is viewed by others as trustworthy, competent, and a good communicator (Harvard Business Essentials, 2003). These persons have the ability to clearly articulate the need for change or, better yet, transition to change. They possess an understanding of the target audience's perspective, can translate intent into action, and foster self-renewal behaviors in their co-workers. Change agents can be viewed as power brokers, because they are the architects of innovative ideas and are dissatisfied with the status quo. They are the minority who actually welcome and do not resist change. Change agents anticipate change rather than simply responding to it. Change agents tend to be of the Lockean School of philosophy, because they are optimists who see the silver lining even in the darkest of times. They identify and track emerging trends, associating them with their core business pursuits. Change agents are masters of adaptation. They are the chameleons of the human species, shaping their products and services around emerging trends in a process that Faith Popcorn (1992) has labeled as "trendbending." The communication skills of change agents allow them to provide for consumers' needs for personalization. Popcorn refers to this as "egonomics." Physical rehabilitation providers possess characteristics that are most congruent with personalization or egonomics. Examples in health care that involve trendbending and egonomics include adult day care centers, specialty centers (e.g., incontinence and Alzheimer's programs), adaptive housing, assistive devices, and disease state management. These service categories require delivery of clinical services in a non-traditional manner and adapted to the incumbent client population. These programs use patient-centric, not department-centered or provider-centric, interventions. Companies with empowered change agents attempt to leverage their skills, competencies, knowledge, and experience.

Change agents appreciate the value of divergent transition strategies including takeover, trade-off, and giving-in and getting out (Lynch & Kordis, 1988). Table 20-3 summarizes circumstances that require different strategies for transitioning to change both at the organizational and personal level. These guideposts can be useful. Providers must recognize, however, that each situation is unique and warrants careful analysis along with malleable transition strategies.

Reece (1988) offers some advice, which may have significance to rehabilitation providers as they continue to face a barrage of changes in how their services are financed and delivered:

> Keep your eyes open, your nostrils flared, your ear to the ground, your options open, and your attitudes about method of payment flexible... don't be too much of a purist—fretting too much about how you're paid, how good were the good old days; or how much this world is changing.

This quotation has as much relevance today as it did in 1988.

Self-Assessment Tool for Transition to Change

Figure 20-12 is a modification of Bridges' original survey. The questions here require introspection regarding how individuals view change and their responses to it from both a personal and organizational perspective (Bridges, 1991). This survey can be a useful tool for rehabilitation professionals as they confront change.

Again, change is external and transition is internal. Thus transition is directly shaped by individual responses.

 Table 20–3 Strategies for Transition to Change

Takeover
- When time is severely limited and a specific outcome is crucial.
- When the relationship is of little importance and a specific outcome is critical.
- When appropriate retaliation is necessary.

Trade-off
- When time is short.
- When the issue is trivial to moderate in importance.
- When others are unwilling to cooperate fully.
- When the relationship is still of primary importance to you.
- When positions are highly polarized but progress is essential.

Give in
- When the issue is trivial but the relationship is crucial.
- When it is presents a good learning experience.
- When it is wise to "buy time" and you do not have a viable exit strategy.
- When compliance is critical during an emergency.

Get out
- When the outcome is of little importance.
- When other priorities demand attention.
- When additional information or resources are required but time does not permit its collection.
- When it is clear that nothing good can come from the situation other than a painful learning experience.

Data from: Lynch D, Kordis PL: Strategy of the Dolphin: Scoring a Win in a Chaotic World. New York, Fawcett Columbine, 1988.

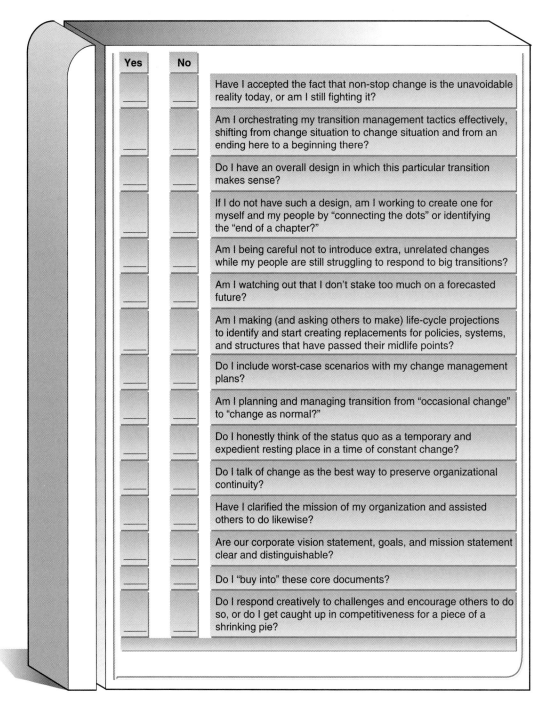

Yes	No	
__	__	Have I accepted the fact that non-stop change is the unavoidable reality today, or am I still fighting it?
__	__	Am I orchestrating my transition management tactics effectively, shifting from change situation to change situation and from an ending here to a beginning there?
__	__	Do I have an overall design in which this particular transition makes sense?
__	__	If I do not have such a design, am I working to create one for myself and my people by "connecting the dots" or identifying the "end of a chapter?"
__	__	Am I being careful not to introduce extra, unrelated changes while my people are still struggling to respond to big transitions?
__	__	Am I watching out that I don't stake too much on a forecasted future?
__	__	Am I making (and asking others to make) life-cycle projections to identify and start creating replacements for policies, systems, and structures that have passed their midlife points?
__	__	Do I include worst-case scenarios with my change management plans?
__	__	Am I planning and managing transition from "occasional change" to "change as normal?"
__	__	Do I honestly think of the status quo as a temporary and expedient resting place in a time of constant change?
__	__	Do I talk of change as the best way to preserve organizational continuity?
__	__	Have I clarified the mission of my organization and assisted others to do likewise?
__	__	Are our corporate vision statement, goals, and mission statement clear and distinguishable?
__	__	Do I "buy into" these core documents?
__	__	Do I respond creatively to challenges and encourage others to do so, or do I get caught up in competitiveness for a piece of a shrinking pie?

Figure 20–12. Self-assessment tool for transition to change. (Modified from Bridges W: Managing Transitions: Making the Most of Change. Reading, MA, Addison Wesley Publishing, 1991, pp 83-85.)

Introspection is the first step to not only survive change but thrive through change.

REFERENCES

Bridges W: Managing transitions: Making the most of change. Reading, MA, Addison-Wesley, 1991, pp 83-85.

Bujak JS: Culture in chaos: The need for leadership and followership in medicine. Physician Executive 25(3):17-24, 1999.

Buckley DS: A practitioner's view on managing change. Frontiers Health Serv Manage 16(1): 38-43, 1999.

Conner DR: Leading at the edge of chaos: How to create the nimble organization. New York, John Wiley and Sons, 1998.

Covey SR: The 7 Habits of Highly Effective People: Restoring the Character of Ethic. New York, Simon and Schuster, 1990.

Davidhizar R & Calhoun D: Understanding the members of your health care "gang:" Seekers and cruisers. Health Care Manage 20(4):40-45, 2002.

Davis W & McCormack A: The Information Age. Reading, MA, Addison-Wesley Publishing, 1979.

Drucker P: Innovation and Entrepreneurship: Practice and Principle, New York, Harper and Row Publishers, 1982.

Flower J: In an era of change...we're changing. Health Forum J 42(2): 66-69, 1999.

Flower J: Is it change? Or is it noise? Physician Executive 24(4):56-59, 1998.

Freudenberger HJ: Burn-Out: The High Cost of High Achievement. Garden City, NY, AnchorPress Doubleday and Company, 1980.

Gold M: The changing U.S. health care system: Challenges for responsible public policy. Milbank Q 77(1):22, 1999, http://www.milbank.org, accessed August 16, 2004.

Gelinas MV & James RG: Learn how to aid organizational change. Healthcare Benchmarks 6(9):105-106, 1999.

Grahame R: The decline of rehabilitation services and its impact on disability benefits. J Royal Soc Med 95(3):114-117, 2002

Greenwald J: HMO cost shifting to continue. Business Insurance 36(20):2, 2002.

Griffith JR: Developing an outcomes approach to health management education. J Health Adm Educ Special No.:125-129, 2001.

Harvard Business Essentials: Managing Change and Transition. Boston, MA, Harvard Business School Press, 2003.

Havighurst CC: American health care and the law—We need to talk! Health Affairs 19(4):84-106, 2000.

Heifetz RA & Linsky M: A survival guide for leaders. Harvard Business Rev 80(6):65-74, 2002.

Izzo J & Klein E: The changing values of workers, organizations must respond with soul. Healthcare Forum J 41(3):62-65, 1998.

Keirsey DM: www.Keirsey.com, accessed August 16, 2004.

Kübler-Ross E: On Death and Dying. New York, MacMillan Press, 1969.

Lawrence PR: How to deal with resistance to change. Harvard Business Rev Jan-Feb:4-12, 1969.

Lynch D & Kordis PL: Strategy of the Dolphin: Scoring a Win in a Chaotic World. New York, Fawcett Columbine, 1988.

McConnell CR: Making change work for you—Or at least not against you. Health Care Manage 20(4):66-77, 2002.

McConnell CR: The manager and the merger: Adaptation and survival in the blended organization. Health Care Manage 19(1):1-11, 2000.

Muller-Smith P: Core culture: The key to successful paradigm shifts. J Post Anesth Nurs 11(1):35-38, 1996.

Naisbett J & Aburdene P: Megatrends 2000. New York, Avon Books, 1990.

Page EP: Tapping the potential in resistance. Semin Nurse Manage 10(3):180-188, 2002.

Peters TJ et al: Circle of Innovation. New York, Random House, 1999.

Peters TJ & Waterman RH: In Search of Excellence. New York, Harper Collins, 1982.

Popcorn F: The Popcorn Report. New York, Bantam Doubleday Dell Publishing Group, 1992.

Reichmann FF: Psychiatric aspects of anxiety. In Stein M et al (eds): Identity and Anxiety: Survival of the Person in Mass Society. New York, The Free Press of Glencoe, 1960.

Schenke R et al: Leading beyond the bottom line: Part 4. The questions it has raised. Physician Executive 27(2): 8-11, 2001.

Secretan LH: Creating organizations that inspire the soul. J Healthcare Design 10:3-6, 1998.

Secretan LH: Managerial Moxie. Rocklin, CA, Prima Publishing, 1993.

Shaw GB: Man and Superman, "Maxims for Revolutionists." Cambridge, MA, The University Press, 1903.

South SF: The secret to successful change: The three D's. Clin Leadership Manage Rev 14(5):216-218, 2000.

Stegall MS: Instilling a soul in your organization without losing yours to it. Clin Leadership Manage Rev 16(2):85-89, 2002.

Talbot JF: Managing for change: Models and questions for group practice leaders. Med Group Manage J 46(5):50-54, 56, 58, 1999.

Tiffan WR: Thriving in change. Physician Executive 26(4):46-51, 2000.

Weber V & Joshi MS: Effecting and leading change in health care organizations. Joint Commission J Qual Improvement 26(7):388-399, 2000.

Wurman RS: Information Anxiety. New York, Bantam Books, 1990.

Suggested Readings

Beer M & Nohria N: Cracking the code of change. Harvard Business Rev 78(3):137, 2000.

Murphy EC & Murphy MA: Leading on the Edge of Chaos. Paramus, NJ, Prentice Hall Press, 2002.

Peters T: Thriving on Chaos. New York, First Harper Perennial, 1991.

Quinn RE: Deep Change. San Francisco, Jossey-Bass, 1996.

CHAPTER 21

Delivery Paradigm Shifts

David W. Clifton, Jr., PT

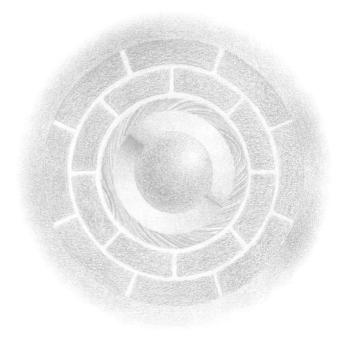

*Their current industry was on a stable even lucrative curve, but around the bend was change
that would transform the business fundamentally, completely, irrevocably.*

- Morrison, 1996, p 6

KEY POINTS

- Traditional health care finance and delivery paradigms must be understood before individuals and organizations can successfully transition to new ones.
- All paradigm shifts present both threats and opportunities depending on how the individual or organization comprehends, interprets, and adapts to them.
- An understanding of the drivers of change is essential for providers to anticipate and transition to change.

Operational Definitions

Change	A modification driven by a factor that is external to the individual or organization.
Paradigm	A paradigm is a pattern, model, example, or set of ideas, principles, or assumptions that standardize and guides human behavior.
Paradigm Shift	The displacement or augmentation of one model by another model(s).
Transition	An individual or organization's response to external changes.

WHAT BUSINESS ARE WE IN?

The quotation by Ian Morrison at the beginning of this chapter speaks of a classic problem associated with industries as they evolve from first-curve companies to second-curve companies. First-curve companies have a traditional business base that represents a majority of their revenues. To survive and thrive, first-curve companies must embrace

second-curve tendencies, especially diversification and entrepreneurialism. Some industries actually begin as second-curve companies, in part because of highly creative innovators operating in unique niche markets. The computer software industry and Silicon Valley come to mind. Second-curve companies do not define their mission solely through the product or service they offer. Instead, these companies take a more global view. For instance, railroads previously viewed themselves as being in the business of transporting goods through rails. This narrow first-curve view nearly led to the collapse of a once powerful industry. The trucking industry held a second-curve belief in its ability to transport goods virtually anywhere. Those railroads that survived did so by viewing their mission as transportation, whatever the means. These second-curve companies collaborated with trucking, maritime, and air transport companies to better serve customer needs.

The I-10 and I-15 corridors in San Bernardino County, California, exemplify the coexistence and, in some instances, collaboration between various transportation sectors. This area boasts one of the world's largest railroad collating sites (e.g., 10 miles long), mega truck stops, and warehousing capabilities. The interaction between different industrial sectors is highly visible.

The title of this text was carefully selected to reflect second-curve tendencies. The term *disability management* is broad enough to avoid pigeon-holing a profession. *Physical rehabilitation* extends beyond the confines of a single discipline, such as physical therapy, occupational therapy, or physical medicine and rehabilitation (PM&R). Using the railroad example, physical therapists are not in the business of only physical therapy. This is only the means and professional designation by which they accomplish their ultimate goal: to prevent, treat, and manage disability. Better yet, physical therapists and occupational therapists are in the business of ability enhancement or functional maximization.

The American health care system today is in the throes of perhaps its most tumultuous time in history, and many of its participants have both first- and second-curve characteristics. Virtually every aspect of health care finance and delivery has undergone some degree of change, with old paradigms yielding to new ones. Hospitals once considered first-curve companies are now "health care systems" with diversified income that transcends their traditional in-patient revenues. Hospitals no longer principally define their service through the number of beds. Clinical services once delivered in separate silos are now provided through vertically and horizontally integrated delivery networks. Figure 21–1 depicts the complexity and diversity of health care organizational and delivery paradigms.

The ever-changing nature and complexity of health care delivery, technology, and information management severely challenges rehabilitation professionals. It seems that the status quo no longer exists, as new developments threaten to alter how care is delivered and by whom. The impact on physical rehabilitation providers is magnified because of their participation in every point on the disability continuum from prevention and wellness to treatment and beyond. Physical and occupational therapists are active in the pre-injury or pre-illness, acute, subacute, and chronic stages of illness and injury. They work in a variety of settings, including home care, employer locations, hospitals, school districts, government agencies, outpatient centers, and extended living facilities. Although their interventions, treatment settings, reimbursement models, patient populations, and clinical documentation requirements may differ, these providers are all in the same business: disability prevention and management. This new paradigm requires that rehabilitation professionals possess a different worldview than traditional providers of care. Perhaps, a Functional Therapy Association will evolve some day?

This chapter strives to equip readers with fundamental knowledge about how to manage change and understand paradigm shifts. Editorial constraints limit the number of paradigm shifts that can be covered in any degree of detail. Therefore readers are encouraged to further explore these issues through suggested readings and other chapters in this text.

Seminal Events in Health Care History

A widely quoted axiom states that *to ignore history is to repeat it*. In this context, it is essential that providers understand the historical events that have led to current challenges.

The current American health care system was forged by a number of key developments, principally guided by three health care benefit cornerstones (Javors & Bramble, 2001). The advent of third-party hospitalization insurance in the 1930s (Blue Cross/Blue Shield plans), the employer-based health benefits of the 1940s, and the establishment of government-based programs (Medicaid and Medicare) in 1965 together led to a fracturing of the

traditional customer-based health care model, otherwise known as private pay. Three distinct participants emerged, the provider as decision-maker, the payer (employer or government), and the consumer (patient). Under managed care, the insurance company serves as intermediary between the patient or consumer and the payer (employer or government). In this role, managed care organizations (MCOs) wield disproportionate power and control over health care spending and delivery while assuming the least amount of financial risk relative to the principal stakeholders: consumer, provider, and employer. As a result, managed care entities may actually be the most expendable stakeholder in the system. This is especially true as more employers continue to self-insure their risks. These employers do not pay an insurance premium. Instead, they set aside funds known as "company reserves" to cover losses on an as-needed basis. This is risky business, so self-insured employers tend to be more interested in injury and illness prevention programs than in non-self–insured employers.

Managed care as a sector is undergoing a great deal of criticism from a variety of health care stakeholders, including consumers, employers, and providers (Larson, 1996; Katz, 2001; Pawlson, 2002; Webb, 2002). Critics of managed care argue that its design is seriously flawed because it treats the payer as the most important component. In terms of control, managed care places insurers at the top and providers at the bottom while excluding the most important party, the consumer or patient. Some assert that since it is the patients who ultimately receive services, they are the most logical locus for financial incentives to facilitate cost-effective care. Patients or consumers in recent years have experienced increasing risk assumption in the form of higher deductibles and co-payments combined with restricted access to services (Javors & Bramble, 2001; Schultz, 2002). When consumers or patients have a financial stake in health care, more prudent use of services often results.

Despite its obvious shortcomings, managed care has driven a number of changes that should enjoy a reasonable degree of longevity. These changes include evidence-based practice (EBP), shared control for treatment choices (between consumer-payer-provider), consumer at-risk contracts (financial risk [e.g., co-payments or deductibles]), provider at-risk contracts (e.g., capitation, discounted fees, prospective payment), and aggregation of providers into discrete units (Javors & Bramble, 2001). Few people can accurately predict, however, which health care finance and delivery model will eventually displace or augment managed care.

PARADIGM SHIFTS: PRODUCTS OF CHANGE

What Is a Paradigm Shift?

When one paradigm displaces, yields to, or augments another, a paradigm shift has occurred. Old paradigms are referred to as the status quo and new ones as innovation. The American health care finance and delivery system(s) has undergone a plethora of paradigm shifts during the past two decades (England, 1997; Bensassat, 1996;

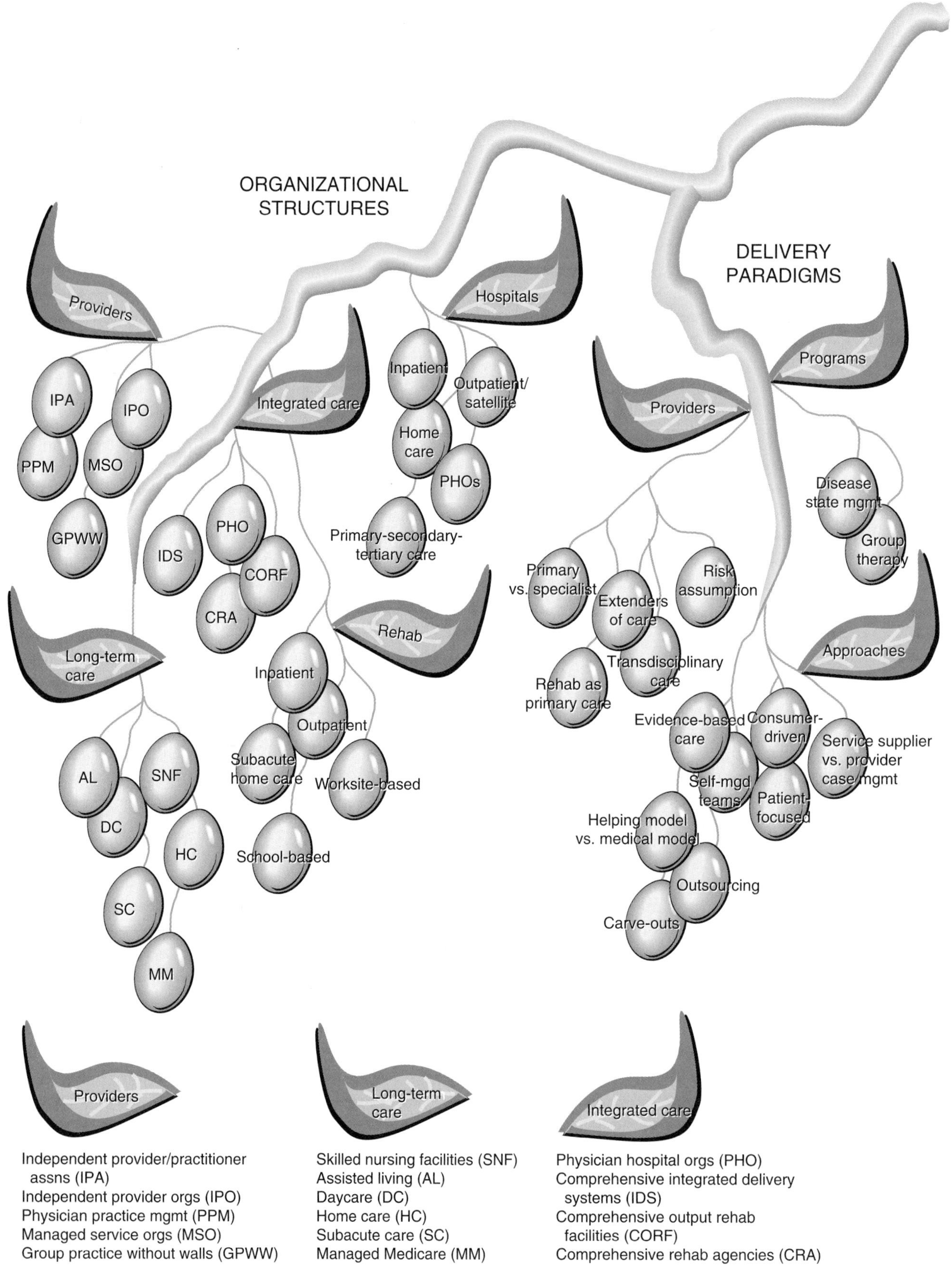
ORGANIZATIONAL STRUCTURES
DELIVERY PARADIGMS
Providers
IPA
IPO
PPM
MSO
GPWW
Integrated care
IDS
PHO
CORF
CRA
Hospitals
Inpatient
Outpatient/ satellite
Home care
PHOs
Primary-secondary-tertiary care
Long-term care
AL
SNF
DC
HC
SC
MM
Rehab
Inpatient
Outpatient
Subacute home care
Worksite-based
School-based
Providers
Primary vs. specialist
Extenders of care
Risk assumption
Transdisciplinary care
Rehab as primary care
Programs
Disease state mgmt
Group therapy
Approaches
Evidence-based care
Consumer-driven
Service supplier vs. provider case mgmt
Self-mgd teams
Patient-focused
Helping model vs. medical model
Outsourcing
Carve-outs
Providers
Independent provider/practitioner assns (IPA)
Independent provider orgs (IPO)
Physician practice mgmt (PPM)
Managed service orgs (MSO)
Group practice without walls (GPWW)
Long-term care
Skilled nursing facilities (SNF)
Assisted living (AL)
Daycare (DC)
Home care (HC)
Subacute care (SC)
Managed Medicare (MM)
Integrated care
Physician hospital orgs (PHO)
Comprehensive integrated delivery systems (IDS)
Comprehensive output rehab facilities (CORF)
Comprehensive rehab agencies (CRA)

Figure 21–1. Organizational and delivery paradigms.

Davidson, 1997). Paradigms incorporate ideas and principles that span intellectual, ideological, ethical, spiritual, and other domains. A paradigm shift does not necessarily imply the replacement of one paradigm with a second. Paradigms do coexist, and they can contain equivalent, if not opposing, worldviews. Paradigms also can merge to form hybrid ones. For instance, extenders of care (new paradigm) did not completely displace more skilled professionals (traditional paradigm), but simply augmented them.

Drivers of Change

Some paradigm shifts have their genesis within the rehabilitation sector itself, and others are associated with changes driven by external factors, especially regulatory activity (Buckley, 1999). Regulatory and compliance issues will not be extensively covered in this chapter. Readers are referred to Chapters 18 and 19 for further discussion of these topics. Although a number of significant paradigm shifts have emanated from the physical rehabilitation sector itself, such shifts typically occur in response to more significant changes at the macroeconomic level. For instance, the role of the gatekeeper effectively rendered rehabilitation a discretionary service, far down on the referral chain of managed care. Primary care physicians' financial incentives resulted in fewer or slower referrals for non-primary services, such as laboratory workups, imaging tests, pharmaceuticals, and ancillary services. Consequentially, physical and occupational therapists see fewer referrals coming from PCPs because they are reimbursed for non-referral through "withhold" pools of capital. The movement toward securing direct access or the ability to evaluate and treat without physician referral is partly a result of the restrictions associated with the gatekeeper role. Physical therapy practice without physician referral, however, has yet to become a dominant paradigm despite the fact that a majority of states allow it within their state practice acts. In addition, consumers (patients), employers, and insurers have not substantially altered their health care selection process as a result of direct access. Direct access has the potential of evolving into a dominant paradigm. However, any evolution likely will be due less to provider advocacy efforts than the result of macroeconomic factors. These factors include better-educated consumers, growth in self-care, restricted health benefit plans, increase in private spending for alternative medicine, growth in medical savings accounts (MSAs), and the assumption by consumers/patients of greater financial risk in the form of co-payments and deductibles.

External drivers of change (outside of one's sector) or those that occur beyond the immediate control of providers must be understood if one is to successfully transition to changes and remain competitive in an ever-evolving health care finance and delivery system. Buckley (1999) cautions that a failure to voluntarily respond or transition to challenges and opportunities will only result in imposed changes in the health care industry.

Some paradigm shifts are major and far-reaching in nature, yet others are limited to one stakeholder group or are of relatively minor significance to society at large.

A Shift from a Deductive Health Care Model to an Inductive Model

A number of major paradigm shifts have significantly altered the clinical reasoning process across all medical professions. For instance, clinical reasoning has shifted from a deductive model to an inductive, probabilistic, or evidence-based approach (Bensassat, 1996). EBP de-emphasizes clinical intuition, unsystematic clinical experience, and pathophysiologic rationale in favor of practice guidelines, standards, treatment protocols and critical pathways of care (Lindberg et al, 1992; Eddy, 1992; Richardson, 1997; Drummond, 1998; APTA, 2001).

A Shift away from the Medical Model of Health Care

A paradigm shift away from the biomedical model that traditionally reduced all diseases to structural or biochemical dysfunctions has significantly impacted today's clinical reasoning.

The new paradigm recognizes the influences of other non-structural or biochemical dysfunctions, such as the psychosocial factors of disease and injury. Rehabilitation professionals should be well-positioned to take advantage of this paradigm, especially in persons with chronic conditions and those needing elder care.

Bensassat (1996) describes a new emphasis on quality-of-life issues versus impairment-based clinical decision making. Rehabilitation providers now routinely use quality-of-life (QOL) measures. QOL instruments now augment traditional impairment measures (e.g., range of motion, muscle performance, balance). However, QOL measures have not completely displaced traditional measures.

Internal and External Forces Align

Some changes that potentially lead to new paradigms are the result of an interaction between internal (within one's sector) and external forces. For example, the use of extenders of care (e.g., physical therapy assistants and certified occupational therapy assistants) by physical therapists and occupational therapists are examples of a potentially new paradigm. New reimbursement incentives, namely lower reimbursement (external driver), have fostered the need for more cost-efficient services that can be accomplished with less expensive staff allocation (internal driver).

Selective contracting fostered by the managed care industry in an effort to restrain health care costs has directly resulted in efforts by providers to become more cost-effective and efficient in the delivery of services.

CYCLES OF CHANGE

Paradigm shifts are obviously the result of change and how persons and organizations adapt to change. Change has been described as constant, complex, and chaotic (Bujak, 1999; Flower, 1998; Flower, 1999). Dramatic societal changes appear to occur every 30 years, or roughly every other generation. The Great Depression occurred 30 years after the turn of the twentieth century. The next 30 years were spent in recovery from the Depression. The infamous 1960s were highlighted by a constellation of social changes, including the social rights movements and the advent of the first government-subsidized health care systems, Medicare and Medicaid. The 1990s were defined by nationwide managed care with a whirlwind of fundamental changes in both health care finance (e.g., at-risk contracts or capitation) and delivery (e.g., primary care physicians or gatekeepers) mechanisms.

The new millennium has begun with a tremendous antimanaged care backlash, and the dust has yet to settle. The Internet promises to compress the 30-year cycles referred to earlier, as data are communicated at breakneck speed. Future health care paradigm shifts are likely to be swifter and, perhaps, more extensive than ever because of an increasingly complex health care sector (Baker, 2002; Beckham, 2001). In an era of business mergers and acquisitions, one can safely predict rapid and, perhaps, profound changes (McConnell, 2000).

Balancing Conflicting Paradigms

It is common for two paradigms to be in conflict with one another. For example, health care organizations that embrace fundamental business principles such as budgeting, resource allocation, and benefit-cost ratios may find it a daunting challenge to balance economic rationality with humanitarian concerns. Because health care is a business, it will be necessary to balance business concerns with health care concerns. This is no easy task for providers who entered the healing arts on the basis of humanitarian motives, not financial ones.

Figure 21-2 depicts the equilibrium that results when business and health care goals, interests, and objectives are in alignment. This figure illustrates two seemingly opposite paradigms. The business paradigm is highly focused on economic incentives and the health care paradigm focuses on humanitarian issues. Opponents and proponents of managed care may frame issues as stark contrasts. For example, antimanaged care sentiment may hold that quality of care suffers under capitation models that reward providers for doing less. However, managed care supporters may contend that economic incentives are essential for those organizations that wish to achieve consistent quality and reduce practice variation.

Change and Transition at the Individual and Organizational Levels

The past decade has seen unparalleled changes in virtually every aspect of health care finance and delivery. Changes have been diverse and frenetic, and have impacted every American in one form or another.

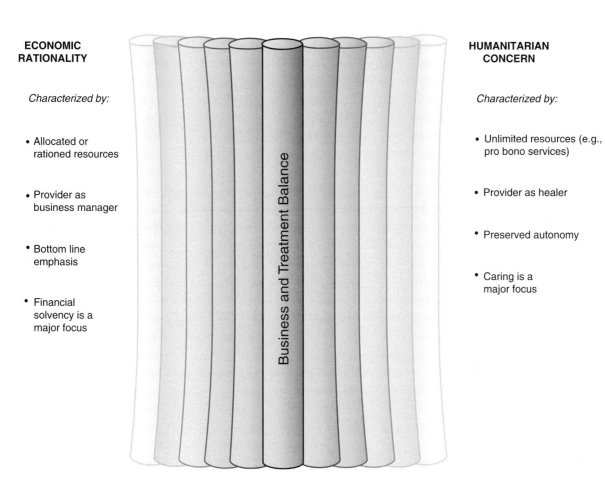

ECONOMIC RATIONALITY

Characterized by:

- Allocated or rationed resources

- Provider as business manager

- Bottom line emphasis

- Financial solvency is a major focus

Business and Treatment Balance

HUMANITARIAN CONCERN

Characterized by:

- Unlimited resources (e.g., pro bono services)

- Provider as healer

- Preserved autonomy

- Caring is a major focus

Figure 21-2. Business-health care equilibrium.

Paradigm shifts elicit a diverse array of responses at both the individual and organizational level (Buckley, 1999; Tiffan, 2000; Hunsaker, 1982; Davidhizar & Calhoun, 2002). Properly managed change can benefit the individual and the organization; however, change will occur whether or not an individual or organization plans for it (Buckley, 1999). Those providers and organizations adept at transitioning to changes that affect an organization's structures, processes, and outcomes are more likely to be successful. Those who resist or deny change will likely be less competitive in a capitalistic system. Successful organizations are those that achieve an alignment of goals, objectives, and understanding between the individuals who compose the organization and the organization's leadership.

Change comes in many forms and either favorably or unfavorably affects providers. The result may have more to do with one's response to change than to the nature of the change itself. Some changes are short-lived and represent fads, yet others result in long-term trends. Providers' understanding of the drivers of change is essential to anticipate and transition to change (Weber & Joshi, 2000).

Flower (1998) provides three filters used by organizations to select a course of action. These questions help to differentiate profound change from what Flower describes as "mere noise."

1. What changes are occurring in the health care industry?
2. Is your organization ready for change?
3. How likely is it that your organization will easily adopt this particular change?

An organization's corporate culture or soul can dictate responses to new paradigms (Talbot, 1999; South, 2000; Heifetz, 2002; Inamdar, 2002; Weber & Joshi, 2000). Successful change depends largely on an organization's ability to identify and respond to what has been described as the "three Ds": discontent, decision, and determination (South, 2000). An organization and its employees may initially feel a degree of discontent when the status quo is challenged. Next a decision has to be made to alter how business is conducted relative to the change. South cautions that decisions alone are insufficient in transitioning or responding to paradigm shifts. Organizations must be determined to execute appropriate responses if they are to remain well positioned. The soul or culture of an organization will dictate how it responds along a continuum from full resistance to total acceptance of change (Izzo & Klein, 1998; Muller-Smith, 1996; Secretan, 1998).

Individuals and corporations both possess egos that serve as obstacles in identifying and responding to paradigm shifts. Egotistical persons and entities often possess the attitude, "it's my way or the highway." These organizations may view changes as incongruent with their current corporate culture and thus resist them (Muller-Smith, 1996).

Other persons and organizations may view change as an aid to business navigation (Gelinas & James, 1999; Tiffan, 2000; McConnell, 2002). In especially turbulent times both optimists and pessimists abound. People fundamentally respond to change through resistance, however, at least until buy-in is achieved (Page, 2002; Hofmann, 2002). Proactive persons and organizations strive to control what they can, leaving less to chance (Tiffan, 2000).

Weber and Joshi (2000) describe the following eight crucial strategies or principles designed for proactive health care organizations:

1. Development of a vision for change.
2. Focus on the change process.
3. Identification or analysis of an organization's potential change agents and internal barriers to change.
4. Building of partnerships between providers and administrators.
5. Creation of a culture of continuous commitment to change.
6. Assurance that change begins at the top with leadership.
7. Assurance that change is communicated well at all organizational levels.
8. Integration of measures of accountability for change at all organizational levels.

TEN PARADIGM SHIFTS IMPACTING PHYSICAL REHABILITATION

Traditional Paradigms Surrender to New Paradigms

Table 21-1 summarizes paradigm shifts that have already significantly impacted or may continue to significantly impact physical rehabilitation providers. This is by no means an all-inclusive list, nor are the paradigms listed in order of importance.

Duncan (1996) outlines a number of traditional rehabilitation paradigms. These have been modified to some degree and are presented here. The "white lab coat syndrome" describes providers' propensity to focus on the biophysical aspects of care such as disease, pathology, physiology

 Table 21-1 Traditional Rehabilitation Paradigm Assumptions

Paradigm	Assumption
"Is my shoulder patient here yet?"	Some therapists are guilty of treating the patient as a body part and offering regionally based treatment. This attitude is similar to the "white lab coat syndrome."
Discipleship	Clinical practice driven by teaching of so-called "experts" or gurus without critical substantiation of claims. A mentality of "This is how so and so does it" prevails.
Father/Mother knows best	Clinical expertise and experience carry the day. Valid treatment guides are developed on the basis of individual clinician expertise only.
White lab coat syndrome	A biophysical emphasis of care (e.g., disease, pathology, physiology, and pathokinesiology) is a sufficient guide in rehabilitation.
Catch as catch can	Unsystematic observations by clinicians used for database development.
The blame game	Excessive use of defense mechanisms. Tendency to see the world not as it is, but as we are (e.g., "Managed care is the root of all evil.")
The Hatfields and McCoys	Turf wars abound. "Other professions are stealing our patients and treatment secrets." "We have seen the enemy and it is everyone but us!"

Based on modified data from Duncan PW: Evidence-based practice: A new model for physical therapy. Phys Ther 4(12):44-48, 1996.

and pathokinesiology. The "father/mother knows best" paradigm is characteristic of providers who believe that their unique clinical expertise and experience will produce reasonable outcomes. These providers tend to ignore or downplay the value of treatment guidelines that are evidence-based. A "catch as catch can" treatment model describes clinicians who fail to systematically capture, analyze, and apply data for clinical decision making purposes. "The blame game" relies on defense mechanisms such as projection. For example, a common provider response may be to cite managed care impositions as the reason for erosion in clinical quality or poor outcomes. "Discipleship" is the practice of following the teachings of so-called experts or gurus who espouse their treatment philosophies in the absence of scientific study or evidence. Depersonalized treatments that focus on body regions instead of the whole person have been a common approach in rehabilitation. Such clinicians may routinely make statements such as "Is my shoulder patient here?" "We operate a hand center" and "My specialty is backs."

Paradigm Shift 1: Outcomes Measures Supplant Process and Structure

Arnold Relman, MD, editor of the American Medical Association's journal during the zenith of managed care growth, described three revolutions impacting American health care (Relman, 1988). The first revolution of health care occurred after WWI with the expansion in medical services, facilities, professions, technology, and funding mechanisms. Medical coverage of Americans peaked in the mid-1960s with the advent of Medicare, Medicaid, and more employer-sponsored plans. The second revolution is depicted as the "revolt of payers" or the "era of cost containment." This era was spawned by an escalation in health care costs as a percentage of gross domestic product. The third revolution is defined by accountability and assessment across all stakeholder groups including employers, traditional insurers, MCOs, providers, and patients. Health care delivery of unknown quality or quantity is no longer acceptable. In this latest revolution, clinical and financial data are addressed through defined treatment protocols, EBP, outcomes measurement, continuous quality improvement (CQI) or total quality management (TQM), and provider profiling. Clinical preferences on the basis of anecdotal evidence only or theory espoused by so-called "experts" is challenged and/or non-reimbursed under this new paradigm.

Paradigm Shift 2: Physical Rehabilitation: Primary Care or Specialty—Which is it?

Physical rehabilitation under managed care is routinely perceived as an elective or discretionary specialty service. Delayed referral or non-referral to rehabilitation by primary care physicians (PCPs) is fairly common. Patients must often convince the "gatekeeper" or PCP of their need for a specialty service, and providers must establish medical necessity and reasonableness of care (Katz, 2001). Some suggest a reduced or eliminated role for PCPs in the next health care paradigm (Larson, 1996; Katz, 2001). A number of factors have weakened the role of PCPs.

Distrust among patients has been documented (Haas et al, 2003). A lack of empirical evidence demonstrating cost savings associated with the gatekeeper model has further contributed to its diminished role (Pati et al, 2003). The growth in Internet use for the purpose of health care information now means that more people have access to data that heretofore was accessible to relatively few (Dickferson & Brenna, 2002). Alternative models (to the PCP model) have not been shown to be more expensive (Escarce et al, 2001). Specialist physicians also have been critical of the gatekeeper model (Pena-Dolhun et al, 2001).

If PCPs continue to lose their grip in managed care, physical rehabilitation professionals may experience a resurgence of referrals similar to when fee-for-service was a dominant model, especially in light of an aging population.

In fee-for-service health care delivery models patients have a choice between primary care and specialist care for entry into the system. This choice is compounded by divergent paradigms, however. Specialists tend to focus on the patient's specific regional or organ-specific problem. These providers have been criticized for a failure to view the patient holistically. In their approach, sparse attention was paid to non-medical aspects of a patient's life that in many cases, were more critical to recovery than treatment of the primary pathology. PCPs tend to possess a more global view of the patient but often lack the requisite knowledge concerning special problems, especially those that are postacute or chronic. PCPs also receive little if any theoretical and didactic training regarding physical rehabilitation. These distinctions have bearing on rehabilitation delivery, because the current health care system is based on a paradigm of predictable acute simple disease (Pawlson, 1994).

Physical rehabilitation providers receive formal training and education that equips them to mange persons with either acute or postacute conditions. Physical rehabilitation providers are positioned as specialists capable of managing persons with unpredictable complex chronic conditions that routinely involve a host of psychosocial issues, but are also capable of offering primary care services. This dichotomy presents a number of questions: *"How do we view ourselves, as specialists or generalists? Are physical rehabilitation providers truly capable of serving a duality of roles? How do rehabilitation providers view themselves, specialists or generalists? How do consumers view rehabilitation providers, specialists or generalists?"*

At least two indicators imply that physical rehabilitation covets specialty status. First, despite the growth in direct access to rehabilitation services, a majority of patients are still referred for rehabilitation. The development of various specialties within rehabilitation suggests that rehabilitation is a primary care service. Thus specialization status is secured for such fields as orthopedics, pediatrics, geriatrics, and sports medicine. Specialty certifications conceivably can render providers as poorly positioned within a managed care structure that rewards primary care and subsequently, non-referral for profit. It is interesting to note that a great deal of focus has been placed on referral-for-profit through physician-owned rehabilitation practices (Office of Inspector General, 1994; APTA, 1993; Medicare, 1995; Johnson, 1992; Mitchell & Scott, 1991).

Physical rehabilitation providers often focus on chronic illness or injury, especially within the Medicare and Workers' Compensation populations. This focus connotes specialty status despite the obvious skill sets directed towards acute conditions.

Rehabilitation's growth has perhaps been hampered to a greater extent by non-referral for profit secondary to PCPs and the managed care sector's perception of physical and occupational therapists as specialists.

Physical rehabilitation providers may need to thoroughly address this issue and reposition themselves as primary care practitioners within managed care structures; otherwise, they risk a reduction in referrals. Of course, underuse of rehabilitation for those who enjoy capitation contracts under managed care may actually be more profitable.

This author is unaware of any published study of consumer perceptions of rehabilitation specialty practice by physical and occupational therapists. Discerning whether consumers view physical and occupational therapists as primary or specialty service providers is a unique and critical research opportunity. Data gained from such a study would be useful from various perspectives, including strategic planning, marketing, entry-level educational program development, and reimbursement. Similarly, payers should be queried regarding their perspectives on physical rehabilitation: primary care or specialty care?

A study sponsored by The U.S. Agency for Health Care Policy and Research revealed that nine of every ten California patients enrolled in managed care plans value the involvement of their primary care physician (Grumbach et al, 1999). However, despite this degree of overall satisfaction, 23% of patients reported difficulty in securing a referral for specialist care.

This finding suggests lost trust and confidence in PCPs. Grumbach et al (1999) concluded that, "Our study shows that patients value having a primary care physician. But they don't want managed care plans to turn their primary care physician into a rationer of specialty care."

High cost is a common argument against referral for specialty services. There is however, some evidence that referrals for specialty do not raise managed care plan costs. In a study supported by the Agency for Healthcare Research and Quality (HS09414), contrary to expectation the overall cost of physician services was 4% higher in a gatekeeper health maintenance organization (HMO) model than in a point-of-service or non-gatekeeper model (Escarse et al, 2000). This study was funded in order to study specialist referral policies on patient health, access to service and health care costs. This finding, coupled with a lack of evidence that gatekeeping keeps costs down, may increase referrals for rehabilitation and other specialty services (Bradford, 1998).

Current delivery models demand that clinical recommendations consider at least three different viewpoints: that of the clinician, the patient, and society (Sharpe & Faden, 1996). Evolving paradigms may demand that the needs and expectations of all stakeholders be met, including the desire of patients to receive specialty services. This challenge is seemingly impossible.

Paradigm Shift 3: From Independent Practice to Collaborative Models of Rehabilitation Delivery

The American health care system has been fragmented for years. This fragmentation has occurred across several spheres: insurance or health benefits, treatment setting, provider type, and irritability stages (acute, subacute, chronic, or postacute).

In the past, rehabilitation providers supplied their care independent of other disciplines. Each discipline was involved in some aspect of disability management yet operated from independent silos. Although providers may have understood their own roles, they generally had little knowledge about other disciplines because of the fragmented nature of care. The patient essentially bounced from department to department, from treatment setting to treatment setting, and from one provider to another to satisfy their clinical needs. Very little coordination existed between parties, and documentation was less than desirable. Professional and educational institutions likewise erected barriers between disciplines and, for the most part, continue to do so (Cooley, 1994; Hilton, 1995; Schmidt, 1994).

Today's market demands the abandonment of discipline-specific models of organization in favor of a programmatic approach that serves the needs of other stakeholders (Smith, 1995).

Dissonance created by service fragmentation is particularly disruptive in rehabilitation because of its protracted nature. If services are not integrated, preferably within the same health care system, results can suffer. No assurance exists of coordinated care, however, even when these services are contained within one health care system through "virtual integration" (Morrison, 1996). Figures 21–3 and 21–4 portray horizontal and vertical integration of services, respectively.

Cross-facility educational programs and staff exchanges are two effective means of coordinating services along a continuum of care. These strategies have been successfully used in persons with spinal cord injuries (Watson-Evans and Sheldon, 1993). Maintenance of a global patient database that spans disciplines and treatment settings provides another means of care coordination and provider collaboration. Patient satisfaction surveys have demonstrated reduced anxiety, enhanced education, and awareness when patients are involved in collaborative care (Watson-Evans & Sheldon, 1993). Results of interdisciplinary models of clinical education also continue to be encouraging (Cox et al, 1999).

Although collaborative approaches differ in many aspects, most require a de-emphasis of the technical skill component of care with a greater emphasis placed on clinical reasoning and reflective practice. Some team approaches currently center around a condition-specific age or gender approach. Wound care teams and women's health care are excellent examples of this collaborative approach.

The composition of a disability management team can further distinguish one program from the next (Bateman, 1999). For instance, a comprehensive wound care team may employ the services of a case manager, home health aide, enterostomal nurse, physical therapist, registered dietician, medical social worker, and occupational therapist.

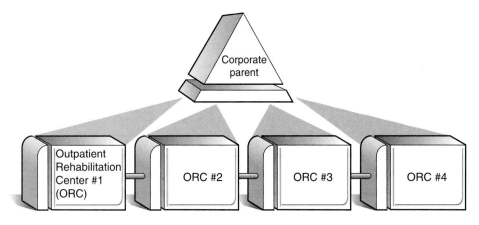

Figure 21–3. Horizontal integration.

Facilitating or providing education of the patient, family, referring physician, and each team member is the keystone of an optimal program (Bateman, 1999; Baranoski, 1996).

Jointly developed critical pathways of care and treatment protocols are essential in a collaborative model. Teams are usually self-governed and devoid of hierarchal structures or line and staff reporting mechanisms. Authority is shared laterally between professionals. Figure 21–5 depicts shared power between disciplines. In this example, the physical therapy clinical manager, occupational therapy clinical manager, and speech and language clinical manager all reside on the same hierarchal level within the organizational chart. Although managers collaborate with other disciplines, they still direct their own discipline-specific subordinates.

Management support and a willingness to surrender authority to the team are vital to success. Team-based performance measures and incentive systems in physical rehabilitation constitute a major paradigm shift away from rewarding individual effort. Communication is the hallmark of team-based care. Self-managed teams are a logical extension of an organization's total quality assurance program (Becker-Reems, 1994). Self-directed teams are not for the faint-hearted because they require a number of process and structure changes (Watson, 1996). Table 21–2 provides a sampling of process and structure elements.

Process-based changes may involve new quality assurance procedures, incentive programs, budgeting policies and procedures, performance appraisal programs, and reporting mechanisms. Examples of structural changes include: job design, budgeting, equipment, job descriptions, facilities, technology, and new information management systems. Self-directed teams necessitate a unique strategic planning process that encourages shared accountability and incentives that are consensual and are aligned with market or consumer needs.

Nomenclature changes accompany the paradigm shift from silo-based (setting- or discipline-specific) to self-managed teams. Products or services are known as programs in a collaborative model. *Product* as a term succumbs to business units and service lines is known as "centers for excellence" (Charns & Smith Tewksbury, 1993).

Effectively managed teams produce lower risk, more efficient care, improved interdisciplinary coordination, higher service quality, and better outcomes. Figure 21–6 illustrates a program-driven collaborative model in which all services are laterally aligned. Staff is allocated depending on the program needs. In this model no physical, occupational, or speech and language departments are delineated.

Paradigm Shift 4: Consumer-Directed and Self-Care

Today a strong trend exists towards consumerism in health care and away from a paternalistic model wherein

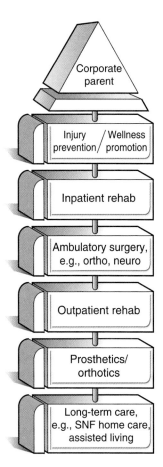

Figure 21–4. Vertical integration.

Figure 21–5. A collaborative model with shared power between disciplines.

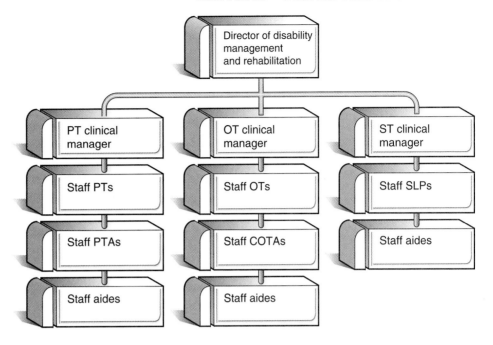

the "doctor knows best" (Campbell, 1991; Emener, 1991; Hagner, 1995; Human Resource Focus, 2002; Waldholz, 2002).

Two changes are necessary in consumer-managed care (Schultz, 2002).

1. Patients must become more personally involved in health care finance.
2. Patients must be educated to appropriately select health care services, to engage in healthy lifestyles, and to manage chronic conditions.

Schultz (2002) notes that 70% of all health care expenditures involve persons with chronic conditions. These persons must be equipped to self-manage various aspects of their condition. Informed choice is the keystone of consumerism and a fundamental covenant of the 1988 Amendments to the Rehabilitation Act of 1973.

The Definition of Consumer-Directed Care

"Philosophy and orientation whereby informed consumers have control over the policies and practices that directly affect their lives. It is a mechanism by which individuals with disabilities can develop the skills to take control of their lives and their environment."

- Kosciulek, 1999

 Table 21–2   A Sampling of Process and Structure Changes

Information management systems
Job design/classification
Job evaluation/performance appraisal
Budgeting
Reporting mechanisms
Quality control processes
Financial compensation
Incentive program
Strategic planning
Reimbursement

Although related, consumer-directed care and self-care have distinct meanings. Consumer-directed care is essentially an issue concerning choice of treatment, whereas self-care involves care that is both supervised and self-administered by the patient or consumer. Self-care is the byproduct of a motivated patient, availability of consumer data, self-funding source and/or dwindling health care funding schemes.

Self-care is the most basic form of primary care, yet little research has been conducted regarding its effectiveness (Padula, 1992). The era of the passive recipient of services is waning in favor of activist patients (DeFriese et al, 1989). Self-care as a new treatment paradigm gained acceptance as an official term in 1983 by Index Medicus, the official publication of the National Library of Medicine (DeFriese et al, 1989). Self-care programs serve as an alternative to clinically based service. This alternative is especially crucial in insurance schemes that minimize access to services. Table 21–3 provides a list of eight purposes of self-care.

The educated consumer's role is so leveraged that it has gone beyond influencing providers. Consumers have become so empowered that some health care experts project a severely diminished role for managed care plans, especially HMOs (Kleinke, 1998; Waldholz, 2002; Anonymous, 2002).

The role of the gatekeeper is diminished under this scenario, as consumers select health care services on the basis of their needs and financial contributions. Managed savings accounts provide a mechanism whereby specific amounts of money are set aside depending on a beneficiary's health status. In an employer-based system, the employer may match an employee's contribution to the managed savings account. The patient is the primary determinant of how and when health care services are purchased. Consumers may elect not to receive provider rendered services and instead, engage in self-care.

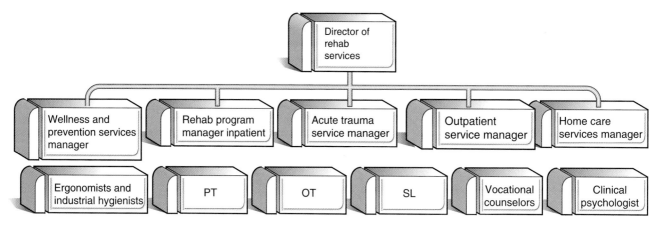

Figure 21–6. Program-driven collaborative model.

The growth in self-care through complementary and alternative medicine or health care is evidence of this paradigm shift. Readers are referred to Chapter 24 for a more detailed exploration of complementary and alternative medicine.

Self-care can be either a complement or substitute for professional services. Persons who engage in self-care typically do so in the early stages of an illness or injury or after discharge from a clinician's care. When self-care proves to be inadequate, a return to professional care may ensue. In rehabilitation it is extremely common to place an individual on a home program of exercise or pain amelioration. These persons may return to a clinical setting if their condition changes or they are in need of additional education and training. Restorative home exercise programs emphasize functionality, but not to the exclusion of home pain modalities. Enhanced home care technology is one of the positive byproducts of Medicare and managed care's "quicker and sicker" discharge policies. A new generation of portable, relatively inexpensive and user-friendly pain modalities and exercise equipment is now available. Restrictive hospital or rehabilitation inpatient policies have also spawned an increase in patient education and caregiver training programs.

Self-care can elicit mixed feelings among providers. Some may view it as a threat to their role and others view it as adjunctive to professional services. Hard data have traditionally been limited as the result of varying definitions of self-care and limited survey instruments, yet

 Table 21–3 Eight Purposes of Self-Care Programs

1. Increase wellness or health status.
2. Reduce risk factors for illness/injury.
3. Prevent the onset of illness/injury.
4. Prevent the spread of disease.
5. Diagnose and assess signs/symptoms of common illnesses.
6. Alleviate or minimize pain, discomfort, or effects of disability.
7. Develop consumer advocacy skills.
8. Prevent iatrogenesis or injury received as a result of treatment.

Data from DeFriese GH et al: From activated patient to pacified activist: A study of the self-care movement in the United States. Soc Sci Med 29(2):195-204, 1989.

government support for this paradigm shift has existed for decades (Gallicchio, 1977).

Self-care programs have a greater emphasis on wellness, health, and lifestyle adjustments than on treatment per se. This approach reduces risk factors associated with illness and injury and in some cases can actually prevent their onset. Self-care can also reduce the risk of spreading contagious disease. Educated consumers can benefit from earlier recognition of symptoms leading to earlier diagnosis. Self-care interventions directed at treatment after onset serve to alleviate or minimize pain and discomfort associated with disability. A heightened consumer advocacy role may help to prevent iatrogenesis or injury received as a result of treatment.

A national strategy for general health improvement may include organized programs to assist consumers in the development of the requisite skills and knowledge to select and/or render much of their own care (Gallicchio, 1977). The Internet may serve as the primary vehicle for this informational exchange. Self-care signifies a paradigm shift from medicalization to a health and wellness model. This new paradigm is an outgrowth of a shift that occurred in the 1970s from public health concerns to individual ones (Kaplan, 1985). Epidemiology moved away from public issues such as immunization to individual lifestyle and behavior issues such as nutrition, driver safety, and smoking cessation. Despite this shift, few studies have proved the effectiveness of self-care (Lorig & Holman, 1989). Health care professions have virtually overlooked this research area, perhaps because they have principally focused on proving that their own interventions work. This focus is understandable as providers struggle for self-survival in an oppressive managed care arena. Rehabilitation providers, however, because of their skills, knowledge, aptitudes, and experience can make substantial contributions to health and wellness in addition to their treatment-based contributions.

Paradigm Shift 5: A Shift from Demand Creation to Demand Management

Demand management is a related concept to self-directed care. Health care as a sector operated for years under an economic model of demand creation. Under demand creation it was the supplier of the service, not the consumer (patient) or customer (employer through insurer), that determined both cost and use rates. Health care and the legal system were two of the few sectors that instructed the patient or customer regarding what they needed, the cost, and how many units (health care visits) were necessary. And there were no guaranteed outcomes!

Demand management is the antithesis of demand creation, because it is predicated on rational decision-making that seeks consumer input. Use or cost reduction is not necessarily the goal of demand management. Demand management involves a rational decision of the patient to self-manage his or her care through education and empowerment (Sternack, 1997). Achievement of a reasonable and appropriate level of care is the primary goal of demand management. Informed choice, a positive by-product, guarantees patient input during care delivery.

Control is the core element that differentiates demand creation from demand management. Choice and control are tandem elements of consumer direction (CD).

The current rehabilitation system erects barriers to CD. Providers who possess the belief that they must "do something to the patient" ignore the value of consumer-directed care. These providers may perceive their patients as passive recipients of their services. Regrettably, this may be a paradox that all hands-on providers face. Duncan notes that provider egos may not be elastic enough to allow sharing of or the transfer of control (Duncan, 1996). The approach whereby the provider assumes total control of disability management creates a paucity of user-friendly information available to their patients or clients. Consequently, many consumers may surf the net for their information, be guided by word-of-mouth advice, or use alternative health care, outside of the medical mainstream.

CD is fueled by three underlying assumptions (Kosciulek, 1999).

Assumption 1: Consumers with disabilities are the experts on their service needs.
Assumption 2: CD should be available to all, regardless of the payer source.
Assumption 3: Choice and control can be introduced into all services and delivery environments.

The United States health care system has been built around an acute care model and therefore grossly lacks the necessary long-term care supports to address chronic disability and an aging population. Consumer-directed initiatives only partially satisfy long-term–care support needs. Patient empowerment is especially crucial in rehabilitation because of the prevalence of chronic long-term conditions (Emener, 1991; Bolton & Brookings, 1996; National Institute on Consumer-Directed Long-Term Services, 1996). Consumer responsibilities under CD include the selection and quality monitoring of services. Patient satisfaction surveys are but one example of this responsibility. Clinical trials, program compliance, and participation in disability research are other expectations of patients. Consumers must also agree to consult with their providers as necessary through communication of their evolving needs. Provider responsibilities include educating patients concerning alternative care choices, ensuring that a maximum range of service options are presented,

respecting patient choices, and recognizing their own delivery limitations. The patient benefits of CD are obvious, but the attitudes and resistance of others has contributed to patients' sense of powerlessness and lack of self-direction.

> *It has become increasingly evident that the powerlessness and lack of self direction often felt by people with disabilities are more frequently related to the attitudes and practices of caregivers, service providers, funding agencies, social institutions, and society in general, rather than to any limitation or impairments resulting from the disability itself.*
>
> *- Parent, 1993*

Providers are obligated by both their professional duty and business contract with the patient to offer clear, accurate, and user-friendly information to the consumer. Informed consent forms must reflect treatment options including the potential benefits and risks associated with choices.

Paradigm Shift 6: Patient-Focused Care/ Consumer-Directed Care

The term "patient-focused care" (PFC) at first glance appears to be a redundancy. After all, is not all care directed at the needs of the patient? PFC speaks to the process and structure of delivery. Traditional systems have incurred organizational fragmentation, specialization, and compartmentalization. Many health care structures and processes were designed with provider or institutional needs in mind rather than those of the patient. For instance, hospitals are traditionally organized around departments that aggregate providers according to their disciplines (e.g., physical therapy or occupational therapy departments) rather than the needs of the patient or client (Table 21–4).

A growing body of knowledge is supportive of PFC (Moore & Komras, 1993; Taffel, 1994; Myers, 1998; McDonagh, 1993; Martin & Cohen, 1995).

Many labels have been applied to the concept of PFC. These labels include pluralistic care, team-directed care, collaborative delivery, and transdisciplinary care. All of these labels flow from the principles supporting CQI and TQI. The foundation of CQI and TQM is outcomes of care versus process and structure. Myers (1998) asserts that balancing decreased costs and enhanced quality serves as the backbone of PFC. PFC is characterized by a number of features, such as patients aggregated into groups that share similar attributes such as diagnoses and care needs

 Table 21–4 Consumer Benefits of Consumer-Directed Care

- Increased autonomy in the decision-making process.
- Enhancement of life management skills.
- Increased feelings of self-worth, confidence, competence, and contribution to society.
- Comfort in knowing that consumers have control over expenditures, especially when co-payments and deductibles are involved.

(Mang, 1995). Disease state management is one example of this strategy. Cross-trained care teams with advanced knowledge of the group's conditions are deployed in a decentralized fashion. By decentralizing their functions, greater efficiency and clinical effectiveness can result. The ultimate goal, however, is to enhance the continuity of care that is commonly lacking. For instance, an average hospital inpatient comes into contact with 55 different people during a typical 4-day stay (McDonagh, 1993). This begs the question, are the needs of the patient or the needs of the provider being considered?

Three common themes surround patient-focused care (Martin & Cohen, 1995).

1. Managed demand: Patients are grouped according to similarities.
2. Redesigned work: Unnecessary work and staff redundancies are minimized or eliminated.
3. Empowered employees: Increased authority as the result of decentralization. Staff possesses authority across tasks.

Promotion of PFC has been hampered by a number of forces. These include licensure and regulatory problems associated with cross-trained teams. Health plans and traditional insurers may place restrictive policies on PFC and even claim duplication of services when multiple providers are involved with one patient. In reality, duplication of services is the antithesis of PFC.

Paradigm Shift 7: Helping Model Versus Medical Model of Care

Every person's response to disability is unique, and emotional issues often assume a disproportionate role in the rehabilitation process. This variable is common knowledge, especially among persons who sustain and providers who manage catastrophic illness or injury such as spinal cord injury, traumatic brain injury, or amputation.

Rehabilitation professionals trained under the medical model approach these cases differently, however, than do those trained under the behavioral sciences (Anderson, 1977).

Anderson notes that physicians and nurses have been traditionally trained under the medical model while social workers and psychologists have been trained under the helping model. Do physical rehabilitation providers fit into the medical model, the helping model, or both?

Goals under the medical model include eradication of disease, cure of the patient, and solution of related problems. Physical rehabilitation providers straddle both models if they address both the biophysical and psychosocial issues confronting their patients. Rehabilitation professionals who value their role as helpers and teachers may offer the best aspects of both models of care. The "helping model" is most consistent with self-care and patient-focused disability management.

Success under the medical model is greatly determined by the degree of trust a patient has in their provider. In the helping model, however, mutuality and nurturing are more critical to success. Providers who are reflective listeners and who design goals on the basis of the patient's needs (versus departmental needs) are more likely to succeed. In the helping model, therapists may serve in a greater capacity as mentor or educator than as treater or provider.

Paradigm Shift 8: Case Management

External case management represents the introduction of a third party into the traditional provider-patient relationship. Case management is a phenomenon associated with managed care and its attempts to curb health care costs. Historically, when cost was not an issue, providers were expected to manage their own cases. Under fee-for-service arrangements, however, little provider incentive existed to manage costs or utilization. Managed care changed the rules and, as a result, aggressively uses case managers (who are usually nurses because of their broad-based knowledge of health care). Case managers are used essentially to monitor and, in some instances, to effect changes in disability management and treatment.

Rehabilitation providers need to become familiar with case management to remain relevant in today's health care delivery system, especially in cases that involve high costs, litigation, vocational issues, protracted length of stay, or catastrophic injury/illness (Table 21–5).

The Definition of Case Management

"Case management is a collaborative process that assesses, plans, implements, coordinates, monitors, and evaluates the options and services required to meet an individual's health needs, using communication and available resources to promote quality, cost-effective outcomes."

- The Commission for Case Manager Certification, 1999

Characteristics of Case Management

Case management is often necessary due to the fragmented nature of American health care. Fragmented care can drive up health care costs and trigger referrals for case management. Case managers serve two fundamental roles that are classified for the purposes of this chapter as medical and vocational. Case managers are engaged to optimize medical outcomes while ensuring expeditious return to gainful employment. Case managers typically serve two masters. They serve as ombudsmen for patients, yet they are paid by a second party. Case managers work in both the private and public sectors and their work is generally funded by insurers, employers, or government agencies. They strive to facilitate the return of injured persons to work across a variety of health benefits systems: workers' compensation, automobile liability, disability (short-term

 Table 21–5 Who Receives External Case Management Services?

- Chronically ill
- High-cost diagnoses
- Multiple trauma
- Selected workers' compensation cases
- Catastrophic injury (e.g., TBI, SCI, AIDS, CA)
- Controversial soft tissue conditions (e.g., LBP, TOS, CTDs)
- Mental health cases (e.g., post traumatic stress disorder)
- Substance abuse

TBI, *Traumatic brain injury*; SCI, *spinal cord injury*; AIDS, *acquired immunodeficiency syndrome*; CA, *cancer*; LBP, *low back pain*; TOS, *thoracic outlet syndrome*; CTD, *cumulative trauma disorders*.

or long-term), Social Security, or other insurance programs. Case managers expedite medical services along the recovery cycle, from the onset of injury/illness to the achievement of maximum medical improvement or optimal functioning. Case managers do not provide direct rehabilitation services. Instead they arrange care at appropriate service sites, secure job analyses, coordinate communication between various stakeholders, and secure additional consultants on an as-needed basis. These professionals may also focus on vocational aspects of a client's case. Vocational functions may include job placement, job retraining or vocational counseling, job referral, on-the-job training or matriculation in structured educational programs (e.g., vocational school). Some case managers are certified vocational counselors and others are not.

Figure 21-7, "A Case Manager's Communication Schematic," provides an overview of essential communication responsibilities that case managers have relative to multiple stakeholders, including the disabled employee, employer representatives, providers, and insurance representatives.

Case Management Professional Designations

Externally provided case management personnel are represented by various professional designations: CIRS (certified insurance rehabilitation counselor), CRC (certified rehabilitation consultant), CRRN (certified rehabilitation registered nurse), CCM (certified case manager) or CDM (certified disability manager). These designations have evolved over the years to describe various forms of certification. Ironically, the case management industry has been until recently as fragmented if not more fragmented than the industry (health care) it was engaged to reign in. Case management as a sector has traditionally been guided by a cacophony of professional trade groups operating without consensual guidelines. It is estimated that more than 150,000 case managers work in the United States (Llewellyn, 1999). These persons belong to a multitude of professional trade groups. These organizations can be found in Table 21-6.

These groups often focus on specific insurance lines. For instance, the Case Management Society of America has historically been most visible in group health and managed care while the Independent Case Management Association focused predominantly on workers' compensation. A relatively recent merger of associations created the Case Management Society of America. This organization has promulgated case management standards and offers a certification through its Commission for Case Manager Certification (http://www.cmsa.org). The Commission for Case Manager Certification is an alliance of 29 organizations united to develop consensus concerning case management philosophy, definitions, standards of practice and voluntary certification. This consortium acknowledges that case management is not a "true" profession in the

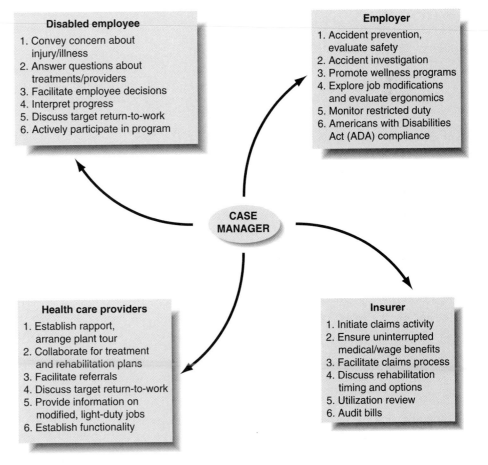

Figure 21-7. A case manager's communication schematic. (Modified from Martin KJ: Workers' compensation: Case management strategies. Case Rev J 43[5]:245-250, 1995.)

Disabled employee
1. Convey concern about injury/illness
2. Answer questions about treatments/providers
3. Facilitate employee decisions
4. Interpret progress
5. Discuss target return-to-work
6. Actively participate in program

Employer
1. Accident prevention, evaluate safety
2. Accident investigation
3. Promote wellness programs
4. Explore job modifications and evaluate ergonomics
5. Monitor restricted duty
6. Americans with Disabilities Act (ADA) compliance

CASE MANAGER

Health care providers
1. Establish rapport, arrange plant tour
2. Collaborate for treatment and rehabilitation plans
3. Facilitate referrals
4. Discuss target return-to-work
5. Provide information on modified, light-duty jobs
6. Establish functionality

Insurer
1. Initiate claims activity
2. Ensure uninterrupted medical/wage benefits
3. Facilitate claims process
4. Discuss rehabilitation timing and options
5. Utilization review
6. Audit bills

Table 21-6 Roster of Case Management Associations/ Societies/Organizations

- Academy of Certified Case Managers (ACCM)
- American Association of Managed Care Nurses (AAMCN)
- American Association Of Occupational Health Nurses (AAOHN)
- American Nurses Credentialing Center (ANCC)
- Association of Rehabilitation Nurses (ARN)
- American Rehabilitation Counseling Association (ARCA)
- Certification of Disability Management Specialists Commission (CDMS)
- Case Management Administrator Certified (CMAC)
- Case Management Society of America (CMSA)
- Disease Management Association of America (DMAA)
- Independent Case Management Association (ICMA)
- International Association of Rehabilitation Professionals (IARP), formerly known as the National Association of Rehabilitation Professionals in the Private Sector or NARPPS

Data from the Case Management Society of America, http://www.cmsa.org/news/newsnew.html, accessed January, 10, 2003.

 Table 21-7 Ten Questions to Ask the Case Manager

1. Who has retained your services (e.g., insurer, employer, patient)?
2. To which professional trade association do you belong?
3. What certification(s) do you have?
4. Do you use treatment protocols, guidelines, or algorithms?
5. If yes to question number 4, how were these developed? By whom?
6. How are you paid for your services? Hourly? Percentage of savings or commission basis?
7. What documentation do you need from rehabilitation?
8. What outcomes measures are of most importance to you?
9. Is an attorney involved in this case?
10. Will you pay for offsite services (e.g., functional job analysis, ergonomic analyses, reasonable accommodations, job retraining?)

purest sense of the word, but rather an area of specialized practice that can include practitioners from a variety of professions (including rehabilitation). The CCM designation serves as an adjunct to a primary professional designation in a health and human services profession. This designation is valid for a 5-year period, after which recertification is required. Physical and occupational therapists who possess the appropriate background may be eligible to sit for the CCM examination and receive certification on receipt of a passing grade.

A Typical Case Manager-Rehabilitation Provider Scenario

A physician may refer an injured worker to physical therapy. The case manager in this scenario must coordinate the flow of information between the physician, therapist, employee, employer, and workers' compensation carrier. Goal alignment is critical between all stakeholders, and individual responsibilities must be mutually understood. For instance, if the employee desires to return to his or her previous job, someone must develop and/or secure a functional job analysis that can be used as a blueprint for the design and execution of a functionally based return-to-work program. A functional job analysis can be crafted by an employer representative, the case manager, an occupational therapist, or a physical therapist. In this example, the case manager must serve as the conductor who coordinates the efforts of an orchestra composed of physicians, therapist, employer's agents, vocational specialists, the employee, and others. In turn, each party owes some degree of accountability to the case manager, who serves the injured worker's needs but is ultimately paid by the employer. Alternative vocational placement may be necessary if the return-to-work program fails. This scenario can become extremely complex, especially when attorneys are involved or a new job position must be considered. It is virtually impossible for a single provider to understand all of the dynamics involved in a complex case (Table 21-7).

Rehabilitation providers should seek additional information from case managers when they are involved in a case. A case manager can be friend or foe to the rehabilitation professional. It is essential that a mutual exchange of information precede any interaction between the therapist and case manager. Table 21-7 provides a series of questions that may be useful to rehabilitation providers in garnering critical information.

Providers as Case Managers

Although the dominant model for case management involves non-providers, this model has its opponents (Issel & Anderson, 1999). Although the external case management model is still prevalent, some believe that providers have the burden of assuring expeditious treatment and that reasonable health care costs have shifted back to the provider, especially in integrated delivery systems. Some provider organizations employ internal case managers for CQI/TQM purposes. A demand for more cost-effective care coupled with optimized outcomes has paved the way for provider-driven case management. Survival under at-risk contracts such as case rates or capitation demands the highest degree of efficiency possible. Such efficiency can be accomplished through the implementation of an internal case management function.

Providers share culpability for market demand for external case management through a collective failure to secure timely and cost-effective outcomes or by ignoring the value of internal case management as a quality assurance tool. Support is growing for providers to perform internal case management to assure that services are medically necessary, reasonable and effective (Fosnaught & Smith, 1996; Shriver, 1999; Shendell-Falik & Soriano, 1997; Fowler, 1995; White, 1999).

Physical and occupational therapists are well suited for internal case management by virtue of their skills, knowledge, and aptitudes. These professionals can offer their expertise across the entire care continuum from acute to subacute and chronic stages of injury or illness. Private practitioners are exceptionally well-qualified, because they often have direct communication with the patient's employer about return to work and vocational issues.

Paradigm Shift 9: Evidenced-Based Practice

EBP, or evidence-based medicine (EBM), perhaps more than any other paradigm shift has impacted health care delivery. EBP provides a vital element towards provider accountability for both clinical and financial outcomes. EBP de-emphasizes intuition, unsystematic clinical experience, and pathophysiologic rationale as insufficient for clinical decision making (Lindberg et al, 1992).

The Definition of Evidence-Based Practice

"The conscientious, explicit, and judicious use of current best evidence in making decisions about the care of individual patients ... evidence-based medicine nears integrating individual clinical expertise with the best available external clinical evidence from systematic research."

- Colyer & Kamath, 1999

The trend toward EBP is undeniable and growing stronger, as evidenced by the profusion of practice guidelines, treatment protocols, and critical pathways of care (Eddy, 1992; Lindberg et al, 1992; Richardson, 1997; Montori & Guyatt, 1997; APTA, 2001)(Table 21–8).

By the end of 1996, more than 75 professional medical organizations had developed more than 2000 practice guidelines (AMA, 1996). The EBP movement is one of a number of efforts designed to teach clinicians how to evaluate and apply published research in practice standards. The quality of clinical practice is only as good as the quality of clinical research that supports it. To be optimally effective, clinicians must learn to separate sound information from disinformation or misinformation. The integrity of the data must be examined and studies published or funded by proponents of their own methodologies must be seriously questioned. Regrettably, many clinicians are ill trained in evaluating the literature with a discerning eye. An inherent lag may always exist, however, between clinical research and clinical practice. Meta-analysis of the literature is one means that providers can use to sort out biases and identify research deficiencies (Ionnides & Lau, 1999). Several recent texts provide useful information for rehabilitation providers as they attempt to digest voluminous amounts of data. These texts include Primer on Measurement: An Introductory Guide to Measurement Issues by Jules M. Rothstein, PhD, PT, and John Echternach, EdD, PT; and Critical Evaluation of Research in Physical Rehabilitation: Towards Evidence-Based Practice by Antoine Helewa, MSc, PT, and Joan M. Walker, PhD, PT.

EBP is not without its critics. A common criticism of EBP is that it places a disproportionate emphasis on the establishment of treatment or test validity without consideration of patient interests, desires, or needs. Stated another way, controlled clinical research in scientific settings is devoid of the human interactions commonly found in disability cases. A myopic focus on biophysical elements at the expense of psychosocial issues reduces the usefulness of practice guides. Early discharge from care is another concern of providers who distrust EBP design motives. Some argue that EBP leads to early discharge because the desire to contain costs outweighs that of enhancing health, especially in an at-risk capitated contract. Other critics fall into the obstructionist category, because they believe that EBP relegates clinical decision making to "cookbook medicine." This is an amusing allegation given that many interventions in physical rehabilitation can be conceived as recipes. Common examples include ultrasound dosage (1.5 W per centimeter squared), therapeutic exercise (3 sets of 10 repetitions), and treatment frequency (three times per week on Monday, Wednesday, and Friday).

The benefit of so-called cookbook medicine is that it standardizes treatment. Treatment variation may be the single biggest reason for the development of managed care strategies. Because cost is driven by use rates defined as visits during a period of time, it is logical to believe that standardization of treatment will allow for better prediction of service costs. This goal can be accomplished, at least in theory, through evidence-based care.

More than 70% of HMOs use practice guidelines, compared with 28% of preferred provider organizations (Physician Payment Review Commission, 1995). By comparison, only 20% of all medical practices were evidence-based by 1992 (Eddy, 1992). Current figures are unavailable.

Payers support EBP for a number of other reasons. EBP allows payers to remain competitive through the generation of plan performance measures, attainment of various accreditations, achievement of regulatory and legislative compliance and, ultimately, by eliminating wasteful health care spending.

Caveats are, of course, associated with payer interest in EBP and clinical guideline development. Plans must frequently modify guides to reflect variations in local markets or patient populations (Government Accounting Office, 1996). The Institute of Medicine supports the use of clinical practice guidelines to determine both the health and cost implications of alternative treatment strategies (Institute of Medicine, 1992).

 Table 21–8 Five Components of the Evidence-Based Practice Diagnostic Process

---

1. **Gathering of clinical data**

   a. Positive presence of a symptom or abnormality.
   b. Negative absence of a symptom or abnormality.

2. **Framing clinical problems**

   a. Synthesize findings into a coherent group or pattern.
   b. Listing "clinical problems" inclusive of biological, psychological, and sociological problems.

3. **Selecting a differential diagnosis**

   a. Identify a range of potential causes.
   b. Generate a short list of feasible causes.
   c. Engage in a process of elimination.

4. **Selecting diagnostic tests**

   a. Confirm the clinical diagnosis.
   b. Consider test reliability, safety, acceptability, availability and cost.
   c. Consider alternative tests from a cost-benefit perspective.

5. **Interpret test results**

   a. Integrate test results with the clinical findings.
   b. Adjust the pretest probability to reflect the test results.
   c. Accept, modify, or reject the diagnosis and test findings.
   d. Design a treatment program commensurate with the diagnosis.

Table 21-9 EBP As a Bridge Between Clinical and Social Ethics

1. Ineffective interventions should be eliminated because they are wasteful.
2. High-cost treatments should be replaced by equally effective but less expensive treatments.
3. Treatment protocols should be developed that encourage consumers and providers to use less expensive procedures as first-line therapies.
4. Reserve higher cost treatments for persons at highest risk or for those who do not respond to less costly first-line interventions.
5. EBP allows all stakeholders, including providers, patients, and payers to make informed health care decisions.

Data modified from Montori VM, Guyatt GH: What is evidence-based medicine and why should it be practiced?, Evidence-based Working Group. JAMA 277(15): 1232-1237, 1997.

Institute of Medicine, Definition of Practice

Guideline "systematically developed statements that assist practitioners in making decisions about appropriate health care for specific clinical conditions." (Institute of Medicine, 1992).

In reality, financial incentives may have a more powerful effect on use rates than EBP (Larson, 1999) (Table 21-9).

In general, guidelines that promote more care are favored by providers, and those with restricted care are favored by payers. Paradoxically, the most effective treatment from a clinical efficacy perspective may not prove to be the most cost-effective (Drummond, 1998). EBP that leads to lower cost services is not a quid pro quo scenario.

Disease State Management

Disease state management (DSM) represents an environment designed specifically for collaborative delivery coupled with EBP. DSM is a program-based and not a discipline-based program to address specific disease states or conditions. Currently at least 50% of all HMOs implement DSM programs (Interstudy, 1997). The pharmaceutical industry pioneered DSM to add value to their products under managed care (Southwick, 1995).

Definition of Disease State Management

"An approach to delivering population-based patient-centered care that is based on a platform of continuous improvement" (Joshi & Bernard, 1999).

Common conditions managed through DSM include those routinely addressed through physical rehabilitation: AIDS, cancer , asthma, diabetes, multiple sclerosis, congestive heart failure, and chronic obstructive pulmonary disease. DSM spans the entire spectrum of health from disease prevention through chronic states. A diverse universe of providers is use that includes both primary care practitioners and specialists. Services are offered through a broad array of settings including hospitals, employer sites, physician offices, skilled nursing facilities, and rehabilitation centers

When DSM programs are designed initially, selected conditions tend to fit one of the following four criteria:

1. High-volume cases
2. High-cost cases
3. Chronic in nature
4. Complex to handle

The physical rehabilitation sector has unlimited opportunity to play a vital role in disease state management. Physical rehabilitation spans all three acuity levels (acute, subacute, chronic) and is rendered in virtually every treatment setting. Lastly, therapists manage innumerable conditions. One of the enormous opportunities that rehabilitation providers have yet to capitalize on involves collaborative research and practice with pharmaceutical companies. Imagine the possibilities of rehabilitation providers working along with drug companies that offer products for wound care, arthritis, circulatory deficiencies, and neuromuscular conditions (Table 21-10).

Rehabilitation providers are uniquely positioned to participate in chronic illness and injury management. In fact, the rehabilitation sector may be the only major group equipped to deal with these cases (Fowler, 1996). The full continuum of rehabilitation services, ranging from hospital-based to home care, positions providers well for full participation.

Some describe DSM as having too narrow a focus, especially because many patients suffer from multiple conditions. For instance, many elderly patients have combinations of problems that cross multiple body systems.

It is not uncommon to see patients with multiple conditions: diabetes, chronic obstructive pulmonary disease, congestive heart failure, amputation, and end-stage renal disease. Does this mean that these patients must seek management of each condition independent of the others? Certainly it challenges a diabetes team if they also have to address a cardiac, pulmonary, or neuromuscular disorder. Multiple diagnoses can shift the focus away from disease-specific management (the very essence of DSM) to a patient-focused management approach. DSM clearly has its critics and shortcomings, but like other paradigms, as it emerges it will be modified over time. Acerbic criticism of this approach remains despite DSM's emergence as a new paradigm.

"Disease management has spilled oceans of ink; it has generated more symposial palaver, more smoke and mirrors (perhaps), more blasts and counterblasts than anything else since "Harry" and "Louise" took their victory lap, having completed the conquest of health care reform." (McCarthy, 1996).

DSM requires a substantial degree of patient compliance and a willingness to help oneself. For those who believe

Table 21-10 Rehabilitation Provider's Role in Disease State Management

- Educate other disciplines about disease-specific interventions.
- Educate patients and their families about disease states.
- Download accurate, reliable and current information on the Internet.
- Evaluate treatment interventions that are selected by patients.
- Develop and provide expertise on how to determine good from bad information.
- Provide collaborative delivery of services that is evidence-based.
- Train extenders of care in treatment interventions.
- Develop working relationships with pharmaceutical companies for research and treatment partnerships.

that humans operate on the principle of expending the least effort possible, this could be another criticism of DSM. For those who believe that personal accountability for health care is noble, this is one of the strengths of DSM.

Technological advances afford patients vastly improved opportunities to self-monitor (Gilbert, 1998). Diabetes and blood sugar tests, home pregnancy tests, and cardiac monitors through computer or telephone link-ups are but a few examples.

Even the harshest critics of DSM must acknowledge that the development of home-based educational programs promises to improve the quality of health, enhance clinical outcomes, and reduce medical resource use (Fries et al, 1997). The World Wide Web offers unparalleled access to data, both good and bad. Applications in DSM are already in existence and target a variety of conditions including asthma, diabetes, multiple sclerosis, HIV/AIDS, hypertension, prenatal care, and dietary issues (Sherter,

 Table 21–11   Summary of Delivery Paradigm Shifts by Stakeholder

Patients	
Old Paradigm	**New Paradigm**
"Patients"	"Consumers"
Passive recipient of care	Engaged in collaborative care
Strictly relied on provider for information	Highly educated with access to data (e.g., Internet)
At little/no financial risk	Co-pays and deductibles
Perception that "more care is better care"	Demand outcome measures
Little informed consent	Strong informed consent
Choice of entry into system	Health plan determines entry into system (e.g., a gatekeeper)

Provider	
Old Paradigm	**New Paradigm**
Component management (e.g., case by case)	Pattern analysis (e.g., EBP)
Clinician's judgment ruled	"In God we trust. All others bring data."
Financially rewarded for doing more	Financially rewarded for doing less
Individual provider silos of care	Collaborative care
Fragmented services	Continuum of care
Specialist-driven	Primary-care driven
"Treatment-driven"	"Management-driven"
Process and structure	Outcomes measures
Idiosyncratic treatment guides	Consensus treatment guides
Random use review	Focuses review (e.g., precertification)
Discipline-driven care	Patient-focused care
Provided a lot of hands-on care	Architect of treatment plan. Carried out by others (e.g., extenders)
Treatment as focus	Consumer education as focus
Impairment focus	Ability/disability focus

Payers	
Old Paradigm	**New Paradigm**
Simply increase the premium when use and costs are high	Can no longer arbitrarily or capriciously raise premiums because of increased competition from self-funded employers and provider-based plans
Assumed control over providers	Returned control to providers in the form of at-risk contracts
Little accountability to employers who purchased health care coverage	Employers demanding accountability
Provided external case management	Providers as case managers
Retrospective denials of services	Precertification/preadmission

Hospitals	
Old Paradigm	**New Paradigm**
Acute care focus	Examining role in chronic care (e.g., disease state management)
Inpatient emphasis	Outpatient, community-based
Minimal focus on wellness (e.g., "medical care" focus)	Heightened focus, "general health focus"
Structured around departmental needs	Structured around consumer's needs
Predominately not-for-profit	Corporate medicine, for-profit
Employed physicians	Partnering with physicians

Employers	
Old Paradigm	**New Paradigm**
Financed but abdicated control over health care to insurers or MCOs	Finance and manage health care through self-funding, demand from MCOs of accountability, purchasing, or business coalitions
Cost-driven (e.g., lowest cost got the contract)	Value-driven, consider benefit-to-cost ratios
Gauged hospital and provider performance through process and structured measures	Demand outcome measures including clinical and financial
Lip service to prevention/wellness	Funding prevention/wellness

1998). Web technologies allow patients to manage secured personal records, diaries linked to health records, access to educational materials, disease-specific chat rooms and support groups, and communication through e-mail with nurses, physicians, and therapists. Rehabilitation providers will serve in a variety of capacities relative to disease state management. But perhaps the greatest challenge will be how to get paid for one's effort. Reimbursement mechanisms for DSM continue to evolve.

Paradigm Shift 10: Extenders of Care

Reimbursement and health care expenditures have led directly to the increased use of extenders of care (Wilson 1998, Sheppard 1994). These persons have traditionally served in support roles, but under the new paradigm they are often the primary care giver.

The use of extenders of care has raised a number of concerns (Robinson et al 1994, Blood & Robinson 1974, Hirsh, 1991). In pure economic terms, extenders are less costly than other licensed professionals. On average they cost 50% to 75% as much as medical professionals. Rehabilitation employs a growing number and variety of extenders, athletic trainers, physical therapist assistants, certified occupational therapy assistants, exercise physiologists, kinesiologists, massage therapists, and strength conditioning coaches. This staffing trend is not without its critics. The widespread use of technicians raises concerns about provider competency, credentials, and clinical outcomes (Salcido, 1996).

Understandably, for some the extender of care paradigm is the "son of Frankenstein," but for others it represents an opportunity (Kuchins, 1999).

The growing support of extenders throughout the health care sector is irrefutable, however. As expected, the use of extenders has been most prevalent in rural settings where access to professionals is limited (Shi et al, 1993).

Government support for this trend is growing, as evidenced by a number of initiatives. At least one initiative by the U.S. Department of Education has attempted to develop skill standards for application to health care workers across the entire sector (Salcido, 1996). Additionally, the National Health Care Skill Standards Project fosters a collaboration between the health care sector, labor entities, and educational organizations (National Health Care Skill Standards Project, 1995). More than 100 major organizations are engaged to develop standards across four service clusters: therapeutic, diagnostic, informational, and environmental. Rehabilitation professionals are ultimately responsible for any and all care that they delegate to others. A number of measures exist that can be used to optimize the use of extenders of care while minimizing any adverse impact. Refer to Chapter 16 for advice on this and other risk management subjects.

WHAT FUTURE PARADIGMS WILL EMERGE?

Some hints exist regarding the future of health care delivery. Emery describes a "production paradigm" that displaces the current "insurance paradigm" (Emery, 1999). In a production paradigm, patients exercise more choice in treatment selection and assume more financial responsibility. A production paradigm is also known as potentiation, because modern technology creates increased potential to prevent many health care problems.

Biotechnology may advance the current health care system beyond disability treatment and management to a true prevention paradigm through genetic manipulation, stem cell research, and an enhanced focus on lifestyle issues such as obesity and fitness levels. In the not so distant future, rehabilitation providers may need to adopt a new paradigm that minimizes their role in treatment and fosters opportunities as mentors, consultants, and educators.

Table 21–11 contrasts "old paradigms" of health care delivery with "new paradigms." Paradigm shifts are listed according to which stakeholder is impacted the greatest. Stakeholders include patients, payers, hospitals, employers, and health care providers. Payers are entities that fund health care including traditional insurance companies, managed care organizations, and self-insured or self-funded employers. It is important to understand that these represent generalizations that allow for exceptions. For instance, under managed care patients/consumers usually have a reduced choice of health care services and providers. This situation may not be true, however, under certain managed care models such as preferred provider organizations.

REFERENCES

American Medical Association (AMA): Directory of Practice Parameters, Chicago, AMA, 1996.

Anderson TP: An alternative frame of reference for rehabilitation: The helping versus the medical model. In Marinelli RP & Dellorto AE (eds): The Psychological and Social Impact of Physical Disability. New York, Springer, 1977.

Anonymous: 2002 Rising health costs signal ominous emerging trends, USA Today, April 22, p A11.

Baker GR: Health-care managers in the complex world of health care. Clin Leadership Manage Rev 16(3):181-186, 2002.

Baranoski S: Partners in healing. Case Rev 2(3):51-53, 1996.

Bateman S: Using a team approach. Rehabil Manage 12(5):48-49, 1999.

Becker-Reems ED: Self-Managed Work Teams in Health Care Organizations. Chicago, IL, American Hospital Pub, 1994, p 231.

Beckham D: Managing complexity. Health Forum J 44(6):41-43, 2001.

Berkowits M: From practice to research: The case for criticism in an age of evidence. Soc Sci Med 47(10):1539-1545, 1998.

Blood H & Robinson HA: Should physical therapists become physician's assistants? Phys Ther 54(4):423-424, 1974.

Bolton B & Brookings J: Development of multifaceted definition of empowerment. Rehabil Couns Bull 39:256-264, 1996.

Bridges W: Managing Transitions: Making the Most of Change. Reading, MA, Addison-Wesley, 1991, p 130.

Buckley DS: A practitioner's view on managing change. Frontiers Health Serv Manage 16(1):38-43, 1999.

Bujak JS: Culture in chaos: The need for leadership and followership in medicine. Physician Executive 24(4):56-59, 1999.

Campbell JF: The consumer movement and implications for vocational rehabilitation services. J Vocational Rehabil 1(30):67-75, 1991.

Charns MP & Smith Tewksbury LJ: Collaborative Management in Health Care. San Francisco, Jossey-Bass, 1993, p 321.

Colyer H & Kammath P: Evidence-based practice. A philosophical and political analysis: Some matters for consideration by professional practitioners. J Adv Nurs 29(1):188-193, 1999.

Cooley E: Training an interdisciplinary team in communicating and decision making skills. Small Group Res 25:5-25, 1984.

Cox PD et al: Interdisciplinary pilot in a rehabilitation setting. J Allied Health 28(1):25-29, 1999.

Davidhizar R & Calhoun D: Understanding the members of your health care "gang"-seekers and cruisers. Health Care Manage 20(4):40-45, 2002.

DeFriese GH et al: From activated patient to pacified activist: A study of the self-care movement in the United States. Soc Sci Med 29(2):195-204, 1989.

DiBella AJ: Reducing health care risk. The challenge is to make everyone feel accountable. Health Forum J 44(4):16-18, 27-28, 2001.

Dickerson SS & Brennan PF: The internet as a catalyst for shifting power in provider-patient relationships. Nurs Outlook 50(5):195-203.

Duncan PW: Evidence-based practice: A new model for physical therapy. Phys Ther 4(12):44-48, 1996.

Eddy DM: Medicine, money, and mathematics. Bull Am Coll Surg 77: 36-49, 1992.

Emener WG: An empowerment philosophy for rehabilitation in the 20th century. J Rehabil 57(4):7-12, 1991.

Escarse JJ et al: Medical care expenditures under gatekeeper and point-of-service arrangements. Health Serv Res 36(6 Pt1):1037-1057, 2000.

Flower J: Is it change? Or is it noise? Physician Executive 24(4):56-59, 1998.

Flower J: In an era of change ... we're changing. Health Forum J 42(2): 66-69, 1999.

Fosnaught M & Smith R: PTs as case managers: An evolving role. PT Magazine 4(6):46-53, 1996.

Fowler FJ: Lowering costs through internal case management. Rehabil Econ Rehabil Manage 3(3):81, 83, 1995.

Fowler FJ: Disease state management. Rehabil Econ Rehabil Manage 9(4):94,96-97, 1996.

Fries JF & Carey C: Patient education in arthritis: Randomized controlled trial of a mail-delivered program. J Rheum 24(7):1378-1383, 1997.

Gallichio JD: Consumer self-care in health, research proceedings series. National Center for Health Services Research, U.S. Department of Health Services Research, U.S. Department of Health, Education, and Welfare, DHEW Pub. No. (HRA) 77-3181.5, 1977.

Gelinas MV & James RG: Learn how to aid organizational change. Healthcare Benchmarks 6(9):105-106, 1999.

Gibert JA: Disease management hits home. Health Data Manage 6(8): 54-59, 1998.

Gold M: The changing U.S. healthcare system: Challenges for responsible public policy. Millbank Q 77(1):1-22, 1999.

Government Accounting Office: Managed Care Plans Customize Guidelines to meet Local Interests, Government Accounting Office Report to the Chairman, Subcommittee on Health, Committee on Ways and Means, House of Representatives, GAO/HEHS-96-95, p 16, 1996.

Grumbach K, Selby JV, Dambery C et al: Resolving the gatekeeper conundrum: What patients value in primary care and referrals to specialists. JAMA 282(3): 261-266, 1999.

Guyatt G: Evidence-based medicine: Teaching the practice of medicine. JAMA 268(17):2420-2425, 1992.

Hagen C: Rehabilitation in Managed Care: Controlling Costs, Ensuring Quality. Gaithersburg, MD, Aspen, 1999, p 323.

Hagner D: Empowerment issues in services to individuals with disabilities. J Disability Policy Studies 6(2):17-36, 1995.

Haas JS et al: Is the prevalence of gatekeeping in a community associated with individual trust in medical care? Med Care 41(5):660-668, 2003.

Heifetz RA & Linsky M: A survival guide for leaders. Harvard Business Rev 80(6):65-74, 2002.

Hilton RW: Fragmentation within inter-professional works: A result of isolationism in health care professional education programs and the preparation of students to function only in the confines of their own disciplines. J Interdisciplinary Professional Care 9:33-40, 1995.

Hirsch HL: Medico-legal considerations in the use of physician extenders. Legal Med 127-205, 1991.

Hofmann P: Confronting the tyranny of conventional wisdom. Health Progress 83(1):63-64, 2002.

Hunsaker PL: Strategies for organizational change: The role of the inside change agents. Personnel 59(5):18-20, 1982.

Inamdar N et al: Applying the balanced scorecard in healthcare provider organizations. J Healthcare Manage 47(3):179-195, 2002.

Institute of Medicine: Guidelines for Clinical Practice: From Development to Use. Washington, DC, National Academy Press, 1992.

Institute of Medicine: Guidelines for clinical practice: From development to use. Washington, DC, National Academy Press, 1992.

Interstudy: The Interstudy Competitive Edge: Part II: HMO Industry Report No. 7.2. Excelsior, MN, 1997.

Ionnides JPA & Lau J: Pooling research results: Benefits and limitations of meta-analysis. J Qual Improvement 25(9):462-469, 1999.

Issel LM & Anderson RA: Avoidable cost of comprehensive case management. Health Care Manage Rev 24(3):64-72, 1999.

Izzo J & Klein E: The changing values of workers, organizations must respond with soul. Healthcare Forum J 41(3):62-65, 1998.

Joshi MS & Bernard DB: Classic CQI integrated with comprehensive disease state management as a model for performance improvement. Joint Commission J Qual Improvement 25(8):383-395, 1999.

Kaplan R: Behavioral epidemiology in health promotion and health services. Med Care 23:564-583, 1985.

Kleinke JD: Bleeding Edge: The Business of Healthcare in the New Century. Gaithersburg, MD, Aspen, 1998.

Kosciulek JF: Implications of consumer direction for disability policy development and rehabilitation service delivery. Lecture delivered at Mary Switzer Memorial Seminar, National Rehabilitation Association, Sept 27-29, 1999, East Lansing, MI, Kosciulekj@Missouri.edu.

Kuchins AA: Finding the silver lining: How the use of non-professional technicians can be an asset to rehabilitation teams instead of a threat. Rehabil Manage 12(4):20-22, 1999.

Larson EB: Evidence-based medicine: Is translating evidence into practice a solution to the cost-quality challenges facing medicine? Joint Commission J Qual Improvement 25(9):448-485, 1999.

Lindberg DA et al: Evidence-based working group: A new approach to teaching the practice of medicine. JAMA 268(17):2420-2425, 1992.

Llewellyn A: The crucial link: The invaluable role of case management in providing quality and cost-effective patient care. Rehabil Manage 12(6):20-22, 1999.

Lorig K, Holman HR: Long-term outcomes of an arthritis self-management study: Effects of reinforcement efforts. Soc Sci Med 29(2):221-224, 1989.

Mang AL: Implementation strategies of patient-focused care. Hosp Health Serv Adm 40(3):426-435, 1995.

Martin T & Cohen M: Patient-focused care: A case study. Rehabil Manage 8(3):67, 70-71, 123, 1995.

Martin KJ: Workers' compensation: Case management strategies. Case Rev J 43(5):245-250, 1995.

McCarthy R: Disease Management: A Critical Look. The 1996 Health Network and Alliance Sourcebook, Vibbert S, Richard J (Eds). New York, Faulkner and Gray Healthcare, 1996.

McConnell CR: The manager and the merger: Adaptation and survival in the blended organization. Health Care Manage 19(1):1-11, 2000.

McDonagh KJ: Patient-Centered Hospital Care, Management Series. Ann Arbor, MI, American College of Healthcare Executives, Health Administration Press, 1993, p 222.

Montori VM, Guyatt GH: What is evidence-based medicine and why should it be practiced?, Evidence-based Working Group. JAMA 277(15): 1232-1237, 1997.

Moore N & Komras H: Patient-Focused Healing: Integrating, Caring and Curing in Healthcare. San Francisco, CA, Jossey Bass, 1993, p 298.

Morrison I: The Second Curve: Managing the Velocity of Change. New York, Ballentine Books, 1996, p 272.

Muller-Smith P: Core culture: The key to successful paradigm shifts. J Post Anesth Nurs 11(1):35-38, 1996.

Myers SM: Focused care: What managers should know. Nurs Econ 16(4):180-188, 1998.

Muller-Smith P: Core culture: The key to successful paradigm shifts. Journal Post Anesth Nurs 11(1):35-38, 1996.

National Institute on Consumer-Directed Long-Term Services (NICDLTS): The benefits of consumer direction. Consumer Choice News 1(2):1-3, 1996.

National Health Care Skill Standard Project home page, http://www.nist.gov/director/quality_program/doc/95_criteria/ A_PUBLIC-PRIVATE-PARTNERSHIP.html, accessed April 12, 2000.

Patterson RF (ed): New Webster's Dictionary. Plantation, FL, Paradise Press, 1998.

Pati S et al: Does gatekeeping control costs for privately insured children? Findings from the 1996 medical expenditure panel survey Pediatr 111(3):456-460, 2003.

Padula CA: Self-care and the elderly: Review and implications. Public Health Nurs 9(1):22-28, 1992.

Parent W: Quality of life and consumer choice. In Wehman P (ed): The ADA Mandate for Social Changes. Baltimore, MD, Brookes, 1993, pp 12-33.

Page EP: Tapping the potential in resistance. Semin Nurs Manage 10(3):180-188, 2002.

Pena-Dolhun E et al: Unlocking specialists attitudes toward primary care gatekeeper. J Fam Pract 50(12):1032-1037, 2001.

Physician Payment Review Commission Survey, 1995, conducted by Mathematica Policy and Research and the College of Virginia, Arrangement Between Managed Care Plans and Physicians: Results from a 1994 Survey of Managed Care Plans. Washington, DC, Physician Payment Review Commission, 1995.

Relman A: Assessment and accountability: The third revolution in medical care. New Engl J Med 319:1220-1223, 1998.

Richardson WS: Evidence-based diagnosis: More is needed. J Evidence Based Med May/June, 1997.

Robinson AJ et al: Physical therapists' perception of the roles of the physical therapist assistant. Phys Ther 74(6):571-582, 1994.

Rothstein J et al: Clinical uses of isokinetic measurements: Critical issues. Phys Ther 67:1840-1844, 1987.

Salcido R: Competence in the new millennium. Rehabilitation Mgmt 9(5):23-24, 1996.

Secretan LH: Creating organizations that inspire the soul. J Healthcare Dissertations 10:3-6, 1998.

Sharpe VA & Faden AI: Appropriateness in patient care: A new conceptual framework. Milbank Q 74(1):115-136, 1996.

Shendell-Falik N & Soriano KB: Managing patient care in a case management model: Elements for success. Semin Nurs Manage 5(1):49-55, 1997.

Sheppard D: Physician extenders in managed care: Reducing risk through supervision and credentialing. J Healthcare Risk Manage 14(4):12-17.

Sherter AL: Disease management on the web. Health Data Manage 6(10):34-38, 1998.

Shi L et al: The determinants of utilization of nonphysician provider in rural community and migrant health centers. J Rural Health 9(1):27-39, 1992.

Shriver D: OTs: The new case managers. Case Rev Rehabil Manage 1(1):25-26, 29, 1999.

Smith R: Erasing turf-lines. Rehabil Manage 8(3):95-97, 1995.

South SF: The secret to successful change: "The three "Ds." Clin Leadership Manage Rev 14(5):216-218, 2000.

Southwick K: Disease management broadens focus of care from episodic to long-term. Strateg Healthcare Excellence 8(6):1-9, 1995.

Stegall MS: Instilling a soul in your organization without losing yours to it. Clin Leadersh Manage Rev 16(2):85-89, 2002.

Sternack J: Demand management the other side of the health care reform equation. Phys Ther 12:24-27, 1997.

Taffel BH: Patient-centered care: An alternative to the traditional doctor-patient relationship. Group Practice J 43(4):78-83, 1994.

Talbot JF: Managing for change. Models and questions for group practice leaders. Med Group Manage J 46(5):50-54, 56, 58, 1999.

Terris M: Crisis and change in America's health system. Am J Pub Health 63:313, 1973.

The Commission for Case Management Certification, CCM, Rolling Meadows, IL, http://www.ccm-commission.org/cert.html, accessed August 16, 2004.

Tiffan WR: Thriving in change. Physician Executive 26(4):46-51, 2000.

Watson-Evans H & Sheldon JA: Interfacility collaboration to enhance spinal cord injury outcomes. Rehabil Manage 6(4):68-69, 1993.

Webb J: Rising costs push employees to pick up slack. Manage Healthcare Executive 12(9):14, 2002.

Weber V & Joshi MS: Effecting and leading change in health care organizations. Joint Commission J Qual Improvement 26(7):388-399, 2000.

White JA: The case manager: To be or not to be. Phys Ther Case Rep 2(3):113-115, 1999.

Wilson D: The BBA expands the role of physician extenders...with major implications for provider-employers. Med Netw Strategy Rep 7(12):8-9, 1998.

Wurman R: Informational Anxiety. New York, Bantam Books, 1989, p 36.

Wynn KE: Hospital restructuring revisited. Phys Ther 5(1):38-50, 1996.

Zabludoff JA: A Conversation with Paul Ellwood, MD. Rehabil Manage 6(4):pg 28, 1993.

SUGGESTED READINGS

Bridges W: Managing Transitions: Making the Most of Change. Reading, MA, Addison-Wesley, 1994, 130 pgs.

Brown M (ed): Integrated Health Care Delivery: Theory, Practice, Evaluation, and Programs. Gaithersburg, MD, Aspen, 1996.

Coile RC: The Five Stages of Managed Care. Chicago, Health Administration Press, 1997.

Freyman JG: The American Health Care System: Its Genesis and Trajectory. New York, Medcom Press, 1974.

Gray JA: Evidence-Based Healthcare. New York, Churchill Livingston, 1997.

Higgs J & Jones M (eds): Clinical Reasoning in the Health Professions. Boston, Butterworth-Heineman, 1995.

Jonas S: Health Care Delivery in the United States. New York, Springer, 1977.

Kongstvedt PR: Essentials of Managed Health Care. Gaithersburg, MD, Aspen, 1997.

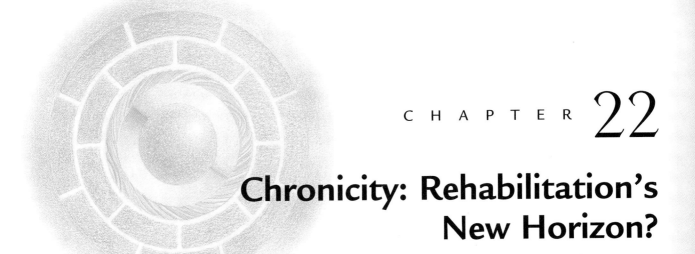

C H A P T E R 22

Chronicity: Rehabilitation's New Horizon?

David W. Clifton, Jr., PT

The United States does not have a coherent approach to caring for people with disabling chronic conditions.

- Hoffman & Rice, 1996

KEY POINTS

- Chronic illnesses and injuries have unpredictable treatment courses and uncertain prognoses relative to acute conditions.
- Chronic conditions usually require a protracted course of treatment.
- The U.S. health care system is fundamentally geared toward acute care and not the management of chronic illness/injury.
- The acute care system is predominantly generalist-driven, while chronic conditions generally require more specialists care.
- Compared with acute illness or injury, chronic conditions tend to involve multiple systems. Persons with chronic conditions face more obstacles to recovery than persons with acute conditions.

Operational Definitions

Chronic Conditions	Ongoing impairment and/or disability because of disease or injury.
Trajectory	The recovery cycle associated with injury or illness expressed as improvement (or lack thereof) over a period of time.
Irritability Stage	The stage of an injury or illness temporarily defined (i.e., acute, duration of less than 2 weeks; subacute, duration of 2 to 12 weeks; chronic, duration of more than 12 weeks).

CHRONIC INJURY/ILLNESS MANAGEMENT: REHABILITATION'S NEXT GOLDEN ERA?

This chapter explores the issue of chronicity in an American health care system that is fundamentally geared toward the care of acute episodic problems. In the current managed care system, rehabilitation is often considered a discretionary service. Many conditions are suitable for physical rehabilitation both before and after chronicity has set in, however. Unfortunately managed care essentially rewards primary care physicians (PCPs) or gatekeepers for non-referral for service, and rehabilitation referrals decline as a result. Few would argue that the prominence of rehabilitation has been diminished under managed care as defined by job growth or lack thereof (American Physical Therapy Association, 1997). Fortunately several trends are at work that appear to be leading to resurgence. For instance, both the prevalence and cost associated with chronic illnesses have exploded in recent years (Hoffman & Rice, 1996).

Many of these conditions require the specialized services of physical rehabilitation experts. In addition, managed care organizations (MCOs) and their gatekeeper model are under enormous siege as evidenced by numerous legislative and regulatory initiatives at the state and federal levels. Employers are more aggressively reasserting their control over health care cost and quality, namely through self-funding. (Figure 22–1).

Rehabilitation providers have begun to produce clinical and financial outcomes data to offset widely published negative publicity regarding the efficacy and cost-effectiveness of services (Agency for Health Care Policy and Research, 1994; Workers' Compensation Research Institute, 1994; Government Accounting Office, 1995).

Estimated number of persons with chronic conditions and direct medical costs for persons with chronic conditions, selected years, 1995–2050

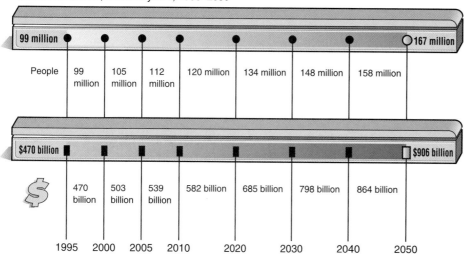

People	99 million	105 million	112 million	120 million	134 million	148 million	158 million	

$	470 billion	503 billion	539 billion	582 billion	685 billion	798 billion	864 billion	

1995   2000   2005   2010   2020   2030   2040   2050

Figure 22–1. The number of persons with chronic conditions is increasing along with the costs of their care. (Data from Hoffman C, Rice DP: Chronic Care in America: A 21st Century Challenge. Princeton, NJ, Robert Wood Johnson Foundation, 1996.)

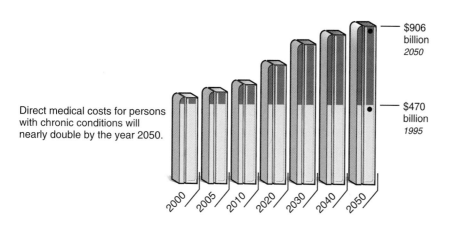

Direct medical costs for persons with chronic conditions will nearly double by the year 2050.

$906 billion 2050

$470 billion 1995

These and other trends may spawn rehabilitation's next golden era. Clinical and consultative opportunities for rehabilitation providers are explored both in this chapter and in Chapter 25. Some opportunities may become quite apparent, but others may require providers to carve out a niche market for their services. Identifying untapped opportunities may require imagination on the part of the rehabilitation provider. Conventional wisdom and treatment paradigms must be challenged if chronicity is to be aggressively managed. This chapter frames some of the issues that providers must understand if they are to be successful, but it by no means offers complete solutions to both this growing challenge and opportunity (Figure 22–2).

HOW IS A CHRONIC CONDITION DEFINED?

Time is the parameter that is most often used to define a chronic condition. This parameter alone, however, fails woefully to explain the complexities associated with chronic conditions. Yet it seems that many providers categorize treatment approaches for chronic conditions by time-driven strategies without examining other variables. Although chronicity is common to many disabling conditions, it may not be the defining feature of an underlying

problem (Sutton & DeJong, 1998). Furthermore, it is not chronicity itself but functional limitations that impact a person's health status.

Treatment approaches may dramatically differ depending on the irritability stage of an impairment or disability.

1990 Personal health care expenditures: $612 billion

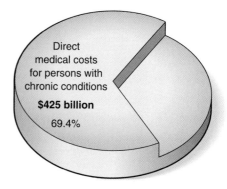

Direct medical costs for persons with chronic conditions
$425 billion
69.4%

Figure 22–2. Direct medical costs of chronic conditions: 1990. Direct medical costs for persons with chronic conditions represent almost 70% of national expenditures on personal health care. (Data from Hoffman C, Rice DP: Chronic Care in America: A 21st Century Challenge. Princeton, NJ, Robert Wood Johnson Foundation, 1996.)

From onset, acute conditions (1 to 2 weeks) are treated with a variety of interventions that are generally not as useful in the management of chronic conditions. For instance, during the acute phase of soft-tissue injury management, a provider might justifiably focus on the use of palliative modalities such as thermal, mechanical, or electrophysiological agents to facilitate tissue healing and earlier movement.

During the acute stage, restorative activities (e.g., work, therapeutic exercise, and kinetic activity) may not be feasible because of increased irritability. Consequently, these activities are generally introduced as the degree of irritability subsides.

As an injury enters the subacute stage, providers may elect to balance palliative and restorative activities. A sandwich approach to treatment (e.g., palliative modalities-exercise-palliative modalities) is quite common during this stage. For example, a patient may be preheated before an exercise regimen to enhance circulation and tissue extensibility. After the exercise session, a clinician may elect to quell symptoms such as pain and swelling through cryotherapy or electrophysiological agents. A sandwich approach may also be used in other irritability stages but is less common during the chronic stage (8 to 12 weeks from onset). A home exercise program is established as quickly as possible along with adjunctive modalities (Figure 22–3).

Chronic conditions usually require a protracted versus episodic treatment. Protracted treatment usually consists of more than a 3-month period or extends beyond the range of normal tissue healing. Restorative activities receive prioritization during the chronic stage and the patient is weaned from palliative modalities, or they are trained to use these modalities as a component in a home exercise program. The provider may simply invert the treatment formula in the chronic stage of soft-tissue injury. This shift in treatment approach often overlooks issues that may be responsible for a patient or patient's failure to improve and that person's resultant disability. A plethora of psychosocial or economic issues might not

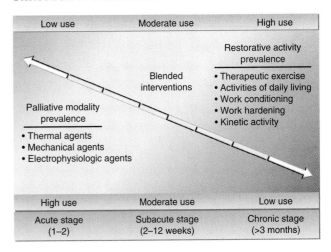

Figure 22–3. Irritability Stages and prevalent interventions: A conceptual model.

be addressed by either palliative or restorative treatment. Chapter 13 examines some of these confounding obstacles to rehabilitation success.

Characteristics of Chronic Conditions

Chronic conditions involve ongoing impairment resulting from disease or injury and have long sequelae (Pope & Tarlov, 1991; Sandy & Gibson, 1996) (Figure 22–4). A number of experts agree that chronic illness or injury is one of the most, if not the most, important issue facing providers, health plans, and policy makers (Larkin, 1987; Lubkin, 1986; Miller, 1992; Murrow & Oglesby, 1996; Newby, 1996). Unfortunately there is a lack of consensus between or within health care stakeholder groups concerning appropriate management of these conditions. Inadequate funding for services compounds the challenge. As a result, successful rehabilitation is far from guaranteed. Some experts have estimated that success rates are 30% or lower (Mayer, 1999).

Figure 22–4. Where are chronic care dollars spent? (Hospital, physician, and other costs from Hoffman C, Rice DP: Chronic Care in America: A 21st Century Challenge. Princeton, NJ, Robert Wood Johnson Foundation, 1996. Nursing costs from Letsch SW, Lazenby HC, Levit KR, et al: National health expenditures, 1991. Health Care Financ Rev 14[2]:1-30, 1992.)

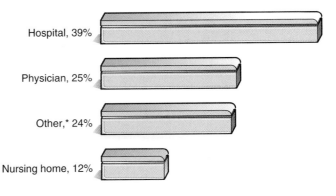

ALMOST TWO-THIRDS OF HEALTH CARE DOLLARS FOR CHRONIC CONDITIONS ARE SPENT ON HOSPITAL CARE AND PHYSICIAN SERVICES

1990 Direct medical costs for persons with chronic conditions: $425 billion

Hospital, 39%

Physician, 25%

Other,* 24%

Nursing home, 12%

*Including prescriptions, dental care, non-physician practitioners, home health care, medical equipment, emergency care.

One of the greatest assessment errors committed by clinicians is a failure to recognize and address the socio-economic factors that impact chronic injury and illness. When applied in the chronic stage, acute care models of delivery may be doomed to failure despite the very best provider motives and skill sets.

PCPs are relatively inexperienced in the management (versus treatment) of persons with chronic conditions (DeJong, 1997; Sutton & DeJong, 1998). Hospitals especially have not proved their efficiency in management of chronic conditions (Millbank Memorial Fund, 1999).

Again, chronic illnesses and injuries have many characteristics apart from the time factor that distinguish them from acute problems and demand a unique rehabilitation approach. These characteristics cross many boundaries including prognosis, social roles, health policy, outcome measures, health care funding, provider roles, psychological impact, and delivery mechanisms. First, most illnesses cannot be cured within our current health care model, which emphasizes acute treatment with a minimal focus on prevention (Morrison, 1993). This situation is likely to change in the future as scientists continue to unlock life's mysteries. The human genome projects (funded by private sector and government initiatives) could conceivably lead to cures for or prevention of chronic conditions such as asthma, arthritis, diabetes, Parkinson's disease, cardiac disease, and multiple sclerosis. Discoveries could lead to dramatic interventions for genetically predisposed persons.

Francis Collins, director of the National Human Genome Research Institute, announced at the White House that, "We have caught the first glimpse of our own instruction book, previously known only to God" (Borenstein, 2000). Stem cell research also offers fascinating possibilities for the management of chronic diseases. For the time being, providers must operate under the premise that chronic conditions are incurable until medical researchers learn to apply this revolutionary information.

Chronic conditions at times become exacerbated and re-enter the acute stage. During these periods of exacerbation, chronic conditions may manifest certain characteristics that are normally associated with acute conditions. Again, providers are therefore cautioned not to inappropriately label a condition on the basis of time elements alone. However, providers may for reimbursement purposes need to explain to claims adjusters or case managers the rationale behind a reapplication of palliative modalities in chronic cases. During exacerbations, treatment versus management may be necessary and treatment may mimic acute care interventions (Table 22-1).

Chronic conditions, unlike acute conditions, have unpredictable treatment courses and uncertain prognoses because of a host of non-biomedical issues. In fact, recovery cycles are analogous to a roller coaster ride. Acute problems follow a steady incline with occasional undulations until they reach the pinnacle of their ascent. At this point, a patient has achieved maximum functional recovery. The application of more treatment is unlikely to result in any significant sustainable functional gains. On the contrary, chronic conditions usually follow a course of exaggerated ups and downs, and at worst they decline when the roller

Table 22-1 Comparison Between Acute and Chronic Care Delivery

Delivery Issue	Acute	Chronic
Goals	To restore a person to their previous level of functioning	To maintain and/or restore functionality. To "habilitate" a person.
Provider(s) and treatment setting	Typically institution-based care provided by skilled professionals	Highly fragmented care, ranging from hospital-based to home care to self-care. Patient and his or her support network provide significant care.
Focus	Biomedical	Psychosocial, vocational and community service
Reimbursement model	Private insurance	Private insurance
	Public financing (e.g., Medicare, Medicaid, social security)	Public financing
Duration of condition since onset	<3 months	>3 months
Disability status	Pathology and/or impairment-based	Disability and/or handicap-based
Delivery paradigm	"Treatment"	"Management"
Service focus	● Diagnostic	● Restorative rehabilitation
	● Surgical	● Vocational
	● Medication	● Disease-state management
	● Palliative rehabilitation	● Transportation services
		● Home health
Demand for rehabilitation	Minimum-to-moderate	Moderate-to-maximum
Prognosis	Generally predictable	Generally unpredictable
Cost to manage	Relatively low	Relatively high
Functional emphasis	Effect a cure	Medical stability
Diagnosis	Typically a single diagnosis	Typically multiple diagnoses, co-morbidities, secondary problems
Prevalence of psychosocial obstacles	Relatively low	Relatively high
Family involvement	Relatively low	Relatively high
Resource use	Relatively low	Relatively high

Data from Clifton, DW: Setting sail on the U.S. chronic care. Rehabil Manage 12(5):20, 22-23, 1999; Grazier, KL: The chronically ill and managed care. J Healthcare Manage 43(6):477-479, 1998; Morrison, MH: Rehab for an aging population. Rehabil Manage 6(4):36-38, 40, 1993; Murrow EJ, Oglesby FM: Acute and chronic illness: Similarities, differences, and challenges. Orthop Nurse 15(5):47-51, 1996; and Sandy LG, Gibson R: Managed care and chronic care: Challenges and opportunities. Managed Care Q 4(2):5-11, 1996.

Table 22–2 Goals of Rehabilitation in Chronic Conditions

- Maintenance of function
- Pain management
- Prevention of co-morbidities or secondary problems
- Client/patient education
- Support staff training and education
- "Habilitation" of the individual to their own unique environment
- Environmental safety through screening or ergonomic analysis
- Reasonable accommodations (e.g., Americans with Disabilities Act compliance)
- Vocational counseling and/or training
- Home exercise program of pain abatement, activities of daily living, and exercise

coaster speeds toward its lowest functional level. This description may be an oversimplification, but it has some merit from a conceptual standpoint. Some individuals with acute problems may also experience a roller coaster ride during the recovery period. These problems tend to be less pronounced and occur infrequently, however. Generally speaking, fewer chronic conditions achieve as rapid and significant functional improvement as do acute cases. In most cases, rehabilitation is geared toward maintenance of function, medical stabilization, prevention of co-morbidities or secondary problems, rehabilitation of the individual to his/her environment, and maximization of function within the constraints of disease processes (Table 22–2).

Trajectory is the term that describes variation in severity over time (Murrow & Oglesby, 1996). Trajectory phases are three-fold and involve the diagnostic phase, during which the medical necessity for care is established. The management (versus "treatment" as in acute care) phase determines priority issues and identifies necessary resources. The third, or "stabilization, phase" describes a condition of remission or stabilization. Chronic conditions may present fourth and fifth phases or loss of function and death respectively (Figure 22–5).

Trajectory is a key concept to understanding the management of chronic conditions (Murrow & Oglesby, 1996). The trajectory of acute conditions requires a focus that is principally aimed at the biophysical aspects of the person's problem. Pathology and related impairments command the clinician's attention, but not to the exclusion of disability. Many of the confounding elements routinely seen in chronic conditions have not had the time or the environment in which to develop, however. Many of the psychosocial or economic issues associated with chronic conditions are routinely absent during the acute phase.

Generally speaking, acute conditions can be managed through primary care, and a relatively low percentage of cases require specialty care (Table 22–3).

Paradoxically, most chronic conditions require specialist intervention and are beyond the scope of a PCP's expertise. A combination of multiple diagnoses and co-morbidities further drives the use of specialists (Figure 22–6). Persons with arthritis are managed by rheumatologists, those with heart disease require cardiologists, and sufferers of demyelinating nerve disorders see neurologists. This begs the question: Is physical rehabilitation a primary service, specialist service, or both? One could reasonably argue that for years the educational emphasis of rehabilitation programs (e.g., physical therapy and occupational therapy) placed a disproportionate emphasis on acute care despite the larger role these professions play in the management of chronic conditions. For example, many physical therapy clinical affiliations or internships focused on hospital-based training. This focus was understandable because hospitals (before managed care) were the principal portal or entry into the health care system for many therapists.

The development of alternative clinical affiliation sites has been a positive by-product of managed care's influence, specifically reductions in hospital inpatient services.

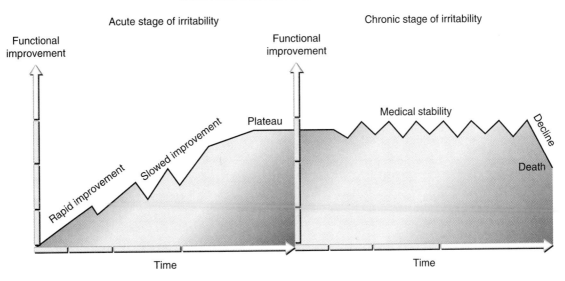

Figure 22–5. Recovery trajectory: Acute conditions versus chronic conditions.

Table 22–3 Top 10 Chronic Conditions Among Older Adults*

	Adults Age 65+	Adults Age 45–64
Arthritis	480	285
Hypertension	394	251
Hearing impairment	296	136
Heart conditions	277	123
Orthopedic impairment	173	162
Sinusitis	169	187
Cataracts	141	21
Diabetes	98	64
Visual impairment	95	46
Tinnitus	85	49

Data from National Center for Health Statistics: Top 10 chronic conditions among older adults. Hyattsville, MD, 1998, http://www.cdc.gov/nchs/, accessed February 3, 2000.

*Prevalence per 1,000 people.

Alternate sites now include long-term–care facilities, private practices, home care agencies, school systems, industrial clinics, health maintenance organization (HMO) departments, wellness centers, faculty-based practices, and employer on-site centers.

Chronic problems, when compared with acute illness or injury, also tend to involve multiple systems. Additionally, the treatment for chronic conditions can create problems in other systems. A classic example involves the person with arthritis who has taken an antiinflammatory medication for years and develops a peptic ulcer as a direct result of the treatment. Other examples exist (e.g., long-term steroid use and osteoporosis or fluid retention). These complications or secondary conditions are relatively rare in acute problems and require an integrated approach to disability management (Moore & Komras, 1993; Satinsky, 1998).

A positive correlation exists between the number of conditions and an increase in disability dependence (Fried et al, 1999; Guralnick, 1989). Fried's study of women between 65 and 85 years of age discovered disabilities in 55% of those reporting three or more chronic conditions, compared with only 13% of women with only one chronic condition.

Chronic conditions often become the principal focus or identity for many, instead of simply a bump in the road of life. Those who suffer from a chronic condition may develop a "diseasecentric" view of themselves. For instance, a person with arthritis may describe himself or herself as an "arthritic" instead of as a person with arthritis. These labels are reinforced by the media and, at times, by providers themselves when they refer to patients in dehumanizing terms such as those found in Table 22–4. It is recommended that rehabilitation professionals, whenever possible, avoid the use of these terms in their departments.

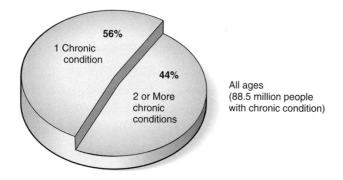

Figure 22–6. Nearly 40 million Americans have more than one chronic condition. (Data from Hoffman C, Rice DP: Chronic Care in America: A 21st Century Challenge. Princeton, NJ, Robert Wood Johnson Foundation, 1996.)

MAJORITY OF PEOPLE WITH MORE THAN ONE CHRONIC CONDITION ARE MIDDLE-AGED OR OLDER

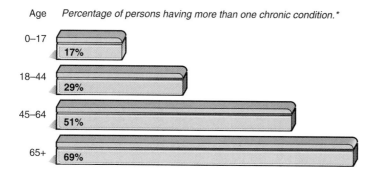

*Rates of co-morbidity by age group, 1987 (Non-institutionalized population)

Table 22–4   Examples of Dehumanizing Terms with Accompanying Phrases for Persons with Chronic Conditions

BY CONDITION

Derogatory Term	Derogatory Phrase
"Arthritics"	We teach joint conservation techniques to our arthritics.
"Diabetics"	Our diabetics receive nutritional counseling.
"Cords"	Recreational activities are offered to our cords.
"Amputees"	We hold a monthly amputee clinic at our center.
"TBIs"	Physical, occupational, and speech therapy is provided to our TBIs (traumatic brain injured)
"Quads"	Quads in our facility receive training in real-life environments.
"Paras"	Paras have more potential for ambulation than do quads.

BY BODY REGION

"Backs"	I specialize in treating backs.
"Knees"	She is a knee surgeon.
"Shoulders"	We use therapeutic bands for strengthening of our shoulder cases.
"Hands"	I work in a hand center.

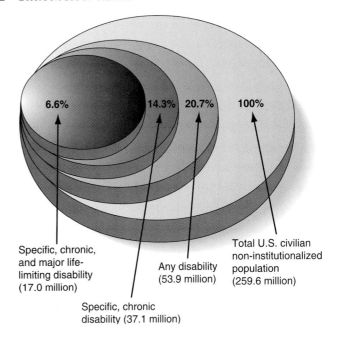

Figure 22–7. Disability Prevalence. (Data from Economic and Social Research Institute, Data from the 1994 National Health Survey, Disability Supplement, Phase 1, April 1999.)

This would represent a first step toward a new paradigm shift in how rehabilitation professionals assist those persons with chronic conditions. Perhaps part of a facility's quality assurance and utilization review program could involve a language cop.

Insurance coverage is abundantly more generous for acute conditions than chronic ones. Acute conditions can be generally handled in one treatment setting or by one professional discipline, and as such, they represent better value in the eyes of an insurer.

Acute conditions typically have a patient-focus, whereas chronic conditions tend to have a family-focus. Acute conditions may marginally involve the patient's family in the care delivery process. In contrast, family or friends may serve as the primary caregivers for those with chronic conditions. There are, of course, many exceptions to these generalizations.

Chronic conditions, when compared with acute conditions, tremendously limit a person's social interaction. Unequivocally, persons with chronic conditions face far more obstacles to recovery than those with acute conditions (Figure 22–7). Many of these barriers are constructed by managed care systems (Brown et al, 1993; Ware et al, 1996; Shaughnessy et al, 1994). Managed care often severs the umbilical cord between the patient and his or her chosen specialist (Riley, 1997). Loss of this tie is especially unfortunate when it has taken a person years and multiple experiments before finally locating a specialist of choice who understands their problem on several planes, including medical, psychological, social, and economic. Few things are more frustrating to a patient than to have to see a PCP just to refill a prescription for a chronic condition with which they have lived for years and taken the same medication. This situation is compounded when a person is confronted with mobility or transportation challenges.

The projected number of persons with chronic conditions continues to increase (Figure 22–8). Managed care

plans for years ignored the chronic illness/injury population in favor of younger, healthier, and more vibrant persons who were devoid of a preexisting injury or illness (Freudenheim, 1996; Gold, 1999; Interstudy, 1999; Newhouse, 1996). This approach gave HMOs an early competitive advantage over traditional Blue Cross plans that openly enrolled these persons. Managed care plans did promote wellness and readily financed preventive programs such as well babies, mammograms, and vaccinations, as long as the individual already had a clean bill of health. The competitive tide changed as the "Blues" restructured and embraced cost-containment strategies, and the HMO population aged, thus ablating the benefits of "patient skimming."

"Patient dumping" is the opposite of patient skimming. This term refers to the referral of a patient or client by one facility or provider to another. This gesture is typically not magnanimous, but rather is designed to transfer a riskier patient to another facility. In these cases, risk could mean a lack of insurance or other problems associated with a particular patient. Unfortunately, this practice seems to occur more frequently with persons with chronic conditions than in those with acute ones (Table 22–5).

Managed care plans have traditionally attempted to force-fit medical solutions to conditions that required social interventions, supports, and structures. Managed care PCPs generally know very little about support systems such as the Veterans Administration, Public Health Service, State Vocational Counseling Agencies, various support groups, and consumer advocacy organizations, because these groups often serve the needs of the chronic and not acute population. Even the most well-intentioned, intelligent, and humane PCP can be at a loss for appropriate placement and referral.

Health care providers need generous clinical, organization, and coordination time to work with chronically ill

PROJECTED NUMBER OF PERSONS WITH ACTIVITY LIMITATION DUE TO CHRONIC CONDITIONS,
SELECTED YEARS, 1995–2050

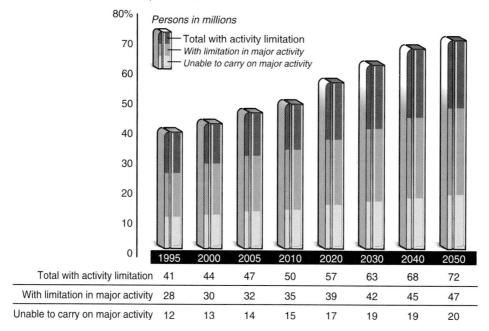

	1995	2000	2005	2010	2020	2030	2040	2050
Total with activity limitation	41	44	47	50	57	63	68	72
With limitation in major activity	28	30	32	35	39	42	45	47
Unable to carry on major activity	12	13	14	15	17	19	19	20

Figure 22–8. Projected number of persons with chronic conditions. (Data from Hoffman C, Rice DP: Chronic Care in America: A 21st Century Challenge. Princeton, NJ, Robert Wood Johnson Foundation, 1996.)

 Table 22–5 Managed Care: Promise versus Reality

The Promise...

Managed care holds great promise for providing the range of integrated services required by people with chronic conditions. One underlying reason for this is the capitation system of financing on which many managed care plans are based, in whole or in part.

The basic idea behind capitation is that each provider receives a pool of funds (a given amount per patient) in advance of treatment. In contrast, more traditional forms of financing—under commercial indemnity insurance or fee-for-service Medicare, for example—use a system in which services are provided on a pay-as-you-go basis.

Under a capitated system, providers should have the flexibility to treat a patient with a chronic condition, or refer him or her to an appropriate mix of medical and non-medical services. Ideally, membership in an HMO or similar prepaid health plan could enable an idividual to have access to an array of services for an single fee.

A capitated system of care has another advantage to a person with chronic conditions. It provides a financial incentive for keeping people healthy and functioning as fully as possible. Hence, managed care programs should and often do emphasize prevention services and attempt to avoid use of emergency rooms and costly acute care services, except when necessary.

The Reality...

In reality, the managed care industry is just beginning to recognize and respond to the needs of people with chronic conditions. Some HMOs do offer important preventive measures for people with chronic conditions. For instance, research has found that some HMOs:

- arrange for handrails to be placed in the homes of people who are frail or disabled;
- create support groups for patients;
- screen enrollees to identify those with chronic problems;
- provide early intervention services.

However, the managed care industry overall has yet to implement these and other practices that would meet the needs of people with chronic conditions. Some spokespeople representing the disability and chronic illness community complain that because they are potentially heavy users of expensive services, they have been shunned from managed care plans. Others who are enrolled in managed care plans report being denied access to treatment and services that they need, and of being assigned to primary care physicians who are not as well-acquainted with their condition as a specialist might be.

The Future Possibilities...

As the population ages, and as managed care spreads throughout the public and private health sectors, the hope is that managed care can evolve to better serve the needs of people with chronic illness and disability. How might it do so? By:

- integrating primary, preventive, and specialty care;
- coordinating medical care with home and community-based services;
- including the patient in the decision-making process;
- responding to the episodic nature of chronic care.

From Hoffman C & Rice DP: Chronic Care in America: A 21st Century Challenge. Princeton, NJ, The Robert Wood Johnson Foundation. 1996.

persons, beyond the time that is provided under the acute medical care model (Jones, 1997).

There is a paucity of research directed at postacute care (Brown et al, 1993; Grazier, 1998). Providers and clinical researchers have invested a disproportionate amount of time and effort studying elements of the acute care system. Again, schools that train physical rehabilitation specialists such as physical and occupational therapists have spent a considerable amount of time preparing their graduates for acute care positions. The traditional focus on hospital-based services is partly at fault in this regard (Figure 22-9). Fortunately a trend appears to be growing toward a more balanced placement of students during their clinical affiliations or internships. This trend may be partially fueled by demographic shifts.

Grazier (1998) opines that "inadequate treatment often results from delays, discontinuity, inaccessibility of specialists of choice, cultural incompetence, or the lack of psychosocial support required to cope with symptoms, treatment, and complications."

DEMOGRAPHICS AND COSTS

Chronic disability is pervasive, accounting for almost 100 million people in the United States alone (Freudenheim, 1996). Chronic conditions are the leading cause of death, illness, and disability. More than 55% of all emergency room visits and almost 7 of every 10 hospitalizations are of persons with chronic conditions (Freudenheim, 1996). Aging baby boomers swell the ranks of those who could benefit for physical rehabilitation services. Reported chronic conditions with the greatest prevalence include sinusitis, arthritis, hypertension, and deformity or orthopedic impairment, which collectively account for 10% of the general population (National Center for Health Statistics, 1998).

It is easy to assume that the majority of persons with chronic disability are elderly (Figure 22-10). This simply is not true! Contrary to popular belief, the vast majority of persons with chronic disability are not elderly. In fact, only 23% of all disability cases involve those older than 65 years of age. (Hoffman et al, 1996; Sandy & Gibson, 1996).

It is equally incorrect to assume that all chronic conditions lead to disability. For instance, not all persons with diabetes suffer from impaired circulation leading to blindness or amputation, although a significant number do.

Estimates of disability vary with one source estimating that 37.7 million people, or 15% of the non-institutionalized U.S. population, have a disability (Trupin & Rice, 1997). These data are based on the 1992 National Health Interview Survey of 49,401 households with 128,412 people surveyed.

The 37.7 million chronically disabled persons reported an average of 1.6 conditions per person, for a total of 61 million limiting conditions (LaPlante, 1997). Almost 42 million chronic conditions were classified as physical impairments and another two million as mental health disorders. The most prevalent conditions were musculoskeletal, representing 17.2% of all functionally limiting conditions. Circulatory conditions were second at 16.7% of the total. These demographics clearly buoy the need for rehabilitation provider involvement in managing persons with chronic conditions. Physical rehabilitation services are clearly needed for every age category. More than 12 million children (<18 years) have at least one chronic condition (Hoffman et al, 1996). Working-age adults (18 to 64 years) account for 60% of non-institutionalized persons with chronic conditions. Chronic conditions across all ages accounted for expenditures of more than $272.2 billion. Broken down, these costs were allocated as follows: persons with one chronic condition, $91 billion; persons with two or more chronic conditions, $181.1 billion; and all persons with acute conditions, $85.7 billion (Hoffman et al, 1996).

These numbers may suggest why managed care plans have not been quick to embrace these populations. As a

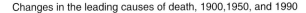

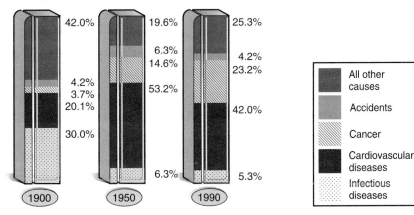

Figure 22–9. The changing nature of illness and death contributes to increased numbers of chronic health conditions. (Data from U.S. Bureau of Census: Statistical Abstract of the United States, 113th ed. Washington, DC, U.S. Bureau of Census, 1993, p 15. In Hoffman C, Rice DP: Chronic Care in America: A 21st Century Challenge. Princeton, NJ, Robert Wood Johnson Foundation, 1996.)

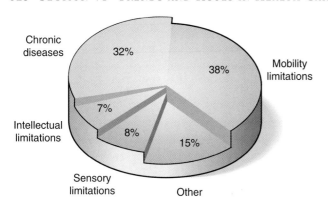

Figure 22–10. Chronic Conditions and Disability Categories. (Data from Pope A, Tarlov A [eds]: Disability in America: Toward a National Agenda for Prevention. Washington, DC, Institute of Medicine, National Academic Press, 1991.)

result, more than 40% of the costs for chronic conditions are borne by public funding sources such as Medicare, Medicaid, and other public assistance programs.

Morbidity, defined as lost workdays, exceeded 4.5 million years of productivity. It is interesting to note that the elderly accounted for only 15% of the total costs associated with chronic conditions (Figure 22–11).

It should be of keen interest to providers involved with workers' compensation that working-age populations (25 to 64 years of age) accounted for 85% of all costs. This fact almost assuredly guarantees a role for physical rehabilitation providers should they offer the right mixture of services supported by evidence-based outcomes. The problem with chronicity will only get worse, with prevalence projected to involve 39 million persons by 2020.

CHRONICITY MANAGEMENT: WHAT IS THE BEST APPROACH?

The most effective treatment for chronicity is to prevent it in the first place. Earlier referral to rehabilitation may reduce the number of conditions that become chronic because of delayed rehabilitation or patient entrenchment in the medical model of care. These persons could benefit from a functionally based model offered by physical rehabilitation providers. Rehabilitation providers can effect earlier referrals through a variety of mechanisms that include:

- Support of direct access legislation that allows patients to receive therapy without a physician's referral. Currently more than 32 states have enacted some form of direct access for physical therapist services.
- Education of PCPs about both the clinical and financial value of rehabilitation. This education will require collection of comparative cost data to demonstrate the value-driven proposition that rehabilitation offers relative to other services.
- Repositioning of rehabilitation as a primary care service versus the specialty that many perceive it to be. To do this, therapists can seek and secure listing on workers' compensation preferred provider panels assembled by employers or insurers. Proposals to MCOs to serve in a triage role for musculoskeletal conditions may be

another example. Opportunities may occur given the current backlash against managed care.

- Direct contracting with employers who finance the majority of health care costs in the United States. This opportunity may be especially ripe if providers can identify self-insured employers or employer purchasing coalitions (Maxwell et al, 1998).
- Engagement in collaborative models of delivery. Rehabilitation private practices have been largely single-service oriented, which tends to place these practices far down on the referral "food chain," especially under managed care.
- Provision of PCPs with the necessary information to make expeditious yet cost-effective referrals for rehabilitation.

Which Provider Group Is Best Suited to Manage Underserved Chronic Populations?

This issue is a source of a great deal of contention among PCPs and specialists (Jeffrey, 1996). Multiple parties, including doctors, health researchers, and even patients themselves, are divided along different fault lines. Specialists may claim that PCPs have a too-limited knowledge of and experience with chronic problems. PCPs may allege that the use of specialists is excessive for many common non–life-threatening or non-surgical cases. In response to this debate, the American Medical Association has lobbied MCOs to allow specialists to treat those who are chronically ill. A designation of "principal care" physician has been suggested by the American Medical Association (Jeffrey, 1996).

To some, physiatrists or physical medicine specialists may appear to straddle both the primary and specialty roles. Some physiatrists are serving in a de facto role by helping former patients manage their postrehabilitation health care (DeJong, 1997). Physical or occupational therapists may view this as a natural extension to their services.

What Is the Role of Physical Rehabilitation Providers?

Rehabilitation is considered an effective approach in creating positive long-term outcomes for the chronically ill individual (Larson, 1995; Jette et al, 1994). Numerous advantages inure to the patient, payer, and other medical providers when physical rehabilitation is aggressively used to manage chronic conditions (Mayer, 1999). Prompt referrals and timely appointments are generally assured. In fact, many rehabilitation centers guarantee expeditious initial evaluations (e.g., within 24 hours of the referral).

This is in contrast to a typical 6-week delay before one can see an orthopedist, neurologist, or neurosurgeon. The largest group of patients in need of care suffers from musculoskeletal conditions. Physical therapists and occupational therapists provide treatment for these conditions, whereas the average general practitioner or PCP, although competent in many areas, possesses minimal theoretical or didactic training in the musculoskeletal system. Therapists also have the luxury (although less so under managed care) of spending more time dealing with psychosocial issues. A rehabilitation visit is easily four to six times longer than a typical physician visit. Therapists receive a broad-based knowledge of multiple body systems and condition-specific treatment methodologies. This knowledge uniquely qualifies therapists to serve in a triage role for patients with

Figure 22–11. Functional limitations and employment status. (Data from McNeil JM: Americans with disabilities: 1991-1993. Data from U.S. Bureau of the Census: Survey of Income and Program Participation. Washington, DC, U.S. Bureau of the Census, 1997, pp 30-33).

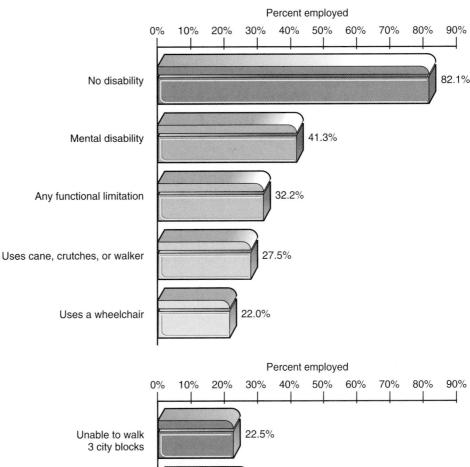

Percent employed

No disability	82.1%
Mental disability	41.3%
Any functional limitation	32.2%
Uses cane, crutches, or walker	27.5%
Uses a wheelchair	22.0%

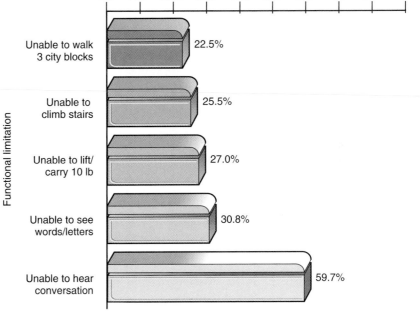

Percent employed

Functional limitation

Unable to walk 3 city blocks	22.5%
Unable to climb stairs	25.5%
Unable to lift/ carry 10 lb	27.0%
Unable to see words/letters	30.8%
Unable to hear conversation	59.7%

chronic conditions that are generally non–life-threatening and patients who are medically stable. This should not be perceived as an attempt by therapists to expand the scope of their practice, because their skills, knowledge, and competencies are already established under the statutes. Instead this presents an opportunity for those with chronic conditions to more readily access the health care systems and work directly with a professional who has an intimate understanding of functionality and the effect of psychosocial issues that are often associated with these conditions (Table 22-6).

Therapists tend to be excellent educators and communicators because they routinely instruct patients and their families as well as extenders of care. Education is the keystone in the management of chronic conditions. Educational programs incorporate a broad spectrum of issues, including self-care, anatomy, ergonomics, physiology, etiology, adaptive equipment, epidemiology, sources of information, support groups, environmental screening, durable medical equipment needs analysis, and patient rights such as "reasonable accommodation" under the Americans with Disabilities Act.

Rehabilitation providers share a common goal with those who suffer from chronic conditions; to achieve the highest level of independence possible, which in turn enhances the quality of life (Larson, 1995). Many persons with chronic disabilities are in need of restorative or

Table 22–6 Do's and Don'ts of Managing Chronic Care

Do's	Don'ts
Empower patients/clients with information regarding prevention, self-care and assistive devices	Continue protracted use of palliative modalities
Identify and address psychosocial obstacles to recovery	Foster a codependent relationship based on "treatment" only
Focus on function	Dwell on pain management alone
Participate in multidisciplinary or collaborative care	Ignore the value of inclusion of the patient's family and friends in care management
Focus on a holistic approach	Attempt to "treat" with a single discipline focus
Serve as a resource for community-based services (e.g., adult day care, vocational counseling, support groups)	Focus on the condition impairment or disease only
Establish a home exercise program as quickly as possible	Emphasize clinically based interventions at the expense of analyzing patient's environmental needs
Wean one's services from patient	Ignore the impact of psychosocial economic, or legal issues
Consider periodic respite from clinical services in order to gauge patient's ability to independently function	Set goals without the patient's and/or family's input
Focus on the patient's environmental needs through habilitation	Underestimate the impact of secondary diagnoses, co-morbidities, and effects of aging on the disability recovery cycle or trajectory

preventive activities such as therapeutic exercise or return-to-work programs. Inactivity is their worst enemy, and provided that their condition is medically stable, restorative activities may very well be the best "medicine." Again, a valuable niche market exists for rehabilitation providers who can position themselves as primary care providers, educators, and enablers of self-care (Clifton, 1999).

Access to a reliable ongoing source of primary health care remains one of the major unresolved issues for people with disabilities, especially among those who are discharged from medical rehabilitation facilities (DeJong, 1997).

Ultimately an effective model of chronic care should contain a number of important characteristics. Sandy and Gibson (1996) provide the following guidelines:

- Integration of both primary and specialty care.
- Integration of medical care with home and community-based services.
- Integration of both patient and family perspectives into the care process.
- Emphasis on functional status and quality of life.
- Delivery of care in multidisciplinary teams.

These services can be paired with three groups of persons with chronic conditions: (1) children with special needs, (2) working-age disabled, and (3) the elderly population.

As the "unfinished business" of medicine, rehabilitation offers restorative care, maintenance services, and preventive strategies, all of which are vital for persons with chronic conditions. Rehabilitation spans these functions through a variety of interventions that include:

- Treatment of functional deficits.
- Stabilization of medical problems.
- Prevention of secondary disabilities.
- Assistance with adaptive interventions.
- Promotion of wellness.
- Patient, family, case manager, and other caregiver education.
- Design of treatment programs for implementation by others in a collaborative model.
- Construction of self-help programs.

- Evaluation of and referral to alternative or complementary health care.

Because MCOs do not relish the added financial risk of chronic populations, "carve-outs" may be feasible. A carve-out involves the segregation of a group of cases from services that are typically capitated. More expensive, prevalent, or poorly understood cases are often considered for carve-out status. Examples include mental health and substance abuse. MCOs also carve-out cases when they lack leverage in a given market of providers.

What Business Is Rehabilitation In?

DeJong (1997) asks, "Are we in the business of rehabilitation or are we in the business of health care for people with disabilities?" This question captures the very essence of how chronicity must be approached. The "business of rehabilitation" is a more restrictive paradigm that implies a treatment-driven, clinician-based model. The "business of health care" invites providers to expand their role on a more global scale by serving as clinician, consultant, and mentor along the entire injury continuum from preinjury to postrehabilitation. "Rehabilitation" implies a return to previous functional levels and quality of life, neither of which may be possible. "Health care" connotes a broader focus but still implies that the provider assumes a hands-on role. Effective management of chronic conditions engages the patient in a collaborative model.

This focus balances three essential elements:

1. Teaching patients to better manage their illness and to prevent secondary illnesses.
2. Tailoring programs to individuals and offering professional support.
3. Following patients throughout the entire injury or illness continuum from prevention to treatment to management (Millbank Memorial Fund, 1999).

Lastly, innumerable opportunities exist for rehabilitation providers, because health education is not tied to any one profession. Perhaps tomorrow's rehabilitation professionals will be the architects of treatment and management programs conducted by others, including patients themselves.

REFERENCES

Agency for Health Care Policy and Research: Acute Low Back Problems in Adults: Clinical Practice Guidelines. Rockville, MD, U.S. Department of Health and Human Services, 1994, Public Health Service, Agency for Health Care Policy and Research (now the Agency for Health Care Research & Quality or AHRQ) Publication No. 95-0643.

American Physical Therapy Association: Workforce Study. Alexandria, VA, Prepared for the American Physical Therapy Association by Vector Research,1997.

Borenstein S: The human "instruction book" is opened. Philadelphia Inquirer, June 27, 2000, p A1.

Brown R, Clement DG, Hill JW et al: Do health maintenance organizations work for Medicare? Health Care Financ Rev 15(1):7-24, 1993.

Clifton DW: Setting sail on the U.S. chronic care. Rehabil Manage 12(5):20, 22-23, 1999.

DeJong G: Primary care for persons with disabilities: An overview of the problem. Am J Phys Med Rehabil 76(Suppl):S2–S3, 1997.

Fried L, Bandeen-Roche K, Kasper JD et al: Association of co-morbidity with disability in older women: The Women's Health and Aging Study. J Clin Epidemiol 52(1): 27-37, 1999.

Freudenheim E: University of California, San Francisco, Institute for Health and Aging, Chronic Care in America: A 21st Century Challenge. Princeton, NJ, The Robert Wood Johnson Foundation, 1996, www.rwjf.org, accessed August 19, 2004.

Gold M: Financial incentives in managed care: Current realities and challenges for physicians. J Gen Intern Med 14(Suppl 1):S6-S12, 1999.

Government Accounting Office: Tighter rules needed to curtail overcharges for therapy in nursing homes. Washington, DC, Office of Health, Education, and Human Services, 1995, Health, Education, and Human Services Pub. 95-23.

Grazier KL: The chronically ill and managed care. J Healthcare Manage 43(6):477-479, 1998.

Guralnick JM et al: Aging in the eighties: The prevalence of co-morbidity and its association with disability. Hyattsville, MD, National Center for Health Statistics, 1989.

Hoffman C, Rice DP: University of California, San Francisco, Institute for Health and Aging, Chronic Care in America: A 21st Century Challenge. Princeton, NJ, The Robert Wood Johnson Foundation, 1996, www.rwjf.org, accessed August 19, 2004.

Hoffman C, Rice D, Sung H: Persons with chronic conditions: Their prevalence and costs. JAMA 276(18):1473-1479, 1996.

Interstudy: The Interstudy Competitive Edge, Part II. HMO Industry Report 9.1. St. Paul, MN, Interstudy Publications, 1999.

Jeffrey NA: Doctors battle over who treats chronically ill. Wall Street Journal, December 11, 1996, B1, B8.

Jette AM, Smith K, Haley SM et al: Physical therapy episodes of care for patients with low back pain. Phys Ther 74:101-105, 1994.

Jones SB: Why not the best for the chronically ill? In Reno VP, Mashard J, Gradison W (eds): Disability Challenges for Social Insurance: Healthcare Financing and Labor Market Policy. Washington, DC, National Academy Press, 1997, pp 101-128.

LaPlante MP: Health Conditions and Impairments Causing Disability No.16. San Francisco, Disability Statistics Center, 1997.

Larkin J: Factors influencing one's ability to adapt to chronic illness. Nurs Clin North Am 22(3):535-543, 1987.

Larson P: Rehabilitation. In Lubkin IM (ed): Chronic Illness: Impact and Intervention, 3rd ed. Boston, MA, Jones and Bartlett, 1995, pp 524-539.

Lubkin IM: Chronic Illness: Impact and Interventions. Boston, Jones and Bartlett, 1986.

Mayer TG: Rehabilitation: What do we do with the chronic patient? Neurol Clin North Am 17(1):131-147, 1999.

Maxwell J, Briscoe F, Davidson S et al: Managed competition in practice: "Value purchasing" by fourteen employers. Health Affairs 17(3):216-226, 1998.

Millbank Memorial Fund: Patients as Effective Collaborators in Managing Chronic Conditions. New York, Center for the Advancement of Health, Millbank Memorial Fund, 1999.

Miller JF: Coping with Chronic Illness: Overcoming Powerlessness, 2nd ed. Philadelphia, FA Davis, 1992.

Moore N, Komras H: Patient-focused healing: Integrating caring and curing in health care. San Francisco, Jossey-Bass, 1993.

Morrison MH: Rehab for an aging population. Rehabil Manage 6(4): 36-38, 40, 1993.

Murrow EJ, Oglesby FM: Acute and chronic illness: Similarities, differences, and challenges. Orthop Nurse 15(5):47-51, 1996.

National Center for Health Statistics: Top 10 chronic conditions among older adults. Hyattsville, MD, 1998, http://www.cdc.gov/nchs/, accessed February 3, 2000.

Newby NM: Chronic illness and the family life cycle. J Adv Nurse 23(4):786-791, 1996.

Newhouse JP: Reimbursing health plans and health providers: Selection versus efficiency in production. J Econ Lit 34(3):1236-1263, 1996.

Pope AM, Tarlov AR: Disability in America: Toward a National Agenda for Prevention, Institute of Medicine (IOM). Washington, DC, National Academy Press, 1991, p 362.

Riley P: Managing care for persons with disabilities: The conflicts between Medicare and Medicaid. In Reno VP, Mashard J, Gradison W (eds): Disability Challenges for Social Insurance, Healthcare Financing and Labor Market Policy. Washington, DC, National Academy Press, 1997, pp 112-118.

Sandy LG, Gibson R: Managed care and chronic care: Challenges and opportunities. Managed Care Q 4(2):5-11, 1996.

Satinsky MA: The foundations of integrated care: Facing the challenges of change. Chicago, American Hospital Publishers, 1998.

Shaughnessy PW, Schlenker RE, Hittle DF: Home health care outcomes under capitated and fee-for service payment. Health Care Financ Rev 16(1):187-222, 1994.

Sutton JP, DeJong G: Managed care and people with disabilities: Framing the issues. Arch Phys Med Rehabil 70:1312-1316, 1998.

Trupin L, Rice DP: Health Status: Medical Care Use and Number of Disabling Conditions in the United States No. 9, Disability Statistics Abstract. San Francisco, Disability Statistics Center, 1997.

U.S. Bureau of Census: Statistical Abstract of the United States, 113th edition, (1980-1990), Washington, DC, U.S. Bureau of Census, 1993.

U.S. Bureau of Census: Historical Statistics of the United States, Colonial Times to 1970, Bicentennial edition, Part I, (1900-1970). Washington, DC, U.S. Bureau of Census, 1975.

Ware J, Bayless MS, Rogers WM et al: Differences in four-year health outcomes for elderly and poor, chronically ill patients treated in HMO and fee-for-service systems. JAMA 276:1039-1047, 1996.

Workers' Compensation Research Institute: Cost drivers in New Jersey. Workers' Compensation Res Brief 10:7, 1994.

SUGGESTED READINGS

Jans L, Stoddard S: Chartbook on Women and Disability in the United States, An Inhouse Report, Washington, DC, National Institute on Disability and Rehabilitation Research, 1999.

Kraus LE, Stoddard S, Gilmartin D: Chartbook on Disability in the United States, 1996, an Inhouse Report (1980-1990), Washington, DC, National Institute on Disability and Rehabilitation Research, 1996.

Lubin IM: Chronic Illness: Impact and interventions. Boston, Jones & Bartlett, 1995, pp 200-217.

Patients as Effective Collaborators in Managing Chronic Conditions. New York, Center for the Advancement of Health, Milbank Memorial Fund, 1999.

Stein REK, Bauman LJ, Westbrook LE: Framework for identifying children who have chronic conditions: the case for a new definition. J Pediatrics 122(3):342-347, 1993.

Stoddard S, Jans L, Ripple JM et al: Chartbook on Work and Disability in the United States, An Inhouse Report (1980-1990), National Institute on Disability and Rehabilitation Research, Washington, DC, H133D50017-96, 1998.

Straus A, Corbin J, Fagerhaugh S et al: Chronic Illness and the Quality of Life. St Louis, Mosby, 1984.

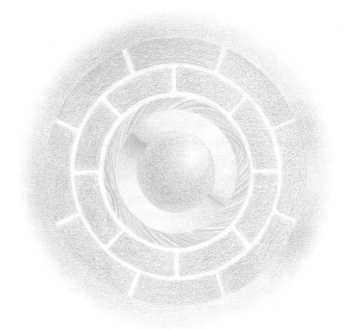

CHAPTER 23

Evolution of Managed Care

Michael R. Burcham, PT, MBA, DHA

The transition to managed care and the increased competition among organized systems of care can be viewed in two ways: (1) through the structure of the arrangements made by managed care plans with providers; and (2) through changes to the form of their practices that providers have made in order to accommodate the plans and to gain more leverage in negotiations with them.

- Gold, 1999

 KEY POINTS

- Today more than 90% of all health insurance sold is some form of managed care.
- Regardless of structure, managed care plans [e.g., health maintenance organizations (HMOs), preferred provider organizations (PPOs), and point-of service (POS) plans] have similar attributes, including arrangements with selected providers, standards of selection of providers, formal quality assurance and utilization management, and financial incentives for membership.
- In the future, rehabilitation services must include on-line medical management, comprehensive data collection, protocol-based treatment approaches, claims management and reporting expertise, and provider training in the fundamentals of managed care.

Operational Definitions

Point-of-Service (POS) Plan	A managed care model in which the individual is given the option of choosing an "in-network" or "out-of-network" provider, although the latter is a more expensive option with higher co-payments and/or deductibles.
Preferred Provider Organizations (PPOs)	An organization that contracts with health care providers who agree to accept discounts from their usual and customary fees.
Exclusive Provider Organizations (EPOs)	A traditional HMO model with a limited provider panel that receives additional patient volume.

FROM TRADITIONAL INSURANCE TO MANAGED CARE

Until the early 1980s, traditional health insurance was the dominant form of health care coverage. Under these plans, individuals had total freedom to choose their physicians, their hospitals, and even their therapists. Very little medical management existed; no one seemed concerned about the length of time an individual was in the hospital or how many visits were incurred during the course of outpatient treatment. Under these medical plans, the patient's liability was rarely more than 20% of the provider's charge.

As costs to employers of medical benefits began to soar, managed care firms formed to assist the employer in reducing health care costs. These firms included a variety of health plans, utilization review firms, and specialty managed care organizations. The basic benefit design began to change, and managed care options slowly replaced the traditional health insurance plan.

Today more than 90% of all health insurance sold is some form of managed care plan (Pretzer, 1994). For most employers, traditional health insurance is simply no longer affordable. These new health plans bring an entirely new set of rules for providers. The patient no longer has the unilateral freedom to choose his or her medical provider, and practitioners are experiencing the tremendous frustration of dealing with a health care system that is completely transformed.

If the truth were known, those who have been in the health care field for any period of time are well aware of the changes around them. Managed care has become the dominant force in the financing of health care, redefining the business, the competitor, and the customer. Managed care has also served as the catalyst for dramatic changes in employee benefits.

The most profound effect of managed care is that it alters the decision making of the practitioner by introducing a myriad of financial incentives and disincentives, policies and procedures, protocols, and processes that serve to quantify, qualify, evaluate, and profile even the most routine decisions. During the next several years, rehabilitation professionals and administrators will be increasingly challenged to validate protocols, measure outcomes, examine the appropriateness of services provided, and demonstrate value to third-party payers (Wolff & Schlesinger, 1998; Government Accounting Office, 1996).

HEALTH INSURANCE

To understand the managed care environment of today, it is helpful to know something of the history of health insurance in the United States.

In the early 20th century, most health care services were private transactions between the patient and the provider. For those who could not afford to pay, hospitals and clinics supported by religious organizations or private philanthropy provided charitable care and many cities and counties maintained hospitals for the care of the poor in their jurisdictions.

In the 1930s, various consumer, employee, and hospital groups created plans that paid their members' hospital expenses for specified services in return for a monthly premium. These plans eventually became Blue Cross plans. Spurred by the success of the hospital insurance plans, physician groups established prepaid plans specifically for physician services that became Blue Shield plans. Private insurance companies created insurance plans which differed from the Blue Cross and Blue Shield plans in that they reimbursed ("indemnified") the policy holder for covered services up to a specified dollar amount. These plans were called "indemnity" plans.

During World War II, health insurance became a popular employee benefit because wages were frozen and workers were in short supply. After the war, organized labor made health insurance a key item in the collective bargaining process. Health insurance coverage grew rapidly during the postwar years and throughout the prosperity of the 1950s. Eventually separate hospital and physician plans gave way to plans that offered coverage for an increasingly comprehensive range of services.

With the founding of Medicare in the 1960s, health care services expanded to cover all individuals. Companies found a reason to invest in medical technology as the customer base grew exponentially. By the early 1970s, for-profit medical providers emerged bringing capital resources to the health care industry. The result was an explosion of medical providers, specialty services, and insurance products. Health care services expanded beyond the city limits. The 1980s brought unprecedented growth with the birth of home health care funding and the migration of surgery from the hospital to the outpatient facility.

The "Old" Environment

For the first three quarters of this century, the central issue in health care policy debate was the expansion of insurance to cover more persons and more services. When the Medicare legislation extending coverage to the elderly and disabled was passed in 1965, national health expenditures accounted for a small percentage only of the U.S. gross national product. In 1970 health care was 7.4% of the gross national product (Bureau of Census, 1980). By 1980, this figure rose to 9.1% and broke double digits (12.2%) by 1990 (Levit et al, 1991).

With the implementation of the Medicare system, large numbers of individuals began to access the health system. This increase led to growing numbers of providers, expanding medical facilities, development of new services, and new technological innovations. During this same period, employers expanded their coverage of health care costs for employees. Health care providers were reimbursed for the majority of their charges, and their bills were rarely questioned.

Cost Emerges as the Dominant Health Care Issue

As health care costs continue to rise, greater portions of state budgets are consumed by Medicaid, and Medicare erodes large portions of the Federal budget. Everyone seems to agree that something must be done to retard the growth in health care costs, but no one seems able to agree on exactly what to do.

Before the economic downturn of the early 1980s, employers had paid relatively little attention to the costs of health benefits. Health benefit costs were not as high as they are today and, because health benefits were not subject to income tax, both employers and employees viewed them as a preferred method of employee compensation. With the recession, some major industrial companies discovered that their employee health benefit costs were greater than their profits. Struggling auto companies learned their foreign competitors had as much as a 5% cost advantage per car solely because of U.S. companies' higher health benefit costs.

Employers analyzed their health costs and found many disturbing facts (Kuttner, 1999). Insurers had no effective mechanisms for restraining increases in providers' fees or in the amount and intensity of services provided to patients. Insurers typically paid according to a "usual, customary, and reasonable" schedule based on analysis of claims from all providers. Providers figured out, however, that by increasing their fees each year they would in time increase the fee limits (called fee "screens"). This system was one of the reasons inflation in medical costs consistently surpassed that of other goods and services.

Numerous seminal studies of health care utilization showed variations ranging from differences in practice style, which could not be explained by differences in medical need, to outright fraud (Chassin et al, 1987, Lewis, 1969;

Wennberg, 1985, 1987, 1991). This was not surprising because most insurers' utilization review efforts were minimal or non-existent.

Some experts contend that 70% to 80% of all medical services meet the criteria for medically necessary and reasonable care (Bluestein & Marmer, 1992). The remaining 20% to 30% of all services may be unnecessary, ineffective, inappropriate, unethical and/or harmful. Debate exists concerning whether or not health care cost containment, medical management, and utilization reviews produce real or imagined savings.

Blustein and Marmer (1992) eloquently summarize the centerpiece of cost containment. "Galvanized by the realization that much medical care is of uncertain value, and bolstered by findings that show significant variation in medical practice patterns, a coalition of policymakers, politicians, and researchers is now actively engaged in seeking to contain costs by eliminating wasteful care."

These authors are quick to note that waste cutting is not synonymous with rationing, which can lead to the denial of necessary services. How to cut wasteful spending remains a controversial issue. A plethora of medical management strategies are used under managed care: clinical guidelines, standards of care, practice parameters, utilization review, provider profiling, and facility benchmarking.

By the mid 1980s, cost emerged as the dominant health care issue. Although before this time few employers had any interest in managed care, employers now took the lead in pushing for more aggressive methods of managing health care costs and encouraging enrollment in various forms of managed care plans. For many small employers, health insurance has become a luxury that the company can no longer afford (Gabel et al, 1997). The result is a growing number of working individuals with no form of health insurance.

Figure 23–1 illustrates the trade-off between cost containment and choice of provider across a diverse health plan spectrum. Cost control is given a higher priority under a group or staff model HMO and given little emphasis under traditional indemnity plans. The consumer's choice of provider is enhanced, however, under a traditional indemnity model when contrasted with a staff model HMO.

Faced with staggering health care costs, employers seem to have little choice but to reexamine their health insurance options. Throughout the private sector, purchasers and consumers are behind the changes in health care delivery and funding (Ladenheim et al, 1994; Marley, 1994; Anonymous, 1994). Rising health care costs, soaring workers' compensation claims, and increased expenditures for retirees have prompted employers to shift from passive purchasers to active consumers.

THE DEFINING FEATURES OF MANAGED CARE

Managed care is defined as systems that integrate the financing and delivery of health care services by means of the following basic elements (Ferrari & Grimes, 1995):

- Arrangements with selected providers
- Standards of selection of providers
- Formal quality assurance and utilization management
- Financial incentives for the membership

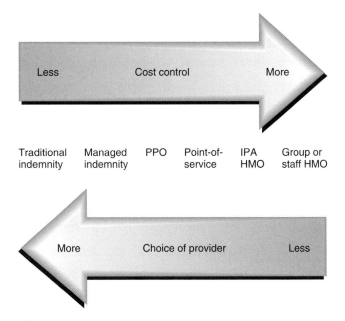

Figure 23–1. Health care plan spectrum. (Data from US General Accounting Office: Managed health care: Effects on employment costs difficult to measure. Washington, DC, GAO/HRD 94-3, 1993.)

Arrangements with Selected Providers

Provider contracting is the most powerful method that MCOs have for controlling cost. Under conventional insurance, no contract exists between provider and insurer. Thus providers are free to set their fees, and insurers have limited leverage in their dealings with providers. By definition, MCOs have contracts with providers (including physical medicine and rehabilitation providers).

Through contracts, MCOs control their costs by having providers agree to accept fees specified by the contract and cooperate with various utilization management features.

In contracting with MCOs, providers agree to accept fees that are almost always lower than their usual fees in return for the flow of patients that they expect to receive from the managed care plan. These MCOs are able to deliver patients to their contracted providers because they contract with a limited number of providers, patients are given financial incentives to only use the contracted providers, and because most plans usually grow their enrollment over time.

Besides discounted fees, provider contracts allow MCOs to control costs by having providers agree to cooperate with medical management, refer to other contracted providers, and adhere to practice guidelines.

When first established, managed care plans usually begin their contracting with hospitals and physicians. In time these plans extend their contracting to encompass other providers such as rehabilitation and other "ancillary services." Sometimes MCOs offer contracts to any provider willing to agree to their contract provisions. Most such plans eventually move to a more selective approach, eliminating providers through fee reductions or more stringent selection criteria.

Standards of Participation for Providers

The methods used to select participating providers are emerging as an area of greater liability risk for MCOs. Traditional insurance plans do not contract with providers and thus make no representations to a practitioner's skill. Managed care organizations not only give enrollees financial incentives to use preferred providers, they often levy financial penalties when members use the physician of their choice rather than the contracted practitioner. These organizations may therefore be said to have a duty to their members to exercise reasonable care in selecting and retaining medical practitioners. Diligent investigation of the provider's licensure and standing, insurance coverage, verification of education, validation of specialty training, and a review of malpractice history have become routine credentialing criteria for MCOs (Carroll, 1997).

Quality Management

As purchasers of health care services seek to control costs through health plans that use cost-containment incentives, concern is growing that the incentives used to influence providers will negatively affect quality of care and access to services (Kahn et al, 1990; Friedman, 1997; Miller & Luft, 1997). As the market evolves and competition among health plans increases, the ability to monitor and assess health plan performance will become an important indicator and measurement of quality in the delivery system.

A quality management plan serves an important purpose in demonstrating the processes that measure treatment results and assure the continuous quality improvement mandated by payers, regulatory agencies, and employer groups. These key customer groups look for documented assurances of quality as well as cost effectiveness. Blustein and Marmer (1992) provide an insightful perspective concerning wasteful spending, appropriate care, and the evolution of interventions designed to control costs. They state that competition, managed care, and prospective payment have not fulfilled their promise, nor have any other panaceas. Paul Ellwood, considered by many to be the grandfather of managed care and the outcomes management approach, asserts, "half of what the medical profession does is of unverified effectiveness" (Ellwood, 1988; Faltermeyer, 1988).

Medical Management

Medical management is the process of evaluating the medical necessity and appropriateness of health care services, frequently by the application of review criteria. Before one can proceed with a discussion of these issues, a proper definition of the terms "medically necessary" and "appropriate care" must be considered. Both of these terms lack universal meanings among various health care stakeholders (Gold, 1999; Clifton, 1995; Charles et al, 1997; Jacobson et al, 1997), yet these concepts remain the centerpiece for reimbursement decision, policy debates and rulemaking initiatives. Wasteful spending, the antithesis of medically necessary and appropriate care, can be segregated into the following four categories (Blustein & Marmer, 1992):

- Ineffective or harmful interventions
- Interventions of uncertain effectiveness
- Ethically troubling practices
- Inefficient allocation of resources

Financial Incentives for Plan Members

During the past several years, the weaving of financial incentives within the patient's benefit plan has become a true art. As a result of the variable co-insurances, co-payments, sliding out-of-pocket limits, and expanded deductibles, very few patients today will knowingly seek care from an out-of-network provider because of the enormous financial cost of such choices. These financial incentive structures have allowed health plans to continue to market their products as "freedom of choice" to consumers, when in reality very few consumers can afford the right to choose (Gawande et al, 1998).

Medical Management: The Centerpiece of Cost Containment

Medical management is often called "the polite art of interference" (Rizzo, 1993). This interference is often the least understood and most frustrating aspect of managed care, yet it provides a framework for therapy organizations to prepare for the coming changes. More than 90% of health insurance plans use utilization or medical management to control costs (Rosenberg et al, 1995). As therapists become more involved in the writing of precise treatment protocols and clinical pathways of care, utilization management will move from an outside influence to an internally driven process. Rehabilitation organizations desiring to survive the changes from fee-for-service to pre-paid, capitated payment systems must develop a thorough understanding of the basic elements of medical management: medical necessity, appropriate setting for services, utilization frequency, and resource management. Once capitated, rehabilitation organizations must operationalize and direct their own medical review programs to successfully manage the patient population.

For all practical purposes, medical management (utilization review) did not exist before 1984. Since that time it has grown into an industry of massive proportions (Government Accounting Office, 1992a). Review firms may work for employers or have contracts with insurers, HMOs, PPOs, and third-party administrators. Insurers and MCOs usually all offer medical review services.

Medical management firms took their cues from Medicare and its professional review organizations (PROs). When Medicare sought to curtail abuse of its system, it developed the PROs (formerly PSROs) as watchdogs for hospitalized Medicare patients (Congressional Budget Office, 1979). The PROs set standards for treating illnesses and began to deny payment for extra treatment that could not be proved to be medically necessary. The practitioner and not Medicare or the PRO, however, remained legally liable for the treatment of the patient. The evolution of utilization review was enhanced as MCOs realized that similar practices would assist them in cost containment.

The result has been phenomenal growth of medical review services. Today it is virtually unheard of for a health plan to not have medical management (utilization review) as a major component of its cost containment strategies.

Review firms initially focused their energies on hospitals (Siu et al, 1984; Payne, 1987). The result has been a dramatic reduction in hospital lengths of stay and admission rates. In the past, preoperative days, when patients were admitted to the hospital the day before surgery, were common; now these are allowed only on rare occasions. Although most inpatient therapy departments were not directly involved in these decisions, they are directly affected by these new policies. The result has been a reduction in the number of therapy professionals needed within the inpatient setting, a redefinition of rehabilitation goals (now "stabilization" replaces "optimum recovery" for most inpatient settings), and the transformation of inpatient rehabilitation from a revenue center to an expense center.

In its brief existence, medical management has gained the enmity of most providers of therapy services. The very idea that some outside individual would have the power to determine whether another therapy visit is necessary or not is abhorrent (Beckley, 1997). Its supporters say, however, that the practice has saved millions for MCOs and employers and helped slow the rising costs of health care for companies of all sizes. An inverse relationship exists between cost control and choice of provider. Greater cost controls tend to lead to less choice of provider, and less rigid health plans foster greater choice of provider.

Medical management can be broken down into five general areas: preauthorization, continued care review, second opinion programs, retrospective review, and case management (Figure 23–2). Managed care programs that remain in Stage I principally focus on securing fee discounts from providers. Savings are then passed on to the payer (at least hypothetically). Other hallmarks of Stage I strategies include shifting care to ambulatory settings (versus inpatient hospitalization) along with strict access controls directed at plan beneficiaries.

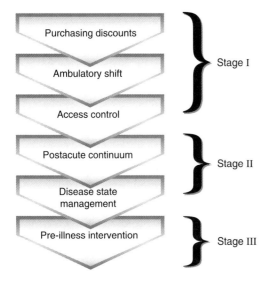

Figure 23–2. Stages of managed care cost strategies. (Data from Fowler: Pricing and managed care. Rehabil Econ/Rehabil Manage 5[1]:88, 1997.)

Stage II MCOs offer services during the postacute phase of the disability continuum compared with hospital-dominated inpatient lengths of stay.

Disease state management (DSM) is a common approach to managing chronic conditions such as asthma, AIDS, cancer, diabetes and heart disease. DSM uses a diversity of services that transcend treatment per se, especially secondary prevention. Unlike the episodic single-service care associated with indemnity plans, DSM uses a systematic team-based approach. DSM includes risk assessment, environmental assessment, field case management, clinical algorithms, and a great deal of patient education.

Stage III MCOs substantially invest in primary prevention services and deemphasize treatment. These organizations provide extensive beneficiary health screenings, lifestyle assistance programs, and heavily empower their insureds to make the right decisions about health care. Prevention of costly health conditions is the credo of third-stage MCOs.

INSURANCE COMPANIES

An insurance company is a corporation licensed under state insurance laws that collects premiums in return for assuming the financial risk for the benefits specified under the insurance policies it issues.

In any health insurance, the following functions may exist:

- Assumption of financial risk for the cost of services used by enrollees.
- Benefit administration such as claims payment and maintenance of eligibility records.
- Marketing the plan to employers and/or individuals.
- Contracting with health care providers.
- Utilization review/case management.

Insurance companies may perform any combination of these functions. Insurance companies and HMOs are the only MCOs licensed under law to collect premiums for employers or individuals in return for the assumption of financial risk for the health care services provider. A significant proportion of insurers' business today, however, consists of administrative services only, in which the risk is retained by the employer (through self-insured plans), and the insurer's role is to administer the claims and/or the cost containment features of the plan.

Not all insurance companies are true MCOs. Although larger insurance companies have developed their own managed care products (HMOs, PPOs, and case management firms), many smaller and medium-sized insurers have not. These other insurers typically enter into arrangements whereby they market products (PPOs and utilization review services) that are actually owned and operated by another organization.

In assessing managed care markets, the rehabilitation marketer should understand that only through the provider contracting function and through case management can a managed care organization deliver business to a rehabilitation company. Consequently, the rehabilitation marketer should focus on insurers' HMO, POS, PPO, and case management units as their relevant target prospects.

Health Maintenance Organizations

HMOs are corporations licensed under the insurance laws of the state in which they operate and which assume financial responsibility for providing a defined set of medical services to their enrollees in return for a fixed premium.

HMOs had their beginnings in the 1930s when several different employers and employee associations contracted with medical groups and hospitals to provide certain services in return for a fixed monthly fee. During the next 30 years, these "prepaid group practices" (as they were called) experienced steady growth in several markets around the country. In the late 1960s, interest in the prepaid model increased because of its potential for controlling cost and for delivering preventive services.

Responding to buyer demands for comprehensive health care covering broader geographical areas, HMOs have been merging, affiliating, and forming joint ventures in record numbers. New corporate combinations have been formed as HMOs enter into alliances with hospitals and other provider organizations. Although the HMO industry is in a state of flux, it appears to be in good financial health with growing enrollment, margins, and cash reserves.

Point-of-Service Structure

In the POS model, the individual is given the option to choose an in-network or out-of-network provider each time the individual seeks medical care. The additional financial costs to the individual who does not seek medical care from the participating primary care physician are significant, however. These additional costs are found in the form of enhanced deductibles, increased coinsurances, and larger co-payments. In addition, the individual's maximum out-of-pocket expenditures for out-of-network providers are twice that for in-network providers.

Origin of the Point-of-Service Plan

Historically, HMO enrollees have had to receive their care from providers under contract to their HMO or their care would not be reimbursed, except for out-of-area emergencies and some other limited exceptions.

To increase their appeal to prospective enrollees and to compete with PPOs, many HMOs have recently implemented new plans called almost interchangeably POS, "open-ended" or "hybrid" plans. In these plans, enrollees can receive maximum benefits (e.g., 100% coverage after any co-pay) by using a plan provider. The enrollee also has the option of going outside the provider panel, however, and still receiving substantial reimbursement (typically in the 50% to 60% range).

Premiums for POS plans are usually higher than those for similar plans without this feature. In some states, POS plans are not licensed as HMOs and are thus regulated under state insurance laws similar to a PPO rather than an HMO.

From a provider's standpoint, a contract with a POS plan will probably translate into less actual volume when compared with a traditional HMO of the same size, because enrollees have the option of using non-plan providers.

For the rehabilitation provider, managed care presents a significant change in referral pattern. In these managed care plans, the primary care physician is now making the decision of whether or not to refer the patient for rehabilitation. The specialists who have long generated the bulk of therapy referrals (orthopedists and neurosurgeons) now find themselves looking to the primary care physician for the approval to treat.

When one considers that these primary care physicians are often given financial incentives to conserve resources and reduce referrals, the potential effect of these changes on the rehabilitation provider becomes clear.

Most health plans that offer an HMO are also moving to offer a POS plan. The POS plan often serves as an opportunity for employers to give employees an incentive (inducement) to try certain attributes of the HMO. It has been shown that individuals who try POS plans will often migrate to the HMO more readily than individuals whose primary managed care network experience is with a PPO.

Preferred Provider Organizations

A PPO is an organization that contracts with health care providers who agree to accept discounts from their usual and customary fees and comply with utilization review policies in return for the patient flow they expect from the PPO. PPOs came into existence because the oversupply of hospital beds and physicians in many areas of the country allowed payers to negotiate discounts with these providers. Essentially, a surplus of providers equates to a buyer's market.

Notice in the above definition that a PPO is an organization that contracts with providers. Although all PPOs contract with providers, PPOs vary considerably as to whether the PPO or another entity processes claims, assumes financial risk, markets to employers, and performs utilization review. Large insurance companies that own PPOs perform all of these functions themselves (e.g., Aetna, Prudential, and Travelers). Many smaller PPO companies, however, mainly develop and maintain provider contracts, and are compensated through "access fees" which they charge insurers and third-party administrators (TPAs) for use of their network in benefit plans marketed by the TPAs and insurers. This arrangement is often referred to as "renting" a network. TPAs are entities that perform insurance functions (e.g., claims administration on behalf of self-insured or self-funded employers). Self-insured employers do not pay insurance premiums to a traditional insurer. Instead, they assume risk and pay on a claim-by-claim basis. They are required to set aside monies into escrow accounts known as "company reserves." Company reserves are calculated as the amount necessary to cover all medical expenses related to a given claim.

Although almost all PPO-based benefit plans include utilization review, not all PPOs perform their own utilization review. These functions may be handled by the PPO, by the insurer or TPA, or by an independent utilization review firm.

Exclusive Provider Organizations

To better compete with HMOs, a number of insurers and other PPO-owning entities have introduced EPOs.

EPOs seek to generate better cost savings than PPOs by eliminating reimbursement for use of non-plan providers. An EPO's benefit design thus resembles that of a traditional HMO. EPOs typically have a more limited provider panel than PPOs, but these providers see more volume for a given number of enrollees as compared with a PPO plan. Forty-four percent of PPOs now offer EPOs, and EPO enrollment is estimated at 8 million employees (not counting dependents).

The Employer's Perspective

Some points should be made about employers. They clearly desire the opportunity to contract directly with health care providers (Clifton, 1996). They are tired of the black box in the middle—employers want to know how the health care system works. They want to know what happens to their health care dollars (e.g., how much of their money goes to somebody's profit margin, and how much goes into operations). Employers strongly desire direct relationships and single source accountability for outcome and service.

The employer is often represented by a consultant organization that the provider never sees. Consultants are used to research the background of various health care entities and to assist the company in its health care purchasing decisions. At the time a health care professional calls on the employer, the health care provider's informational packet ends up on the consultant's desk for consideration. So it should be understood that most employers, savvy employers at least, are going to have a consultant behind the scenes who will recommend a provider or not. An organization is much more likely to succeed if the consultants in the provider's market are known.

Companies are becoming more nationally oriented, and they want options in multiple locations. In addition, the payer is looking for a single source for local contracting. These desires are not opposites but rather points along a continuum. The health care provider should first give the payer local market density and a single point of service. Next the provider should give that same level of local density across multiple geographic locations.

CHARTING A COURSE FOR MANAGED CARE

Employers have set the managed care playing field in motion. By allowing their employees to choose among competing health plans, companies are keeping the pressure on health plans to lower costs and improve services (Daniels & Sabin, 1998; Gossfield, 1998). When a plan becomes too expensive, employees avoid it and eventually it is dropped. For vendors to keep enrollees, they must stay competitive. Most employers feel that they do not have more money to give to the health system.

Recognizing the considerable strength in numbers, businesses continue to join together to form purchasing cooperatives. Coalitions of large and small employers that negotiate fees directly with HMOs, hospitals, and physicians are finding they can leverage volume discounts on their health care, educate and empower their workers, and hold health care providers accountable for procedures

and practices. The result: local group purchasing is changing the market and setting a course for managed care.

Marketing to Managed Care Organizations

Compared with traditional therapy referrers, marketing, promoting, and selling rehabilitation services to managed care is a much more complicated process for reasons that include the following:

- Identifying and qualifying prospects requires understanding managed care.
- Decision-makers can be difficult to identify and access.
- Multiple decision-makers often exist.
- Information demands by prospects can be challenging.
- Criteria used by prospects can be unclear or complex.
- Sales cycles are typically long.

Three basic steps can assist the administrator of therapy services to position his or her organization for the managed care environment.

Step I: A thorough assessment of the current market.
Step II: Design and development of a managed care strategy.
Step III: Evaluation of strategic partnerships.

Step I: Assessing the Market

In developing a specific managed care strategy for rehabilitation services, one must begin by conducting a market assessment. This process includes a strategic analysis of therapy costs, normative outpatient visits per case, the referral patterns of local health plans, and one's own position within the market. Information gained from the market assessment is used to customize the network to meet the contracting objectives of area payers.

A market assessment forms the basis of strategic decision-making whether one is trying to develop a strategic plan for a major hospital or trying to determine the business opportunity for private practice therapy.

Relevant data should be collected and analyzed according to the following guidelines. The results of this analysis will be used to determine the nature and scope of the strategic plan. The analysis should accomplish the following goals

- Determine the location, affiliation, and scope of existing providers.
- Identify market locations with limited access to rehabilitation.
- Delineate the current basis of reimbursement in the market.
- Project emerging rehabilitation pricing and reimbursement trends.
- Determine the level of physician involvement in rehabilitation ownership.
- Quantify the degree of integration of physical medicine and rehabilitation services within the local market.
- Assess the potential for affiliations and strategic partnerships.
- Identify existing payers and their product types.
- Quantify the payers' scope of rehabilitation benefits and benefit limitations.

- Determine the payers' current level of medical management expertise in rehabilitation and the types of medical reviews being conducted.
- Construct profiles of health plan business cycles and market position.
- Identify those health plans that form managed Medicare and Medicaid products.
- Identify firms that are forming workers' compensation networks in the market.
- Assess the historical charge patterns of one's own facility.
- Determine the size of the therapy market and ownership of market share.

Variables such as area employer presence, market cost comparisons, managed care competition, the rehabilitation market size, market opportunity and one's own historical cost experience will provide important information to the development of the strategic plan.

Before a strategic plan is formulated, a review should be done of the business objectives of the organization and proper parameters set to ensure that the managed care strategic plan fits within the overall strategy of the organization and is consistent with the mission and desired direction of its rehabilitation services.

Step II: Designing the Plan

A strategic plan creates the structural basis of organizational direction and growth. The strategic plan design should accomplish the following goals:

- Define the roles of all parties (e.g., manager, staff, development department).
- Delineate communication lines and processes.
- Delineate organizational issues.
- Determine the type of legal considerations as one determines the specific strategies/network (e.g., independent practitioner or provider network [IPA], MSO, PPO).
- Quantitate contracting risks and capitation strategies.
- Define the organization's product(s).
- Delineate the rehabilitation services needed to complement one's facility.
- Establish the quantity of sites for inpatient, subacute, and outpatient services to entirely serve the market.
- Craft competitive pricing strategies including financial impact of pricing.
- Determine a managed care marketing strategy.
- Define a structured bidding process for health plans.
- Determine the physicians who will be impacted by the plan.
- Establish the communication process with medical staff.
- Construct a timeline for completing the tasks identified within the plan.

Step III: Exploring Strategic Partnerships

Therapy managers should carefully evaluate the potential of developing strategic partnerships with other complimentary organizations. A single therapy organization will rarely be positioned well on all points of the rehabilitation continuum. Strategic partnerships enable the organization to secure providers throughout the full scope of rehabilitation services.

In choosing to create strategic partnerships, providers should complete the following steps:

- Analyze existing operations to evaluate managed care readiness.
- Determine the types of systems needed for data collection and information management.
- Determine the number of provider sites needed for inpatient and outpatient care.
- Identify gaps in network services and locations.
- Develop policies and procedures for delivery system providers.
- Craft medical management policies, procedures, and services.
- Establish a professional advisory board.
- Determine quality, utilization, and cost controls and measures.
- Develop incentive mechanisms.
- Build outcomes tracking and reporting systems.
- Construct provider and payer profiling reports.
- Develop payer contracting components.
- Determine claims flow and payment flow.
- Develop contractual instruments.
- Complete provider contracting and strategic partnering throughout inpatient rehabilitation, subacute and/or skilled nursing facility (SNF), home health, and outpatient settings.
- Develop delivery system provider orientation and education plan.

It should be remembered that every health care market is different and involves a dynamic process. Providers who merely imitate a process or strategy from another market have little chance for success. For instance, workers' compensation represents a patchwork quilt of 50 statutes. What is permissible or acceptable in one workers' compensation market may not be acceptable in another. What is acceptable in workers' compensation may or may not be acceptable in a group health environment. It is incumbent on rehabilitation providers to fully understand the insurance rules, regulations, policies and procedures, process, and structural elements of each insurance system with which they interface.

For many therapy providers, the formation of strategic alliances will be centrally linked to the organization's managed care strategy, delivering any facet of rehabilitation care necessary, promoting the proper utilization of health care resources, and providing information to all providers for the purposes of self-analysis and solution development.

SUMMARY

In the future, the administrative infrastructure of therapy services must include on-line medical management, comprehensive data collection, protocol-based treatment approaches, claims management and reporting expertise, and provider training in the fundamentals of managed care.

Intensive managed care programs may carve out costly services including physical rehabilitation. Figure 23–3 depicts a managed care continuum that encompasses a variety of cost-containment strategies.

Administrators of therapy departments clearly hold in their hands the opportunity of a lifetime. Therapist managers

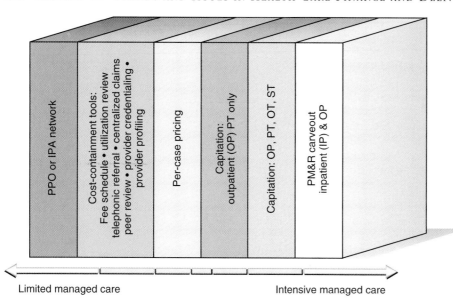

Figure 23–3. The managed care continuum. (Redrawn with permission from Burcham MP: Managed care: Surviving utilization review. Rehabil Manage 7[5]:102-103,125, 1995.)

Limited managed care

Intensive managed care

who choose to pursue this managed care strategy of market integration and continuum management may find themselves influencing and directing therapy activity for their entire communities.

REFERENCES

Anonymous: An overview of the predominant health care reform. Medical Interface 7(8):113, 116-117, 1994.

Beckley NJ: Rehab under managed care: The influence of managed care on rehab providers and programs. Rehab Manage 10(1):105, 116, 1997.

Blustein J, Marmer TR: Cutting waste by making rules: Promises, pitfalls and realistic prospectives. Univ Pennsylvania Law Rev 148(5): 1571-1572, 1992.

Bureau of Census, U.S. Department of Commerce: Statistical abstract of the United States 1990, 110th ed. Washington, DC, Government Printing Office, 1990.

Carroll R: Risk Management Handbook for Health Care Organizations, 2nd ed. Chicago, American Hospital Publications, 1997.

Charles C, Lomas J, Giacomini M et al: Medical necessity in Canadian health policy: Four meanings and ... a funeral? Millbank Q 75(3): 365-394, 1997.

Chassin M, Kosecoff J, Park R, et al: Does inappropriate use explain geographic variations in the use of health care services? A study of three procedures. JAMA 258:2533-2569, 1987.

Clifton DW: Payor-provider alliances. Rehabil Manage 9(5):100-102, 1996.

Clifton DW: Legal issues in peer review and utilization: Part I. PT Magazine 3(12):77-79, 1999.

Congressional Budget Office: The effects of PSROS on healthcare costs: Current findings and future evaluations. Washington, DC, Government Printing Office, 1979.

Daniels N, Sabin J: The ethics of accountability in managed care reform. Health Affairs 17(5):50-64, 1998.

Ellwood PM: Shattuck lecture–Outcomes management: A technology of patient experience. New Engl J Med 318:1549-1551, 1988.

Faltermeyer E: Medical care's next revolution. Fortune Oct. 10, p 126, 1988.

Ferrari BT, Grimes S: Will HMOs pass their physical? McKinsey Q (3):79-89, 1995.

Freidman E: Managed care, rationing and quality: A tangled relationship. Health Affairs 16(3):174-182, 1997.

Gabel JR, Ginsburg PB, Hunt KA: Smaller employers and their health benefits, 1988-1996: An awkward adolescence. Health Affairs 16(5): 10-110, 1997.

Gawande AA, Blendon RJ, Brodie M et al: Does dissatisfaction with health plans stem from having no choices? Health Affairs 17(5): 184-194, 1998.

General Accounting Office Medicare Part B, inconsistent denial rates for medical necessity across six carriers. Washington, DC, General Accounting Office, 1992, GAO/T-PEMD-94-17.

General Accounting Office: Utilization review: Information on external review organizations. Washington, DC, General Accounting Office, 1992a, GAO/HRD-93-22FS.

General Accounting Office: Practice guidelines: Managed care plans customized guidelines to meet local interests. Washington, DC, General Accounting Office, 1996, GAO/HEHS-96-95,

Gold M: The changing U.S. healthcare system. Millbank Q 77(1):3-37, 1999.

Gosfield AG: Who is holding whom accountable for quality? Health Affairs 16(3):26-40, 1997.

Grogan C, Feldman R, Nyman J et al: How will we use clinical guidelines? The experience of medical carriers. J Health Polit Policy Law 19:7-26, 1994.

Jacobsen PD, Asch S, Glassman PA et al: Defining and implementing medical necessity in Washington State and Oregon. Inquiry: The Journal of Health Care Organization Provision and Financing 34: 143-154, 1997.

Kahn K, Rogers W, Rubestein L et al: Measuring quality of care with explicit process criteria before and after implementation of the DRG-based prospective payment system. JAMA 264:1969-1973, 1990.

Kuttner R: The American health care system: Employer-sponsored health coverage. New Engl J Med 340(3):248-252, 1999.

Ladenheim K, Lipson L, Markus A, et al: Health Care Reform: 50 State Profiles, 3rd ed. Washington, DC, Intergovernmental Health Policy Project at the George Washington University, July 1994.

Levit KR et al: National health expenditures 1990. Health Care Financ Rev 13(1):29-54, 1991.

Lewis CE: Variations in the incidence of surgery. New Engl J Med 281: 880-884, 1969.

Marley S: Healthcare reform coup. Bus Insur 28(33):9, 1994.

Miller RH, Luft HS: Does managed care lead to better or worse quality of care? Health Affairs 16(5):7-25, 1997.

Moorehead JF, Clifford J: Determining medical necessity of outpatient physical therapy services. Am J Med Qual 7(3):81-84, 1992.

Payne SMC: Identifying and managing inappropriate hospital utilization: A policy synthesis. Health Serv Res 22:709-769, 1987.

Pretzer M: Will fee-for-service go the way of Marcus Welby? Med Econ 71(4):144-148, 150-152, 1994.

Rizzo J: Physician uncertainty and the art of persuasion. Soc Sci Med 37:1451-1459, 1993

Rosenberg SN, Allen DR, Handte JS et al: Effect of utilization review in a fee-for-service health insurance plan. New Engl J Med 333: 1326-1330, 1995.

Siu AL, Sonnenberg FA, Manning WG et al: Inappropriate use of hospitals in a randomized trial of health insurance plans. New Engl J Med 315:1259-1266, 1984.

Wennberg J: Variations in medical practice and hospital costs. Conn Med 49(7):444-453, 1985.Wennberg JE: The paradox of appropriate care. New Engl J Med 258:2568-2569, 1987.

Wennberg JE: Unwanted variations in the rules of practice. JAMA 265(10):1265-1270, 1991.

Wolff N, Schlesinger M: Risk, motives and styles of utilization review: A cross-condition comparison. Soc Sci Med 47(7):911-926, 1998.

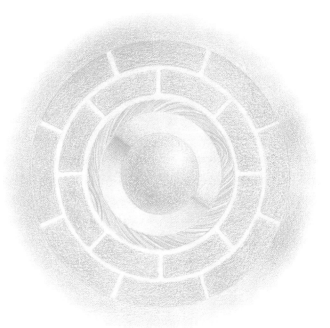

CHAPTER 24

Complementary and Alternative Health

David W. Clifton, Jr., PT

Complementary and alternative medicine [health] comprises those practices used for the prevention and treatment that are not widely taught in medical schools, nor generally available in hospitals.

- Jonas & Jacobs, 1996

KEY POINTS

- Consumer use of complementary and alternative health (CAH) interventions is growing faster than conventional interventions despite the fact that most are not covered by insurance.
- A comprehensive disability management program may be incomplete without selected CAH interventions.
- There is potential for collaboration between rehabilitation providers and CAH proponents because many patients use both. CAH and physical rehabilitation share a number of attributes.
- Successful integration of conventional and unconventional therapies will depend on how CAH practitioners address a host of issues across a number of spheres: ethical, legal, clinical outcome measures, regulatory, risk management, and reimbursement.

 Operational Definitions

Complementary and Alternative Health (CAH)	Any intervention not embedded in the biomedical model or promoted by medical association. Also known as unconventional therapies.

WHY CONSIDER COMPLEMENTARY AND ALTERNATIVE HEALTH?

Any discussion of disability management would be incomplete without addressing CAH. For the purpose of this chapter, CAH, or complementary and alternative health,

has displaced the term CAM, or complementary and alternative medicine, a term that permeates the clinical literature. CAH embraces many preventive strategies that are wellness-based, whereas the term "medicine" implies treatment after injury or disease.

There is No Alternative Medicine

Fontanarosa and Lundberg (1998) contend that there is no alternative medicine, but only scientifically proven, evidence-based medicine that is supported by sound data and unproven medicine, for which scientific evidence is lacking. These authors consider it irrelevant to make a distinction based on "Eastern" versus "Western," unconventional versus mainstream, or mind-body versus molecular genetics.

All medicine should subscribe to the same levels of evidence that a given intervention targets a specific disease or condition both safely and efficaciously. Angell and Kassirer (1998) also assert that there cannot be two forms of medicine—conventional and alternative. They contend that interventions are adequately tested or not and they either work or do not work. Once a treatment regimen has been rigorously tested, it becomes a moot point whether it is labeled conventional or alternative. These distinctions may only be important from an historical or cultural perspective.

Effective disability management demands a variety of interventions and a diversity of providers. Some of these interventions fall within mainstream health care, and others do not. CAH represents those unconventional therapies not universally embraced by the medical establishment. Some CAH therapies, however, have gained increasing acceptance.

For instance, both chiropractic and acupuncture straddle conventional and unconventional therapies (Meeker, 2002; Smith et al, 2002).

The purpose of this chapter is to introduce a general overview of CAH and to pose the question, *Are certain CAH therapies complementary to or an alternative to physical rehabilitation?* It is incumbent on rehabilitation professionals to enhance their understanding of CAH, especially those techniques that have been validated. To blatantly reject what CAH selectively offers could be a dereliction of one's professional duty. A number of conventional practitioners have attempted to learn more about CAH and to apply this knowledge in their practices (Gellman & Kennedy, 2002; Berman et al, 2002; Bottomley, 2000, Dalen, 1998; Kronenberg et al, 1994).

Integration of conventional and unconventional interventions is a hotly debated issue (Dalen, 1998; Eisenberg, 1997; Hastings Report, 2000; Kronenberg et al, 1994).

Interestingly, users of CAH and physical rehabilitation share several characteristics. These persons often suffer from conditions that are poorly managed within the traditional biomedical system partly because of the system's emphasis on acute care. Second, many of these conditions are deemed incurable through surgery, medication, or other means. CAH and rehabilitation patients are often dissatisfied with conventional medicine and its organ-based paradigm. (Gevitz, 1988; Paramore, 1997; Weil, 1995) These persons often seek a holistic approach to their problems. CAH practitioners understand a basic philosophy of health care espoused by Hippocrates, "*It is more important to know what sort of person has a disease than to know what sort of disease a person has.*"

Patient dissatisfaction with conventional medicine is not the only reason why CAH is sought (Swartzman et al, 2002). At least one study has failed to demonstrate a correlation between patient dissatisfaction with conventional treatment and increased use of unconventional therapies (Astin, 1998).

WHAT IS COMPLEMENTARY AND ALTERNATIVE HEALTH?

A cacophony of terms is used to describe those interventions that do not fall within the biomedical model of medicine (Silenzio, 2002). A sampling of these is found in Table 24–1.

Biomedicine has represented the dominant health care model in the United States during the past century (Silenzio, 2002). Any intervention not embedded in the biomedical model or promoted by medical associations is considered complementary, alternative, unorthodox, or unconventional.

What Conditions are Treated by Complementary and Alternative Health?

A multitude of conditions are addressed through CAH. Typically, incurable or difficult-to-manage conditions account for many patient visits (Wooten, 2001). Chronic conditions top the list, including AIDS, cancer, multiple sclerosis, digestive problems, back pain, anxiety, headache, and chronic pain syndromes (Wootton & Sparber, 2001; Sparber & Wootton, 2001; Medical Letter on the CDC and

Table 24–1   Terms to Describe Unconventional Health Care

- Alternative medicine
- Alternative health
- Alternative therapies
- Complementary and alternative medicine
- Holistic health
- Holistic medicine
- Unconventional care
- Unconventional medicine
- Unorthodox medicine
- Unorthodox therapies

Data from Astin JA: Why patients use alternative medicine: Results of a national study. JAMA 279:1548-1553, 1998; Borkan J, Neher JO, Anson O et al: Referrals for alternative therapies. J Fam Pract 39:545-550, 1994; Ernst E: Prevalence of use of complementary/alternative medicine: A systematic review. Bull World Health Organ 78(2):252-257, 2000; Eisenberg DM: Advising patients who seek alternative medical strategies. Ann Intern Med 127:61-69, 1997; Gevitz N (ed): Other Healers: Unorthodox Medicine in America. Baltimore, MD, Johns Hopkins University Press, 1988; Kaptchuk TJ, Eisenberg D: The persuasive appeal of alternative medicine. Ann Intern Med 129(12):1061-1065, 1998; Micozzi MS: Foreword. Orthop Phys Ther Clin North Am September:xi-xii, 2002; and Hastings Center Report: Alternative and complementary medicine: What's a doctor to do? Hastings Center Report 30(1):47-48, 2000.

FDA, 2000b; Shiflett, 1999; Arnold, 1999; Berman & Swyers, 1997). Table 24–2 lists 10 conditions commonly treated with CAH.

Diversity of Complementary and Alternative Health Interventions

Editorial restraints and the sheer volume/variety of CAH prevent an exhaustive discussion of every CAH therapy. The following examples demonstrate the diversity of both CAH and target conditions, however, Individuals with cancer routinely seek and receive CAH therapies (Patterson, 2002; Medical Letter on the CDC and FDA, 2002b; Cassileth, 2000). Likewise persons with various musculoskeletal ailments are also frequent CAH users (Berman et al, 1998; Astin et al, 2002; Michalsen et al, 2002;

Table 24–2   Ten Conditions Commonly Treated with Complementary and Alternative Health Care

Condition	Percentage of Population with Condition
Back problems	32%
Chronic pain	29%
Neurological conditions	27%
Insomnia	20%
Severe headaches/migraine	19%
Depression	19%
High blood pressure	17%
Arthritis/rheumatism	17%
Neurological paralysis (e.g., cerebral vascular accident [CVA])	17%
Urinary problems	13%

Data from Kraus HH, Godfrey C, Kirk J et al: Alternative health care: Its use by individuals with physical disabilities. Arch Phys Med Rehabil 79(11):1440-1447, 1998.

Hinman et al, 2002; Vallbona & Richards, 1999; Casimiro et al, 2002; Jensen et al, 2002; Kasahara et al, 2002). Chiropractic services, acupuncture, and electromagnetism are routinely incorporated into treatment plans for chronic pain especially, pain of a musculoskeletal nature (Vallbona & Richards, 1999; Berman et al, 2002; Arnold & Thornbrough, 1999; Davis & Rawls, 1993).

Sherman et al (2002) report on the effectiveness of maggot therapy in 18 of 21 patients receiving wound care treatment. Arnold and Thornbrough cite the effectiveness of traditional Chinese herbal medicine as a valuable primary or adjunctive therapy (Arnold & Thornbrough, 1999). A number of studies have demonstrated the use of prayer and meditation in the management of a variety of conditions (Matthews & Larson, 1997; Matthews et al, 1998; Matthews & Clark, 1998).

Evidence-Based Complementary and Alternative Health

Mainstream support is growing for selective CAH therapies as evidenced by systematic analyses that transcend single clinical studies. For instance, a National Institute of Health (NIH) consensus document supports the role of acupuncture for a host of conditions including (NIH, 1997):

- Low-back pain
- Tennis elbow/lateral epicondylitis
- Carpal tunnel syndrome
- Headache
- Fibromyalgia
- Osteoarthritis degenerative joint disease
- Cerebral vascular accident
- Menstrual cramps
- Asthma

A Cochrane Database Systematic Review of the clinical literature has been conducted on the use of acupuncture and electro-acupuncture in the treatment of rheumatoid arthritis (Casimiro et al, 2002).

One of the most comprehensive surveys to date regarding CAH involved 223 professional organizations devoted to unconventional therapies (Long et al, 2001). The purpose of this survey was to determine the appropriateness of various therapies for selected conditions. Treatment prevalence, costs, contraindications, and practitioner training/education were also examined. The top seven most common conditions in order of frequency were as follows:

- Stress/anxiety
- Headaches/migraine
- Back pain
- Respiratory problems
- Insomnia
- Cardiovascular problems
- Musculoskeletal problems

Complementary and Alternative Health User Profile

CAH users span every socioeconomic, ethnic, racial, educational, and occupational group, however, middle-aged and well-educated white females represents the most common CAH user profile (Eisenberg, 1993). Interestingly, 72% of users do not inform their medical physicians about their choice of unconventional therapies. This is another reason for providers to remain open-minded about CAH therapies. This lack of disclosure presents rehabilitation professionals with a unique opportunity to reach out to patients in an effort to understand their unmet wants, desires, and needs. It is incumbent on rehabilitation providers to develop a strengthened rapport with their patients who consider CAH use (Eisenberg 1997; Kraus et al 1998, Pappas & Perlman 2002). Rehabilitation providers may wish to redesign initial evaluation forms to reflect inquiry about CAH therapy use. A simple checklist patterned after Table 24-1 may serve this purpose.

Persons who use unconventional therapies do so for a variety of reasons (Ernst, 2000; Kaptchuk & Eisenberg, 1998). A national study revealed that many persons use unconventional treatment because it is more consistent with their values and beliefs than traditional medicine (Astin, 1998). Some view CAH as being more wholesome or natural than conventional medicine. For these persons, dissatisfaction with the conventional biomedical model of health care delivery drives CAH prevalence (Berman et al, 1998). Rehabilitation providers can learn lessons from these observations. CAH offers a greater opportunity for the patient to exercise more control over health care decisions and to collaborate with their providers (Astin, 1998). Astin (1998) opines that CAH therapies versus conventional medicine tend to be viewed as pure versus toxic, organic versus synthetic, low technology versus high technology, and coarse versus processed. CAH therapies are viewed as less invasive and as natural, which becomes the defining metaphor for some users. This view is most often associated with the use of dietary supplements, vitamins, aromatherapy, herbal medicines, saunas, and mud packs.

Although the physical being or state is important, much of CAH focuses on the relationship of mind and spirit (Kaptchuk & Eisenberg, 1998). Unconventional therapies are viewed as a means of calling on the body's natural healing mechanisms, vital energy, or life-supporting cosmic forces (Jonas & Jacobs 1996).

Why Do Consumers Use Unconventional Therapies?

- Consumers are dissatisfied with conventional treatment.
- CAH offers more personal autonomy and control.
- CAH is more consistent with the patient's values, beliefs, and worldview.
- CAH is viewed as less invasive.
- CAH is more natural/less toxic.
- CAH recognizes the mind-spirit relationship.

CONVENTIONAL MEDICINE BEGINS TO EMBRACE CAH

CAH interventions have spawned dialogue within the conventional medical community. Boucher and Lent (1998) surveyed physicians' attitudes regarding unconventional medicine. Dalen (1998) explored the integration of conventional and unconventional medicine. Murray 1993) addressed alternative medicine's role in general practice. O'Brien (2002) examined the benefit and risk associated with CAH.

Schoenberger et al (2002) describe the opinions and practices of medical rehabilitation providers regarding prayer and meditation. Conventional medical physicians have been generally slow in accepting unconventional therapies (Lee, 1993). This reticence is the result of a constellation of factors beginning with the educational system. The selection process for medical students places a premium on stellar grades. Lee (1993) asserts that "students get high grades when they simply repeat their tests exactly what the teacher wants them to say." As a result, Lee contends that medical schools are populated with students who are adept at absorbing information but not necessarily wisdom that is based on independent questioning and thinking processes. Lee further asserts that medical schools dispense data that focus on "rescue" medicine or interventions that treat symptoms. This approach is reinforced by a reimbursement system that rewards providers for organ classification of injury or disease, specifically the International Classification of Diseases system. Economic reward under this and other reimbursement systems demands an organ-based approach to health care delivery. Last, professional liability concerns inhibit adoption of CAH because malpractice may be defined by the comparison of one's treatment approach to a community standard of care. A community standard of care typically describes conventional biomedical or "in-the-box" interventions. Development of a community standard of care also requires consensus-building of a large provider universe over a protracted period of time. Paradoxically, although many CAH techniques (e.g., herbal treatment, acupuncture) have existed for 1000 years, CAH as a collection of interventions is a relative newcomer.

In fairness to conventional medical physicians, a patient's personal belief system triggers choices between conventional and unconventional interventions. Autonomy, a longstanding general ethical principal holds that the person's beliefs and choices should be respected provided they pose no harm or risk to the patient or others (Johnson, 1986). The choice to use unconventional therapies elicits a potentially heated debate between conventional practitioners and their patients and between providers and payers. The provider-patient relationship serves as the foundation of sound medical care (Pappas & Perlman, 2002). Mutual understanding between providers and their patients produces benefits while minimizing risks to both parties. Conventional medicine providers must respect the choices made by their patients and educate them in order to prevent adverse effects from these choices. Patients must feel comfortable speaking with their conventional providers about CAH therapies. Of course, this respect and comfort level can be attained only if conventional providers covet knowledge/wisdom concerning CAH and can convey it in a non-judgmental manner. A systematic presentation of CAH information in medical and allied medical schools is essential to accomplish this goal (Konafel, 2002; Martin, 2001; Bates & LoRe, 2000).

Brokaw et al (2002) report the findings of a survey of 53 medical schools offering courses in unconventional therapies. Only 17.8% of respondent schools offered unconventional therapy courses that emphasized a scientific or evidence-based approach. This finding is interesting considering that one of the chief criticisms of unconventional therapies centers on the paucity of evidence that supports CAH (O'Brien, 2002; Miller et al, 2002).

Park (2002) cites four reasons for the incorporation of CAH into medical school curriculum:

1. Medical schools are embracing an integrative medicine movement with an underlying holistic philosophy.
2. Clinical decision making requires the ability to handle uncertainty whether it involves conventional or unconventional interventions.
3. A growing societal interest in treatment diversity.
4. CAH will help to direct biomedical, psychological, and sociomedical research agencies.

Mainstream medical journals now include a representative sampling of unconventional medicine articles. More than 80 articles had appeared in American medical journals by 1998 (Okie, 1998). At least 34 of the nations' 125 medical schools offer elective courses in CAH (Millbank & Fox, 1998). Table 24-3 contains a roster of CAH courses taught in U.S. medical schools.

Sixty percent of medical schools have integrated CAH practices in core curriculum (Wetzel, 1998). The MEDLINE database contains more than 1500 articles on CAH annually (Ernst, 2000).

Despite CAH's shortcomings, a number of medical specialty groups have seized opportunities of leadership in unconventional therapies. Monkman (2001) provides instruction in how to explore the internet for CAH data. Physical medicine and rehabilitation physicians or physiatrists have been especially involved in CAH therapies (Kronenberg et al, 1994; Ko & Brebrayer, 2000). Of Canadian physiatrists, 72% refer patients for alternative medicine therapies (Ko & Brebrayer, 2000). Acupuncture (85%), biofeedback (81%) and chiropractic (80%) are the most frequently used interventions by percentage of respondents. Only 7% of physiatrists believe that CAH presents a threat to their patients.

The absence of evidence-based clinical trials does not dissuade some providers, who believe that clinically sound and ethical alternative health therapies can target individual patient needs (Adams et al, 2002). Some alternative health practitioners are quick to point out that "conventional medicine like CAM [CAH] is fraught with uncertainty" (Park, 2002). Nearly 80% of therapies in conventional medicine have not been proved through rigorous scientific study, according to the United States Office of

Table 24-3 Complementary and Alternative Health Care Course Taught in U.S. Medical Schools

• 76.7%	Acupuncture
• 69.9%	Botanicals
• 65.8%	Meditation and relaxation
• 64.4%	Spirituality/faith/prayer
• 60.3%	Chiropractic
• 57.5%	Homeopathy
• 50.7%	Nutrition and diet

NOTE: Data represent a percentage of 73 course directors or respondents representing 53 medical schools.
Data from Brokaw JJ, Tunnicliff G, Raeses BU et al: The teaching of complementary and alternative medicine in U.S. medical schools: A survey of course directors. Acad Med 77(9):876-881, 2002.

Technology Assessment (OTA, 1994). However, the Office of Technology Assessment no longer exists.

Critics of CAH cite treatment variation or lack of standardization in spite of the fact that conventional medicine too suffers from this problem. In a watershed study that examined 75 million physician claims under Medicare Part B (Chassin et al, 2002), a large degree of variation was shown in the prevalence of medical and surgical services. These variations were geographically-driven.

The best medical wisdom will be required to determine the indications for which services are provided to patients and to evaluate the appropriateness of performing procedures for these indications. Interpretation of the results of such an effort may be difficult and at times may not favor the medical profession.

- Chassin et al, 2002

Both conventional and unconventional therapies share at least one attribute: both use a similar approach based on practitioners' clinical experience in the absence of evidence-based practice (Park, 2002). Both conventional and unconventional medicine continue to strive for evidence-based practice (Sackett et al, 1996; McAlister et al, 2000; Ray, 2002).

A number of controversies surround CAH despite its astronomical growth both in terms of prevalence and expenditures (Ramos-Remus & Russell, 1997; Angell & Kassirer, 1998; Fontanarosa, 1998; Schneiderman, 1998; Tillman, 2002). Some mainstream providers do not recognize the synergies that exist between conventional and unconventional therapies (Ramos-Remus & Russell, 1997).

Acceptance of CAH can be seen in selected initiatives, however. On April 27, 2002 the Federation of State Medical Boards (FSMBs) adopted its "Model Guidelines for the Use of Complementary and Alternative Therapies in Medical Practice" (Horrigan et al, 2002). The genesis of this document was the FSMB's convening of a "Special Committee for the Study of Unconventional Health Care Practices" (Health and Medicine Week, 2002). This committee produced a seminal document that provides physicians with greater latitude in selecting, referring to and using unconventional therapies. The document contains safe harbor language that insulates physicians from charges of unprofessional conduct stemming from the selection of unconventional therapies over conventional treatment choices. The FSMB document covers the following areas: consultation and/or referral to licensed or otherwise state-regulated health care practitioners, clinical evaluation, treatment plan development, provider education, sale of goods, and clinical integration. Perhaps, physical rehabilitation professionals could benefit from adoption of a similar document?

WHAT IS THE GOVERNMENT'S ROLE IN COMPLEMENTARY AND ALTERNATIVE THERAPIES?

The federal government has a significant financial stake in health care finance and delivery because of its program sponsorship, including Medicare, Medicaid, Civilian Health & Medical Program of the Uniformed Services (CHAMPUS), and workers' compensation (e.g., railroad

workers, longshoremen). The United States government recognized the growing role of alternative medicine when in 1992 when it established The Office of Alternative Medicine (OAM). OAM is a component of NIH and commands a budget in excess of fifty million dollars (NIH, 1994). OAM has since been renamed the National Center for Complementary and Alternative Medicine (NCCAM). The NCCAM Website is http://www.nccam.nih.gov. The NCCAM is the federal government's lead agency conducting scientific inquiry into unconventional therapies. Established in 1998, its stated purpose is to "facilitate the evaluation of alternative medical treatment modalities and their effectiveness." A 2-year study by the Institute of Medicine (IOM) will use content experts from a broad range of unconventional and conventional disciplines including: internal medicine, behavioral science, nursing, epidemiology, pharmacology, educational research and administration. This task force is charged with three main responsibilities: first, to provide a comprehensive overview of unconventional therapies currently in use by the American public; second, to identify unconventional therapy scientific and health policy issues, regulation, integration, training, and practitioner credentialing/certification; and third, to assist in decision-making through the development of a conceptual framework. The IOM study has a number of prestigious sponsors (Table 24–4).

Complementary and Alternative Health Databases

There are a number of databases incorporating CAH literature. NCCAM and the National Library of Medicine (NLM) have created a partnership, "CAM on PubMed," as a subset of the National Library of Medicine's PubMed database (http://www.nlm.nih.gov/nccam/camonpubmed.html).

The MEDLINE database contains approximately 1500 articles devoted to alternative health per year (Ernst, 2000).

Alternative health interventions must meet the scientific standards of NCCAM in order to be recognized by any federal agency. Top ratings are received by those interventions that have undergone controlled randomized double blind clinical trials. Sixteen federal agencies or

Table 24–4 Federal Government Co-Sponsors of Institutes of Medicine Complementary and Alternative Medicine Study

- Agency for Health Care Research and Quality
- John E. Fogarty International Center
- National Cancer Center
- National Center for Complementary and Alternative Medicine
- National Center for Research Resources
- National Institute on Aging
- National Institute on Alcohol Abuse and Alcoholism
- National Institute on Arthritis, Musculoskeletal, and Skin Diseases
- National Institute of Dental and Craniofacial Research
- National Institute of Diabetes, Digestive, and Kidney Diseases
- National Institute of Mental Health Diseases
- National Library of Medicine
- National Institutes of Health Office of Behavioral/Social Science Research
- National Institutes of Health Office of Dietary Supplements

organizations support the IOM's effort to study the efficacy and safety of complementary and alternative medicine. The NCCAM web site has a page that lists all of the current clinical trials being performed involving complimentary and alternative medicine and funded by the NCCAM. This listing is available at the following address: http://nccam.nih.gov/clinicaltrials/treatmenttherapy.htm.

PREVALENCE OF COMPLEMENTARY AND ALTERNATIVE THERAPIES

In general, Americans use fewer CAH services than do Europeans, Asians, or Australians (Ko & Brebrayer, 2000). Estimates of CAH utilization vary depending on the source and range from 9% to 65% of the United States population (Eisenberg et al, 1998; Maclennon et al, 1996). There is clearly a growing trend in the use of CAH, however (Borkan et al, 1994; MacLennan et al, 1996; Perkin et al, 1994). Alternative health use has risen by 30% to 60% in the United States (Mills et al, 2002).

Trends Associated with Complementary and Alternative Health

The growth of CAH can be gauged through the following five trends:

1. within conventional medical institutions (Bates & Lore 2000; Brokow et al 2002; Boucher 1998; Konafel 2002).
2. The increase in government funding (NIH, 1999).
3. The increase in public and private insurance funding or reimbursement of CAH. (Kaltsas, 2000; Altshul, 2002, Wolsko et al, 2002).
4. The increase in utilization of CAH.
5. CAH achieves public health agenda status (Bodeker & Kronenberg 2002).

Americans made an estimated 629 million visits to CAH providers in 1997 (Wolsko et al, 2002). This figure greatly surpasses the number of visits for conventional medicine through primary care physicians, which accounted for

Table 24–5 Utilization of Conventional Versus Unconventional Therapies by Persons with Disabilities

Condition	Conventional Therapy	Unconventional Therapy
Anxiety	13.1%	42.1%
Depression	25.0%	33.9%
Headache	18.9%	51.4%
Insomnia	16.1%	32.3%
Pain	33.9%	51.8%

Data from Kraus HH, Godfrey C, Kirk J et al: Alternative health care: Its use by individuals with physical disabilities. Arch Phys Med Rehabil 79(11):1440-1447, 1998.

243 million visits (Eisenberg, 1993). Nearly 9% of the U.S. population or 17.5 million adults accounted for more than 75% of the 629 million visits. On average, 19 visits per year were made to CAH providers by Americans with costs exceeding $500 per capita (Eisenberg et al, 1993). Unconventional services are more prevalent in western states (Barnes et al, 1999; Ernst, 2000). Persons with physical disabilities select CAH more often than conventional therapies (Kraus et al, 1998).

In a survey of 502 hospitals (158 respondents), only 6% offered unconventional therapies in 1998 (Horrigan & Block, 2002). This number had dramatically increased to 15% of hospitals by 2000. The five most popular hospital-based CAH interventions include pastoral care, massage therapy, guided imagery, and therapeutic nutrition. Table 24–5 compares conventional versus unconventional therapies for five conditions.

Figure 24-1 depicts the relationship between persons with a principal diagnosis (expressed by percentage) who use medical care only, medical care and alternative care combined, and alternative care only. Through the NCCAM, the federal government has increased funding for CAH analysis from $2 million in 1992 to $113.2 million in 2003 (Health and Medicine Week, 2002). This is a phenomenal increase in funding at a time when other government

Figure 24–1. Patterns of treatment: Medical doctor, alternative health provider, and both. (Data from Kraus HH, Godfrey C, Kirk J et al: Alternative health care: Its use by individuals with physical disabilities. Arch Phys Med Rehabil 79[11]:1440-1447, 1998; and Eisenberg DM, Kessler RC, Foster C et al: Unconventional medicine in the United States. New Engl J Med 328:246-252, 1993.)

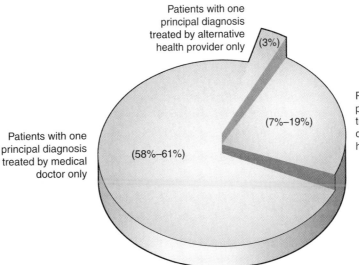

initiatives are drastically slashing funding (e.g., Balanced Budget Act, Medicare).

FUNDING OF COMPLEMENTARY AND ALTERNATIVE THERAPIES

Self-Pay

CAH services are predominantly funded through consumer out-of-pocket or self-payment, so in this regard CAH remains outside of mainstream medicine that enjoys reimbursement across multiple insurance lines (Eisenberg et al, 1993; Astin, 1998; Bodeker & Kronenberg, 2002). Seventy-six percent of patients private pay for their CAH services (Horrigan & Block, 2002). This is a significant percentage, and some would argue an endorsement for CAH. Would 76% of conventional medicine pay for it if insurance was unavailable? Americans spend more on CAH than for all hospitalizations combined (Eisenberg et al, 1993; Astin, 1998).

Public and Private Funding

Public and private funding sources are increasing coverage for CAH. At least six states mandate coverage for acupuncture: California, Florida, Nevada, New Mexico, Texas, and Washington (Altshul, 2002). Three states mandate naturopathic coverage: Arkansas, Utah, and Washington. In 2000, 70% of all employee-sponsored programs covered chiropractic service followed by 12% for massage (White House Commission on Complementary and Alternative Medicine Policy, 2002). Pelletier and Astin (2002) provided the most comprehensive overview of CAH reimbursement to date by managed care organizations and traditional insurers.

Government funding for CAH is increasing especially in the areas of outcomes research and practitioner training/education (McCarthy, 2002). A United States Presidential Commission final report on "Complementary and Alternative Medicine Policy" outlines 29 recommendations and more than 100 action items to be undertaken by federal agencies (Gordon, 2002). The report's approach involves pluralistic guidance for the integration of CAH and conventional medicine through respectful interdisciplinary collaboration. This involves application of biomedical research principles to CAH. The final report outlines 10 guiding principles that include the following examples: "wholeness approach in healthcare delivery," "evidence of safety," "evidence of efficacy," "the healing capacity of the person," "the right to choose treatment," and "an emphasis on health promotion and self-care." These examples appear to be consistent with some basic principles of physical rehabilitation. The report also promises to advance funding for unconventional therapies and is available at http://www.whccamp.hhs.gov/finalreport.html.

WHO ARE THE PROVIDERS OF COMPLEMENTARY AND ALTERNATIVE HEALTH CARE THERAPIES?

Myriad CAH therapies and associated practitioners exist (Cherkin et al, 2002). More than 1100 professions and occupations are regulated by statute, approximately 600

Table 24–6 Eight Most Common Complementary and Alternative Health Therapies

	Percentage of Persons Who Use Each Alternative Health Service
● Chiropractic	42%
● Massage	32%
● Herbal medicines	30%
● Megavitamins	24%
● Meditation	21%
● Homeopathy	10%
● Naturopathy	10%
● Acupuncture	10%

Data from Eisenberg DM, Kessler RC, Foster C et al: Unconventional medicine in the United States. New Engl J Med 328:246-252, 1993.

of them through state licensure (Millbank & Fox, 1998). The number of CAH practitioners is exponentially higher than those of regulated medical professions such as physicians, nurses, and therapists.

Professional practice guidelines or standards are not currently available for the vast majority of CAH therapies (Millbank & Fox, 2001; Angell & Kassirer 1998). Professional practice standards are necessary for CAH providers if they are to be fully accepted within the mainstream health care sector. Standards address provider training, education, licensure, and ethical conduct. These attributes at least theoretically ensure the safety, effectiveness, and efficacy of these interventions. Without these oversight mechanisms, consumers are less certain about the credentials of CAH practitioners and the safety of therapies. It is conceivable that when conventional medical providers leverage their licensure by offering CAH, consumer confidence should improve. As previously discussed, however, there is a paucity of evidence-based clinical trials regardless of who is the actual provider of service.

Some providers of CAH straddle both conventional and unconventional interventions. (Meeker & Haldeman, 2002; Schoenberger et al, 2002; Smith et al, 2002) Chiropractic therapy is the best example of this connection because of two relatively recent developments. Chiropractors achieved heightened recognition secondary to a successful lawsuit against the American Medical Association and, as a result, this profession gained more acceptance from insurers through reimbursement (Congressional Quarterly Researcher, 1992). Despite victories in both the legal and reimbursement arenas, chiropractic treatment is still considered by some as an alternative intervention to the medical model of health care delivery (Eisenberg, 1993). Chiropractic therapy is the most prevalent CAH service and is used by 42% of unconventional therapy consumers (Table 24–6).

WHAT IS THE ROLE OF PHYSICAL REHABILITATION PROVIDERS IN ALTERNATIVE HEALTH?

Should Rehabilitation Embrace Complementary and Alternative Health?

At least four reasons exist why rehabilitation providers may desire to learn more about CAH.

1. Selected CAH techniques may augment traditional rehabilitation services and potentially enhance clinical outcomes.
2. Rehabilitation providers may elect to collaborate with CAH providers in the management of complex cases.
3. Many patients of rehabilitation services also participate in CAH interventions. It is essential that providers learn more about these techniques to gauge their effects, both good and bad, on rehabilitation services. This education is akin to therapist understanding of pharmacological or chiropractic interventions and their impact on recovery cycles.
4. A paucity of data exists to support many conventional rehabilitation interventions, and to summarily reject CAH without thoughtful study would be the equivalent of living in a glass house while throwing stones. Rehabilitation providers are encouraged to maintain an open yet critical mind while further exploring the integration of CAH into their practices.

There is evidence that physical rehabilitation providers have begun to selectively embrace non-conventional interventions (Cromer, 1998; Massy & Perlman, 1999). A number of authors have addressed the synergistic opportunities that exist between CAH and physical rehabilitation (McCloy, 2000; Taylor & Majundmar, 2000; Bottomely, 2000; Stephens, 2000; Anderson, 2000; Deutsch et al, 2000). However, at present no systematic study exists of collaboration between CAH and rehabilitation.

An entire issue of *Orthopaedic Physical Therapy Clinics of North America* (a conventional rehabilitation journal) was devoted to the exploration of complementary and alternative interventions (Gallantino, 2000). This issue provides further support for collaboration between conventional and unconventional therapies.

Some view non-conventional therapies as new age-old approaches to human healing (Miccozzi, 2000). Miccozzi opines that many people are more desirous of "high touch" than "high tech." These persons view the biomedical model of care as too impersonal. Because physical rehabilitation has its roots in high touch through hands-on treatment, it is well positioned to seize opportunities to address unmet needs.

Rehabilitation and CAH appear to be most congruent in therapies such as acupuncture, magnet therapy, acupressure, rolfing, chiropractic, Feldenkrais, tai chi, myofascial release, craniosacral therapy, traditional Chinese herbal medicine, myofascial therapy, the Pilates method, and the Alexander method. (Shiflett, 1999; Anderson & Spector, 2000; Arnold & Thornbrough, 1999; Berman et al, 1988; Bottomley, 2000; Hinman et al, 2002; Massy, 1999; Taylor & Majundmar, 2000).

In a survey of 1221 medical professionals including physical and occupational therapists, a majority endorsed prayer and meditation but placed greater belief in meditation (Schonberger, 2002). Nurses and occupational therapists responded with more support of meditation and prayer when compared with physicians and physical therapists. Interestingly, although they expressed belief in CAH, a majority of conventional providers did not refer for these services. This finding suggests a need for more involvement in CAH by rehabilitation providers. This goal can be accomplished through the following mechanisms:

1. Secure additional training and education in unconventional therapies.
2. Collaborate with CAH practitioners.
3. Refer patients for CAH services on a selective basis.
4. Participate in research on CAH efficacy and safety.
5. Provide patients with accurate and timely consumer information that allows them to make intelligent and informed decisions.

It is especially important to appreciate that patients are selecting CAH therapies over mainstream medicine, and by doing so they often shift from an insurance-covered service to one that requires private payment. This situation illustrates the depth of patients' belief in and passion for unconventional care.

The contention that CAH is more closely aligned with a person's value and belief system (when compared with conventional treatment) should suggest several things to rehabilitation professionals (Astin, 1998; Kaptchuk, 1998; Kraus et al, 1998). First, patients need to be more engaged in the design and execution of their rehabilitation programs. Second, rehabilitation providers may need to better connect with the mind-spirit philosophy if they are to better understand their patients. Rehabilitation needs to carefully balance technological innovation with a high touch approach. Third, rehabilitation providers may wish to explore additional training and education in unconventional therapy and consider the integration of these services into conventional practice.

Complementary and Alternative Health and Rehabilitation Studies

The NIH sponsors a multitude of studies that specifically target rehabilitation interventions (http://www.clinical-studies.info.nih.gov). These studies focus on both conventional and unconventional therapies. For instance, protocol number 98-N-0115 is a study of whether amphetamines along with standard rehabilitation hasten recovery after stroke (NIH, 1998). Protocol 96-CC-0040 studied the use of personal computers in occupational therapy as a means to develop work skills and to improve concentration (NIH, 1996). As a result of its studies, NIH has endorsed certain alternative therapies. Meditation, hypnosis, and biofeedback were among the unconventional treatments the NIH endorsed in 1995 (NIH, 1999). A 12-member panel at a conference titled "Integration of Behavioral and Relaxation Approaches into the Treatment of Chronic Pain and Insomnia" (NIH, 1999) came to the following conclusions.

- Relaxation approaches are effective in treating a variety of chronic conditions, including low back pain, arthritis, and headache.
- Hypnosis is effective in alleviating chronic pain associated with various cancers, irritable bowel syndrome, temporomandibular disorders, and tension headaches.
- Biofeedback is effective in relieving pain, tension headache, and insomnia.

The NIH (1999) panel recommended insurance reimbursement for psychosocial therapy for chronic pain and insomnia as a component of comprehensive medical services.

Alternative health should enjoy continued growth as both government research support and payer reimbursement continues. Physical rehabilitation providers must individually, and perhaps collectively through national professional organizations, determine whether and how they will integrate conventional services with unconventional services.

WHAT DOES THE FUTURE HOLD FOR UNCONVENTIONAL THERAPIES?

CAH, as it continues to evolve, will undergo many changes and challenges, not unlike other emerging technologies. There will always be naysayers, proponents, and fence sitters. The reality is that conventional medicine has yet to eliminate human suffering or to dramatically contain health care costs. Managed care has not fulfilled its early billing and as such continues in its own evolution, facing its own brisk challenges. Table 24-7 provides a summary of 10 challenges that confront unconventional therapies.

The ultimate success of CAH may hinge on the integration of conventional and unconventional therapies. This will require that its practitioners address a host of issues across a number of spheres: ethical, licensure, liability, clinical outcome measures, management, government regulation, and reimbursement. The World Health Organization has articulated a number of challenges relative to CAH. These are found in Table 24-8. The World Health Organization breaks these challenges to action into four major areas: access; rational use; national policy and regulation; and safety, efficacy, and quality.

Providers are challenged to lobby their professional organizations to adopt a position on CAH research, referral, and use. Equally, professional organizations need to engage in active dialogue and collaboration if the benefits of CAH are to outweigh the risks.

Table 24-9 highlights 12 reasons why CAH reimbursement is projected to grow. Once funding mechanisms are in place, little can slow the momentum of CAH.

Table 24-8 World Health Organization Complementary and Alternative Medicine Challenges for Action

National policy and regulation

- Lack of official recognition of CAM
- Lack of regulatory/legal mechanisms
- Lack of integration into the national health care system
- Equitable distribution of benefits
- Inadequate allocation of CAM development and capacity building

Safety/efficacy/quality

- Inadequate evidence base for CAM
- Lack of national or international safety standards
- Lack of adequate regulation of herbal medicines
- Lack of CAM provider regulation
- Lack of standardized research methodology

Access

- Lack of data measuring access levels and affordability
- Lack of official recognition of CAM providers' role
- Need to identify safe and effective practices
- Lack of cooperation between CAM practitioners
- Unsustainable use of medicinal plant resources

Rational use

- Lack of training for CAM providers
- Lack of CAM training for allopathic practitioners
- Lack of information for the public on rational CAM uses
- Lack of communication between CAM and allopathic practitioners and between allopathic practitioners and consumers

Data from World Health Organization: WHO Traditional Medicine Strategy 2002-2005, Geneva, Switzerland, May 16, 2002 http://www.who.int/medicines/organization/trm/orgtrmain.shtml, accessed December 4, 2002.

Rehabilitation providers must decide whether they are going to respond to the demand of consumers/patients for alternative and complementary interventions. To ignore CAH may result in the abdication of a significant role in the future of prevention, wellness and health care

Table 24-9 12 Reasons Why Complementary and Alternative Health Reimbursement is Projected to Grow

1. Increasing use of CAH by consumers who currently predominantly self-pay.
2. Increasing diversity of CAH providers, especially conventional medical providers who are already currently reimbursed under employer-based or government-based benefits programs.
3. Growth in CAH within conventional medical education institutions.
4. Strengthened licensure, certification, registration, and accreditation.
5. Growing support at the federal government level (e.g., NIH/National Center for Complementary and Alternative Medicine).
6. Consumer antimanaged care backlash and a trend toward a friendlier generation of managed care.
7. Growing paradigm shift from medical care to health/wellness.
8. More educated consumers.
9. Enhanced information technology and communication (e.g., Internet).
10. A paradigm shift regarding patients from "giving them fish" to "teaching them to fish."
11. Increasing funding of CAH by some managed care organizations may have a domino effect on others.
12. Some conventional therapies continue to be a source of dissatisfaction among consumers because of their loss of autonomy and collaboration in treatment.

Table 24-7 10 Weaknesses Associated with Complementary and Alternative Health Therapies

1. Poor regulatory oversight
2. Practitioners too diverse
3. Paucity of clinical outcomes measures
4. Relatively weak reimbursement
5. Relatively few traditional medical and health care providers are formally trained/educated in complementary and alternative health care
6. Paucity of validation studies in refereed/peer reviewed journals
7. Broadly labeled cluster of services
8. Practitioners without standardized credentials, certifications, licensure, and examining boards
9. Absence of professional liability insurance protecting the public to some degree
10. CAH interventions do not undergo safety screening (e.g., FDA)

Data modified from Milbank SL, Fox DM: Enhancing the accountability of alternative medicine. New York, The Milbank Memorial Fund, 1998, p 35, http://www.med.harvard.edu/publications/milbank, accessed December 5, 2001.

in the future. Inversely, to blindly accept CAH without methodical study and research may represent an abdication of one's professional ethics, (e.g., the dictum to do no harm).

REFERENCES

Adams KE, Cohen MH, Eisenberg D, Jonsen AR: Ethical considerations of complementary and alternative medical therapies in conventional medical settings. Ann Intern Med 137(8):660-664, 2002.

Altshul S: Get your treatments insured. Prevention 54(4):57, 2002.

Anderson BD, Spector A: Introduction to Pilates-based rehabilitation. Orthop PT Clin Am 9(3):395-410, 2000.

Angell M, Kassirer J: Alternative medicine: The risks of untested and unregulated remedies. New Engl J Med 339(12):839-841, 1998.

Anonymous: Complementary and alternative medicine: More extramural scientists needed to bolster information on CAM. Health and Medicine Week November 4, p 6, http://www.proquest.umi.com, accessed December 2, 2002a.

Anonymous: Complementary and alternative medicine: More than 70% of adults with cancer use alternative therapies, Medical Letter on the CDC and FDA. Health and Medicine Week October 6, http://www.proquest.umi.com, accessed December 2, 2002b.

Arnold MD, Thornbrough LM: Treatment of musculoskeletal pain with traditional Chinese herbal medicine. Phys Med Rehabil Clin North Am 10(3):663-671, 1999.

Astin JA: Why patients use alternative medicine: Results of a national study. JAMA 279:1548-1553, 1998.

Astin JA, Beckner W, Soeken K et al: Psychological interventions for rheumatoid arthritis: A meta-analysis of randomized controlled trials. Arthritis Rheum 47(3):291-302, 2002.

Barnes J et al: Articles on complementary medicine in the mainstream medical literature, Arch Intern Med 59: 1721-1725, 1999.

Bates B, LoRe F: Teaching complementary and alternative medicine in residency programs. Arch Phys Med Rehabil 81(9):1256-1257, 2000.

Berman BM, Bausell RB, Lee WL: Use and referral patterns for 22 complementary and alternative therapies by members of the American College of Rheumatology: Results of a national survey. Arch Intern Med 162(7):766-770, 2002.

Berman BM, Jonas WS, Swyers JP: Issues in the use of complementary/alternative medical therapies for low back pain. Phys Med Rehabil Clin North Am 9(2):497-513, 1998.

Berman BM, Swyers JP: Establishing a research agenda for investigating alternative medical interventions for chronic pain. Primary Care 24(4):743-758, 1997.

Bodeker G, Kronenberg F: A public health agenda for traditional, complementary, and alternative medicine. Am J Public Health 92(10):1582-1591, 2002.

Borkan J, Neher JO, Anson O et al: Referrals for alternative therapies. J Fam Pract 39:545-550, 1994.

Bottomley JM: The use of Tai Chi as a movement modality in orthopaedics. Orthop Phys Ther Clin North Am 9(3):361-373, 2000.

Boucher T, Lent S: An organizational survey of physicians' attitudes about and practice of complementary and alternative medicine. Altern Ther 4(6):61-62, 1998.

Brokaw JJ, Tunnicliff G, Raess BU et al: The teaching of complementary and alternative medicine in U.S. medical schools: A survey of course directors. Acad Med 77(9):876-881, 2002.

Casimiro L, Brosseau L, Milne S et al: Acupuncture and electro-acupuncture for the treatment of RA. Cochrane Database Syst Rev (3):CD0037898, 2002 (Review).

Cassileth BR: Complementary therapies: The American experience support care. Cancer 8(1):16-23, 2000.

Chassin MR, Brook RH, Park RE: Variations in the use of medical and surgical services by the Medicare population. New Engl J Med 314(5):285-290, 2002.

Cherkin DC, Deyo RA, Sherman KJ et al: Characteristics of licensed acupuncturists, chiropractors, massage therapists, and naturopathic physicians. J Am Board Fam Pract 15(5):378-390, 2002.

Anonymous: Congressional Quarterly: Congressional Quarterly Inc., in conjunction with EBSCO Publishing, 2(4):73-9, 1992.

Cromer M: Medicine or magic?: Alternative medicine's impact on rehabilitation. Rehabil Manage 11(2):56, 58-59, 1998.

Dalen GE: Conventional and unconventional medicine: Can they be integrated? Arch Intern Med 158(9):2179-2181, 1998.

Davis A, Rawls W: Magnetism and Its Effects on the Living System. Kansas City, MO, Acres U.S.A., 1993.

Deutsch JE, Derr LL, Judd P, Reuven B: Treatment of chronic pain through the use of structural integration (Rolfing). Orthop Phys Ther Clin North Am 9(3):411-425, 2000.

Eisenberg D et al: Trends in alternative medicine use in the United States 1990-1997. JAMA 280:1569-1575, 1998.

Eisenberg DM, Kessler RC, Foster C et al: Unconventional medicine in the United States. New Engl J Med 328:246-252, 1993.

Eisenberg DM: Advising patients who seek alternative medical strategies. Ann Intern Med 127:61-69, 1997.

Ernst E: Prevalence of use of complementary/alternative medicine: A systematic review. Bull World Health Organ 78(2): 252-257, 2000.

Ernst E: Prevalence of complementary/alternative medicine for children: A systematic review. Eur J Pediatr 158:7-11, 1999.

Ernst E et al: Complementary medicine—A definition. Br J Gen Pract 45:506, 1995.

Fontanarosa PB, Lundberg GD: Alternative medicine meets science. JAMA 280:1618-1619, 1998.

Fugh-Berman A (ed): Alternative Medicine: What Works? Tucson, AZ, Odonian Press, 1996.

Gallantino ML (ed): Preface. Orthop Phy Ther Clin North Am 9(3):275-40, 2000.

Gellman H, Kennedy C: Orthopaedic medicine: Complementary and alternative medicine has its place. Obesity, Fitness and Wellness, March 24; http://www.proquest.com, accessed December 2, 2002.

Gevitz N (ed): Other Healers: Unorthodox Medicine in America. Baltimore, MD, Johns Hopkins University Press, 1988.

Gordon JS: The White House Commission on Complementary and Alternative Medicine Policy: Final report and the next steps. Altern Ther Health Med 8(3):28-31, 2002.

Hastings Center Report: Alternative and complementary medicine: What's a doctor to do? Hastings Center Report 30(1):47-48, 2000.

Hinman MR, Ford J, Heyl H: Effects of static magnets on chronic knee pain and physical function: A double-blind study. Altern Ther Health Med 8(4):50-55, 2002.

Horrigan B, Block B: CAM insurance coverage on the rise. Altern Ther Health Med 8(4):30, 2002; http://www.proquest.umni.com, accessed December 2, 2002.

Jensen OK, Rasmussen C, Mollerup F: Hyperhomocysteinemia in rheumatoid arthritis: Influence of methotrexate treatment and folic acid supplementation. J Rheumatol 29(8):1615-1618, 2002.

Johnson PR: Patient autonomy in decision making: Recent trends in medical ethics. Linacre Q 53(2):37-46, 1986.

Jonas WB, Jacobs J: Healing with Homeopathy: The Natural Way to Promote Recovery and Restore Health. New York, NY, Warner Books, 1996.

Kaltsas H: Help get acupuncture covered under Medicare. Altern Med 36(20):22, 2000.

Kaptchuk TJ, Eisenberg D: The persuasive appeal of alternative medicine. Ann Intern Med 129(12):1061-1065, 1998.

Ko GD, Berbreyer D: Complementary and alternative medicine: Canadian Physiatrists attitudes and behaviors. Arch Phys Med Rehabil 81:662-667, 2000.

Konafel J: The challenge of educating physicians about complementary and alternative medicine. Acad Med 77(9):847-850, 2002.

Kraus HH, Godfrey C, Kirk J et al: Alternative health care: Its use by individuals with physical disabilities. Arch Phys Med Rehabil 79(11):1440-1447, 1998.

Kronenberg F, Mallory B, Downey JA: Rehabilitation medicine and alternative therapies: New words, old practices. Arch Phys Med Rehabil 75(8):928-929, 1994.

Lee SI, Khang YH, Lee MS et al: Knowledge of attitudes toward, and experience of complementary and alternative medicine in Western medicine—and Oriental medicine—trained physicians in Korea. Am J Public Health 92(12):1494-2000.

MacLennan AH, Wilson DGH, Taylor AW: Prevalence and costs of alternative medicine in Australia. Lancet 347:569-573, 1996.

Martin JB: Historical and professional perspectives of complementary and alternative medicine with a particular emphasis on rediscovery and embracing complementary and alternative medicine in contemporary Western society. J Altern Complement Med 7(Suppl 1): S11-S18, 2001.

Massy PB, Perlman A: Lasting resolution of chronic thoracic neuritis using martial-arts-based physical therapy. Altern Ther Health Med 5(3):103-104, 1999.

Matthews DA, Larson DB: Faith and medicine: Reconciling the twin tradition of healing. Mind/Body Med 2:3-6, 1997.

Matthews DA, et al: Religious commitment and health status. Arch Fam Med 7:118-124, 1998.

Matthews DA, Clark C: The Faith Factor: Proof of the Healing Power of Prayer. New York, NY, Viking Press, 1998.

McAlister FA, Straus SE, Guyatt GH: Integrating research evidence with the care of the individual patient: user's guide to the medical literature. JAMA 283:2824-2836.

McCarthy M: U.S. panel calls for more support of alternative medicine. The Lancet 359(9313):1213, 2002; http://www.whccamp.hhs.gov, accessed December 2, 2002.

McCloy CM: Nutritional considerations in orthopaedic physical therapy. Orthop Phys Ther Clin North Am 9(3):321-339, 2000.

Meeker WC, Haldeman S: Chiropractic: A profession at the crossroads of mainstream and alternative medicine. Ann Intern Med 136(3):216-227, 2002.

Michalsen A, Moebus S, Spahn G et al: Leech therapy for symptomatic treatment of knee osteoarthritis: Results and implications of a pilot study. Altern Ther Health Med 8(5):84-88, 2002.

Micozzi MS: Foreword. In Galantino ML (ed): Preface. Orthop Phys Ther Clin North Am Sept 9(3):xi-xii, 2002.

Milbank SL, Fox DM: The Milbank Memorial Fund, Enhancing the accountability of alternative medicine. New York: The Milbank Memorial Fund, 1998; http://www.med.harvard.edu/publications/milbank, accessed December 5, 2001.

Miller EJ, Hollyer T, Guyatt G et al: Teaching evidence-based complementary and alternative medicine: A learning structure for clinical decision changes. J Altern Complement Med 8(2):207-214, 2002.

Mills EJ, Hollyer T, Guyatt G et al: Teaching evidence-based complementary and alternative medicine: A learning structure for clinical decision changes. J Altern Complement Med 8(2):207-214, 2002.

Monkman D: Educating health professionals about how to use the web and how to find complementary and alternative medicine (CAM). Information Complement Ther Med 9(4):258, 2001.

Murray J, Shepherd S: Alternative or additional medicine?: An exploratory study in general practice. Soc Sci Med 37:983-988, 1993.

National Center for Complementary and Alternative Medicine (NCCAM); http://www.nccam.nih.gov, accessed November 18, 2002.

National Institutes of Health: NIH panel endorses alternative therapies for chronic pain and insomnia. http://www.nccam.nih.gov/nccam/cam/1995/dec/4.htm, accessed August 2, 1999.

National Institutes of Health and Prevention: Practice and Policy Panel, Office of Alternative Medicine, Clinical Practice Guidelines in Complementary and Alternative Medicine: An Analysis of Opportunities and Obstacles. Arch Fam Med 6:149-154, 1997.

National Institutes of Health: Expanding medical horizons. A report to the National Institutes of Health on alternative medical systems and practices in United States. NIH publication # 94-0066, Bethesda, MD, National Institutes of Health, 1994.

National Institutes of Health: National Institutes of Health Alternative Medicine Clearinghouse, Bethesda, MD, National Institutes of Health, 1997.

National Institutes of Health and Prevention: National Center for Complementary and Alternative Medicine (NCCAM), 2002, http://www.nccam.nih.gov, accessed December 2, 2002.

National Institutes of Health: Neuroanatomical and neurophysiological basis of motor recovery associated with treatment of recent stroke using amphetamine and physical therapy. Clinical Research Studies, NIH Protocol Number: 98-N-0115.

National Institutes of Health: Linking occupational therapy process and patient performance: the personal computer activity in occupational interventions. Clinical Research Studies, Protocol Number 96-CC-0040, Washington, DC, NIH, 2000.

O'Brien K: Problems and potentials of complementary and alternative medicine. Intern Med J 32(4):163-164, 2002.

Pappas S, Perlman A: Complementary and alternative medicine. The importance of doctor-patient communication. Med Clin North Am 86(1):1-10, 2002.

Paramore LC: Use of alternative therapies: Estimates from the 1994 Robert Wood Johnson Foundation National Access to Care Survey. J Pain Symptom Manage 13:83-89, 1997.

Park CM: Diversity, the individual, and proof of efficacy: complementary and alternative medicine in medical education. Am J Public Health 92(10):1568-1572, 2002.

Patterson RE: Complementary and alternative medicine: More than 70% of adults with cancer use alternative therapies. http://www.proquest.umi.com, accessed December 2, 2002.

Pelletier KR, Astin JA: Integration and reimbursement of complementary and alternative medicine by managed care and insurance providers: 2000 update and cohort analysis. Altern Ther Health Med 8:38-39, 2002.

Perkin MR, Pearcy RM, Fraser JS: A comparison of the attitudes shown by general practitioners, hospital doctors, and medical students towards alternative medicine. J Rehabil Soc Med 87:523-525, 1994.

Ramos-Remus C, Russell AS: Alternative therapies-medicine, magic or quackery? Who is winning the battle? J Rheumatol 24: 2280-2282, 1997.

Ray JG: Evidence in upheaval: incorporating observational data into clinical practice. Arch Intern Med 162:249-254.

Sackett DL, Rosenberg WMC, Muir Gray JA et al: Evidence-based medicine: What it is and what it isn't. Br Med J 312:71-72, 1996.

Schneider RH, Alexander C, Salerno JW et al: Disease prevention and health promotion in the elderly with a traditional system of natural medicine. J Aging Health 14:57-58, 2002.

Shiflett SC: Overview of complementary therapies in physical medicine and rehabilitation Phys Med Rehabil Clin North Am 10(3):521-529, 1999.

Silenzio VMB: What is the role of complementary and alternative medicine in public health? Am J Public Health 92(10):1562, 2002.

Schoenberger NE, Mattheis RJ, Shiflett SC, Cotter AC: Opinions and practices of medical rehabilitation professionals regarding prayer and meditation. J Altern Complement Med 8(1):59-69, 2002.

Smith M, Greene BR, Meeker W: The CAM movement and the integration of quality health care: The case of chiropractic. J Ambul Care Manage 25(2):1-16, 2002.

Sparber A, Wootton JC: Surveys of complementary and alternative medicine. Part II: use of alternative and complementary cancer therapies. J Altern Complement Med 7:281-287, 2001.

Swartzman LC, Harshman RA, Burkell J, Liundy ME: What accounts for the appeal of complementary/alternative medicine, and what makes complementary/alternative medicine "alternative"? Medical decision making. Int J Soc Med Decision Making 22(5):431-450, 2002.

Taylor MJ, Majundmar M: Incorporating Yoga therapeutics into orthopaedic physical therapy. Orthop Phys Ther Clin North Am 9(3):341-359, 2000.

Tillman R: Paying for alternative medicine: The role of health insurers. Ann Am Acad Pol Soc Sci 583:64-75, 2002; http://www.proquest.umi.com, accessed December 2, 2002.

U.S. Congress, Office of Technology Assessment: Identifying health technology assessment, identifying health technologies that work: Searching for evidence. Washington, DC, US Office of Technology Assessment, 1994.

Vallbona C, Richards T: Evolution of magnetic therapy from alternative to traditional medicine. Phys Med Rehabil Clin North Am 10(3): 663-671, 1999.

Weil A: Natural Health, Natural Medicine. New York, Houghton Mifflin, 1995.

Wetzel MS, Eisenberg DM, Kaptchuk TJ: Courses involving complementary and alternative medicine at U.S. medical schools. JAMA 280: 784-787, 1998.

White House Commission on Complementary and Alternative Medicine Policy, Final Report, March 2002, http://www.whccamp.hhs.gov/finalreport.html, accessed December 4, 2002.

Wolsko PM, Eisenberg DM, Davis RB et al: Insurance coverage, medical conditions, and visits to alternative medicine providers: Results of a national survey. Arch Intern Med 162(3):281-287, 2002.

Wootton JC, Sparber A: Surveys of complementary and alternative medicine, Part IV: Use of alternative and complementary therapies for rheumatological and other diseases. J Altern Complement Med 7:715-721, 2001.

Wootton JC, Sparber A: Surveys of complementary and alternative medicine, Part III: Use of alternative and complementary therapies for HN/AIDS. J Altern Complement Med 7:371-377, 2001a.

World Health Organization: WHO launches the first global strategy on traditional and alternative medicine. http://www.who, accessed September 14, 2002.

SUGGESTED READINGS

Cooter R (ed): Studies in the History of Alternative Medicine. New York, St. Martin's Press, 1998.

Gordon JS: The White House Commission on Complementary and Alternative Medicine Policy: Final Report and Next Steps, Altern Ther Health Med 8(3):28-31, 2002.

Jonas AR, Siegler M, Winslade WJ: Clinical Ethics, 3rd ed, New York, McGraw Hill, 1992.

Long L, Huntley A, Ernst E: Which complementary and alternative therapies benefit which conditions? A survey of the opinions of 223 professional organizations. Complement Ther Med 9(3):175-185, 2001.

National Center for Complementary and Alternative Medicine Website, http://www.nccam.nih.gov, accessed August 21, 2004.

Shiflett SC: Overview of complementary therapies in physical medicine and rehabilitation. Phys Med Rehabil Clin North Am 10(3):521-529, 1999.

Weil A: Natural Health, Natural Medicine: A Comprehensive Manual for Wellness and Self-Care. Boston, Houghton Mifflin, 1995.

CHAPTER 25

Beyond Managed Care: A Vision of the Future

David W. Clifton, Jr., PT

"Although predicting is perilous, not predicting is even more perilous. It leaves us unprepared for the changes going on right under our noses, confronts us with recurrent surprises, and most problematic, makes us reactive to change instead of agents of change."

- Jerome P. Kassirer, 1999

KEY POINTS

- Rehabilitation providers must look beyond their own clinical paradigm if they are to understand and fully participate in future health care paradigms.
- Change is imminent and, at times, rapid.
- People and organizations generally resist change.
- Change is external and situational, whereas transition reflects a person's or organization's response to change.

Operational Definitions

Change	External situations that affect persons and organizations.
Paradigm	A pattern, a model, or an example.
Transition	A person's or organization's internal responses to change.

TRANSFORMATIONS IN AMERICAN HEALTH CARE

The health care sector is in the midst of one of its most tumultuous periods in history (The Pew Health Professions Commission, 1998). Forces driving health care have become increasingly complex and diverse. A rehabilitation provider's practice is profoundly impacted by social pressures, technological advances, legal precedence, economic realities, ethical dilemmas, political shifts, and a plethora of other environmental change agents. As a result, today's providers have surrendered a significant

degree of autonomy. However, this may be an ideal time for rehabilitation providers to serve as change agents.

Drivers of change will demand that providers possess an unparalleled degree of comprehension if they are to contribute and not simply respond to changes. Figure 25–1 depicts a variety of external forces that directly or indirectly shape rehabilitation practice. These extrinsic forces promise to persist beyond the managed care era. Those that have predicted the demise of managed care may be overlooking a fundamental observation concerning health care. Rarely is a finance or treatment paradigm completely supplanted by another one. Instead, hybrid models tend to evolve that incorporate elements of the old with those of the new. For instance, MRI and CT scans did not supplant plain film x-rays as a diagnostic tool, they simply augmented existing technologies. Capitation did not completely obliterate fee-for-service reimbursement; it simply augmented it. Primary care physicians did not supplant the need for specialists; they simply augmented these services. There are many other examples of coexistence of seemingly disparate and, perhaps, competing paradigms (Table 25–1).

Regulatory and legislative initiatives will continue to influence health care. Perhaps the next major health care transformation will involve a form of socialized health care? Financial and reimbursement challenges will facilitate the development of more cost effective, value-driven alternatives. Managed care represents denial or selective rationing of care; however, the next generation may involve the substitution of more efficient and cost-effective interventions, not the denial of services. Competitive and professional issues such as multidisciplinary or collaborative

Figure 25–1. Drivers of change.

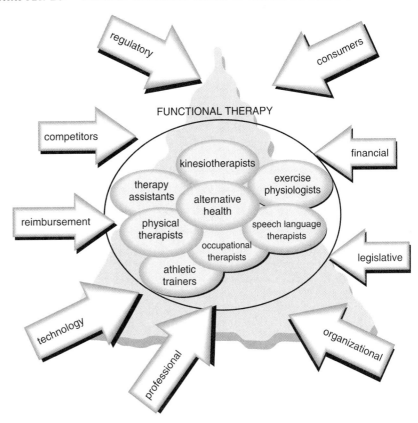

FUNCTIONAL THERAPY

Table 25–1   Health Care Drivers of Change

Type	Driver
Social	1. Population growth and redistribution
	2. Aging and chronicity
	3. Growth in alternative therapies
	4. Concern for underinsured and uninsured
Technology	1. Information technology explosion
	2. Genetics research and unlocking of human genome
	3. Telemedicine
	4. Self-care innovations
	5. Blending of financial and clinical data
	6. Improved health screenings
Economic	1. Alteration of managed care
	2. Growth in employer control of health care
	3. Shift from public to private financing
	4. Focus on "value purchasing"
	5. Reapportionment of providers
	6. Continued closings of hospitals
	7. Growth in provider networks
Political	1. Managed care reforms, state and federal
	2. Growth in consumer special interest
	3. Professional association reforms
	4. Shift from consumer protection to enhancement of health
Legal	1. Tort cases and unfavorable verdicts
	2. Continuous assault on ERISA protections (Employee Retirement Income Security Act)
Environmental	1. Focus on health and wellness, not medical
	2. Integrated benefits
	3. Growth in prevention focus
	4. Focus on management versus treatment

Data modified from Jamison: Chronic illness management in the year 2005. Nurs Econ 16(5):246-253, 1998.

care are sure to modify how clinicians render their services. Again, a provider's actions or inactions will to some degree be driven by forces beyond their immediate control. Therefore, it is incumbent on providers to think outside of the clinical box, to explore beyond their profession's boundaries, and to participate in and adapt to new paradigms. A paradigm is a model, pattern, or example (Patterson, 1998). Participation in new paradigms will require a greater understanding of other health care stakeholders and their perspectives as well as a heightened ability to track and respond to macrotrends and countertrends.

Ultimately, rehabilitation providers must expeditiously transition to change by embracing new paradigms. Otherwise, providers run the risk of exclusion while others fill the void. The purpose of this chapter is to encourage providers to take a long view in a world of uncertainties and tendencies toward short-term gratification. The title of the chapter "Beyond Managed Care" implies several things. One, managed care is an interim step to the next major transformation of health care. Two, managed care will be fundamentally restructured. This view is shared by those who consider managed care as an interim stage of development (Kleinke, 1999; Morrison, 1996). There is strong evidence that a new transformation has begun (Clifton, 1996). However, managed care (according to some) has left some permanent structural changes to American health care (Reece, 1988).

In order to know, even remotely, where health care is going, one must first understand from whence it came. Chapters 20, 21, and 23 provide a historical perspective concerning issues that contributed to the direction in which health care is now headed. A combination of these and other forces create "scenarios," which are instruments that allow us to take the long view in a world of uncertainty (Schwartz, 1996). Scenarios can be referred to as "myths of the future," but they have utility in considering the possibilities and necessary steps for future action (Schwartz, 1996). This chapter will outline a number of likely scenarios based on the historical pathway of health care, current trends and countertrends, evolving paradigms combined with educated guessing and speculation. As Yogi Berra is said to have quipped, *"the future is hard to predict because it isn't here yet."*

Stages of Transformation

Predicting the future of health care may be perilous; however, much can be learned by examining the past. Reece described three "Great Transformations in American Health Care" (Reece, 1988).

The first transformation was the "scientific" one, marked by significant advances such as anesthesia, asepsis, radiology, and intravenous fluids. This was followed by a "social" transformation defined by the advent of health care funding sources in the form of employer provided care (group health and workers' compensation) and government sponsored health care (Medicare and Medicaid). This second transformation, identified by fee-for-service (FFS), led to an open-ended spending policy and, consequently, escalating health care costs. These spiraling costs ushered in the third transformation known as managed care. This third transformation is quickly evolving into a yet unknown fourth transformation. Although a completely new health care paradigm or transformation has not yet fully evolved, there are hints to its components. Growing antimanaged care sentiments reveal less about what this new transformation will include and more about what it will exclude (Clarke, 2000; Millenson, 1998; Paris & Hines, 1995; Savage, et al, 2000).

Control has been methodically wrested from managed care organizations (MCOs) through an array of legislative, litigatory, economic, and consumer-driven mechanisms. One example involves the abolishment of "gag clauses" in managed care contracts, which had prevented physicians and other providers from disclosing to patients information concerning the financial incentives built into managed care contracts. Critics of managed care claim that it does little to actually "manage" the process or outcome of care because it focuses on cost control through at-risk provider contracts, patient co-payments, deductibles, and restricted access to care (Houck, 1997). Managed care's ability to trim perceived and/or real excessive costs from the system has apparently run its course as costs have again begun to spiral out of control. It is estimated that by the year 2008, health expenditures will exceed $2.2 trillion (Smith et al, 1999). These data will lead to innovations in health care finance and delivery. Efficiency and customer value are predicted to supplant managed care's cost fixation. Efficiencies are realized in a mature market through a number of mechanisms:

- Expanded use of care extenders
- Increased patient responsibility

- Evidence-based interventions
- Nurse triage via telephonic online client support call centers
- Automated office functions
- Customized patient educational materials
- Collaborative care models

A mature managed care market will see a major transition from a dependent patient model to a more independent patient role (Houck, 1997). Managed care organizations will continue attempts to regain consumer trust that has been seriously eroded over the past decade (Millenson, 1998).

Although it is doubtful that all components of managed care will become extinct, enough may disappear to make it unrecognizable by today's generation. Clearly, new paradigms will emerge and provide rehabilitation providers with both threats and opportunities. Those who view the glass as half full rather than half empty may be the ones who prosper through the next millennium.

Getting a Glimpse of the Future

Clues to the future of health care, especially rehabilitation, can be found through an analysis of trends/countertrends. Trends and countertrends can be identified in a variety of data sources. A number of these resources are included in the Appendix as well as Chapter 15.

Foundations and independent think tanks are good sources of data. Foundations such as the Robert Wood Johnson, Pew Charitable Trust, John Hartford Foundation, Kellogg Foundation, and Milbank Memorial Fund publish outstanding works that can enlighten providers concerning the future of health care delivery and finance. For example, publications of the Milbank Fund address salient issues:

- *Better Information, Better Outcomes?: The Use of Health Technology Assessment and Clinical Effectiveness Data in Health Care Purchasing Decisions in the United Kingdom and the United States*, The Milbank Fund, 2000
- *Evaluating the Quality of Health Care: What Research Offers Decision Makers*, The Milbank Fund, 1996
- *Patients as Effective Collaborators*, The Milbank Fund, 1999
- *Enhancing the Accountability of Alternative Medicine*, The Milbank Fund, 1998

Government entities are sources of trend data. The "Healthy People 2000" initiative is a good example of a coordinated and comprehensive assessment of disease prevention needs conducted by the U.S. Public Health Service (US Public Health Service, 2000). This project has three goals: (1) increase the span of healthy life for Americans, (2) reduce health disparities among Americans, and (3) achieve access to preventive services for all Americans.

The Pew Health Professions Commission (1998) promulgated an insightful listing of "Twenty-One Competencies for the 21st Century." Please refer to Table 25–2.

This document provides a template for rehabilitation professionals in understanding their future role, expectations, and competency needs as expressed by an independent, outside-the-box source. Of course, rehabilitation providers must also look to their peers and professional associations for additional direction.

Table 25–2 21 Competencies for the 21st Century

1. Embrace a personal ethic of social responsibility and service
2. Exhibit ethical behavior in all professional activities
3. Provide evidence-based, clinically competent care
4. Incorporate the multiple determinants of health in clinical care
5. Apply knowledge of the new science
6. Demonstrate critical thinking, reflection, and problem-solving skills
7. Understand the role of primary care
8. Rigorously practice preventive health care
9. Integrate population-based care and services into practice
10. Improve access to health care for those with unmet health needs
11. Practice relationship-centered care with individuals and families
12. Provide culturally sensitive care to a diverse society
13. Partner with communities in health care decisions
14. Use communication and information technology effectively and appropriately
15. Work in interdisciplinary teams
16. Ensure care that balances individual, professional, system and societal needs
17. Practice leadership
18. Take responsibility for quality of care and health outcomes at all levels
19. Contribute to continuous improvement of the health care system
20. Advocate for public policy that promotes and protects the health of the public
21. Continue to learn and help others learn

Data from The Pew Health Professions Commission: Recreating Health Professional Practice for a New Century. The Pew Charitable Trusts, administered by the University of California Center for the Health Professions, 1998, http://www.futurehealth.ucsf.edu/pewcommm.html, accessed September 5, 1999.

NEW PARADIGMS

The following vignettes describe new health care paradigms that are based on historical patterns, current evidence, logic, and a significant degree of speculation. Rehabilitation providers will command an invaluable role in virtually every one of these evolving paradigms. This of course, assumes a certain degree of provider buy-in, innovation, and tolerance for risk taking (Table 25–3).

Table 25–3 Paradigm Shifts: A Sampler

Old Paradigm	New/Future Paradigm
Single discipline focus of rehabilitation	Functional teams in collaborative model
Patients referred to rehabilitation by other medical personnel	Patients/consumers self-refer
Clinician directly renders care	Patients or other support staff render care or patient engages in self-help
Physical plant-based services	Cyberspace-based services (e.g., telemedicine, consumer education)
Education supplements care	Education is care
Payer-provider tension or competition	Partnerships between providers-payers
Patient-focused	Consumer-focused
Rehabilitation-focused	Habilitation-focused

NOTE: There is no clear temporal demarcation between "old" and "new/future" paradigms. Some old models are carried forward and some future models of delivery have already begun.

Paradigm Shift No. 1: Medical to Health Focus

Current insurance plans and health care organizations are principally structured around the idea that medical care will be provided after injury or illness afflicts people. Although there are some preventive health programs, the health care system in America is fundamentally treatment-centered. In the next transformation of health care, treatment will be secondary to prevention of injury and illness. Under this new model, hospitals and physicians will continue to lose a degree of control as other participants play roles that are more pivotal. This can only benefit physical rehabilitation providers. Continued expansion in the application of extenders of care, community-based services, consumer education, and information technology will relegate physicians to a lesser role.

This is especially true of those physicians who continue to restrict their focus on an impairment or pathology level and fail to assess function. The reality is that many of the specific services physicians currently perform will be done by physician assistants, nurse practitioners, and perhaps physical and occupational therapists.

Telemedicine that uses online communication and remote testing capabilities exemplifies a trend that will potentially reduce the amount of time patients directly spend with practitioners. This too reflects a health-focused versus medical-focused approach.

Paradigm Shift No. 2: Demand-Driven Versus Supply-Driven Providers

In 1998, The Pew Health Professions Commission published a 142-page report entitled "Recreating Health Professional Practice for a New Century." This thoughtful report is essential reading for both the entry-level rehabilitation provider as well as advanced clinicians. The report concludes that professional health education has traditionally expanded on its own accord, irrespective of emerging market forces or health care sector direction. Essentially, providers and their professional organizations determined whether more therapists should be trained and released into the market. It is quite obvious that the supplier-driven approach has not succeeded (The Pew Health Professions Commission, 1998).

One excellent example of this can be found in physical therapy. The American Physical Therapy Association (APTA) actively encouraged the development of new schools producing master's degree, entry-level practitioners. Leaders in this profession had proclaimed a severe shortage of physical therapists throughout the 1980s and most of the 1990s. The response was an explosion of physical therapy and physical therapist assistant programs throughout the United States. This trend was in direct opposition to a study indicating no shortage, but an actual surplus of physical therapists (APTA, 1997).

This supply-driven strategy resulted in unprecedented cutbacks in PT staff nationwide as managed care had diminished its role through various mechanisms such as "gatekeepers," reduced benefit structures and beneficiary financial risk-sharing in the form of higher deductibles or co-payments. It could be argued that the drop in PT utilization was part of the natural cycle following zealous growth in the 1980s. Fortunately, with every change there are opportunities.

The Pew Health Professions Commission published a number of useful recommendations that set a vision for tomorrow's health care providers:

1. *"Change professional training to meet the demands of the new health care system."*

A failure to subscribe to a market-driven approach will result in reduced autonomy and influence within the emerging health care system. Health professionals will need to continually consider how they add value to the system. Professions must be aligned in size and scope to meet public needs, not solely personal or professional needs. Otherwise, there will undoubtedly be a shortage of customers and a surplus of providers. Schools that prepare future rehabilitation professionals must continue to reassess their role in an evolving health care system. This may require abandonment of past preferences.

The new health care paradigm will not restrict services but focus on substituting better processes that are evidence-based and more promising in terms of outcomes, both functionally and financially (Entoven & Vorhaus, 1997).

2. *"Ensure that the health profession workforce reflects the diversity of the nation's population."*

The next generation of health professionals should represent the nation through a diversity that allows it to reach the populations that bear the greatest burdens of poor health and non-access to care. A diverse provider pool will facilitate a greater understanding of cultural differences, especially as they pertain to behavioral responses to illness and injury.

3. *"Require interdisciplinary competencies in all health professionals."*

A strong trend currently exists and is expected to continue for interdisciplinary or multidisciplinary teams of providers working in integrated health delivery systems. A collaborative approach that is patient-focused, not departmentally or disciplinarily focused, will be required. This will require a de-emphasis on professional titles and a shared interdisciplinary vision of care.

4. *"Continue to move education into ambulatory practice."*

This recommendation is an easy one for physical rehabilitation providers because many of them have served internships or affiliations in non-hospital settings. This will represent a greater challenge for physicians and other ancillary staff that are traditionally hospital-trained or institutionally based. Because hospitals no longer render a majority of services, this shift in clinical internship focus is a logical extension.

As more rehabilitation is moved into alternative settings, educational training programs will follow the lead until interns or affiliates are found in home care, subacute, employer onsite centers, schools, private practices, government facilities, and other nontraditional settings.

 Table 25-4 Core Elements of a Public Health Service

- Prevent epidemics
- Protect food/water supply
- Promote healthy behavior
- Serve the needs of high-risk persons
- Disaster responses
- Protection of the environment
- Development of health policy
- Foster health research
- Monitor public's health

From US Centers for Disease Control and Prevention: Core Functions of Public Health. Atlanta, GA, Centers for Disease Control and Prevention, 1991.

5. *"Encourage public service of all health professional students and graduates."*

Few physical rehabilitation providers have any experience in the arena of public or community-based health delivery. This will become increasingly important as the trend towards community health and self-care continues to grow. This will be an especially important goal consistent with provider diversity, preventive-focused, and community-based efforts.

Table 25-4 describes the basic elements of a public health service. A growing role for public health services is predicted especially, targeting vulnerable populations (Wall, 1998).

Unlike medicine's focus on "treatment," public health focuses on health promotion. The Institute of Medicine (IOM) has defined three core elements of public health as:

1. Assessment
2. Policy development
3. Policy assurance

All three of these areas invite rehabilitation provider participation (IOM, 1988).

Paradigm Shift No. 3: From Acute Care to Post-Acute Care

Many acute conditions resolve with or without treatment, are adequately managed with current methodologies, or go on to become chronic or post-acute conditions. An entire chapter of this book is devoted to the issue of chronicity. Rehabilitation providers are perhaps the best clinicians in managing chronic conditions due to intimate knowledge of clinical and psychosocial issues. To date, managed care has done a modest job at best and a poor job at worst in managing chronic illnesses and injuries.

Paradigm Shift No. 4: Providers as Mentors or Partners in Patient Self-Care

Teaching is the profession at the very core of all professions and trades. Teachers prepare others to apply knowledge and skill sets. Why should rehabilitation professionals not serve a similar role with persons who must learn to self-manage chronic or incurable conditions such as diabetes, arthritis, or heart disease? These people live with their conditions 24/7 and are better served when receiving information and skill sets that promote self-help. Rehabilitation providers are uniquely positioned to convert their knowledge into educational and training modules for patient consumption. Disease state management programs serve as current examples wherein education is the keystone that supports other services. Tomorrow's rehabilitation programs must be designed as turnkey approaches to facilitate patient empowerment. The former "treatment" paradigm implies a laying on of hands that will effect a change or, optimally, a cure. The new paradigm values self-sufficiency over treatment.

Habilitation of the client is a more appropriate goal than *re*habilitation that implies a return to one's previous level or state of wholeness.

Providers must be cognizant that patient education and empowerment may be predicated on a minimal baseline of literacy and comprehension. Recent evidence provides disturbing evidence that many patients lack the fundamental and assumed ability to understand information and instructions necessary to effectively self-manage their health (Gasmararian, 1999). Illiteracy is a genuine obstacle facing this paradigm shift. Could it be that only those with an adequate degree of education are candidates for self-empowerment and self-care?

The human and capital costs of health illiteracy are staggering. Over 44 million Americans are considered functionally illiterate, with another 53 million marginally illiterate (Friedland, 1998). These persons have an inability or great difficulty in understanding the simplest instructions for medication prescriptions, informed consent, and comprehending laboratory results. This problem is in direct conflict with the need to promote self-help, patient responsibility, and empowerment. Rehabilitation professionals, because of their potentially significant role in chronic care management, can take the lead in educational programs. Should they accept this challenge, rehabilitation providers can ameliorate the effects of non-access to care, poor care, or the unnecessary development of chronic conditions.

This system (public health) remains essentially fragmented with enormous variations in service scope, quality, and outcomes. Rehabilitation professional associations need to take a more aggressive, participatory role in the standardization of this sector.

Government entities must rededicate themselves to a full commitment as a mere one percent of the national health care dollar is spent on local, state, and federal programs (Center for Studying Health System Change, 1996). In 1993 public health programs accounted for $18.4 billion dollars in spending, which at first glance appears to be quite significant; however, this is miniscule when compared to the aggregate dollars spent on treatment (Wall, 1998).

Paradigm Shift No. 5: Telehealth or Telemedicine Augments Hands-on Rehabilitation

Telemedicine, telehealth, and telerehabilitation involve the use of electronic communication and information technologies to provide or support clinical care without a physical presence or hands-on involvement. Support for telehealth appears to be growing (Bauer, 2002; Kelly, 2002). Telehealth serves a number of purposes, including the following:

- Provider continued education
- Independent consultation

- Diagnostic image assessment
- Direction of care
- Patient monitoring
- Patient instruction/education
- Family instruction/education

The use of the Internet will continue to grow and augment current hands-on treatment. Net-based educational materials will play an instrumental role, especially in chronic disease management. This trend parallels the growth in self-help for conditions such as neurological disorders (e.g., multiple sclerosis, Parkinson's disease), arthritis, cardiopulmonary conditions, and diabetes.

Chapter 12 provides greater detail in terms of the various applications in information technology that will evolve and have direct bearing on how rehabilitation providers manage care.

Presently, telemedicine enjoys greater use in Europe than in the United States (Couturier et al, 1998; Lemaire & Jeffreys, 1998; Riva & Gamberini, 2000; Samad et al, 2002). A wide range of applications have been reported in the literature. Telemedicine has been applied in the management of leg ulcers, pediatric cardiology, spinal cord trauma, stroke, adult cardiac conditions, geriatric rehabilitation, and orthotic assessment (Ades et al, 2000; Couturier, 1998; Lemaire & Jeffreys, 1998; Phillips et al, 2001; Sable, 2002; Samad et al, 2002; Sparks et al, 1993; Tran et al, 2002).

Telerehabilitation with post-CVA patients may prevent delayed or fragmented rehabilitation services, especially in rural populations. Additionally, physical therapy exercises have been communicated through virtual reality technology (Popescu et al, 2000).

The telemedicine market continues to grow with the prospects for a bright future (Bauer, 2002; Hospital Case Management, 1999; Popescu, 2000; Temkin et al, 1996). Telemedicine guidelines of a clinical, operational, and technical nature continue to develop but remain in its infancy (Loane & Wootton, 2002). Some advocate the development of international guidelines. Savings from telemedicine consultations have been reported (Brunicardi, 1998).

Telemedicine, despite its promise, is not without its challenges (O'Brien, 2002; Riva & Gamberini, 2000). Reimbursement mechanisms have yet to be fully developed and may be problematic (Jacobsen, 2002).

Paradigm Shift No. 6: Increased Access to Health Care

The shell game of cost shifting will cease if we as a society agree that a reasonable degree of universal health care coverage is a right accorded to all Americans. The current system of resource distribution and allocation is predicated on denial of service access to select groups of patients. Managed care has served to heighten consumers' awareness of access to health care restrictions and, consequentially, has resulted in tremendous antimanaged care backlash. A majority of Americans (52%) believe that the federal government should regulate managed care organizations (Blendon et al, 1998).

The current health care debate is framed by two opposing schools of thought: "medicalists" and "marketists"

(Glied, 1997). Glied describes "medicalists" as those persons or entities that view health care as a right, equity as a goal, and government as the solution to health care distribution and financing challenges. "Marketists" to the contrary, view health care as a commodity to be purchased and sold through the same market forces that impact on other goods and services. Marketists generally prefer voucher or medical savings accounts (MSAs) over guaranteed health care.

Some believe that the current medical model in America is based upon the false hope that medical science can master death and illness (Callahan, 1998). Callahan proposes "sustainable medicine" that possesses the following attributes:

> *"It will, first, provide the people of a society with a level of medical and public health care sufficient to give them a good chance of making it through the life cycle and of functioning at a decent level of physical and mental competence. It will, second, be a medicine that can be equitably distributed without undue strain, affordable to the society. It must be, third, be a medicine that has, with public support embraced finite and steady-state health goals and has limited aspirations for progress and technological innovation."*

Rehabilitation providers are well positioned in Callahan's alternative health care delivery model. Any model that proposes universal coverage can only benefit rehabilitation providers who currently reside well down the managed care referral chain, often rendering discretionary services versus essential ones. However, rehabilitation providers must alter their current paradigm of "rehabilitation" in favor of "habilitation" if they are to seize new opportunities presented by equitable health care financing and delivery models.

Paradigm Shift No. 7: Habilitation Supplants Rehabilitation as the Dominant Model of Delivery

Has rehabilitation operated on the false pretense that persons will be *r*estored or *r*ehabilitated to their pre-morbid, pre-injury, or pre-illness state? Perhaps the term rehabilitation sets providers up for failure in a system of limited resources, particularly for chronic or catastrophic conditions that generally cannot be cured? Rehabilitation providers must accept the reality that habilitation is the reality, not rehabilitation. Is it not the ultimate goal of all physical and occupational therapy to facilitate a patient's adaptation or habilitation to their own unique environs, whether it is work, school, home, sports, or the community at large?

This paradigm shift is consistent with the shift from a medical model to a health model to an independent living model described in the Americans with Disabilities Act of 1990 (ADA) (ADA, 1990). Because individual functioning is largely mediated by the environment, new measures will evolve to describe environmental barriers (National Center for Dissemination of Disability Research). Tomorrow's therapists may focus more on environmental issues. A person's condition may be viewed less from a medical-centric position and more from an environmental perspective.

 Table 25–5 A Sampler of Veterans Affairs Technology Initiatives: Human-Environment Interfacement

"A self-adaptive digital processor for prosthesis control"
"Body powered toddler hands"
"Obstacle avoidance training with computer simulated environments: A pilot study"
"FES-aided paraplegic cart using a controllable friction brake"
"Paraplegic walking made practical with FNS and orthoses"
"Minimizing falls in the elderly"
"Trans-train: Transdisciplinary training of rehabilitation personnel in assistive technology"
"Force sensors for control of power wheelchairs"
"The determination of environmental accessibility and wheelchair user proficiency through virtual simulation"

Specifically, providers will attempt to facilitate adaptive features, both behavioral and technological, with the goal of inclusion and productivity of persons with disabilities. Evidence of this shift is strong and represented by broad research addressing human-environment matching (Department of Veteran Affairs, 1997).

The federal Department of Veteran Affairs periodically publishes research projects focusing on assistive devices designed to overcome environmental barriers while maximizing individuals' functioning. Table 25–5 portrays a sampler of technology initiatives that show promise in disability prevention and management (US Department of Veterans Affairs).

The future beyond managed care looks very bright for physical rehabilitation providers who possess additional credentials in biomedical engineering, human factors, ergonomics, industrial engineering, and adaptive or assistive technology.

Figure 25–2 depicts an independent living paradigm for rehabilitation that attempts to balance the triad of client functionality, assistive technology, and environmental adaptations. Reasonable accommodations under ADA exemplify this approach to rehabilitation or, better yet, habilitation. Reasonable accommodations attempt to facilitate a safe match of the worker to the worksite through a combination of administrative or engineering controls.

Administrative controls include rest breaks, job rotation, job sharing, additional training, and policy/procedure revisions. Engineering controls include assistive or adaptive

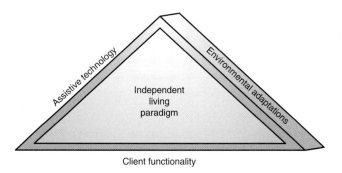

Figure 25–2. Independent living paradigm.

devices, environmental modifications, powered mobility, prosthetics/orthotics, visual aids, and tool redesign that maximize function while avoiding exacerbations of one's condition.

Paradigm Shift No. 8: Rehabilitation Selectively Embraces Alternative Health

A paradigm shift related to the medical-focus to health-focus involves the increasing use of complementary and alternative medicine (CAM) or alternative health interventions. Readers are referred to the separate chapter on CAM for more details.

CAM is aggressively sought, especially by persons with chronic conditions who do not perceive or enjoy the benefits of traditional medical interventions. These users are willing to pay privately for services that are often not supported by clinical research or other forms of evidence. This observation alone should speak volumes to those who fail to address the holistic needs of these persons. On balance, CAM also offers its users more self-help options than does traditional medicine.

Medical providers, including physical rehabilitation professionals, should explore the possibilities of carefully incorporating selected CAM interventions into their traditional practices or run the risk of losing these patients to other practitioners. Those who have been in practice long enough recall the days when osteopathic doctors (DOs) were frowned upon by medical doctors (MDs), when chiropractors were considered empirics with little of value to offer, and when physical therapy was struggling for recognition and validation by others in the medical community. Today, all three of these professions are widely embraced, receive reimbursement for their services, and are considered mainstream practitioners. Should medical providers criticize CAM practitioners in light of the fact that many so-called mainstream practices are without appropriate levels of validation? Based upon these observations, should not an open mind be maintained by traditional providers when considering CAM interventions? Should these providers consider augmenting services either through referrals to CAM providers or by adopting some of the more promising techniques? Physical rehabilitation and CAM share a number of notable attributes. Both value a holistic approach, both focus on function, both emphasize self-help, and both serve as alternatives to medication and invasive procedures.

Paradigm Shift No. 9: Rehabilitation Providers' Professional Health Education

Providers, their educational institutions, and professional organizations have a choice of either responding to change or becoming agents of change themselves. One means of accepting the role of change agent is to reconfigure how it is we educate and train rehabilitation providers. Traditional professional education expanded on its own accord, often without regard for market-demands. The Vector study regarding the oversupply of physical therapists exemplifies this tradition. Data suggest that a supplier-driven approach has been unsuccessful (The Pew Health Professions Commission, 1998). An oversupply of physical therapists was created at a time when managed care reduced the need for therapy through financial disincentives (e.g. non-referral for profit by primary care physicians or PCPs and through the promotion of extenders of care who were less expensive).

Educational programs for allied health professionals were traditionally discipline-focused. Physical therapists were trained to go into physical therapy centers, occupational therapists into occupational therapy settings. There is now a strong trend toward interdisciplinary or team-based practice. Some schools have responded by integrating selected coursework and affiliations across various disciplines.

A new paradigm has emerged in the form of problem-based learning (PBL) (Bruhn, 1992). Problem-based learning organizes curriculum based upon clinical problems. This is a departure from subject or theoretical-based curriculum. Problem-based learning values analytical and cognitive skills more than knowledge for knowledge's sake. The trend towards holistic health care supports PBL as both promote a dynamic, versus a static, approach to care delivery. Today's clinician must be more adaptable and amenable to change. He or she must understand the paradigms of multiple health care stakeholders and be willing to collaborate, even when it means teaching or instructing others to perform their previous job tasks.

The Pew Health Professions Commission's (1998) "Twenty-One Competencies for the 21st Century" (see Table 25-2) provides a template of trends that need to be considered when designing and implementing educational programs.

The following competencies directly relate to educational program design:

- Provide evidence-based, clinically competent care
- Embrace a personal ethic of social responsibility and service
- Incorporate the multiple determinants of health in clinical care
- Demonstrate critical thinking, reflection, and problem-solving skills
- Understand the role of primary care
- Partner with communities in health care decisions
- Work in interdisciplinary teams
- Ensure care that balances individual, professional, system, and societal needs
- Continue to learn and to help others

Paradigm Shift No. 10: Rehabilitation-Educated Medical Students

Retooling rehabilitation professional education is only part of the formula geared towards collaborative care. Rehabilitation providers must assist others in understanding their specialty, particularly about when and how to refer for services. Medical students have traditionally received very little didactic or theoretical education/training specific to disability and rehabilitation. The aging of Americans coupled with exponential growth in chronic illness are two trends certain to spawn more educational modules specific to rehabilitation's role in disability prevention and management.

Crotty et al (2000) describe an effective approach to educating medical students and physical rehabilitation and disability management. This training involves four activities, including following a patient through his or her inpatient rehabilitation multidisciplinary program. Next, medical students visit two patients who are living with disabilities in the community. During these visits they assess the patients' physical, mental, and social status. The third cog in the wheel involves visitation of a community-based service directed at those with disabilities. Simulating a person by randomly assigning a specific disability case to constitutes the last and perhaps most important stage of their four-week training module.

Flax acknowledges limitations of physiatrists in a presentation entitled "The Future of Physical Medicine and Rehabilitation" (Flax, 2002). Flax describes holistic care as a first for physiatry and acknowledges that accomplishment of this goal requires the following elements: ancillary medical personnel or rehabilitation team, physiatrist as the primary care physician, and residency programs that prepare physical medicine and rehabilitation (PMandR) physicians as primary care clinicians. Flax notes that only twenty-eight percent of all physiatrists work in rehabilitation units.

Paradigm Shift No. 11: Rehabilitation-Educated Extenders of Care

Extenders of care such as physician assistants, nurse practitioners, physical therapist assistants, and certified occupational therapist assistants have become a prevalent force in health care (Managed Care Interfacement, 1998). This trend promises to continue into the foreseeable future. The need to offer efficient, cost-effective care under managed care at-risk reimbursement schemes (e.g., capitation, case rates) directly fuels the growth in extenders of care (Managed Care Interfacement, 1998; Sheppard, 1994). However, the Balanced Budget Act (BBA) has an equally, if not more, profound effect because of mandated cost cuts or quotas across various treatment settings (Wilson, 1998).

The goal of cost effectiveness has been reported with the use of extenders (Managed Care Interfacement, 1998). Controversy has swirled around the use of extenders over the past half century (Curry, 1953; Gray, 1964; Moyer, 1972; Nickelson, 1996; Perry, 1966; Robinson et al, 1994; Sheppard, 1994).

The use of physician extenders, including nurse practitioners and physician assistants, means that rehabilitation providers must focus some of their educational efforts towards this highly influential group in addition to primary care physicians and physical medicine and rehabilitation (PMandR) physicians or physiatrists. One cannot assume that this latter group is sufficiently educated in rehabilitation practices and principles or possessive of intimate knowledge of physical or occupational therapy interventions, despite the fact that they are often the trigger for rehabilitation referrals.

Physician extenders of care and primary care physicians (PCPs) must be trained to recognize candidates for rehabilitation, command a working knowledge of admission criteria, and comprehend physical rehabilitation documentation, assessment tools, treatment interventions, outcome measures, and discharge criteria.

Physician assistants acknowledge the need for more information about physical rehabilitation (Saladin et al, 1999). Again, this presents physical rehabilitation providers with a unique opportunity to collaborate in the development of education/training tools that are beneficial to all parties, but especially patients.

Paradigm Shift No. 12: Collaborative Care Delivery Model

Various terms are used both interchangeably and distinctly to describe situations in which multiple providers coordinate their services: interdisciplinary, multidisciplinary, interprofessional, and integrated care. Review of the clinical literature requires that clinicians carefully evaluate operational definitions before drawing conclusions about collaborative care.

There appears to be a strong and growing trend concerning the use of collaborative care for a multitude of conditions (Hankin et al, 2001; McCallin, 2001). A multidisciplinary approach for upper extremity conditions successfully utilized physiatry, OT, PT, pain psychology, and vocational counseling services (Tong, 2001). Chronic pain has been managed with improvements found in cognition and coping mechanisms (Jensen et al, 2001). Post-stroke care has been reported to be successful with fewer complications when using a multidisciplinary model (Ozdemir et al, 2001). Maximization of functional outcomes in persons with cerebral palsy has been reported secondary to a multidisciplinary approach (Gormely, 2001). Similar reports have been published regarding sub-acute services in low back pain, (Karjalainen et al, 2001), proximal femoral fractures (Cameron et al, 2000), leg ischemia (Tomlinson, 2000), chronic low back pain (Geddes & Chamberlain, 2001), diabetic-related foot amputations (Apelquist & Larson, 2000), cancer (Cole et al, 2000), congestive heart failure (Kasper et al, 2002), and following total replacement surgery (Ridge & Goodson, 2000).

Comparative studies of multidisciplinary service versus primary care have yielded mixed results. Grahn et al (2000) found that multidisciplinary rehabilitation programs for a variety of musculoskeletal disorders (MSDs) were more effective than primary care only. Geddes and Chamberlain (2001) reported more than 86% of 912 post-stroke patients returned to community living following a general practitioner oriented program. Cameron et al (2000) in a study of 1069 patients with post-operative hip fractures, did not find a multidisciplinary approach to be conclusively effective. Yet some have found multidisciplinary community-based rehabilitation to be effective even years after initial traumatic brain injuries (Powell et al, 2002).

Benefits to patients, referral sources, and managed care organizations attributed to an integrated delivery approach has been reported (Matalon et al, 2002). Multidisciplinary disability management services have been cost-effective and efficient when a four-step strategy is employed (Clanet & Brassat, 2000):

1. Multidisciplinary assessment
2. Identification of potential areas of functional improvement
3. Short-term and long-term goal setting
4. Outcomes measurement

Questionable benefits have been associated with the use of multidisciplinary services in the management of selected conditions. Karjalainen et al (2000) conducted an analysis of 1808 abstracts related to the management of fibromyalgia. Only seven abstracts met their inclusion criteria. They concluded that there is little scientific evidence to support the use of multidisciplinary services in the management of fibromyalgia. There is a clear need for controlled clinical trials (CCTs) and random controlled trials (RCTs) relative to collaborative models of health care delivery (Karjalainen et al, 2000).

Collaborative care models are often physician-dominated (Gair & Hartery, 2001). Physiatrists or physical medicine and rehabilitation physicians commonly direct health care teams and determine the following attributes of a given case:

- Admission criteria
- Diagnostic work-up
- Treatment setting
- Prescribed services
- Treatment modifications
- Assistive technology prescriptions
- Mobility technology prescriptions
- Discharge criteria

A medical-dominant model tends to reduce participation of other team members, particularly non-physician team members, and can be the antithesis of a collaborative model. Non-physician team members such as occupational or physical therapists may actually possess more clinical expertise in dealing with functionality, disability determination, and patient-worksite accommodations.

Gair and Hartery (2001) advocate a reduction in the level of medical dominance, which leads to a greater contribution among all team members as well as patient care quality and outcomes enhancement. Education and training of all team members is critical to success. Evidence suggests that shared learning models between professional disciplines enhances one's appreciation of other team members (Partis, 2001). One survey of 588 students representing 8 different professions gauged perceptions professionals held about others (Hawk et al, 2002). Physician assistants were found to possess the most positive attitudes towards other professionals, whereas chiropractors held others in the lowest esteem. Physical therapists, osteopathic physicians, nurses, and podiatrists were all fairly consistent in their opinions of other medical professionals.

A common functional language is another prerequisite for successful collaboration (Berman et al, 2000). A language that describes impairment, disability, and handicap supports a multidisciplinary approach because disability management and physical rehabilitation require functional assessments rather than standard clinical and laboratory assessments used by physicians (Clarke et al, 1999).

Consensus documents pertaining to the management of specific conditions can also serve to span the chasm that exists between divergent groups (Johnson et al, 2000). There are a number of examples of multidisciplinary consensus documents produced by the Agency on Healthcare Quality and Research, AHCPR, the Cochrane Reviews, and the Institute of Medicine (IOM) (AHCPR, 2004; Doyle et al 2003; Gatchel & McGeary, 2002; IOM, 1992).

Despite its obvious advantages, multidisciplinary or collaborative care does have its critics (Illman, 2002). A number of authors have reported no significant benefits to early interdisciplinary rehabilitation in whiplash-related disorders (Sterner et al, 2001).

Paradigm Shift No. 13: Strategic Alliances Between Employers-Providers

The assault on managed care coupled with employers' reassertion of control over not only the financing but also the delivery of health care services will present many opportunities for rehabilitation professionals. Providers may enjoy opportunities for direct contracting with employers through a number of services, including prevention, treatment, and disability management (Clifton, 1996; Kennedy & Jennings, 1998).

Figure 25-3 contrasts the current prevalent triad model for health care delivery with a direct contracting model. In the triad model, a provider can only access the employer via the insurer or managed care organization. This will be displaced by an ability to directly contract with employers across the entire injury continuum from prevention to treatment to disability management services.

Employers' most compelling reason for direct contracting is to secure more control over their health care expenditures. The obvious benefit to providers will be removal of a middleman or intermediary in the form of the insurer/MCO. Health maintenance organizations themselves have acknowledged that ancillary services (including physical rehabilitation) are an "employer phenomenon" (Milliman & Robertson, 1995).

Business coalitions or purchasing alliances directly purchase health care services. These networks are similar to provider networks in that they forge partnerships among members in order to gain critical mass, economies of scale, lobbying strength, market share, and leverage in managed care negotiations. There are nearly 100 business coalitions in the United States, with many of them members of a mega-coalition, the National Business Coalition on Health located in Washington, D.C.

There is also a national health care purchasing coalition created by large multi-state employers. The National HMO Purchasing Coalition was formed by eight members, including American Express and Marriott International (Vibbert, 1996). This coalition represents over 600,000 people in more than 27 cities from coast to coast. Unlike many of their local counterparts, this coalition was created as a for-profit operation of William Mercer, Inc. The coalition negotiates significant insurance premium reductions from managed care organizations or MCOs.

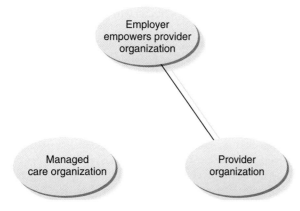

Figure 25–3. Triad model of health care delivery yields to a direct contracting model.

Currently, most business coalitions represent larger employers, but there is good reason to believe that small to mid-sized employers will consolidate in the future in order to enjoy similar advantages. Readers are encouraged to refer to Chapter 27 for an exploded view of other employer-specific opportunities.

Paradigm Shift No. 14: Value Purchasing

Value is in the eye of the beholder and may have little to do with price per se. Because managed care has served to aggregate providers into accountable units, transferred financial risk to both the patient (co-pays, deductibles) and providers (capitation, case rates), and has restrained both unit costs and the number of units purchased (utilization rate), providers must differentiate their services from those of others. *How does one differentiate clinical services?* The facetious response is, "*any way you can!*" However, in a competitive service sector like health care, differentiation comes from demonstrating value to the customer whether that be the patient, employer, third party casualty insurer, or managed care organization. Price alone is typically a losing proposition in a service industry where customer service is the key to business success. Tomorrow's rehabilitation provider will need to demonstrate a value proposition to his or her customers. This value proposition may vary depending on whom one is serving at the time. Employers, insurers, case managers, referring physicians, and patients covet highly unique attributes in their relationship with the physical rehabilitation professional. The provider must discern what is of most value to the particular stakeholder with whom they are dealing in a given situation.

There are many examples of diverse expectations based on a specific stakeholder's unique perspective. For example, although there is currently a strong trend toward delivering evidence-based care, this may be of little interest to the patient, especially a private pay patient.

The surge in alternative health use, which for the most part is without clinical validation, clearly demonstrates that patients are willing to spend money on anything that promises to alleviate human suffering whether or not it is evidence-based. A peer reviewer, payer, professional colleague, or utilization review expert, on the other hand, may rightfully demand evidence to support a particular treatment regime. It is safe to assume that there are some providers who do not perceive the need for evidence-based interventions, provided they adopt a humanitarian approach to patient care.

Table 25-6 contrasts how different issues may have a business-bias or clinical-bias depending upon the stakeholder's particular perspective.

Table 25–6 Stakeholder Issue-Domain Relationship

Stakeholder	Issue	Business	Clinical
Patient/Client	Access to care	X	
	Affordability	X	
	Accurate diagnosis		X
	Medically necessary		X
	"Do no harm"	X	X
	Confidentiality	X	X
	Informed consent	X	X
Providers	Optimal reimbursement	X	
	Paperwork reduction	X	X
	Preauthorization	X	X
	Diagnostic workup		X
	Autonomy	X	X
	Shared risk	X	
Employer	Cost	X	
	Productivity	X	
	Product quality	X	
	Risk management	X	
	Healthy workforce	X	X
Insurer	Cost	X	
	Profit	X	
	Risk management	X	
Investors	Profit	X	
Public/community	Cost on system	X	
	Tax base	X	
	Public health	X	X
	Disease prevention	X	X

NOTE: This table demonstrates how each issue may have a business and/or clinical primary significance depending upon the individual stakeholder and their particular paradigm or focus. Striking a balance between business and clinical aspects of care is essential to success in the emerging community context of health care.

Value is a derivative of the relationship between benefit and cost. Elements that define value purchasing of health care services can be divided into two general categories, administrative and clinical. Administrative elements do not directly contribute to clinical success but are enablers of clinical success. For instance, accessibility to health care, affordability, confidentiality covenants, and informed consent are facilitators of value-driven care. Diagnostic acumen, medical necessity, and reasonable treatment exemplify clinical components of the value statement. There are some components that bridge both clinical and administrative domains. A provider's oath to do no harm illustrates an issue that spans both domains.

Paradigm Shift No. 15: Continued Growth of Rehabilitation Networks

Rehabilitation networks should continue to grow if they provide value to their multiple customers: patients/clients, employers, insurers, case managers, disability managers, government, and others. These networks are not truly national, but are state, local, or regional in scope. This is due to a number of variables, including state professional regulations, the patchwork quilt of workers' compensation laws, local geopolitical influences, and the fact that the majority of employers are small to mid-sized, and not national in scope. There is relatively little demand for national companies in a business sector dominated by small businesses. Even once-large insurance companies have reduced their scale and empowered local offices to make selective contracting decisions. The lesson here is that local culture cannot be ignored when offering health care services.

Despite the torrid consolidation activity within rehabilitation, the market remains fundamentally fragmented. Large publicly traded corporations have consolidated roughly 10% of the market. In some locales, however, they dominate market share. The past five years have not been kind to these efforts as corporate stock values plummeted after their intoxicating rise during the late 1980s and early 1990s. Large publicly traded rehabilitation companies commonly market that they are "fully integrated networks" when in reality, only the business-side (e.g., financial pages) is truly integrated. Few have truly integrated their clinical services, especially across treatment settings (e.g., from inpatient to outpatient). Again, local cultural differences often dictate how services are rendered.

Rehabilitation networks must possess certain attributes if they are to be successful in the emerging health care economy. A comprehensive system for grading networks has been proposed (Clifton, 1998). This system examines attributes across three spheres: structure, process, and outcome. Networks are given an "A" (excellent), "C" (average), or "F" (failure) under this schema. Tables 25–7 through 25–13 contain criteria divided into the following:

- Network credentialing and recredentialing
- Continuum of care
- Technology requirements
- Treatment protocols and guidelines
- Outcome measures
- Documentation standards
- Risk assumption

This grading scheme is based on common sense and utility, not empirical research.

Paradigm Shift No. 16: Chronic Illness and Injury

Managed care has essentially wrung much of the excess cost out of the system in mature markets. We are now in a new cycle of rising medical costs and elevated insurance premiums. Much of this has to do with managed care's early focus on the easy target of reduced cost—acute care. Chronic care will surely drive the next era of health care, given the shifting population demographics. However, to date, managed care has had a minimal impact on these costs. Further, the cost controls of HMOs have come at a price for patients (Cadette, 1998).

It is estimated that by the year 2008 health expenditures will exceed $2.2 trillion (Smith et al, 1999), calculated at an annual rate increase of 6%. This represents 16.2% of the gross domestic product. These data mimic the 1980s, a decade of spiraling costs, and will inevitably lead to new innovations in health care finance and delivery. The number of underinsured and uninsured are projected to escalate well into the next decade. This population is rife with chronic conditions and, if a mechanism can be created to afford them care, this may be a boon for rehabilitation, given its prominence in the management of these conditions. (Refer to Chapter 22 for a more detailed examination of this issue.) Medicare spending will continue to climb despite the cost-reduction quotas tied to the Balanced Budget Amendment (BBA). The decline in hospital use will only represent 30% of national health care expenditures, down from 37% in 1997 (Smith, 1999).

There is a common misconception that the American health care system is an employer-sponsored or employer-based system. Yes, it may be true that employers pay the insurance premiums to third party insurers and MCOs, but it is the employee who ultimately pays (Cadette, 1998; Kuttner, 1999). Employees pay through wage and benefit concessions. In today's managed care market, with higher co-payments and deductibles, enrollees actually take a triple hit. They receive lower wages in lieu of health insurance, are at greater financial risk via co-payments or deductibles and must endure restrictive benefit structures that tell which service they qualify for (access), how much of it they can receive (utilization rates), the cost of the service, and from whom they must receive it. Insult is added to injury when employees must self-purchase supplemental medical benefits, especially for coverage of their families. This has partly contributed to the groundswell of anti-managed care sentiment. This practice is considered to be reprehensible as "virtually all ethicists have condemned America's private, voluntary purchase approach to health insurance *as a national disgrace*" (Banja, 2000).

This system leaves many underinsured or uninsured and usurps those that are insured of their freedom of choice and autonomy. Yet, in 1998, over 160 million Americans received employer-sponsored health insurance (US Bureau of the Census, 1999). Rehabilitation providers will directly benefit when the underinsured and uninsured

Table 25-7 Networking Credentialing and Recredentialing

A Grade:

1) Providers compare outcome measures, patient satisfaction surveys and other performance measures to normative database (recredentialing only).
2) All providers, eg, PTs, OTs, practice their discipline at least 20 hours/week.
3) All practitioners have functioning knowledge of managed care strategies—this way require that a "pretest" be administered with a minimal passing grade established.
4) Providers are certified by the federal Medicare program as either freestanding rehab agencies or as independent physical therapy practices.
5) Support personnel (assistants, aides) are on-site supervised and guided by licensed personnel.
6) Provider ratios do not exceed two full-time support staff per licensed professional, eg, two physical therapy assistants per one PT, two certified occupational therapy assistants per one OT.
7) Providers demonstrate at least 3 years of experience in the treatment of specific patient population, eg, age group, diagnostic conditions.
8) Providers apply well-referenced treatment protocols for specific conditions.
9) Providers are willing to accept risk for payment based on outcome measures that have been coestablished by health plan and provider organization.
10) Networks have a track record of expelling members who:
    a) do not meet optimal standards of care (versus minimal standards as in a "C" grade).
    b) have treatment durations and costs that exceed central tendency measures (eg, median) by more than two standard deviations.
    c) promote services for which they are not equipped (from a technology or expertise standpoint) to cost-effectively deliver.
    d) have been convicted of a felony.
    e) have had their licensure revoked and/or suspended.
    f) have been convicted of an ethical violation.
    g) have balanced billed patients under at-risk contracts (including Medicare).
    h) have had their Medicare certification revoked.
11) Providers participate in the network's internal or external quality assurance utilization review program.
12) Professional liability policy is of an occurrence basis (versus claims-made).
13) Individual providers are capable of participating in electronic claims submission.
14) Providers compare their individual clinical outcomes and patient (consumer) satisfaction surveys to comparative database adjusted by geography, severity indices, age, etc.
15) Providers are willing to accept reasonable levels of "pro bono" service, eg, <5%.

C Grade:

1) Therapists or providers are graduates of an accredited school.
2) Therapists or providers successfully passed the appropriate state licensure examination.
3) Providers have a minimum of 3 years of clinical experience (in any specialty area).
4) Providers possess minimum professional liability insurance thresholds of $1,000,000 single occurrence, $3,000,000 aggregate. Policy is minimally a claims-made policy.
5) Providers adhere to minimally acceptable clinical documentation standards as promulgated by their professional trade association, eg, American Physical Therapy Association, American Occupational Therapy Association.
6) Providers minimally track clinical outcome measures manually.
7) Only licensed professionals evaluate, revaluate, and modify treatment plans, and engage in discharge planning activities.

F Grade:

1) Networks fill their provider roster based on which providers offer discounted fees (common among worker's compensation preferred providers organizations).
2) Networks are developed strictly out of the need for geographic coverage and nothing more.
3) Facilities and providers are purchased to fill a specific service or geographic need irrespective of quality indicators.
4) Networks offer services rendered by nonprofessional persons primarily for the sake of cost-containment versus "value purchasing."
5) Networks are devoid of those attributes listed under grades "A" and "C."

Reprinted with permission. DW: Making the grade. Part II. Case Review/Rehab Manage 4(5):18-24, 1998.

finally receive adequate health care for a variety of chronic conditions.

RESPONDING TO CHANGE

"There is nothing more difficult to take in hand, more perilous to conduct, or more uncertain in its success, than to take the lead in the introduction of a new order of things."

- Niccolo Machiavelli

Health care providers have been both witness to and subjects of unparalleled change over the past decade. The pace of change shows no signs of slowing. Double-digit medical inflation has returned, a patient's bill of rights continues to be debated, Medicare reimbursement policies continue to shift, and a plethora of managed care bills exist. If managed care is an interim step, then what is next as health care continues its transformation? How will rehabilitation providers then deal with change?

The first step in dealing with change is to acknowledge it. Changes have impacted virtually every realm of physical rehabilitation, from ownership to clinical practice.

All change, both good and bad, creates a certain degree of stress, uncertainty, and fear. Typical responses to change are not dissimilar to stages of grieving: denial, anger, bargaining, disorientation, depression, and sadness (Blendon et al, 1998). Bridges asserts that "it isn't the changes that do you in, it's the transitions." Change is situational and external to a person, whereas transition is the psychological process people go through in coming to terms with the new situation.

Table 25-8   Continuum of Care

Grade A:

1) Physical rehabilitation services are offered at various treatment settings including inpatient, outpatient, home care, skilled nursing facilities, on-site.
2) Rehab services include physical therapy, occupational therapy, speech and language, and respiratory therapy.
3) Rehab services include physiatry/physical medicine and rehabilitation, and chiropractic care.
4) Rehab services involve alternative health care when necessary and considered a covered expense.
5) Preventive services offered include ergonomic screenings, postoffer or preemployment examinations, nutritional counselling, home environmental screens, etc.
6) Patient, payer, referring physician, case manager, and employer educational programs are offered.
7) Independent physical therapy evaluations are available.
8) Disability evaluations or functional capacity evaluations are available.
9) Providers are willing to offer a case or episodic rate irrespective of how many and which treatment setting are required to produce the desired clinical outcome.
10) Providers participate in "disease state management" through the following mechanisms:
    a) disease mapping
    b) treatment based on condition, not available reimbursement
    c) diversified treatment settings
    d) ability to "carve-out" portions of care
    e) Proven cost-effective treatment/management interventions
    f) Strong educational elements for all stakeholders

Grade C:

1) Network provides two or more rehab services.
2) Network provides two or more treatment settings.
3) Providers are willing to attend team conferences or multidisciplinary rounds.
4) Network accepts all insurance lines including workers' compensation, disability, group health, auto liability, Medicare, Medicaid, managed Medicare.
5) Network is able to treat two or more of the following: Medicare population, workers' compensation, pediatric, sports medicine.
6) Network has educational programs for two or more of the following: patients, patient's family, case managers, employers, claims adjusters.
7) Network accepts cardiac (stable, nontelemetry), musculoskeletal, neurological case load.

Grade F:

1) Network has only one rehab service.
2) Network has only one treatment setting.
3) Network offers patient education only or has no educational components.
4) Network does not accept all insurance lines.
5) Network serves a narrow or one patient population only.

Reprinted with permission. DW: Making the grade. Part II. Case Review/Rehab Manage 4(5):18-24, 1998.

Table 25-9   Technology Requirements

Grade A:

1) Appointments are made within 24 hours of referral.
2) The rehabilitation network engages in precertification of services.
3) Electronic transmission of claims is available.
4) Clinical outcome measures are tracked via computer with comparison to a national and/or regional database with the ability to segregate data based on age, gender, zip code, treatment setting, condition, and discipline.
5) The patient's condition is described through objective functional measures with timetables for goal achievement.
6) Providers are capable of predicting within reasonable certainty the following treatment costs, duration, and disability status at program's completion for a host of conditions.
7) The rehab network has the necessary equipment and facility orientation to manage musculoskeletal, neurological, and cardiac (stable, nontelemetry) patients.
8) Objective valid/reliable baseline measures of impairment and disability are utilized. These are supported by the following peer consensus, clinical research literature, clinical curriculum and peer review organizations.
9) The provider/facility is willing to execute termination of services clause (preferably "with cause").
10) The network has an internal case management director that coordinates with the employer/health plan case management staff.

Reprinted with permission. DW: Making the grade. Part II. Case Review/Rehab Manage 4(5):18-24, 1998.

Change involves three stages: endings, a neutral zone, and beginnings (Bridges, 1996). A failure to transition to change generally occurs because mistakes are made in the "neutral zone." The neutral zone is a period of time when opportunity can flourish but danger lurks. Bridges describes this period as "an emotional wilderness," "like being between two trapezes," and the "nowhere between two somewheres." All of these terms convey a sense of ambivalence. Figure 25-4 depicts the stages of change and transition.

A failure to bring full closure is one of the biggest reasons why companies and their employees fail when responding to change (Bridges, 1996). Endings occur with virtually every change. Ownership shifts present one of the most challenging changes to rehabilitation providers. Ownership changes in health care occurred frequently throughout the 1980s and 1990s. There are few changes that affect providers more than when their private practice, hospital, or long-term care facility is acquired by a competitor. Changes inherent in mergers and acquisitions are both profound and diverse. In this scenario, a rehabilitation provider has inherited a new employer, co-workers, political structure, corporate mission and vision, and a whole new way of conducting business. Since many

Table 25–10 Treatment Protocols and Guidelines

Grade A:

1) Protocols are tied to current clinical literature.
2) Protocols have been approved by a panel of experts in each specialty area.
3) Protocols are transdisciplinary.
4) Protocols transcend insurance lines and patient populations.
5) Protocols are utilized as part of the network's internal quality assurance utilization review program.
6) Protocols are updated at least annually. The network receives an A+ grade if these are updated on a semiannual basis.
7) Protocols cover at least the top 10-15 conditions managed by the network.
8) Protocols are "condition-specific" versus ICD-9 specific whereby multiple diagnostic codes are collapsed into manageable conditions, eg, low back pain without neurological signs, nonoperative shoulder impingement.
9) Protocols are readily distributed and not kept in a "black box." Networks receive an A+ if protocols are endorsed/accepted by national professional associations.
10) Protocols are adjusted with provider feedback and beta-site testing.
11) Protocols provide a narrow range of visit and disability or treatment durations adjusted for severity, existence of comorbidities, or secondary diagnoses.

Grade C:

1) Protocols are ICD-9 or code driven.
2) Protocols are not beta-site tested.
3) Protocols describe a narrow patient population.
4) Protocols are updated annually.
5) Protocols are applicable to one discipline only.

Grade F:

1) Protocols are based on anecdotal information, not hard data, eg, appropriate clinical literature.
2) Protocols are site-specific and not correlated with existing treatment protocols used by other institutions.
3) Protocols are not shared with providers, case managers, health plans, and referring physicians.
4) Protocols are used only to maximize reimbursement versus improve cost-effectiveness and treatment outcomes.
5) No attempt is made to adjust protocols secondary to patient populations, age, gender, severity indices, comorbidities, and secondary diagnoses.
6) Treatment or disability durations are so broad as to render the protocol useless.

Reprinted with permission. DW: Making the grade. Part II. Case Review/Rehab Manage 4(5):18-24, 1998.

 Table 25–11 Outcome Measures

Grade A:

1) Clinical outcome measures link "impairment" (eg, pain, range of motion, muscle performance, edema) with disability or functionality (eg, return-to-work status, activities of daily living, sports participation).
2) Outcomes link "days (visits/units)-dollars (case cost)-disability (functional outcome)."
3) Outcome system is user-friendly and available at the individual clinic level.
4) Outcome system provides a national, regional, and local database against which a given provider or facility can be compared, eg, facility benchmarking, provider profiling.
5) Outcomes are linked to interventions so these may be modified when necessary.
6) Outcomes reports are concise and understandable to all stakeholders including employers, payors, case managers, and others.
7) Outcome measures adjust for severity and other aggravating circumstances.
8) Outcomes are used to improve performance, not just for reimbursement purposes.
9) Outcome measures describe a diverse patient/condition population.
10) Outcome measures can be linked to other databases, eg, disease state management.
11) Outcome measures program includes patient and consumer satisfaction surveys.

Grade C:

1) Outcome measures describe a narrow patient population.
2) Outcome reports are meaningful to providers only.
3) Outcome measures are not adjusted sufficiently for severity and, therefore, serve only as general quality indicators.
4) Outcome reports address clinical measures, but are devoid of financial data.

Grade F:

1) Outcome measures fail to link impairment and disability.
2) Outcome measures are used for reimbursement purposes only and not continuous quality improvement.
3) Outcome measures are not user friendly or available at the individual clinic level.
4) Outcome measures provide no comparative database or ability to benchmark facilities and profile providers.

Reprinted with permission. DW: Making the grade. Part II. Case Review/Rehab Manage 4(5):18-24, 1998.

Table 25-12 Documentation Standards

Grade A:

1) Network members' clinical documentation exceeds the minimum national standard of care.
2) All centers are standardized documentation procedures.

Grade C:

1) Network's clinical documentation meets national standards.

Grade F:

1) Network's clinical documentation is substandard to published guidelines.
2) Inconsistent documentation standards are used throughout network.

Note: As with all categories or grades, there may be some individuals who score well despite an aggregate poor score for the network. Obviously, these persons should be the standard bearers for others.

Reprinted with permission. DW: Making the grade. Part II. Case Review/Rehab Manage 4(5):18-24, 1998.

 Table 25-13 Risk Assumption

Grade A:

1) Rehabilitation networks are willing to alter their reimbursement model depending on a health plan's needs.
2) Networks demonstrate significant financial reserves and cash flow to offset unanticipated losses.
3) Networks are willing to secure necessary surely bonds in order to demonstrate financial capacity.
4) Networks have the ability to link financial data with clinical data.

Grade C:

1) Networks are able to engage in capitation only, but not case or episodic rates.
2) Networks collect, but cannot link financial and clinical data.

Grade F:

1) Networks are unwilling to enter into any at-risk contract.
2) Networks are unable to demonstrate adequate financial reserves to offset unanticipated losses.
3) Networks reimburse their provider members before the network itself receives payment.

Reprinted with permission. DW: Making the grade. Part II. Case Review/Rehab Manage 4(5):18-24, 1998.

Figure 25-4. Stages of change and transition. (From Bridges: Managing Transitions: Making the Most of Change. Reading, MA, Addison-Wesley Publishing, 1991, p 130.)

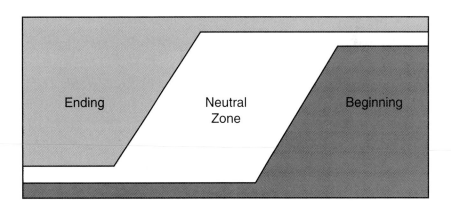

changes are beyond the control of the provider, learning how to transition to changes is a valuable adaptation strategy. Perhaps the most important tool in dealing with change is to secure information, and then get more of it. This describes the very essence of this book.

REFERENCES

Ades PA, Pashkow FJ, Fletcher G et al: A controlled trial of cardiac rehabilitation in the homesetting using electrocardiographic and voice transtelephonic monitoring. Am Heart J 139(3):543-548, 2000.

Ad Hoc Committee on Health Literacy for the Council on Scientific Affairs, American Medical Association: Health literacy. JAMA 281(6):552-557, 1991.

Agency for Health Care Policy and Research, http://www.ahcpr.gov, accessed May 12, 2002.

American Physical Therapy Association: Workforce Study, conducted by Vector Research, Inc, executive summary. Alexandria, VA, American Physical Therapy Association, 1997.

Americans with Disability Act of 1990 (ADA), Public Law 101-336, 42 U.S.C. 12101.

Anonymous: Telerehabilitation may be in future of rehab care. Hosp Case Manage 7(12):213-214, 1999.

Applequist J, Larson J: What is the most effective way to reduce incidence of amputation in the diabetic foot? Diabetes/Metabolism Res Rev Sept-Oct, 16(Suppl):s75-83, 2000.

Banja JD: The improbable future of employment-based insurance. The Hastings Center Report 30(3):17-25, 2000.

Bauer JC: Insights on telemedicine: How big is the market? J Healthcare Information Manage 16(2):10-11, 2002.

Berman S, Miller AC, Rosen C: Assessment training and team functioning for treating children with disabilities. Arch Phys Med Rehabil 81(5):628-633, 2000.

Blendon RJ, Enthoven AC, Singer SL et al: Understanding the managed care backlash. Health Affairs 17(4):80-94, 1998.

Bridges W: Managing Transitions: Making the Most of Change. Reading, MA, Addison-Wesley Publishing, 1991, p 130.

Bruhn JG: Problem-based learning: An approach toward reforming allied health education. J Allied Health 21(3):161-173, 1992.

Brunicardi BO: Financial analysis of savings from telemedicine in Ohio's prison system. Telemedicine J 4(1):49-54, 1998.

Cadette WM: Regulating HMOs: An ethical framework for cost-effective medicine. Public Policy Brief No. 47. Annandale-on-Hudson, New York, Jerome Levy Economics Institute of Bard College, 1998.

Callahan D: False Hopes: Why America's Quest for Perfect Health Is a Recipe for Failure. New York, Simon and Schuster, 1998, p 336.

Cameron ID, Handoll HH, Finneson TP et al: Coordinated multidisciplinary approaches for inpatient rehabilitation of older patients with proximal femoral fractures. Cochrane Database System Rev 4: CD000106, 2000.

Center for Studying Health System Change: Teaching Changes in the Public Health System. Issue Brief. Washington, DC, Center for Studying Health System Change, 1996.

The figure shows three stages: **Ending**, **Neutral Zone**, **Beginning**.

Clanet MG, Brassat D: The management of multiple sclerosis patients. Current Opinion Neurol 13(3):263-270, 2000.

Clarke RL: Beyond managed care. J Healthcare Financial Manage 54(7):16, 2000.

Clifton DW: A friendlier managed care. PT Magazine 4(12):24-26, 1996.

Clifton DW: Making the grade, part I. Case Rev 4(4):16-19, 1998.

Clifton DW: Making the grade, part II. Case Rev 4(5):18-24, 1998.

Cole RP, Scialla SJ, Bednarz L: Functional recovery in cancer rehabilitation. Arch Phys Med Rehabil 81(5):623-627, 2000.

Couturier P, Tyrrell J, Tonetti J, Rhul C: Feasibility of orthopaedic tele-consulting in a geriatric rehabilitation service. J Telemed Telecare 4(Suppl 1):85-87, 1998.

Crotty M, Finucane P, Ahern M: Teaching medical students about disability and rehabilitation: Methods and student feedback. Med Education 34(8):659-64, 2000.

Curry FV: Role of nonprofessional assistants: A survey of physical therapy departments in California. Phys Ther 33:587-588, 1953.

Doyle J, Waters F, Jackson N: New developments for effectiveness of systematic review in health promotion. Cochrane Health Promotion and Public Health Field, Promotion Ed 10(3):118-119, 2003.

Entoven A, Vorhaus C: A vision of quality in health care delivery. Health Affairs 16(3):44-57, 1997.

Flax H: The Future of Physical Medicine and Rehabilitation. Washington, DC, Department of Veteran Affairs Medical Center, http://www.pmr.vcu.edu, accessed February 14, 2002.

Friedland R: New Estimates of the High Costs of Inadequate Health Literacy. Proceedings of "Promoting Health Literacy: A Call to Action," Washington, DC, October 7-8, 1998.

Gair G, Hartery T: Medical dominance in multidisciplinary teamwork: A case study of discharge decision-making in a geriatric assessment unit. J Nurs Manage 9(1):3-11, 2001.

Gatchel RJ, McGeary D: Cochrane collaboration-based reviews of health care interventions: Are they unequivocal and valid scientifically or simply nihilistic? Spine J 2(5):315-319, 2002.

Gazmararian JA et al: Health literacy among Medicare enrollees in a managed care organization. JAMA 281(6):245-551, 1999.

Geddes JM, Chamberlain MA: Home-based rehabilitation for people with stroke: A comparative study of six community services providing coordinated multidisciplinary treatment. Clin Rehabil 15(6):589-99, 2001.

Glied S: Chronic Condition: Why Health Reform Fails. Cambridge, MA, Harvard University Press, 1997, p 545.

Gormley ME: Treatment of neuromuscular and musculoskeletal problems in cerebral palsy. Pediatr Rehabil 4(1):5-16, 2001.

Grahn B, Ekdahl C, Borquist L: Motivation as a predictor of changes in quality of life and working ability in multidisciplinary rehabilitation: A two-year follow-up of a prospective controlled study in patients with prolonged musculoskeletal disorders. Disabil Rehabil 22(15):639-654, 2000.

Gray JM: Function of nonprofessional physical therapy personnel. Phys Ther 44:103-109, 1964.

Greenfield L, Colen BD, Cleary PD, Greenfield S: Evaluating the quality of health care: What research offers decision makers. New York, Milbank Memorial Fund, 1996, p 25.

Hankin HA, Spencer T, Kegerreis S et al: Analysis of pain behavior profiles and functional disability in outpatient physical therapy clinics. J Orthop Sports Phys Ther 31(2):90-95, 2001.

Houck S: The myth of managed care moving beyond managing cost to really managing care. Cost Quality 3(1):1-6, 1997, http://www.cost-quality.com, accessed March 15, 2002.

Illman J: U.K.'s effort to improve multidisciplinary care criticized. J Natl Cancer Institute 94(3):163-4, 2002.

Institute of Medicine (IOM): Guidelines for Clinical Practice: From Development to Use. Washington, DC, National Academy Press, 1992.

Institute of Medicine (IOM): The Future of Public Health. Washington, DC, National Academy Press, 1988.

Jacobsen KR: Space-age medicine, stone-age government: How Medicare reimbursement of telemedicine services is depriving the elderly of quality medical treatment. Specialty Law Digest, Health Care Law Feb 274:9-37, 2002.

Jamison M: Chronic illness management in the year 2005. Nurs Econ 16(5):246-253, 1998.

Jensen MP, Turner JA, Romano JM: Changes in beliefs, catastrophizing, and coping are associated with improvement in multidisciplinary pain treatment. J Consult Clin Psychol 69(4):655-62, 2001.

Johnson MV, Wood K, Stason WB: Rehabilitative placement of post-stroke patients: Reliability of the clinical practice guidelines of the Agency for Health Care Policy and Research. Arch Phys Med Rehabil 81(5):539-548, 2000.

Karjalainen K, Malmivaara A, Van Tulder M: Multidisciplinary biopsychosocial rehabilitation for subacute low back pain in working-age adults: A systematic review within the framework of the Cochrane Collaborative Back Review Group. Spine 26(3):262-269, 2001.

Kasper EK, Gerstenblith G, Hefter G: A randomized trial of the efficacy of multidisciplinary care in heart failure outpatients at high risk hospital remission. J Am Coll Cardiol 39(3):471-80, 2002.

Kassirer JP: The next transformation in the delivery of health care. New Engl J Med 332(1):52-53, 1999.

Kelly B: Telemedicine begins to make progress. Health Data Manage 10(1):72-76, 78, 2002.

Kennedy V, Jennings MC: Beyond HMOs: Trends in employer contracting. Healthcare Financial Manage J 52(8):45-48.

Kleinke JD: The U.S. Health Care System after the Managed Care Revolution. Harvard School of Public Health, Center for Continuing Professional Education, The Harvard Conference on Strategic Alliances in Healthcare: Redefining Healthcare, October 14-15, Boston, Harvard School of Public Health, 1999.

Kuttner R: The American health care system: Employer-sponsored health coverage. New Engl Med 340:248-252, 1999.

Lemaire ED, Greene G: Continuing education in physical rehabilitation using Internet-based modules. J Telemedicine Telecare 8(1):19-24, 1998.

Lemaire ED, Jeffreys Y: Low-bandwidth telemedicine for remote orthotic assessment. Prosthet Orthot Int 22(2):155-167, 1998.

Loane M, Wooton R: A review of guidelines and standards for telemedicine. J Telemed Telecare 8(2):63-71, 2002.

Machiavelli N, The Prince. WK Marriott trans-ed. London, England: J.M. Dent & Sons, 1908.

Matalon A, Nahmani T, Rubin S: A short-term intervention in a multidisciplinary referral clinic for primary care frequent attenders: Description of the model, patient characteristics and their use of medical resources. Fam Pract 19(3):251-6, 2002.

McCallin A: Interdisciplinary practice—a matter of teamwork: An integrated literature review. J Clin Nurs 10(4):419-428, 2001.

Milbank Fund: Patients as Effective Collaborators in Managing Chronic Conditions. New York, Milbank Fund, 1999, p 25.

Milbank Memorial Fund: Enhancing the Accountability of Alternative Medicine. New York, Milbank Fund, 1998, p 35.

Milbank Memorial Fund: Better Information, Better Outcomes? Milbank New York, Milbank Fund, 2000, p 29.

Millensen ML: Stand by me: To thrive as the new American health care system managed care will have to go beyond consumer satisfaction and once again earn the public's trust. Healthplan 39(6):56-61, 1998.

Milliman & Robertson Co: HMO's managed workers' compensation strategies and products. San Francisco, Milliman & Robertson Co, 1995.

Morrison I: The Second Curve: Managing the velocity of change. New York, Ballantine Books, 1996, p 272.

Moyer CF: No need for assistant? Phys Ther 52(12):1326, 1972.

National Business Coalition on Health, Washington DC, http://www.NBCH.org, May 12, 2002.

National Center for Dissemination of Disability Research (NCDDR), http://www.ncddr.org, May 12, 2002.

Nickelson DE: Physician extenders: a wave of the future or a passing fad? NAHAM Manage J 22(3):26, 1996.

O'Brien LA: Telemedicine is not needed. Texas Medicine, Texas Medical Association 98(2):9, 2002.

Ozdemir F, Birtane M, Tabatabaei R: Comparing stroke rehabilitation outcomes between acute inpatient and non-intense home settings. Arch Phys Med Rehabil 82(10):1375-1379, 2001.

Paris NM, Hines J: Payer and provider relationships: The key to reshaping health care delivery. Nurs Adm Q 19(3):13-17, 1995.

Patterson RF: New Webster's Expanded Dictionary. Plantation, FL, Paradise Press, 1998.

Perry J: Responsibilities in patient care. The need for non-professional assistants in physical therapy. Phys Ther 46(3):250-255, 1966.

Phillips VL, Vesmarovich S, Hauber R et al: Telehealth: Reaching out to newly injured spinal cord patients. Public Health Reports 116(Suppl)1:94-102, 2001.

Popescu VG, Burdea GC, Bouzit M: A virtual-reality-based telerehabilitation system with force feedback. IEEE Trans Inf Technol Biomed 4(1):45-51, 2000.

Powell J, Heslin J, Greenwood R: Community-based rehabilitation after severe traumatic brain injury: A randomized controlled trial. J Neuro Neurosurg Psychiatry (England), 72(2):193-202, 2002.

Reece RL: And who shall care for the sick? Minneapolis, MN, Media Medicus, 1988, p 278.

Ridge RA, Goodson AS: The relationship between multidisciplinary discharge outcomes and functional status after total hip replacement. Orthop Nurs 19(1):71-82, 2000.

Riva G, Gamberini L: Virtual reality as telemedicine tool: Technology, ergonomics and actual applications. Technol Health Care 8(2):113-127, 2000.

Robinson AJ, McCall M, DePalma MT: Physical therapist's perceptions of the roles of the physical therapy assistant. Phys Ther 74(6):571-582, 1994.

Saladin LK, Morrisette DC, Brotherton SS: Making the physical therapy referral. J Am Acad Physician Assistants 12(2):18-20, 23, 27-32, 1999.

Samad A, Hayes S, Dodds S: Telemedicine: an innovative way of managing patients with leg ulcers. Br J Nurs 11(6)Suppl:S38-S52, 2002.

Savage GT, Campbell KS, Patian R et al: Beyond managed costs. Healthcare Manage Rev 25(1):93-108, 2000.

Schwartz P: The Art of the Long View: Planning for the Future in an Uncertain World. New York, Currency Doubleday, 1996.

Sheppard D: Physician extenders in managed care: reducing risk through supervision and credentialing. J Healthcare Risk Manage 14(4):12-17, 1994.

Smith S et al: The next decade of health spending: A new outlook. Health Affairs 18(4):86-95, 1999.

Sparks KE, Shaw DK, Eddy D et al: Alternatives for cardiac rehabilitation patients unable to return to hospital-based program. Heart Lung: J Crit Care 22(4):298-303, 1993.

Spitzer WO, Skouron ML, Salmi LR et al: Scientific monograph of the Quebec Task Force on Whiplash-associated Disorders: Redefining "whiplash" and its management. Spine J 20(8 Suppl):15-73S, 1995.

Sterner Y, Lofgrin M, Nyberg V et al: Early interdisciplinary rehabilitation programme for whiplash associated disorders. Disabil Rehabil 23(10):422-429.

Temkin AJ, Uliicny GR, Vesmarovich SH: Telerehab: A perspective of the way technology is going to change the future of patient treatment. Rehabil Manage 9(2):28-30, 1996.

The Pew Health Professions Commission: Recreating Health Professional Practice for a New Century. The Pew Charitable Trusts, administered by the University of California Center for the Health Professions, 1998. http://www.futurehealth.ucsf.edu/pewcommm.html, accessed September 5, 1998.

Tran BQ, Buckley KM, Prandoni CM: Selection and use of telehealth technology in support of homebound caregivers of stroke patients caring. National Association for Home Care Magazine 21(3):16-21, 2002.

US Bureau of the Census: Current Population Reports, Series P60-202. Washington, DC, Government Printing Office, 2000.

US Public Health Service: For a Healthy Nation: Returns on Investment in Public Health. Rockville, MD, Public Health Service, 1994.

US Centers for Disease Control and Prevention: Core Functions of Public Health. Atlanta, GA, Centers for Disease Control and Prevention, 1991.

US Department of Veteran Affairs: Research and Design Progress Report Services, vol 34. Baltimore, MD, Veterans Health Administration Rehabilitation Research and Development Service, Scientific and Technical Publications Section (122), 1997.

Vibbert S (ed): The 1996 Health Network and Alliance Sourcebook. New York, Faulkner and Gray, 1996.

Voelker R: Do consumers "get" quality? In Service R (ed): The State of Health Care in America. Business & Health 17(6)Suppl A:14-18, 1999.

Wall S: Transformations in public health systems. Health Affairs 17(3):64-80, 1998.

Wilson D: The BBA expands the role of physician extenders ...with major implications for provider-employers. Med Network Strategy Rep 7(12):8-9, 1998.

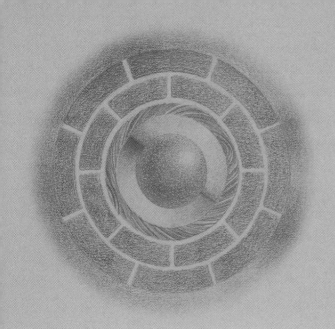

From Clinicians to Consultants

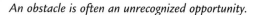

CHAPTER 26

Profiles in Disability Management

David W. Clifton, Jr., PT

An obstacle is often an unrecognized opportunity.

- David W. Clifton

If challenges are the catalysts for change and innovation, then what a grand time to be involved in disability management! The convergence of new technology and medical interventions coupled with the most educated consumers in history and access to immediate information has enabled a number of entrepreneurial individuals and their organizations to carve unique market niches. These niches are located at various points along the health and disability continuum as depicted in Figure 26–1. The continuum ranges from disability prevention and wellness through disability treatment/management to postdisability consultation.

This chapter profiles a small sampling of the diverse entities that address unfulfilled needs within the disability management area. Each of the profiled entities occupy one or more positions along the continuum depicted in Figure 26-1. Readers should appreciate, however, that most entities provide comprehensive services that span the entire continuum.

Other chapters in this text have extensively covered disability prevention, treatment, and management literature, practices, and principles. This chapter brings to life some disability management practices and principles through real world applications. Profiled entities have developed and continue to develop market-driven strategies that differ in nature and scope but share the following common goals:

● Minimize the pain associated with impairment and disability.
● Reduce cost associated with disability.
● Eliminate or reduce suffering (psychological/social/ economic) associated with disability.
● Reserve and/or restore independence and human dignity.

All of these entities have directly or indirectly contributed to disability management. Profiles run the gamut from small to large organizations, well-known organizations to obscure entities, individuals, publicly traded corporations to privately held companies, and local to international organizations.

Finally, inclusion in this chapter does not constitute any type of endorsement of any product or service, person, or organization. Inclusion is simply intended to provide readers with applied examples of disability prevention, treatment, and management. It should be understood that many other entities offer unique contributions to disability prevention and management. Editorial restraints do not permit their inclusion here.

DISABILITY PREVENTION AND WELLNESS SERVICES

Although prevention and wellness services predominantly reside on the far left side of the continuum, it is important to understand that these activities traverse the entire continuum from pretreatment to posttreatment. For example, ergonomic analysis can function as a primary or secondary prevention of injury or illness.

Ergonomics may be used during the initial design phase of a tool, workspace, or piece of equipment. Ergonomic analysis can also be vital in safely returning the injured worker to gainful employment. Ergonomics can serve as the compliance link between workers' compensation and the Americans with Disabilities Act (ADA) and the Occupational Safety and Health Administration (OSHA). Recommendations that result for ergonomic controls (administrative and engineering) may produce the blueprint for "reasonable accommodations" under ADA or OSHA injury/illness abatement requirements.

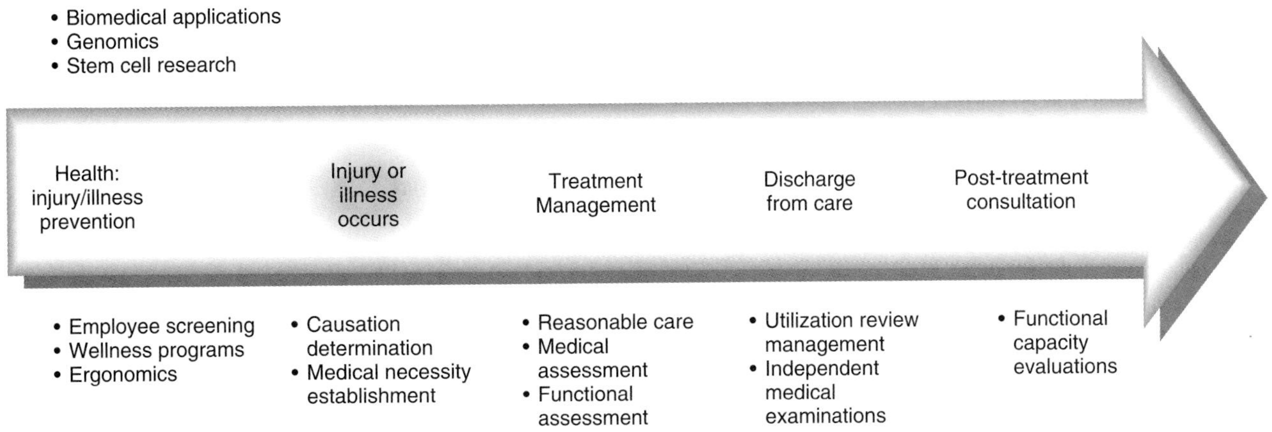

- Biomedical applications
- Genomics
- Stem cell research

| Health: injury/illness prevention | Injury or illness occurs | Treatment Management | Discharge from care | Post-treatment consultation |

- Employee screening
- Wellness programs
- Ergonomics

- Causation determination
- Medical necessity establishment

- Reasonable care
- Medical assessment
- Functional assessment

- Utilization review management
- Independent medical examinations

- Functional capacity evaluations

Figure 26–1. Disability continuum.

The following disability management profiles of organizations or entities can be described as preventive in nature, but not exclusively so.

Applied Ergonomic Technology

Jenkintown, PA
Contact: David Ridyard, CIH, CSP; dridyard@home.com.

Applied Ergonomic Technology (AET) is a firm that offers ergonomics, industrial hygiene, and safety services to employers. Ergonomic services include developing practical solutions for manual materials handling problems to reduce back and cumulative trauma disorders; designing office, computer, and industrial workstations; and developing comprehensive ergonomics programs for compliance with OSHA guidelines and the ADA. AET considers education to be a keystone of an ergonomic program and provides ergonomics awareness training for engineers, managers, production employees, and office employees.

AET applies a five-step model for ergonomic assessments. Figure 26–2 describes this process through a flow diagram. Step one involves the identification of risk factors, both human and environmentally based. These risks are then quantified (step two) in terms of severity, and controls are considered. Step three, analysis of business factors, is often lacking in many ergonomic and for that matter injury prevention programs. AET defines "business factors" as factors that determine whether the proposed ergonomic controls are accepted by management and employees. Typical business factors can involve labor-management rapport, personnel issues such as seniority, labor organizations, and budget impact items. Budget impact items involve cost-effectiveness of controls, productivity impact, product quality impact, waste minimization, and the cost of injuries, especially for self-insured employers. Typical personnel issues include acceptance of controls by end users, implementation time, reliability/maintainability of controls, upper management-employee support, and

regulatory impact. Ergonomic controls can be of an administrative or engineering nature or both.

Administrative controls attempt to alter human behavior in a positive manner to reduce the risk of injury/illness. Examples of these controls include job sharing, extra rest breaks, warmup exercises, two-person lifts, and job rotation.

Engineering controls attempt to alter the job task itself, the worksite, tools, or equipment.

Step four involves the implementation of ergonomic controls that are identified through a combination of risk quantification with an understanding of business factors. Step five represents the quality assurance stage when implementation of controls, testing effectiveness, and follow-up are conducted to determine if additional risk factors have been identified. This continuous improvement model eliminates the common hit or miss approach to injury prevention consultation. Political conflict and labor relations problems often associated with consultation initiatives can be minimized (Shrey & LaCerte, 1995).

AET's principal, David Ridyard, CIH, CSP, outlines the keys to success of an ergonomic program (Ridyard, 1990). Ergonomic programs that subscribe to these principles have been proven to reduce injury rates, severity, and lost-time incidents (Table 26–1).

DISABILITY TECHNOLOGY INNOVATIONS

The following profiles address organizations that have made a significant impact on the treatment and management of disability after the individual has sustained the disability. Although one could argue that secondary prevention is a byproduct of their technologies, it is not the primary focus of this discussion.

Editorial restrictions do not allow for an extensive exploration of these entities and their products/services. Readers are encouraged to contact the Websites listed here for additional data and product/service samples.

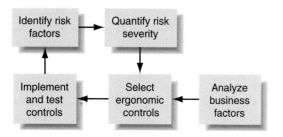

Figure 26–2. Applied Ergonomics Technology's ergonomic process.

 Table 26–1   Ergonomic Assessment Keys to Success

- Follow a proven ergonomics process
- Quantify injury risk levels thoroughly and consistently
- Determine critical business factors:
  - Understand company culture and climate
  - Determine what will drive ergo process
- Implement controls that reduce injury risk levels and optimize business factors
- Provide appropriate level of engineering design and support
- Test effectiveness of controls
- Fine-tune controls to increase effectiveness
- Establish a system to manage the ongoing ergonomics process:
  - Good engineering design
  - Ergonomics team involvement
  - Employee involvement and feedback

From: David Ridyard, CSP, CIH, CPE, Applied Ergonomic Technology, Jenkintown, PA.

Genzyme

Genzyme Corporation
Cambridge, MA 02139
http://www.genzyme.com

Genzyme is a highly diversified biotechnology company that uses a wide range of technologies to develop human health care products and services. The four divisions of the company all have their own common stock and are traded on the NASDAQ stock exchange. Genzyme General develops and markets health care products and services, including therapies for rare genetic diseases and diagnostic products. Genzyme's suite of products/services address a patient population well known to physical rehabilitation providers. Genzyme Tissue Repair is a leading developer of biological products geared toward the orthopedic market. Some therapists may be familiar with this division, which develops and markets a product for knee cartilage damage and for severe burns. Genzyme Molecular Oncology develops therapies that target cancer through genomics or gene therapy. Genzyme Surgical Products develops instruments, devices, biomaterials, and biotherapeutics for use in cardiothoracic and general surgery. Genzyme is a pioneer in the area of "biosurgery," which combines mechanical with biological agents in surgery or other interventional procedures.

Carticel and Epicel are perhaps the two most well-known products to those in the rehabilitation profession. Carticel are autologous cultured chondrocytes that are used in the repair of clinically significant cartilaginous defects of the femoral condyle. A patient's cartilage cells are removed, sent to a lab for culturing, and returned to the patient's joint surface. This implantation procedure is performed to restore a normal joint surface in chronic conditions such as arthritis. Genzyme's literature reports that approximately 200,000 total knee replacements are performed annually at a cost of $25,000 each. Approximately 4000 patients have received Carticel treatment. Epicel involves skin grafts for the treatment of severe burns. These new technologies are certain to affect how physical rehabilitation is performed, particularly under a disease state management model. Therapists will require additional knowledge relative to biotechnologies that impact shared patient population, especially those with chronic disease, injury, and illness.

Moore Design Associates

Phoenix, AZ, and New York City

Patricia Moore is an internally recognized gerontologist and industrial designer. She is the founder of Moore Design Associates and serves as an adjunct professor at Arizona State University. She is a proponent of "universal design" methodology. Universal design attempts to meet the lifespan needs of all consumers, regardless of ability levels, by affording access to different environments. Dr. Moore has worked with a diverse client base with an emphasis on transgenerational design. Her functional designs range from kitchen products to railroad cars. Moore Design clients include AT&T, Bell Communication, Canada-Air, Corning Glass, OXO International, Proctor & Gamble, Searle, Sun Beam, and 3-M Corporation. Valley Metro Rail retained Moore Design Associates to design the interior of rail cars to make them more accessible for disparate populations who must use public transportation.

Dr. Moore is the author of *Disguised: A True Story*, published in 1985 (Moore & Conn, 1985). This book describes the experience of Dr. Moore when between 1979 and 1982 she disguised herself as an 80-year-old woman and traveled to more than 100 cities. During this journey, she glazed her eyeglasses with Vaseline to simulate cataracts and feigned arthritis. This experience made her acutely aware of the challenges faced by elders in navigating common environments. She has dedicated an entire career to the design of tools, equipment, and environments that allow persons of diverse anthropometric and functional ability levels to use them. Dr. Moore was recently honored by the Industrial Designers Society of America when her peers elected her as a Fellow.

Rehabilitation professionals may be quite familiar with Dr. Moore's work. In 1991 she partnered with David Guynes of Guynes Design Inc., an architectural firm. This collaboration resulted in the design of health care and rehabilitation facilities that encouraged independence and community reintegration. "Easy Street" was one of the first products designed as a microcosm of a local environment for training patients in reacclimation. Figure 26–3 depicts a variety of environments designed by Guynes Design. Other products include Family Road, Independence Square, Our Town, Rehab 123, and Worksymes. Even though the Guynes-Moore collaboration has since dissolved, Moore continues to work on a variety of projects using the "universal design" methodology.

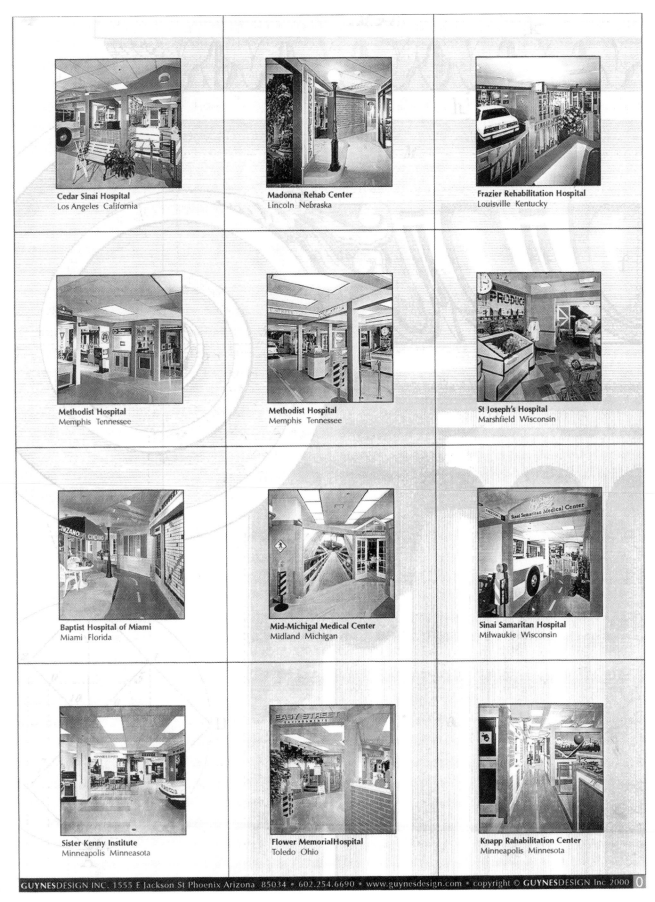

Figure 26–3. Guyne's sample environments.

Independence Technology L.L.C.

Independence Technology L.L.C. (a division of Johnson & Johnson)
Warren, New Jersey
Website: http://www.independencenow.com

Independence Technology is a company created to empower individuals through cutting-edge technology. Their mission is "to help people with disabilities achieve even more" and "to help people with disabilities live their lives with greater freedom" (Independence Technology, 2003). Independence Technology is a relatively new division of Johnson & Johnson, a universally recognized healthcare products/service company. In 1995 Johnson & Johnson assembled health care professionals who were recognized experts and thought leaders in the disability world. By 1999, Independence Technology, L.L.C., was formed to focus on meeting the needs of people with disabilities. In partnership with Deka, Independence Technology developed the INDEPENDENCE iBOT Mobility System. Deka is a company founded and operated by Dean Kamen, the inventor of the IT or personal transport system that is currently undergoing testing by the United Postal Service and other entities. Johnson & Johnson gathered a small group of people to form a professional exploratory products group to assess the disability market and to focus on unmet needs. The iBOT had been classified as an investigational medical device, but recently a U.S. advisory panel unanimously voted to urge Food and Drug Administration approval. The iBOT is available by prescription only and features of the device will be set to the size, weight, and ability of the user. Users include persons with disability who are dependent on power mobility. The iBOT Mobility System is designed to use its four wheels on rough terrain and to rise vertically to eye level while balancing on two wheels. The iBOT Mobility System functions are made possible by gyroscopes

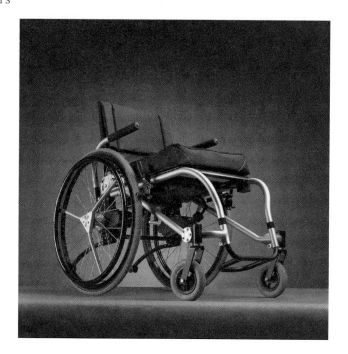

Figure 26–5. Independence Technology: iGLIDE Manual Assist Wheelchair.

that are computer programmed to create balancing capabilities on the basis of the user's center of gravity. In effect, the gyroscopes operate on the same principle by which humans are able to stand, balance, and navigate around various environments including stairs. This mobility unit enables the user to safely ascend and descend stairs, a capability not offered by traditional power wheelchairs.

Independence Technology has also recently introduced a new manual wheelchair called the iGLIDE This device provides the freedom associated with a manual wheelchair with a subtle source of automated power, hence its name, iGLIDE Manual Assist Wheelchair. This wheelchair allows transport over hills, grass, carpet, and ramps with a push of the hand rim.

Figures 26–4 and 26–5 feature two of Independence Technology's mobility devices designed to enhance functionality and independence for their users.

DISABILITY DATA MANAGEMENT

Chapter 12 of this book is dedicated to information technology in disability management. The following profiles augment this chapter by describing how some organizations have effectively used data management in their management of key aspects of disability management.

CareScience

CareScience
Philadelphia, PA
Website: www.carescience.com

CareScience is a publicly traded company (it trades on NASDAQ under the symbol CARE) with offices in Philadelphia, San Francisco, and Triangle Park, North Carolina. The company is a leading provider of care management services to hospitals, health systems, and

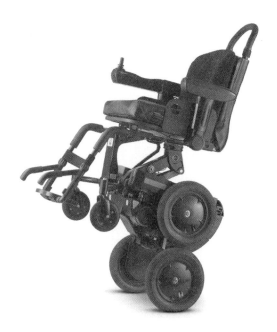

Figure 26–4. Independence Technology: iBOT 3000.

pharmaceutical and biotechnology companies. CareScience has partnered with more than 160 hospitals and health care systems and 45 pharmaceutical companies nationwide. CareScience specializes in clinical knowledge and informed decision making. It offers a systematic approach to identifying and quantifying improvements in clinical outcomes through a suite of programs.

"Care Data Exchange" involves clinical data integration and results reporting that offers a single-portal view of clinical data from multiple data sources both within an enterprise and between enterprises. "Care Management System" or "CaduCIS" is a suite of Internet-based solutions that uses cutting-edge research and methods to assist health systems in improving quality, care management, and clinical performance. To date rehabilitation services are not included, however. Optimum treatment patterns are identified along with protocols designed to minimize complications. Data are collected from within an organization and through public data sources. Statistical methodologies for risk adjustment used by CareScience were developed at the University of Pennsylvania through a unique collaboration between medicine (School of Medicine) and business (Wharton School of Business). CaduCIS supports providers' efforts to monitor performance, develop protocols, profile individual providers, educate providers, and augment accreditation and compliance.

CareScience provides consultants (onsite and offsite) who assist health care systems to monitor and manage care. These consultants also conduct Clinical Strategy Retreats that assist groups to facilitate a common vision about successful clinical care management strategies. These strategies link clinical to financial management.

CareScience contends that their Care Data Exchange enables providers to secure information through the Internet without the need to invest in expensive servers or central computers This program addresses a common obstacle to rendering quality health care: getting the data to make informed decisions. Subscribers of this service can pull data from the individual computers of other providers involved in the patient's care and access it through the Internet.

Informed consent of the patient is the keystone to this data exchange similar to paper exchanges.

Focus on Therapeutic Outcomes

Focus on Therapeutic Outcomes
Knoxville, TN
http://www.fotoinc.com

Focus on Therapeutic Outcomes (FOTO) is one of the nation's largest physical rehabilitation outcomes databases and report services companies. Its mission is to "reach excellence in efficient and accurate collection and analysis of data for the medical rehabilitation industry that exceeds customer expectations for comparative outcomes information, research, and consultation" (http://www.fotoinc.com, accessed May 12, 2002).

In 1992 six national rehabilitation companies began what today is known as FOTO. These companies included MedRehab (merged with Mariner, Prism, Rehability, Healthsouth), Rehabworks, also known as Continental (now SelectMedical), Healthsouth, Caremark (merged with Healthsouth), RehabClinics, also known as Novacare (now a division of Select Medical), and Rehability (merged with Healthsouth). By 1994, FOTO became independently owned and operated with a mission of serving the post-acute rehabilitation industry. FOTO strives to achieve the following goals:

- Develop and maintain provider databases.
- Remain independent of both providers and payers.
- Establish standard outcomes systems.
- Promote validation of therapeutic intervention.
- Promote improvement in patient care.

FOTO measures functional outcomes for musculo-skeletal, industrial, neuromuscular, cardiopulmonary, and pediatric patients. Provider clients include physical and occupational therapists, orthopedists, chiropractors, and orthotists and prosthetists. FOTO has 54 measures approved by the Joint Commission for Accreditation of Healthcare Organizations through its ORYX initiative. FOTO's suite of products/services includes a variety of reports designed to assess clinical efficiency, outcomes, and patient satisfaction. Participants in this database receive a nationally benchmarked outcomes profile each quarter that compares their clinic's efficiency and effectiveness with the national aggregate data. FOTO's "Outcomes Profiles" are divided into eight impairment categories and five types of outpatient care to track and compare the following data sets:

1. Efficiency: average number of visits, average duration, and average net revenue per episode.
2. Outcome indexes: outcome index, functional change in patients; value index, functional change per dollar; and utilization index, functional change per visit.
3. Other Information: patient satisfaction, reason for discharge, and therapist functional goals at discharge.

FOTO's Outcome Index represents an average change across the following six functional scales: physical functioning scale, role limitation because of physical problems, bodily pain, mental health, energy/fatigue, and social functioning. A clinic or clinician's percentile ranking is calculated on the basis of these data ranging from 0 to 99. The higher the score, the better. For example, if a clinician's percentile ranking for similar cases or conditions treated is 65%, then 65% of the provider population treating similar cases had outcome indices below this clinician's.

Customized optional reports are available that sort data by International Classification of Diseases (ICD)-9 codes, therapist identifiers, referral sources, payment sources, geographical regions, and body parts or regions. Sample FOTO reports can be found in Figures 26-6, 26-7, and 26-8.

Smart Tracks

Smart Tracks
Stillwater, MN

SmartTracks "Care Management System" was created out of market demand for effective care management.

Text continued on p. 383.

Efficiency Statistics and indices risk-adjusted by Age, Severity, and Acuity

Efficiency Statistics

Patient Satisfaction

Therapist Functional Goals at Discharge

Risk-Adjusts scores for Outcome (Functional Change), Value (Change per Dollar), and Utilization (Change per Visit). These Risk –Adjustment Factors impact change the most.

Outcome Profile (Quarter 3, 1999) – Risk Adjusted with Acuity
Results of data based on last 12 months

Reporting Unit: Any Therapy Clinic
Care Type: Orthopedic

Practice ID: 00-000-00-0
Impairment Category: All Categories

Severity Level: Slight   UNIT

	Age<45 ACUITY				Age<45 ACUITY				Age<45 ACUITY				Age<45 ACUITY		
#Days	0-21	22 – 90	90+	#Days	0-21	22 – 90	90+	#Days	0-21	22 – 90	90+	#Days	0-21	22 – 90	90+
# Pts	35	45	60	# Pts	35	45	60	# Pts	35	45	60	# Pts	35	45	60

Outcome Profile (Quarter 3, 1999)
Results of data based on last 12 months

Reporting Unit: Any Therapy Clinic
Care Type: Orthopedic

Practice ID: 00-000-00-0
Impairment Category: All Categories

	UNIT	
Statistics:		
# Patients:	964	112,032
Visits:	6.98	9.47
Duration (in days):	33.01	34.85
Dollars:	850.33	796.69
Outcome Indexes		
# Patients:	690	79,087
Outcomes: (OI)	89.63	56.02
Percentile Rank:	88**	
Value: (OI/Net Rev):	150.95	116.39
Utilization: (OI/Visits)	168.34	78.3
Satisfaction:	97.36%	94.79%
Reason for Discharge:		
% Goals Met:	64.75%	58.23%
% Goals Not Met (Pt reached maximum benefit):	11.75%	16.38%
% Non-Compliant:	12.05%	12.42%
% No Progress/ No Goals Met	11.45%	12.97%
Therapist Functional Goals at Discharge:		
% All Goals Met:	52.00%	44.07%
% Some Progress / Partial Goals Met:	42.50%	48.55%
% No Progress / No Goals Met:	5.50%	7.38%

Outcome Indices

Risk Adjusted Values

Severity Level:	UNIT					
Slight	All Ages	Age<45	Age>=45	All Ages	Age<45	Age>=45
# Patients*	195	93	106	19,978	8,791	11,369
Outcome:	48.04	53.20	44.89	22.80	28.25	35.33
Value:	101.31	120.92	69.91	62.38	81.87	45.38
Utilization:	113.07	134.36	100.97	40.36	51.86	30.23
Moderate						
# Patients*	187	93	93	19,420	8,489	10,996
Outcome:	99.70	97.79	105.13	63.72	71.93	58.90
Value:	174.39	172.26	179.53	143.32	168.55	123.25
Utilization:	200.76	204.48	198.95	96.25	115.37	50.95
Severe						
# Patients*	144	72	65	20,198	8,658	10,967
Outcome:	168.60	170.71	164.19	101.51	114.63	96.55
Value:	290.38	284.47	305.92	218.02	252.74	183.35
Utilization:	309.03	334.25	288.65	144.53	171.99	124.60
Very Severe						
# Patients*	164	78	90	19,491	8,590	11,327
Outcome:	276.55	298.82	254.39	161.35	177.21	148.71
Value:	422.56	474.54	359.71	295.90	341.36	268.98
Utilization:	478.57	570.80	379.99	201.29	235.75	175.07

Figure 26–6. FOTO sample report.

Resource Predictor

The Patient Resource Predictor provides a risk-adjusted prediction of the results of patient care. It also provides a comparison of the patient to the national aggregate for the six functional scales - Physical Functioning, Role Physical (work related tasks), Pain, Energy, Mental, and Social.

Employment Status

Patient Intake

The Patient Intake report includes subjective comments, made by the patient, about their general health.

Patient Intake

09/28/1999

Reporting Unit:	Any Therapy Clinic	Practice Id:	00-000-00-0
Patient Id:	000-11-2222	Onset:	91 Days - 6 Months
Name:	PATIENT	Initial Date of Service:	9/1/1999

Initial Employment Status: Restricted Duty

RISK ADJUSTMENT CRITERIA:

Impairment Category:	Lumbar Spine / Sacrum	Severity:	Very Severe
Care Type:	Orthopedic	Age:	35

History
General Health: Patient reports general health is fair and somewhat worse now than one year ago. Patient generally completes 20 minutes of exercise once or twice a week.

Patient Reports:
This condition began 91 days - 6 months.
An employment status as restricted duty working full-time (40+ hours a week), and is with the same employer and is performing the same job.
Having been off work and requiring treatment for the same problem requiring current treatment within the past six months.
Having previously received Workers' Compensation benefits.
Prescription medication is being taken for this condition.
Patient has had one surgery for this primary condition.

Subjective Comments
In the past week patient reports:
Very Severe bodily pain that interfered quite a bit with normal work activities.
Physical health resulted in fewer accomplishments at work or activity and the kind of work or other regular daily activities has been limited.
Felt calm and peaceful a little of the time.
Had lots of energy a little of the time.
Felt downhearted and depressed most of the time.
Problems interfered with social activities most of the time.

Health now limits the following activities a lot:
Lifting or carrying groceries
Climbing one flight of stairs
Walking several hundred yards
Walking one hundred yards
Lifting overhead to a cabinet

Patient Tracking Number: 100

Patient Specific Resource Predictor

Reporting Unit:	Any Therapy Clinic	Practice Id:	00-000-00-0
Patient Id:	000-11-2222	Onset:	91 Days - 6 Months
Name:	PATIENT	Initial Date of Service:	9/1/1999

Initial Employment Status: Restricted Duty working Full-time (40+ hours a week)

RISK ADJUSTMENT CRITERIA:

Impairment Category:	Lumbar Spine / Sacrum	Care Type:	Orthopedic
Age: 35		Severity:	Very Severe

FUNCTIONAL SCORES

	Phys Funct	Role Phys	Pain	Energy	Mental	Social
Admission	20.00	0.00	25.00	20.00	20.00	25.00
FOTO Mean	27.63	10.53	10.53	17.89	31.58	36.84

FOTO
Mean Resource Utilized (Risk Adjusted)

FOTO patients with similar functional admission scores have utilized resources as indicated below: The probability is that the patients results will be near the mean. The number of risk adjusted patients during the last 12 months in the FOTO database is: 412

Statistics:		MEANS
	Visits	7.57
	Duration	27.36
	Dollars	$875.40

Outcome Index:		
	Outcome	219.25
	Value	333.47
	Utilization	325.26

Satisfaction:		
	Satisfaction	98.10%

Reasons for Discharge:		
	% Goals Met	60.00%
	% Goals Not Met (Pt reached maximum benefit) :	13.33%
	% Non-Compliant	13.33%
	% Other	13.33%

Patient Tracking Number :100

Results for other patients who are similar to this patient

Figure 26–7. FOTO sample report.

Discharged Patient Activity Summary

This report provides a similar comparison to the Trend Report, summarizing the results of care for this patient as compared to the results for similar patients in the national aggregate.

Treatments Provided

Trend Report

The Trend Report summarizes the progress of the patient in comparison to other similar patients across the country. The higher the score, the better.

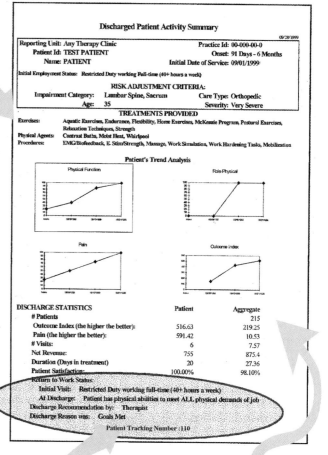

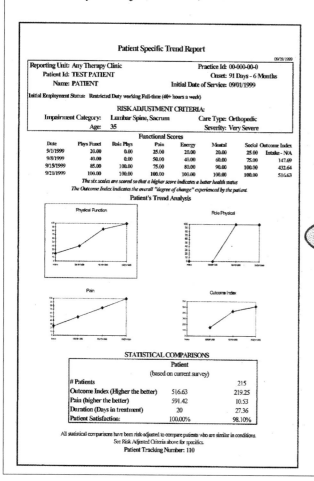

Employment Status

Results for other patients who are similar to this patient

Figure 26–8. FOTO sample report.

SmartTracks is a home-grown product of Orthopaedic Sports, Inc. (OSI), a private outpatient physical and occupational therapy practice located in the highly managed St. Paul, Minnesota, market. This profile illustrates the ability of relatively small organizations to meet the challenges of a rapidly evolving healthcare sector.

SmartTracks had the following initial four goals:

1. To serve as a patient categorization or guideline process through the collection of meaningful and manageable patient outcomes. These data assist therapists in accurately predicting the number of visits and consumed resources associated with a given case. Table 26–2 illustrates SmartTracks "Utilization/Functional Outcomes Totals Report," a component of the company's "OUTCOMES TODAY" product.

2. Serve as ongoing care management tools to ensure that treatment interventions are consistently applied across providers, thereby inducing variation which is at the core of virtually every managed care strategy.

3. Use as training tools to assist rehabilitation providers in understanding this organization's philosophy of care, clinical expectations, and encouraging participation in critical decision making and problem-solving exercises.

4. SmartTracks also serves as a marketing tool for its proprietor by demonstrating a commitment to total quality management. The SmartTracks system contains a suite of components that include the following:

   - Clinical guidelines described by case definitions.
   - Documentation process and forms.
   - Patient educational materials.
   - Internal review guidelines.
   - Referral source reference.
   - Outcomes software.
   - Continued education enhancement.

Figure 26–9 depicts a sample patient educational piece provided by OSI (the parent company of SmartTracks). This example addresses shoulder impingement. Figures 26–10 and 26–11 are examples of OSI's daily treatment and management and reevaluation documentation tools. Both of these documents identify data elements critical to standardization of service or, inversely, reduction in treatment variation between providers who are treating/managing similar cases.

Solucient

Solucient
Corporate Headquarters
Evanston, IL

Solucient is an international company formerly known as HCIA-Sachs. Solucient is an industry leader in providing payers, providers, employers, consultants, and pharmaceutical companies with relevant strategic intelligence. Solucient equips its clients with data that can be applied to growing revenues, benchmarking, measuring results, and better understanding consumers of health care services. Well-known Solucient publications include the following:

- *Length-of-stay* series
- *The Directory of Health Care Professionals*
- *The DRG Handbook: Comparative Clinical and Financial Benchmarks*
- *The Comparative Performance of U.S. Hospitals: The Sourcebook*
- *Profiles of U.S. Hospitals*
- *The Strategic Use of Data*
- *Guide to the Managed Care Industry*
- *Market Profiles for Medicare Risk Contracting*

Solucient offers an extensive suite of services and has recently worked with the National Council on Compensation Insurance in the development of a workers' compensation data warehouse. Solucient's goal is "to provide its client base with the best patient-focused information on the purchase, use, and outcome of various healthcare services" (http://www.hciasachs.com, accessed April 15, 2000).

Solucient is perhaps best known to providers because of its publication of the *100 Top Hospitals* beginning in 1993. This initiative led to the study and publication of the 100 Top Hospitals Orthopedic Benchmarks for Success, a collaborative effort with the Human Motion Institute[SM]. *Orthopedic Benchmarks for Success* uses Medicare-based data to compare performance across four medical procedures: total knee replacement, total hip replacement, partial hip replacement, and intertrochanteric fracture. The methodology applied in the calculation of orthopedic benchmarks was based on a computerized review and analysis of more than 700,000 Medicare

Table 26–2 Outcomes Today SmartTracks Utilization/Functional Outcomes Totals Report

NON-OP SHOULDER IMPINGEMENT-I

Number of Cases:	206	Average Duration-In-Days:	35	Average Number-Of-Visits:	4

NON-OP SHOULDER IMPINGEMENT-II

Number of Cases:	122	Average Duration-In-Days:	51	Average Number-Of-Visits:	5

NON-OP SHOULDER IMPINGEMENT-III

Number of Cases:	151	Average Duration-In-Days:	53	Average Number-Of-Visits:	6

NON-OP SHOULDER IMPINGEMENT-IV

Number of Cases:	40	Average Duration-In-Days:	62	Average Number-Of-Visits:	7

NON-OP SHOULDER IMPINGEMENT-V

Number of Cases:	35	Average Duration-In-Days:	48	Average Number-Of-Visits:	7

Text continued on p. 387.

What is shoulder impingement?

Impingement is an overuse problem of the shoulder that results in pinching of the rotator cuff or biceps tendon between the arm bone (humerus) and the tip of the shoulder (acromion). The tendons then become inflamed, swollen, and painful.

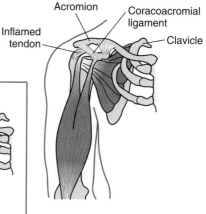

Acromion
Coracoacromial ligament
Inflamed tendon
Clavicle

Causes of shoulder impingement

- Poor posture
- Repetitive overhead activities
- Muscle weakness
- Loss of shoulder range of motion
- Shoulder instability ("Looseness")
- Trauma

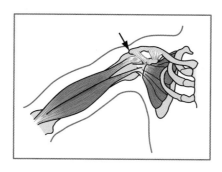

What you can expect from physical therapy

- You may be more sore after your first visit from the evaluation.
- Your shoulder pain may not be completely eliminated by the end of your physical therapy but you will be educated in how to continue making progress after you are discharged.
- It may take up to 2–3 months to gain full benefit from your exercise program.
- The longer your symptoms have been present affects the length of time for optimal recovery.
- A higher demand for function may result in need for an ergonomic work site evaluation, extended treatment, and/or work conditioning prior to return to work.
- The number of visits in physical therapy will be determined by your physical therapist and physician. On average, patients are seen 4–12 visits depending on the severity of the symptoms.

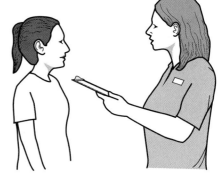

Physical therapy goals

- Decrease your pain and improve your ability to perform normal daily activities.
- Learn what activities to modify or avoid while your shoulder is healing.
  1. Avoid overhead activities.
  2. Sleep positions–avoid arms overhead at night.
  3. Avoid poor postures.
  4. In general, avoid any painful movements of the shoulder. This only causes more irritation to the already inflamed tendons.
- Understand the importance of following your physician's instructions regarding your medication.
- Learn and demonstrate the appropriate exercises for strength, flexibility, and postural connection.

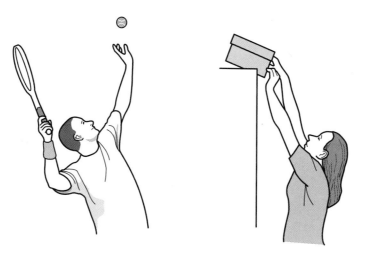

Figure 26–9. SmartTracks educational piece: Shoulder impingement.

ORTHOPAEDIC SPORTS, INC.

DAILY TREATMENT & MANAGEMENT	NON-OPERATIVE SHOULDER IMPINGEMENT SYNDROME

Patient Name:

VISIT	DATE:	VISIT	DATE:

SUBJECTIVE: Exercise Compliance ❏ Yes ❏ No

Relative to last visit, pain is ❏ Less ❏ More ❏ Same
Explain:

Other:

FUNCTIONAL CHANGES:	Patient Reports	Therapist Observes	Improved	Worse

SUBJECTIVE: Exercise Compliance ❏ Yes ❏ No

Relative to last visit, pain is ❏ Less ❏ More ❏ Same
Explain:

Other:

FUNCTIONAL CHANGES:	Patient Reports	Therapist Observes	Improved	Worse

OBJECTIVE need not measure all at every visit

ASSESSMENT Progressing as Expected

AROM/PROM: Flexion	°	°	❏ Yes ❏ No
Abduction	°	°	❏ Yes ❏ No
ER	°	°	❏ Yes ❏ No
IR	°	°	❏ Yes ❏ No
Arm Behind Back			❏ Yes ❏ No
	°	°	❏ Yes ❏ No
Strength/MMT:	P F G N Pain		❏ Yes ❏ No
	P F G N Pain		❏ Yes ❏ No
	P F G N Pain		❏ Yes ❏ No
	P F G N Pain		❏ Yes ❏ No
Scapular Control: Can control eccentric lowering	❏ Yes ❏ No		❏ Yes ❏ No
			❏ Yes ❏ No
			❏ Yes ❏ No

OBJECTIVE need not measure all at every visit

ASSESSMENT Progressing as Expected

AROM/PROM: Flexion	°	°	❏ Yes ❏ No
Abduction	°	°	❏ Yes ❏ No
ER	°	°	❏ Yes ❏ No
IR	°	°	❏ Yes ❏ No
Arm Behind Back			❏ Yes ❏ No
	°	°	❏ Yes ❏ No
Strength/MMT:	P F G N Pain		❏ Yes ❏ No
	P F G N Pain		❏ Yes ❏ No
	P F G N Pain		❏ Yes ❏ No
	P F G N Pain		❏ Yes ❏ No
Scapular Control: Can control eccentric lowering	❏ Yes ❏ No		❏ Yes ❏ No
			❏ Yes ❏ No
			❏ Yes ❏ No

ASSESSMENT:

ASSESSMENT:

TREATMENT TODAY	PLAN OF CARE (POC)	TREATMENT TODAY	PLAN OF CARE (POC)
❏ Therapeutic Exercises ** ❏ Neuro Re-ed ** ❏ Therapeutic Activities** ❏ Joint Mobilization _____ ❏ Ultrasound _____ ❏ Massage _____ ❏ Ice ❏ Heat ❏ E-Stim (unattended)_____ ❏ _____	❏ Continue ❏ Change (explain):	❏ Therapeutic Exercises ** ❏ Neuro Re-ed ** ❏ Therapeutic Activities** ❏ Joint Mobilization _____ ❏ Ultrasound _____ ❏ Massage _____ ❏ Ice ❏ Heat ❏ E-Stim (unattended)_____ ❏ _____	❏ Continue ❏ Change (explain):

SIGNATURE:	LIC #:	SIGNATURE:	LIC #:

** SEE THERAPEUTIC PROCEDURES/SELF MANAGEMENT SHEETS   KEY: AROM=Active Range of Motion; PROM=Passive Range of Motion; IR=Internal Rotation; ER=External Rotation; P=Poor; F=Fair; G=Good; N=Normal; L=Left; R=Right; MMT=Manual Muscle Testing; E-Stim=Electrical Stimulation-

Figure 26–10. SmartTracks sample evaluation form: Non-operative shoulder impingement syndrome.

ORTHOPAEDIC SPORTS, INC.

RE-EVALUATION	NON-OPERATIVE SHOULDER IMPINGEMENT SYNDROME

Patient Name:	Visit#	Date: ___ / ___ / ___

SUBJECTIVE: Is Patient Satisfied With: Service? ❑ Yes ❑ No _____ Progression? ❑ Yes ❑ No _____

Relative to 1st visit, is pain ❑ Increased ❑ Decreased ❑ No Change _____

Exercise compliance ❑ Yes ❑ No _____

Other: _____

FUNCTIONAL STATUS:	Must Refer to Initial Problems/Expected Outcomes	Progressing Toward Expected Outcome

1. _____ ❑ Yes ❑ No ❑ Outcome Met
2. _____ ❑ Yes ❑ No ❑ Outcome Met
3. _____ ❑ Yes ❑ No ❑ Outcome Met
4. _____ ❑ Yes ❑ No ❑ Outcome Met

OBJECTIVE: Need not measure all			ASSESSMENT Progressing as Expected	OBJECTIVE: Need not measure all		ASSESSMENT Progressing as Expected
AROM/PROM: Flexion	°	°	❑ Yes ❑ No	**Palpation:**		❑ Yes ❑ No
Abduction	°	°	❑ Yes ❑ No	Tissue Quality:		
ER	°	°	❑ Yes ❑ No	Patient's Pain Response to Palpation:	Min Mod Sev	
IR	°	°	❑ Yes ❑ No	**Palpation:**		❑ Yes ❑ No
Arm Behind Back			❑ Yes ❑ No	Tissue Quality:		
Painful Arc:	°	°	❑ Yes ❑ No	Patient's Pain Response to Palpation:	Min Mod Sev	
Strength/MMT: Flexors	P F G N Pain		❑ Yes ❑ No	**Flexibility:** Latissimus	°	❑ Yes ❑ No
Abductors	P F G N Pain		❑ Yes ❑ No	Pectoralis Minor	cm	❑ Yes ❑ No
ER	P F G N Pain		❑ Yes ❑ No	**Posture:**	P F N	❑ Yes ❑ No
IR	P F G N Pain		❑ Yes ❑ No	**Posterior Capsule Tightness:**	N Min Mod Sev	❑ Yes ❑ No
Supraspinatus	P F G N Pain		❑ Yes ❑ No	**Scapula:** Can control eccentric lowering	❑ Yes ❑ No	❑ Yes ❑ No
Serratus Anterior	P F G N Pain		❑ Yes ❑ No			❑ Yes ❑ No
Lower Trapezius	P F G N Pain		❑ Yes ❑ No			❑ Yes ❑ No

ASSESSMENT: Therapy has been effective to date: ❑ Yes ❑ No Effective = Has shown progress in 2 of 3 (subjective; objective; and/or functional) **If "No", see comments below.**

❑ Patient has met all expected functional outcomes ❑ Patient is progressing adequately toward expected functional outcomes
❑ Patient is not progressing as expected - Explain why: _____
Comments: _____

New /or Modified Expected Functional Outcomes:
1) _____
2) _____

TREATMENT TODAY:	❑ Re-evaluation ❑ Therapeutic Exercise** ❑ Neuromuscular Re-education**
	❑ Therapeutic Activities** ❑ Joint Mobilization _____
	❑ Massage ❑ Ultrasound _____
	❑ Ice/Heat ❑ _____ ❑ _____

TREATMENT PLAN:	EXPECTED VISITS/TIME FRAME:
❑ Continue plan of care	❑ Modify plan of care _____

Therapist Signature:	License #:

**SEE THERAPEUTIC PROCEDURES/SELF MANAGEMENT SHEET KEY: N=Normal; Min=Minimal; Mod=Moderate; Sev=Severe; P=Poor; F=Fair; G=Good; L=Left; R=Right; IR=Internal Rotation; ER=External Rotation; MMT=Manual Muscle Testing; AROM=Active Range of Motion; PROM=Passive Range of Motion;

Figure 26–11. SmartTracks care management in physical therapy.

Table 26–3 2001 National Utilization Rates by Service Line

Solucient product line	Discharge rate per 1000	ALOS	Days rate per 1000
Cardiology	17.6	3.8	67.5
OB/delivery	13.4	2.5	33.6
Pulmonary	10.9	5.3	58.0
Normal newborns	9.7	2.0	19.4
Orthopedics	8.4	4.4	37.4
Gastroenterology	8.0	4.1	32.8
General surgery	7.6	6.8	51.9
Psych/drug abuse	6.0	7.6	45.8
Neurology	5.1	4.9	25.3
General medicine	4.6	7.4	34.3
Neonatology	4.4	6.1	26.7
Gynecology	3.2	2.9	9.3
Endocrine	3.0	4.2	12.6
Oncology medical	2.5	6.6	16.5
Nephrology	2.4	5.0	12.0
Urology	2.2	4.0	8.7
Vascular surgery	1.7	6.4	11.0
Open heart	1.6	8.9	14.2

Data from Solucient: Inpatient Estimates, 12th edition, Evanston, IL, 2002.

orthopedic cases. This study considered risk-adjusted mortality rates, risk-adjusted complications rates, average length of stay, and cost per patient adjusted for illness severity, among other variables. On a broader note, Solucient also publishes national utilization rates by service line. Table 26–3 provides an overview of the 2002 inpatient estimates for multiple medical specialties including cardiology, orthopedics, neurology, pulmonary, and 14 others. For instance, the average length of stay for orthopedics is 4.4 inpatient hospital days compared with 7.7 days for general medicine and 8.9 days for open heart surgery.

Solucient blends clinical, financial, and patient data in developing integrated analyses of healthcare information. These analyses allow for physician or provider profiling, health plan member profiling, disease management, quality management, and provider network management that collectively facilitate balancing cost, risk, and quality. Solucient's goals are to improve health plan member satisfaction, improve provider and plan performance, and lower costs. Figure 26–12 demonstrates Solucient's *Integrated Managed Care Solutions.*

Solucient's Webpage provides an overview of its "Provider Business Decision Suite" and at least 19 different data warehouses that can be used for strategic planning, sales and marketing, and/or quality improvement purposes (Solucient, 2001).

Although Solucient's efforts are not currently directed at physical rehabilitation, a strong likelihood exists that a trickle-down effect will occur, especially given physical rehabilitation's high profile in workers' compensation.

DISABILITY TREATMENT AND MANAGEMENT SERVICES

The following entities provide an array of disability services that fall within the treatment range of the disability continuum. These organizations make the distinction between disease and impairment, impairment and disability, and disability and handicap. Their services are based on enhancing functionality, emphasizing ability versus disability, and returning their patients/clients to activities of daily living.

Easter Seals

Easter Seals
Chicago, IL
Website: http://www.easter-seals.org

Easter Seals is a not-for-profit organization created in 1919 to help children and adults with disabilities gain greater independence. Easter Seals offers extensive services that span the entire disability continuum at more than 400 sites across the United States and Puerto Rico. Principal programs include:

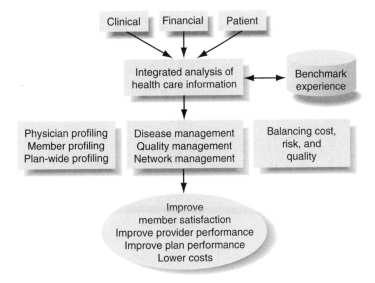

Figure 26–12. Solucient's integrated managed care solutions.

- Children services: 311 sites provide developmental monitoring, early childhood services, inclusive child care, developmental preschool programs, and services for school-aged children. Easter Seal's goal is to become the nation's premier provider of inclusive child care (for children 6 months to 5 years of age). Easter Seals serves the needs of more than 20 million children and their working parents.
- Physical medicine and rehabilitation: 212 sites provide physical, occupational and speech-language therapies, audiology, social work, rehabilitation engineering, recreational therapy, and other support services. Easter Seals is the nation's largest provider of pediatric rehabilitation and early intervention.
- Camping and recreation programs: 125 programs exist nationwide including day camps, recreation programs, and residential camping for adults and children. Easter Seals is the largest provider of these services in the United States.
- Job training and employment services: 104 service sites provide evaluation and assessment, work adjustment/ employee development, job placement, employment planning, occupational skills training, school-to-work transitions, and assistive technologies for community-based and supportive employment.
- Adult and senior service programs: 78 adult day care services are offered along with assisted living programs, and in-home care.
- Residential housing programs: 33 programs support individuals with disabilities to live with greater independence in their communities.

Easter Seals addresses the needs of persons with disabilities whether they are congenital conditions, the result of injury or illness, or functional limitations experienced in aging. Easter Seals' operations are decentralized and managed by chief executive officers at the local level. Figure 26–13 depicts the decentralized corporate structure of Easter Seals across five service domains. These five domains are rehabilitation, inclusive child care, job training, adult day services, and camp and recreation. They represent a consolidation of services that once numbered 20. Easter Seals

today does not have a single corporate structure, rather each of its 100 organizations (15,000 employees) represents its own 501C(3) not-for-profit entity. Easter Seals overcame structural barriers by lining up services along a vertical axis with all five services available to each individual location. The individual strengths of each organization are highly prized by Easter Seals. Local fundraising efforts are bolstered by ensuring that funds derived from local sources are expended locally. Networks that comprise individual organizations range from loose affiliations to franchise models. This restructuring has also facilitated multidisciplinary programs.

Donald Jackson, a physical therapist who serves as chief operating officer at Easter Seals corporate offices, sums up the contribution of Easter Seals.

The rate of incidence of many disabling conditions has doubled over the last decade and the number of babies born and living with physical or mental disabilities is twice what is was 25 years ago. In addition, demographic projections predict a tremendous increase in the number of senior citizens, particularly, the frail elderly, age 85 and over. Our greatest strength is that we're able to help people of all ages and with a wide range of disabilities. No one is refused service because of financial difficulties and fees for service are based on a family's ability to pay.

- Daus, 1998

Isernhagen Work Systems

Isernhagen Work Systems
Duluth, MS
Contact: Margot Miller
Website: http://www.iws.workwell.com

Susan Isernhagen is considered one of the nation's pioneers of functional capacity and evaluation and work hardening services beginning with her tenure at the Polinsky Institute in Minneapolis, MN. Isernhagen Work Systems (IWS) provides disability-related services across the entire continuum from injury prevention to post-treatment consultation. IWS services are principally geared towards disability management within the workers' compensation sector. A menu of their services can be found in Table 26–4. These services fall under a program called "work injury management and prevention." This program strives to match workers to their worksite to effect safe yet expeditious return to work, maintenance of gainful employment, or exploration of new employment.

IWS provides services that are congruent with the ADA and with OSHA and Equal Employment Opportunity Commission policies. In fact, the IWS Web site has links to ADA, OSHA, and the Equal Employment Opportunity Commission. Figure 26-14 depicts a flow diagram of the IWS work injury management program. An emphasis is placed on function and injury or disability prevention. In this schematic, a functional job analysis (FJA) plays a vital role in the development of a functional job description to aid in the hiring or return-to-work processes. The FJA also serves as an underpinning of ergonomic programs that are consistent with ADA and OSHA. FJAs are also used in

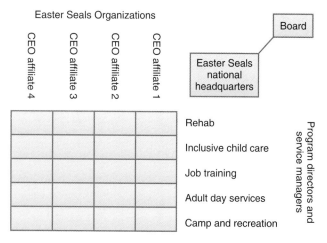

Figure 26–13. Easter Seals: Decentralized corporate structure. (Data from Easter Seals, Chicago.)

Table 26-4 Isernhagen Work Systems Work Injury Management and Prevention Services

- Functional job analysis
- Functional job description
- Ergonomic evaluations of work site
- Education for injury prevention
- Work technique training
- Stretch therapy
- Prework screening
- Prework conditioning
- Early intervention
- Aggressive rehabilitation onsite or offsite
- Work rehabilitation
- Functional capacity evaluation
- Return-to-work coordination

Data from Isernhagen Work Systems Website: http://www.iws.workwell.com, accessed February 26, 2003.

the prevention and education sphere for safety and ergonomic training of employees or management.

National Rehabilitation Hospital

National Rehabilitation Hospital
Washington, DC
Website: http://www.nrhrehab.org
Contact: Cathy Ellis, PT

The National Rehabilitation Hospital (NRH) was established in 1986 as a private not-for-profit inpatient rehabilitation facility. NRH has 128 licensed beds and employs approximately 787 people throughout its primary inpatient site and 18 outpatient sites. The NRH Medical

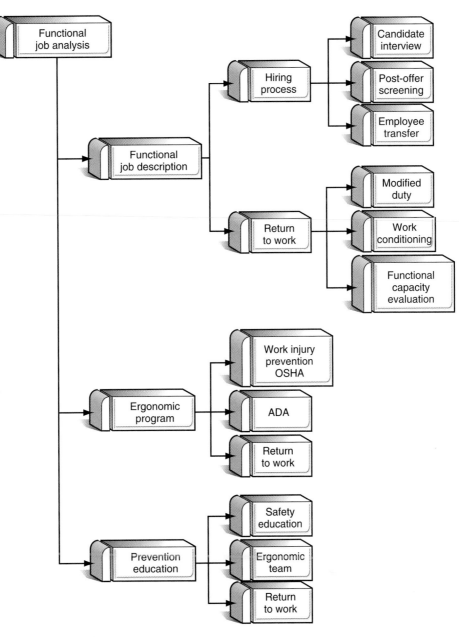

Figure 26-14. Isernhagen Work Systems: Work injury management and prevention.

Rehabilitation Network's mission is to serve the community as a regional and national leader in rehabilitation by targeting the following five goals:

1. Provide quality patient care in inpatient, outpatient, transitional, and home care programs.
2. Conduct rehabilitation research.
3. Provide education and training of rehabilitation professionals and the community.
4. Promote assistive technology that helps persons with disabilities in living productive lives.
5. Serve in an advocacy role by working with persons with disabilities in communicating their needs to policymakers at a local, state, and national level.

NRH offers services along the entire continuum of care, and patients can enter the continuum at any point. Table 26–5 provides an extensive service capability across diverse treatment settings. The breadth of NRH's programs and services prohibits any detailed coverage. Readers are encouraged to peruse NRH's Website, marketing and collateral materials, and extensive research roster.

Regional Rehabilitation is a network that provides outpatient services in Northwest Washington and Maryland. This network is a subsidiary of NRH, however, a number of centers are joint ventures between NRH and Suburban Hospital.

Vocational rehabilitation services offered by NRH include the following:

- Comprehensive vocational assessment
- Individual/group counseling
- Career development
- Situational assessment
- Job-seeking skills
- Job analysis
- Worksite assessment
- Job development
- Selective job placement
- School reentry
- Employer education
- Work adjustment training
- Industrial rehabilitation consultation
- Volunteer employment

In part because of its Washington location, NRH provides services through its International Program. The center's multicultural and multilingual staff provide rehabilitation to persons from around the world in collaboration with various embassies. This feature differentiates NRH from many rehabilitation systems.

NRH's Telehealth Center uses cutting-edge technology that extends NRH's reach to remote sites around the world. NRH medical and rehabilitation staff provide live, interactive diagnostic and consultation services for patients who have needs because of a variety of conditions. Customized training courses for health care providers are also provided through the Telehealth Center. Additionally, the Telehealth Center provides homebound clients with monitoring and early interventional services. These services are provided through state-of-the-art televideo conferencing capabilities that involve the patient's telephone, television monitor, and a camera. Equipment, installation, and necessary training are provided by NRH.

 Table 26–5 National Rehabilitation Hospital's Service Capabilities

- Acupuncture
- Amputee clinic
- Aquatic therapy
- Arthritis program
- Audiology services
- Augmentative communication clinic
- Back injury prevention/treatment
- Biofeedback
- Brain injury prevention/treatment
- Breast cancer rehabilitation
- Cardiac rehabilitation program
- Continence training
- Driver's evaluation
- Ergonomics assessment & worksite analysis
- Fall prevention program
- Fertility clinic
- Foot and running clinic
- Functional capacity evaluations
- Golf performance enhancement
- Hand therapy
- Independent medical evaluations
- Intraoperative short-stay elective procedures, or SSEP, monitoring
- Lymphedema program
- Memory evaluation and neurobehavioral treatment
- Neuropsychology services
- Neurological services
- Occupational rehabilitation
- Orthopedic and musculoskeletal disorder programs
- Pain management
- Pediatric speech and language services
- Pelvic pain services
- Performing arts medicine
- Physical therapy
- Postconcussive syndrome care
- Postpolio care
- Prosthetics and orthotics training
- Psychology services
- Rehabilitation needs assessment
- Repetitive motion disorders
- Reflex sympathetic dystrophy (RSD) evaluation/treatment
- Seating and mobility evaluation
- Speech and language services
- Spinal cord injury prevention/treatment
- Sports medicine
- Stroke prevention/treatment
- Swallowing evaluation/treatment
- Vestibular rehabilitation
- Vocational evaluation services
- Work hardening
- Wound and skin care

The NRH Research Center conducts research that is funded by federal and private agencies including the National Institutes of Health, the National Institute on Disability and Rehabilitation, The Department of Defense, the Robert Wood Johnson Foundation, and the Multiple Sclerosis Society. The NRH Research center is also the host site for the Research and Training Center on Medical Rehabilitation Services and Health Policy, which is funded by the National Institute for Disability and Rehabilitation Research (NIDRR). The NRH Website has an extensive listing of various research projects as well as an alphabetized search selection of clinical programs and services.

OUR System

OUR System
c/o Norman Peterson & Associates
Ashland, OR
Website: http://www.returntowork.com

OUR System is an acronym for optimum utilization of resources system. This workers' compensation consulting company was founded by Norman Peterson in 1985. The OUR System is a proactive transitional work program that places injured workers at the job site through a series of temporary jobs that aid their recovery. This program is geared towards workers' compensation and disability management. OUR adheres to the following principles:

1. To delay rehabilitation is to compromise rehabilitation. Working can be a form of functional rehabilitation given careful matching of the worker to the worksite.
2. The longer a worker remains off the job, the less likely he or she will return to gainful employment.
3. Psychosocial factors can affect the outcome of work-related conditions when injured workers remain out of work.

The OUR System tailors its program to each industry or employer with whom its works, but the following goals are consistent:

- Increase the injured employee's physical capacities.
- Assist in early return to work within the employee's physical abilities.
- Lessen the employee's financial concerns.
- Maintain productivity and decrease workers' compensation costs.
- Provide all concerned parties with a uniform approach to rehabilitation.

OUR involves a five-step disability management process designed to safely but expeditiously return injured workers to gainful employment.

1. **Review.** Review the employer's workers' compensation history by using available claims data. These data provide clues to which workstations/worksites should be evaluated.
2. **Proposal.** Present a plan for the identification and documentation of bridge assignments, which are then customized to the employer's needs. Bridge assignments are transitional or temporary work positions that may match the injured employee's functional abilities.
3. **Documentation.** Once a proposal has been accepted, trained consultants visit the worksite to research work needs, organize tasks into transitional bridge assignments, draft detailed functionally based bride assignments and assemble operating manuals that describe employer policies, procedures, bridge job matrices, and bridge assignment descriptions. The OUR System manual and photos of bridge jobs for workers potentially enables offsite physicians to make more informed decisions when making return-to-work decisions. These manuals provide physicians with options for job placement during the recovery stage of an injury or illness. Each job has been analyzed with detailed specifications documented.
4. **Training.** Multiple stakeholders are assembled for training in the use of the OUR System. These persons include employees, health care providers, attorneys, safety officers, risk managers, human resource and third-party health plan administrators.
5. **Evaluation.** Quarterly visits are made to the worksite after program implementation.

Norm Peterson & Associates, the purveyor of the OUR program, also offer employer services designed for the early identification of potentially problematic cases. The critical claims management program gives the following definition of a critical claim: "A critical claim is any injury claim which may be identified, according to agreed upon criteria, as likely to have a costly and/or negative outcome for the employer, the employee or both."

This service involves an employer-selected critical claims management team that typically includes risk manager, human resource director, third-party administrator, benefits coordinator, medical providers including therapists, and a company nurse. These persons receive training and a manual that outline claims management policies and procedures, rehabilitation services, and transitional duty programs. This manual is co-drafted by team members and revised when necessary. Team members then periodically meet for discussion of critical claims and/or to revise policies and procedures. This approach is similar to a healthcare organization's monthly Medicare meeting, physician rounds, or case management round-ups.

Figure 26–15 demonstrates a 5-year follow-up study of lost time claims costs and resultant cost savings produced through the use of transitional duty as a form of work rehabilitation.

Physical Therapy Provider Network

Physical Therapy Provider Network
Calabasa, CA
Website: http://www.ptpn.com

Physical Therapy Provider Network (PTPN) is the nation's oldest and largest independent physical therapy network founded in 1985. PTPN operates in 23 states with more than 1100 clinical sites and approximately 3000 therapists (physical, occupational, and speech). PTPN was created in response to the rapid growth of managed care in Southern California. Today it boasts more than 500 managed care contracts with approximately 4000 payers. Ninety percent of PTPN's managed care contracts are with preferred provider organizations. Member therapist practices empower PTPN to market and negotiate managed care contracts on their behalf. PTPN members offer a constellation of services that span the entire disability continuum from prevention/wellness through treatment to posttreatment. PTPN is included in this chapter's disability treatment and management section, however, because of its extensive network capabilities. PTPN was created to give independent private practitioners leverage when negotiating managed care contracts and as an alternative to selling their practices to gain critical mass. PTPN markets itself to payers as a "one-stop" opportunity that can meet all of their therapy needs through one contact point. PTPN offices must meet stringent membership requirements.

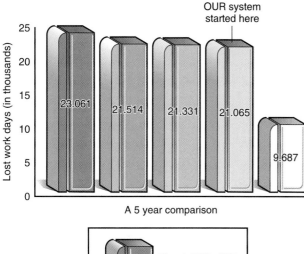

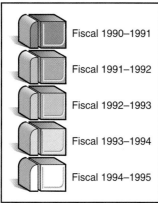

Figure 26–15. OUR System: 5-year comparison of lost work days. (Data from Norm Peterson and Associates, Ashland, OR.)

Table 26-6 describes PTPN's Membership Criteria. No corporate or physician-owned practices are enrolled in PTPN. Only independent therapists can belong to PTPN. Members are initially credentialed and thereafter recredentialed on a biannual basis. PTPN asserts that its credentialing process exceeds the National Committee on Quality Assurance (NCQA) requirements. Biannual visits to member sites are also conducted. PTPN's quality assurance program includes the following elements:

- Practice profiling
- Peer review
- Retrospective case review
- Site surveys for compliance with Membership Standards
- Patient satisfaction surveys
- Discharge surveys
- Continued education requirement of 15 contact hours (patient care related) annually

In 1990, PTPN began to expand nationally through a franchise program, beginning with Michigan. Additional franchises were established in Connecticut, Florida, Louisiana, Massachusetts, New Hampshire, New York, Rhode Island, and Tennessee.

PTPN's co-founder and president, Michael Weinper, MPH, PT, forecasts growth in opportunities beyond treatment including fitness, wellness women's health, ergonomics, job site analysis, prevention and evaluation programs (Weinper, 1999).

Therapeutics Associates, Inc.

Therapeutic Associates, Inc.
Seattle, WA
Website: http://www.tairehab.com

Therapeutic Associates, Inc. (TAI) is a rehabilitation company with a 40-year history serving 48 locations in the

 Table 26–6 Physical Therapy Provider Network Membership Criteria

1. Member is licensed by the State or is otherwise permitted by the standards established by Corporation, to provide the services specified in this Agreement without the requirement of supervision by another person. The persons so qualified to render services are hereinafter referred to as "Practicing Therapists."
2. Member is owned in the majority by Practicing Therapists. A minority interest in the Member may be held by natural persons who are not Practicing Therapists; however, such persons shall not refer to the Member for profit. In no event shall any interest in the Member be held by Physicians, Doctors of Osteopathy, Dentists, Chiropractors, Podiatrists or others with similar credentials as may be designated by the Corporation.
3. Member renders services on its own responsibility and is free from the administrative control of an employer.
4. Member treats individuals as its own patients for whom it has the right to collect a fee or other compensation for services rendered.
5. Member maintains, at its own expense, an office space and the necessary equipment to provide an adequate program of services.
6. Member is engaged in the practice of services on a regular basis. Office must be open for at least three days per week and a minimum of twenty hours per week.
7. Member and their Practicing Therapists are graduates of an accredited educational program pertaining to the services specified in this Agreement as conducted by an organization formally recognized by Corporation as qualified to conduct such programs.
8. Member is certified by the Federal Medicare Program as a participating provider. Corporation may at its sole option waive such a requirement.
9. Practicing Therapists who have a majority interest in the Member practice must each have a minimum of three (3) years clinical experience.
10. Member uses Practicing Therapists to perform and document all patient evaluations, treatment plans and patient reevaluations.
11. Member patient treatments are performed by Practicing Therapist or are performed under the supervision of a Practicing Therapist by an assistant or aide who meets the requirements of Corporation.
12. Member continually maintains the ratio of Practicing Therapists to assistants and aides specified by Corporation. In no event shall ratio be less than that specified by state law or regulation.

Note: This list represents a partial listing of Physical Therapy Provider Network Membership Criteria, Calabasa, CA.
Data with permission from Physical Therapy Provider Network.

western states. TAI is a physical therapist-owned company that employs physical, occupational, and speech therapists. TAI was one of the first rehabilitation companies in the United States to recognize the need for both fiscal and clinical accountability. TAI's Therapy Referral Handbook, now in its second edition, provides single-page treatment summaries for 89 diagnoses. This handbook is used by therapists, referring physicians, case managers, claims adjusters, and others. Figure 26–16 provides a sample page or diagnosis from the handbook. Handbook pages list the ICD-9 codes that fall within the treatment/management guidelines. These codes or conditions drive key evaluation components, treatment goals, length of stay expressed in visit number, and discharge criteria for physical therapists. These elements represent the efforts of TAI clinicians who conducted extensive literatures searches before arriving at a consensus on how to manage different conditions. The handbook describes circumstances that may require additional visits and/or alteration of the treatment plan. This is in recognition that although standardization of treatment is a worthy goal, in reality every case has unique elements that require flexibility.

TAI offers physical rehabilitation providers a diagnosis-based functional outcome system called Therapeutic Associates Outcomes System (TAOS). Currently more than 320 facilities in 25 states use TAOS. TAOS provides five data points including utilization, functional index, perceived pain, perceived improvement, and work days lost. Outcome data are warehoused in a national database for comparative information. TAI's Website states various uses for these data, including the following:

- Identification of efficacy of treatment
- Quantifiable patient progress for referrers
- Identification of best practice/therapist for overall education
- Data for referrers and payers on effectiveness of treatment
- Marketing and contract negotiations
- Performance appraisals

TAOS is approved by the ORYX initiative of the Joint Commission for Accreditation of Healthcare Organizations. TAOS data are collected through patient worksheets on initial evaluation and again on discharge from services. Office staff score the patient-completed worksheets and enter the data on TAOS' online Webpages. Quarterly TAOS reports are made available to subscribers. Customized reports can segregate outcomes data by category [e.g. by ICD code, anatomic area, insurance group, and referring physician (Tables 26–7 and 26–8)].

DISABILTY CONSULTATION

The Foto Group

San Bernadino, CA
Website: http://www.rtw.org

The Foto Group is a multidisciplinary rehabilitation company that offers services along the entire disability continuum. This group is a highly diversified disability management and rehabilitation company that applies its resident knowledge and talents in a variety of areas. Customers (aside from the patient) include traditional insurance companies, managed care organizations, Medicare intermediaries and healthcare providers and/or systems. The Foto Group should not be confused with Focus on Therapeutic Outcomes (FOTO) of Knoxville, Tennessee. The FOTO Group is discussed here under disability consultation because of its success in converting clinical knowledge, aptitudes, experience, and skill sets into non-treatment offerings to other customers.

The Foto Group: RTW, Inc.

Mary Foto, OTR, past president of the American Occupational Therapy Association, is the sole proprietor of The Foto Group. Return-to-Work (RTW) is the clinical piece of this entity. Founded in 1993, RTW is a 20,000-square-foot independent therapist-owned state-of-the-art outpatient care practice and research laboratory. RTW employs more than 25 people and specializes in providing individually tailored rehabilitation therapy for postoperative patients, injured workers, and athletes.

RTW uses a partnering paradigm when dealing with workers' compensation cases and disability management. RTW's approach to disability management is established in three steps (Foto & Niemeyer, 1993).

STEP ONE: FOCUS ON OUTCOME OVER PROCESS. Outcomes management is based on data gathering and management. This process begins with a unique intake process that includes initial comprehension screening to identify potential psychosocial barriers to rehabilitation. Areas of focus include the following:

- Client's educational history
- Client's occupational history
- Social functioning
- Problems with customary roles
- Vitality or fatigue level
- Bodily pain
- General perceptions of physical and mental health
- Job satisfaction
- Use of alcohol or other substances
- Expectations regarding therapy outcome and return-to-work

This approach is a dramatic departure from traditional rehabilitation's focus on physical impairments and functioning only. This paradigm recognizes the influence of psychosocial and other non-physical factors on recovery cycles and functional outcomes. RTW conducts a second level of screening if psychosocial barriers appear to be present. A second screening level assesses variables such as depression, somatization, quality and intensity of pain, personality factors, and life stressors. The purpose of this screening level is to predict which cases are likely to be most costly to the provider and payer. On the basis of this prediction, clients are profiled on the complexity of their needs and allocation of resources necessary to overcome rehabilitation barriers. Again, these barriers are often non-physical or clinically based. Each client is assigned

ICD-9: 722.0 723.4 722.71
APTA MUSCULOSKELETAL Preferred Practice Pattern: A, B, F, G, H, J
APTA NEUROMUSCULAR Preferred Practice Pattern: F

CERVICAL DISC PATHOLOGY

EXAMINATION

History and systems review

Tests and measures:
- Cervical/thoracic ROM
- Passive intervertebral mobility
- Neurological examination
- Posture assessment
- Upper extremity functional ROM
- Craniovertebral stability tests
- Pain
- Strength

Establish plan of care

GOALS AND OUTCOMES

- Centralized pain: 2/10 or less with alleviation of any radicular signs and symptoms
- Cervical/thoracic ROM: 80% of AMA guides and equal bilaterally

Cervical			
Flexion	50°	Extension	60°
Rotation	65°	Sidebend	35°
Thoracic			
Flexion	32°	Extension	*
Sidebend	8°	Rotation	24°

- Grip strength 90% of uninvolved extremity
- Restore balanced posture (head position, shoulder position, spinal curvatures)
- Spinal strength and stability to prevent reinjury: 4+/5 manual muscle test of the cervical and scapular muscles
- Return to previous functional status for ADL, vocational, recreational and sport activities as identified by patient
- Independence in a progressive home exercise program emphasizing function

NUMBER OF VISITS: 7-14

Circumstances requiring additional visits
- Persistent functional strength deficit or ≤ 3/5 on manual muscle test
- History of previous injury/surgery to related area
- Persistent radicular symptoms or neurological deficit
- Severe deconditioning
- Special occupational needs requiring extensive fitness/strengthening
- Restriction in segmental joint mobility
- Surgery is indicated, however the patient is not a surgical candidate due to risk factors
- Bilateral upper extremity radiculopathy
- Presence of fracture

DISCHARGE

Home program
- Flexibility
- Self-mobilization
- Home traction PRN
- Monitoring
- Strengthening
- Modalities PRN
- Cardiovascular conditioning

Criteria for discharge
- Patient displays understanding of the role of proper posture and body mechanics in the prevention of reinjury
- All rehabilitation goals have been achieved with the exception of previous functional status for recreational and sport activities

THERAPY REFERRAL HANDBOOK • Cervical/Thoracic   55

Figure 26–16. TAI: Therapy Referral Handbook sample page.

Table 26-7   Sample Facility Profile Report

	Facility 1Q-2002	Facility 2Q-2002	Facility 3Q-2002	Network 3Q-2002	TAOS 3Q-2002
CERVICAL/THORACIC					
Number of patients	15	33	26	762	2,198
Functional improvement	56.73%	57.74%	60.08%	46.88%	49.60%
Decrease in pain	57.16%	59.19%	62.73%	54.90%	57.82%
Perceived improvement	70.33%	72.27%	74.62%	72.61%	72.28%
Number of visits	7.5	8.8	8.6	9.7	10.1
Work days lost	2.5	4.2	3.9	4.8	6.8
LUMBAR					
Number of patients	19	20	29	1,066	3,217
Functional improvement	54.28%	52.04%	51.35%	43.76%	48.24%
Decrease in pain	68.97%	66.65%	64.75%	51.64%	57.46%
Perceived improvement	76.32%	75.50%	69.66%	69.88%	71.70%
Number of visits	6.3	6.9	8.2	9.3	8.9
Work days lost	0.0	0.0	2.3	7.6	10.7
LOWER EXTREMITY					
Number of patients	15	13	22	1,199	4,077
Functional improvement	73.09%	66.51%	61.99%	60.57%	53.99%
Decrease in pain	75.25%	68.72%	57.14%	54.66%	59.25%
Perceived improvement	75.71%	71.46%	65.45%	72.63%	73.63%
Number of visits	6.6	6.2	9.3	9.9	10.1
Work days lost	0.8	0.0	1.3	8.8	11.7
UPPER EXTREMITY					
Number of patients	11	17	18	888	3,113
Functional improvement	56.11%	67.45%	75.76%	56.83%	49.10%
Decrease in pain	65.76%	71.54%	79.23%	65.08%	57.93%
Perceived improvement	74.55%	77.50%	79.41%	71.28%	72.52%
Number of visits	8.1	6.9	10.9	11.0	10.8
Work days lost	0.0	0.0	6.7	11.5	11.1

With permission from Therapeutic Associates, Inc, Portland, OR.

one of three levels of care driven by projections related to treatment course, outcome, and need for service. For example, Level I clients are expected to return to their former vocational or avocational activities. These persons have minimal tissue damage and pain, are within 14 days of injury or surgery, and have missed little work time. Level II clients are predicted to return to work after 5-8 weeks of treatment, because their residual impairments are of a mild nature, tissue damage is minimal to moderate, and 6 weeks or more have lapsed between symptom onset and interventions. These persons may also have signs of depression. Level III persons represent the most intensive group that may require 9-12 weeks of care. Interventions for this group include psychological counseling, work capacity evaluation, work hardening, job site modification, job coaching, and/or alternative work placement. These persons have sustained severe tissue damage, suffer from severe depression and may have decreased cognitive skills.

STEP TWO: INTERNAL UTILIZATION MANAGEMENT. An internal utilization management protocol compatible with external utilization management is established (Niemeyer et al, 1994). This process monitors client needs and subsequent progress. Referrals are screened to prospectively determine the medical necessity for rehabilitation services, the intensity of service, cost and length of stay.

STEP THREE: DEVELOPMENT OF INTERNAL CASE MANAGEMENT. A case management protocol is developed that aligns with and supports the workers' compensation carrier's case management program, if available. Activities that fall within the internal case management program are depicted in Table 26-9. The case management data when combined with utilization management data (especially outcomes data) allows RTW to structure case or episodic rates for rehabilitation.

The Foto Group: Treat-it.com, Inc.

RTW is also an information technology research as well as a clinical site. RTW generates data that it houses within Treat-it, a separate corporation within The Foto Group that provides time and cost-efficient solutions to non-physician healthcare professionals, most notably physical and occupational therapists. Available through either a wireless personal digital assistant or personal computer with an Internet browser, the company provides clinicians nationwide with a point-of-care, turnkey clinic/patient management solution that includes patient scheduling, authorization and intake, diagnostic plans, outcome reports, and electronic billing and remittance. Provider users pay for Treat-it data management through

Table 26–8   Sample Facility Profile Report

	Facility 1Q-2002	Facility 2Q-2002	Facility 3Q-2002	Network 3Q-2002	TAOS 3Q-2002
PATIENT POPULATION					
Number of patients	61	84	96	3,915	13,995
Male	42.52%	46.43%	39.58%	42.64%	42.00%
Female	57.38%	53.57%	60.42%	57.36%	58.00%
AGE RANGE					
Under 21	6.56%	357%	3.13%	8.38%	9.19%
21-35	36.07%	23.81%	26.04%	19.50%	18.37%
36-49	27.87%	34.52%	28.13%	29.53%	29.40%
50-65	13.11%	21.43%	26.13%	26.07%	25.82%
Over 65	16.39%	16.67%	14.58%	16.52%	17.23%
INSURANCE					
HMO/PPO	75.41%	65.48%	64.58%	43.85%	35.54%
Medicare	8.20%	14.29%	14.58%	12.86%	13.57%
Medicaid	0.00%	0.00%	2.08%	1.85%	1.82%
Worker's comp	6.56%	4.76%	6.25%	15.26%	16.92%
Auto	9.84%	15.48%	12.50%	9.70%	7.18%
OUTCOMES					
Functional improvement	62.31%	66.85%	67.05%	66.65%	58.53%
Decrease in pain	53.41%	54.09%	66.13%	63.58%	56.33%
Perceived improvement	75.17%	75.60%	69.79%	71.30%	71.98%
Number of visits	9.8	9.5	9.0	10.0	9.85
Work days lost	0.6	2.8	3.2	8.4	10.4
ACUITY					
0-15	24.07%	10.67%	18.18%	26.05%	27.02%
16-30	20.37%	16.00%	27.27%	18.19%	19.98%
31-60	27.78%	29.33%	18.18%	19.19%	18.37%
61-90	3.70%	8.00%	11.69%	9.19%	9.09%
91-120	22.22%	33.33%	18.18%	5.00%	4.95%
Over 120	1.85%	2.67%	6.49%	21.66%	20.58%

With permission from Therapeutic Associates, Inc, Portland, OR.

Table 26–9   Return-to-Work (The Foto Group) Internal Case Management Elements

- Early screening for and identification of biomedical or psychosocial barriers to recovery and return to work.
- Assessment of obstacles to recovery.
- Development of a plan of action to address these obstacles or barriers.
- Coordination of interventions with other providers.
- Coordination with insurance representatives.
- Coordination with employers.
- Maintenance of a client database to identify recurrent patterns, monitor treatment effectiveness, and identify best practices.

installation fees, recurring monthly payments, or a percentage of total billings.

The Foto Group: External Utilization Management

External utilization management is the third installment in The Foto Group's offerings. The Foto Group was the first therapist-owned company in the nation to offer peer review of rehabilitation therapies, assistive technology, durable medical equipment, and prosthetics and orthotics in Medicare cases. The Foto Group has served as a disability consulting firm since 1969, providing rehabilitation expertise to California Blue Cross/Wellpoint.

This organization offers a myriad of services including utilization management, case management, independent review decisions, appeals and reconsiderations, policy research and development, provider education and training, payer training, coding and billing analysis, documentation expertise, patient advocacy, and communication networking.

Numerous physical, occupational, and speech-language therapists review reimbursement claims for payers and advise Medicare and Blue Cross/Wellpoint on electronic billing solutions involving medical necessity and acceptable standards of practice. Foto group therapists developed the first online model for coding and classifying therapy services for prospective payment (the 700-701 form). The Foto Group also developed the first paperless medical information system for the assessment of rehabilitation claims.

FINAL CAUTIONARY NOTE

The data provided in this chapter are substantially derived from Webpages, marketing and collateral materials provided by each profiled entity. Readers are strongly encouraged to further investigate the validity and potential applications of their innovations, products, and services within a disability management and physical rehabilitation framework. Some of these technologies (e.g., CareScience's Care Data Exchange do not currently apply to physical rehabilitation, but may offer future applications. All of these entities continue to act as change agents, and readers are encouraged to follow their progress. The diversity of offerings described should serve as an inspiration for those rehabilitation professionals who wish to explore entrepreneurial tracks or to think out-of-the-box.

REFERENCES

CareScience: http://www.carescience.com, accessed March 3, 2003.

Daus C: Your neighborhood Easter Seals, home health care dealer. J Home Med Equipment Services/Supplier 10(4):111, 1998.

Focus on Therapeutic Outcomes (FOTO): http://www.fotoinc.com, accessed February 25, 2003.

Foto M, Niemeyer LO: Working partners. Risk & Benefits J 3(3):24-25, 30-31, 1993.

Guynes Design: www.guynesdesign.com/clients/clients.html, accessed October 18, 2000.

Independence Technology Website: http://www.indetech.com/index.html, accessed February 2, 2003.

Isernhagen Work Systems Web site: http://www.iws.workwell.com, Accessed February 26, 2003.

Moore P, Conn CP: Disguised: A True Story. Nashville, TN, Thomas Nelson Inc., 1985.

National Rehabilitation Hospital: collection of marketing and collateral materials, http://www.nrhrehab.org, accessed September 16, 2000.

Neimeyer LO, Foto M, Holmes-Enix: Implementing managed care in an industrial rehabilitation program. WORK 4(1): 2-8, 1994.

Physical Therapy Provider Network: http://www.ptpn.com, accessed October 22, 2000.

Return-to-Work: http://www.rtw.org, accessed March 5, 2003.

Ridyard D: A Successful Applied Ergonomics Program for Preventing Occupational Back Injuries, Advances in Industrial Ergonomics and Safety, II. Philadelphia, Taylor & Frances, 1990.

Shrey DE, LaCerte M: Principles and Practices of Disability Management in Industry. Winter Park, FL, GR Press, Inc., 1995.

Solucient (formerly HCIA-Sachs) Website, http://www.hciasachs.com, accessed October 29, 2000.

Solucient Website, http://www.solucient.com/soluitions/provider.shtml, accessed July 29, 2001.

Therapeutic Associates Inc: http://www.tairehab.com, accessed March 3, 2003.

Weinper M: PTPN: Looking to the future (white paper), December 1999, www.ptpn.com.

CHAPTER 27

Consulting Opportunities for Rehabilitation Providers

David W. Clifton, Jr., PT

"In times of turmoil, those who succeed are usually those who are willing to experiment, take risks and adapt."

- Threlkeld et al, 1999

KEY POINTS

- Physical rehabilitation providers possess the requisite knowledge, experience, and skill sets transferable to service as consultants.
- Formal education and training of rehabilitation professionals generally fails to address the vital role of these professionals as consultants to insurance companies, managed care organizations, employers, third-party administrators, government agencies, consumer/advocacy groups, and the legal community.
- Various resources exist that can assist rehabilitation providers in positioning themselves as consultants.
- Opportunities abound for those clinicians who can make the transition from clinician to consultant.
- A customer-driven approach is more effective than a technology-driven approach to disability management consulting.

Operational Definitions

Business Coalitions	A collection of employers that pool their resources in order to address issues related to disability management/prevention; also known as purchasing cooperatives or business alliances.
Consultant	A person who provides technical or professional advice in an outsourced manner not generally associated with treatment or patients per se.
Primary Prevention	Interventions that target risk assessment designed to prevent the initial onset of disease and injury.
Need Analysis	The process of ascertaining the specific needs of a potential user of consulting services; the needs analysis identifies the scope of a problem/challenge and may offer a hint at solutions as well.
Secondary Prevention	Early warning systems designed to detect and treat disease or injury before they become full blown clinical presentations.
Stakeholder	Any person or entity involved in the finance and delivery of health-related services to selected individuals or groups.
SWOT Analysis	An analysis of an individual's or organization's strengths, weaknesses, and threats or opportunities relative to the environment in which they operate.
Tertiary Prevention	Strategies that attempt to minimize the effects of disease or injury after it has occurred.

WHY CONSULT?

Consultation in the context of this discussion refers to those services that are non–treatment-oriented and generally not directed at patients per se. Clinicians who serve as consultants derive a number of benefits from the experience. When a provider ventures into various worksites, his or her understanding of injured employees may grow and translate into improved clinical performance. For example, a therapist who performs a functional job analysis as an employer consultant can become more effective as a clinician when designing work conditioning, work hardening, or functional capacity evaluations. When therapists perform medical record review, their own clinical documentation and use of evidence-based practice may improve.

Consulting also provides a means for both individuals and organizations to diversify revenue sources beyond care provision. When clinicians serve as consultants they begin to better appreciate the perspectives held by others who are direct or indirect stakeholders in health care. These may include employers, insurers, labor organizations, government agencies, school districts, or the legal community.

Times of rapid and profound change can produce threat or opportunity depending on a number of factors, including a person's or organizations' positioning, risk aversion, skill sets, and response to change. Consultation can serve as a hedge against difficult clinical times, defined by lower and slower reimbursement, job layoffs, uncertainty, and the imposition of change by external forces (e.g., regulatory activity).

Rehabilitation providers are endowed with inherent skills and knowledge to serve as outstanding consultants to industry (Clifton, 1993; Reis, 2003). Yet despite the obvious and growing demand for their knowledge, relatively few rehabilitation providers offer consultation services to business and industry. The reason for this is unclear but evidence suggests that a lack of formal training and education plays a role (Bryan et al, 1994) (Table 27-1).

Competencies Required of Consultants

Little has been written about the core competencies required of rehabilitation providers who wish to serve as consultants.

Bryan et al (1994) conducted one of the earliest surveys of clinicians for the purpose of identifying non-clinical competencies reported by a group of occupational health physical therapists. This survey, although admittedly flawed in design, offers useful information about how consultants to industry perceive their individual competencies versus the importance of certain attributes and skill sets. Respondents were asked to rate their competence in the performance of specific services relative to the importance of these services in serving client companies. Areas of self-perceived competence included:

- Understanding of key concepts and variables within business and industry organizations
- Understanding of federal and state laws and regulations that affect business and industry and their implications to consultants
- Understanding of the basic legal aspects of contractual law to which business and consultants are subject
- Awareness of current trends and issues impacting on business and industry relative to occupational health
- Development of marketing materials
- Maximization of marketing opportunities through the use of appropriate personal marketing skills
- Knowledge of the expected consultant's role within industry
- Knowledge of business safety and risk management concerns
- Development of expert witness expertise

These and other competencies (total N = 35) were rated by respondents on a Lickert scale of 1–4, with 1 representing a low level of individual competence, and 4 the highest level of competence. Surveyed therapists also rated these competencies with regard to their importance in serving as consultants. The mean value for individual competence in all 35 areas was lower than the mean value of perceived importance of these competencies to business needs. In summary, respondents who served as consultants consistently reported a gap between their competence and the importance of possessing certain knowledge levels and skill sets. Key areas of provider weakness included competencies centering around financial issues such as the computation of cost-benefit ratios and return-on-investment (ROI) formulae. Additionally, consultant's competency in regulatory and legislative issues codified by the Occupational Safety and Health Administration (OSHA) and the Americans with Disabilities Act (ADA) was self-reported as "limited." These deficiencies may partly explain why relatively few providers serve as consultants.

A second survey of California physical therapists identified a relatively small percentage of providers involved in the following consulting areas: industrial rehabilitation (8.6%); federal, state, or local government (6.5%); school districts (6.5%); and wellness or prevention programs (1.3%) (McGinty et al, 2001). These figures are especially low given that California is generally viewed as a progressive state regarding health and wellness innovations.

Bryan et al (1993) reported that consultants to industry acquired their competence through a variety of mechanisms. These are summarized in Table 27-2.

Table 27-1   Why Clinicians Should Consider Consulting

- Enhancement of professional status
- Enhancement of one's personal and professional competencies
- Contribution to health and wellness of society
- Provision of service in underserved areas
- Fusion of clinical and business knowledge
- Public relations tool when treating an employer's injured workers
- Potential entry for on-site rehabilitation services
- Enhancement of one's clinical understanding of work-related injury/illness
- Revenue enhancement
- Practice diversification

Table 27-2   Where Do Physical Therapists Gain Consulting Expertise?

Physical therapy schools	1.64%
Continuing education course	15.50%
College coursework	5.16%
Networking with colleagues	8.10%
Practical experience	59.87%
Other	9.71%

From Bryan JM, Geroy GD, Isernhagen SI: Nonclinical competencies: A survey of occupational health physical therapists. J Orthop Sports PT 19(5):305–311, 1994.

A mere 1.64% of respondents indicated that they acquired their consultative services through formally structured programs such as physical therapy educational programs. The majority of respondents (59.87%) reported that practical or hands-on experience was the primary mode for development of consultative expertise and competence. This observation is not an indictment of educational institutions as much as it is a plea for alternative sources of data. This is precisely the goal of this and other chapters; to contribute to the current body of knowledge designed to encourage more active participation of rehabilitation providers in non-treatment venues.

Who Are the Customers of Consultative Services?

Rehabilitation providers have traditionally viewed the patient as their primary customer and the referring physician as a secondary customer. While this may be true in a treatment relationship, consultation involves diversification in terms of both service offerings and customers. For the purpose of this chapter, a customer is any person, organization, or entity that is in a position to potentially purchase and/or directly consume consulting services from a provider outside of the patient-provider relationship. Table 27–3 lists potential customers for non-clinical consultation. Identification of potential customers, transferable skills, knowledge, and aptitude demands that providers view cases with an eye toward diversification (Clifton, 1995).

Some consulting opportunities may spring from a patient-provider relationship whereas others are secured through prospecting leads or via a request for proposal (RFP). Of course, clinicians must consider the legal and ethical ramifications of converting a patient encounter into a consulting possibility, especially in light of HIPAA compliance requirements (www.cms.hhs.gov/hipaa). However, common examples of consultation services that flow from patient encounters may include:

- Performance of a functional job analysis in advance of work hardening, work conditioning, or a functional capacity evaluation
- Ergonomic analysis of a job station from which employees have developed carpal tunnel syndrome
- Education and training of employers in appropriate job-jobsite matching, OSHA compliance, and modified or transitional duty development
- Employee back school

Table 27–3 Consulting Opportunities by Sector

Health Plans	Government
1. Develop peer/utilization review criteria	1. Serve as content expert for Social Security and Medicare
2. Develop treatment guidelines in cooperation with preferred providers	2. ADA consultant to local municipalities
3. Provider relations and education	3. Serve on community boards of health
4. Conduct provider credentialing	4. Serve on employers' WC panels as content expert
5. Assist plans in selecting acceptable outcome measures	5. Veteran's Administration expert on assistive technology

Utilization Management	School Districts
1. Conduct medical record review	1. Content expert for intermediate units regarding children with disabilities
2. Telephonic case management	2. Health and physical education regarding adaptive equipment
3. On-site or field case management	3. Sports medicine with athletic teams
4. Independent patient evaluations, disability assessments	4. Student screenings, (e.g., posture, scoliosis)

Legal Community	Long-Term Care
1. Expert testimony in professional liability, workers' comp, automobile liability, and disability insurance	1. Design specialty programs for specific groups
2. OSHA abatement in cumulative trauma	2. Quality assurance for skilled nursing facilities, home care, subacute care facilities
3. ADA expertise	3. Serve as Medicare auditor

Employer-Based	Unique Opportunities
1. Ergonomics	1. Consultation with pharmaceutical companies
2. ADA compliance	2. Consultation with physician practice management organizations on rehabilitation issues
3. Functional job analysis	3. Consultation with employee benefit assistance (EAP) firms
4. Wellness/health promotion	4. Collaboration with alternative health practitioners (e.g., chiropractors)
5. OSHA abatement	5. Mobile health screening
6. On-site rehabilitation	6. Consultation with labor organizations
7. Management training	7. Consultation with durable medical equipment manufacturers and dealers
8. Employee training and education	8. Design ergonomic tools/utensils for manufacturers

Internet	Sports Organizations
1. Consumer education	1. Consult with professional teams
2. Durable medical equipment assessment	2. Consult with collegiate teams
3. Consultation with manufacturers	3. Consult with exercise equipment
4. Preferred provider posting and referral service	4. Consult with athletic shoe manufacturers

PREVENTION: THE LAST FRONTIER?

Unimaginable resources and billions of dollars are expended annually in the "treatment" of disability, yet relatively little is spent on the prevention side of the equation. Similarly, providers (including physical and occupational therapists) have traditionally received incredible education and training in disability treatment, but relatively little in prevention services. However, professional organizations are addressing this need through a variety of mechanisms. For example, the American Physical Therapy Association's *Guide to Physical Therapist Practice* acknowledges that practice must transcend treatment alone and encourage participation in diverse health and wellness programs (APTA, 2001). Specific recommendations include:

- Identification of lifestyle factors (e.g., stress, obesity)
- Exercises to increase bone mass and/or density
- Endurance exercise programs (e.g., cardiovascular)
- Consumer education

Prevention may be the last frontier in disability management. However, this will require that both the supply-siders (providers) and demand-siders (payers) go beyond lip service and plunge into this arena bringing with them every resource available. There is a growing demand for health promotion programs. A Hewitt Associates survey revealed that 92% of all U.S. companies currently provide some form of health promotion, 71% offer employee education/training, 74% use health screenings, and 77% encourage disease management and wellness programs (Hewitt Associates, 2001). Physical and occupational therapists are uniquely qualified to fully participate in a prevention paradigm (Rothman & Levine, 1992).

The number and diversity of potential consulting venues are only hampered by one's lack of imagination or inability to transfer skill sets and knowledge. A sampling of potential consulting venues can be found in Figure 27–1.

Primary-Secondary-Tertiary Prevention

There are essentially three categories of prevention activities: primary, secondary, and tertiary (Rhomberg, Wolf, Evanoff, 1995). *Primary prevention* targets risk assessment designed to prevent disease and injury through a variety of preemptive measures. These include workstation evaluation, job redesign, employee preplacement screenings or evaluations, ergonomic task forces/committees, employee and management education/training, and environmental screenings. *Secondary prevention* incorporates early warning systems designed to detect and treat disease or injury before they become full clinical presentations or have heightened severity and consequence (both human and financial suffering). Blood sugar testing for diabetes, bone densimetry for osteoporosis detection and pulmonary testing represent examples of secondary prevention initiatives. *Tertiary prevention* strategies attempt to minimize the effects of disease or injury after it has occurred. Disease state management strategies involve primary, secondary, and tertiary interventions. Examples include blood pressure screenings for those with diagnosed high blood pressure (HBP), range-of-motion assessment for arthritics, and postural screenings in persons with scoliosis or kyphosis. It is common for one stage of consulting

Figure 27–1. Consulting continuum.

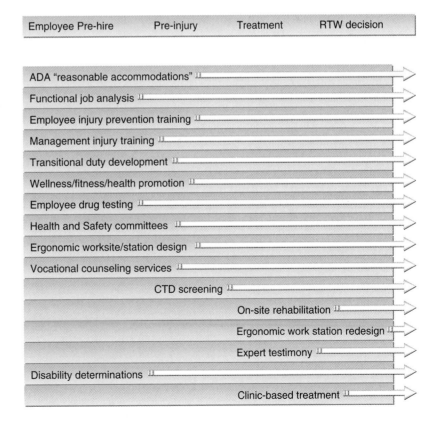

to lead to the next in a natural progression. For instance, if a therapist is managing a patient within the workers' compensation (WC) system, a number of spin-off services may naturally evolve. Performing a functional job analysis to serve as a blueprint for functional capabilities testing is one example of the connectivity between levels (Shrey & LaCerte, 1995; Isernhagen, 1995; Miller, 1996). Ergonomic analysis of an injured worker's job station or work site is another example of a consultation service that can be a design element of the discharge or RTW plan (Wiersma, 1996; Lunda, 1996). Again, physical and occupational therapists possess skill sets amenable to ergonomic consultation (Jacobs, 1999). Rehabilitation providers are ideally suited—on the basis of their extensive knowledge of anatomy, physiology, movement analysis, injury mechanisms, and human performance—to serve as ergonomic experts. This service would entail knowledge and skill sets separate and aside from, but still related to, clinical expertise.

CONSULTING VENUES

Government Consulting

Government consulting opportunities abound and are too numerous to cover in any detail. Governments at every level, local, state, and federal, are potential recipients of consulting services. Governments paradoxically drive many consultation programs through legislative actions while serving as employers themselves.

The Americans with Disabilities Act (ADA), WC, and Social Security represent three large opportunities for providers with the requisite knowledge and skill sets. Disability assessment under Social Security and WC (state and federal plans) affords unique consulting opportunities. Therapists who can perform valid physical functioning testing can play a vital role in key areas:

1. Determination of disability status under various benefit structures
2. Matching an injured worker to a potential job or vocation
3. Determination of a patient's candidacy for vocational counseling
4. Determination of the need for and type of alternative treatment program
5. Performing peer or utilization review for various government health plans (Medicare, Medicaid, CHAMPUS)

Service as a content expert on various panels charged with developing disability management policies, procedures, and guidelines represents another potential consulting venue. Those providers with occupational medicine or ergonomics experience may discover opportunities working with the Occupational Safety and Health Administration (OSHA) or the National Institute of Occupational Safety and Health (NIOSH). The Veterans Administration is always in need of rehabilitation, assistive technology, and disability management expertise. The U.S. Public Health Service employs thousands in service of its mission to keep America healthy.

The Federal government through a number of agencies needs content experts in rehabilitation and disability management. For instance, the Social Security Administration has attempted to identify those persons who no longer qualify to be on disability rolls. This requires functional testing that falls within the expertise of therapists. Federal fraud and abuse initiatives, such as "Operation Restore Trust" (ORT), also require content experts. This program was a two-year demonstration project that focused on long-term-care costs in five states: California, Florida, Illinois, New York, and Texas (Office of Inspector General, 1997). This project involved cooperation between federal and state agencies. Participating agencies and entities included the Federal Bureau of Investigation, U.S. Postal Service, Railroad Retirement Board, OIG, Defense Criminal Investigative Service, State Attorneys General offices, Health Care Financing Administration (now the Centers for Medicare & Medicaid, Administration on Aging), state survey and certification agencies, Medicaid agencies, Medicare contractors, and the U.S. Department of Justice. This initiative resulted in $23 of savings for every $1 spent on ORT. Clearly, there are opportunities for rehabilitation experts if they seek them out.

Payer Consulting

The term "payer" describes any entity that finances health care services, including traditional casualty/indemnity insurance companies, disability insurance companies, group or general health insurers, self-insured or self-funded employers, third party administrators (TPAs), and a host of managed care entities such as HMOs, Preferred Provider Organizations, and Point-of-Service (POS). Employer consultation needs are described separately, as they ultimately finance more than 80% of all health care in the United States. Insurers predominantly hire non-medical staff to manage claims and reduce risk. For instance, an average claims adjuster lacks medically based education/ training, but must manage complex medical claims with few resources available to him or her. Health plans and insurers have an insatiable need for content experts who have a command of the rehabilitation body of literature, prevailing clinical practices, and standards of care. This knowledge can be applied in the development of peer or utilization review criteria, treatment protocols, early intervention programs, clinical pathways of care, provider credentialing or re-credentialing criteria, disability determinations, and the development of outcome measures tools. Clinicians-turned-consultants can also collaborate with health plans in the development of educational materials for patients/enrollees, primary care physicians (PCPs), employers, and clinicians. Provider-relations positions would be well served if clinicians/ consultants were to fill them. Companies such as Unum (a disability insurer), Liberty Mutual (WC), PMA Insurance Group (WC), Standard Insurance (disability insurer), Prudential (Group and Life Insurer), Sun Life of Canada (disability insurer), and Mutual of Omaha (disability insurer) have developed support services that facilitate disability prevention and management (Scott 2000).

Readers may find Jan Tecklin's chapter (Chapter 11) to be of interest. This chapter describes in detail a physical rehabilitation case management program offered to a large WC company by a utilization review company owned by a physical therapist.

Legal Consulting

The legal sector has many uses for rehabilitation provider knowledge and skill sets. Rehabilitation professionals can enjoy participation as experts in professional liability cases, WC, disability insurance, general liability insurance, OSHA compliance activities, ADA compliance, and other venues. Plaintiff and defense lawyers in WC, automobile liability, disability insurance, and Medicare cases commonly require clinical expertise not available through traditional expert physicians. A number of federal initiatives, including ADA and OSHA, demand rehabilitation expertise for reasonable accommodations of persons with disabilities to the workplace. The ADA demands a provider paradigm shift from directly serving persons with disabilities to providing technical assistance to employers relative to "reasonable accommodations" (Mullins et al, 1996; Kornblau & Ellexson, 1991; Hablutzel & McMahon, 1992; U.S. Office of Disability Employment Policy, 2002).

Lawyers handling professional liability cases need experts who can compare the facts of a given case to the professional or community standard of care as either a plaintiff or a defense witness. For instance, only physical therapists may be qualified to interpret the physical therapy community standard of care.

Virtually every insurance company and managed care organization has a special investigative unit, or SIU, whose principal responsibility is to investigate potential fraud cases. In-house attorneys and fraud investigators routinely require the services of rehabilitation professionals as content experts to conduct research and testify in cases of alleged fraud. This type of consultation can help to preserve the integrity of a profession by purging it of unscrupulous and fraudulent providers. Postal inspectors often uncover evidence of suspected fraud in cases wherein the Postal Service has been used to submit fraudulent bills to insurance companies. Again, rehabilitation providers may be required as content experts in these cases. Providers who offer expert testimony in these instances should not perceive it as "dirty business." Professional or expert testimony serves several vital roles: it provides a means for consumer protection against fraud and abuse, preserves the integrity of a profession, and represents one of the hallmarks of professionalism—peer review.

School District Consulting

School districts are increasingly required by law (e.g., ADA) to accommodate students with disabilities. Mainstreaming children—the process of integrating students with physical or mental disabilities into the general student population—spawns consultation opportunities for entrepreneurial-minded therapists. Intermediate units or special education units serve as portals for exploring these services. Increased funding of services for children with special needs should facilitate the use of physical and occupational therapists for assessment, treatment, and reasonable accommodation purposes. This need is especially great in adolescents who must transition from school to work (Chandler et al, 1996). A "reasonable accommodation" under ADA involves any modification or adjustment to a job, workstation, worksite, or environment that enables a qualified candidate, applicant, or employee with a disability to participate in the performance of essential functions (Lunda, 1996).

Long-Term Care Consulting

Shifting demographics, such as the aging population, fuel the need for innovative services within the long-term care sector that includes prevention programs, specialty programs for persons with Alzheimer's disease, cancer, osteoporosis, and other age-specific conditions (Clifton, 1999). Environmental screening, barrier removal, bone densiometry assessment, and adaptive equipment consultation opportunities are certain to grow as America ages. Workers no longer retire on their 65th birthdays, and many remain valued employees. Coy and Davenport (1991) assert that older employees are susceptible to afflictions associated with aging: decreased endurance, flexibility, strength, reaction time, and accuracy.

Internet Consulting

The Internet is still in its infancy but is certain to present unique opportunities for those providers who can match their competencies to evolving market needs and trends. Consumer health care information, provider consultation, telemedicine or telehealth, assistive device consultation, and self-help programs may all require the specialized knowledge and skill sets of rehabilitation providers.

Conventional health care providers' collaboration with alternative health providers (AHPs) or complementary and alternative medicine providers (CAM) may also manifest itself through the Internet. Additionally, this vehicle facilitates provider collaboration with other stakeholders, including labor organizations, employee assistance programs, practice management, and pharmaceutical firms. Readers are encouraged to refer to Chapter 12 for an expanded view of Internet opportunities.

Rehabilitation Engineering

Niche markets can be developed, particularly when one technology is applied to another. Rehabilitation engineering represents a synergy between applied technology and rehabilitation principles. As the rehabilitation sector continues to address the evolving needs of populations (e.g., baby boomers and disease state management), rehabilitation engineering will play a vital role. Rehabilitation engineering credentials generally involve five key components (Winters, 1995):

1. Experience in the core sciences, including engineering
2. Problem solving skills
3. Hands-on design experience
4. Knowledge of rehabilitation practices and principles
5. Clinical internship service

Rehabilitation engineering requires quantitative analysis and evaluation of human performance and function. Physical and occupational therapists covet core skill sets, knowledge, and aptitude conducive to rehabilitation engineering. The design of adaptive equipment, mobility devices, and new treatment technologies represent areas of emerging opportunity.

Rehabilitation engineering received great impetus through the Assistive Technology Act of 1998. This act fostered the development of 56 assistive technology (AT) projects (one in every state and territory). The Department of Veterans Affairs, through its Rehabilitation RandD Progress Reports, has further promoted the value of AT. This publication is available free of charge from the Veterans Health Administration (VHA) and is distributed annually. Rehabilitation RandD Reports summarize a plethora of research projects, many of which are related to rehabilitation engineering. The following major subject headings illustrate areas of potential interest to rehabilitation professionals:

- Amputations and limb prostheses
- Biomechanics
- Functional assessment
- Functional electrical stimulation
- Geriatrics
- Head trauma and stroke
- Independent living aids
- Muscles, ligaments and tendons
- Neurological and vascular disorders
- Orthopedics
- Orthotics
- Psychological and psychosocial disorders
- Sensory, cognitive, and communication aids
- Spinal cord injury and related neurological disorders
- Wheelchair and powered vehicles
- Wound and fracture healing
- Miscellaneous

The Rehabilitation Engineering and Assistive Technology Society of North America (RESNA) is an interdisciplinary association for the advancement of rehabilitation and assistive technologies (AT). RESNA's mission is "to improve the potential of people with disabilities to achieve their goals through the use of technology" (http://www.resna.org). Rehabilitation providers may benefit from tracking RESNA research initiatives or participating as members.

EMPLOYER-FOCUSED CONSULTING

Employer Support of IDM

Employers represent the largest potential market for disability prevention and management programs (Fernberg, 1999; Gilpin, 2000). A 1995 survey of 135 HMOs conducted by Milliman & Robertson, a Seattle-based health care actuarial firm, reported that a demand for ancillary services is an "employer phenomenon" (Milliman & Robertson, 1995). Physical and occupational therapy are components of ancillary services.

Employers are increasingly investing in integrated disability management (IDM) programs that focus on absence management. IDM programs transcend clinical treatment per se and involve injury/illness prevention, medical case management, and return-to-work programs (RTW) (Darphin, 1995; Fitzpatrick & King, 2001; Hochanadel & Conrad, 1993; Watson Wyatt Worldwide, 1999). For consultants, self-insured or self-funded employers are a prime target as they continue to shed conventional WC coverage. Employers with reasonable loss records (low injury/loss frequency and/or low payouts versus premiums collected) can select self-insurance as a means of avoiding high premium payments. This employer-centric model is founded on several disability management principles: workplace safety, early intervention, and expedient RTW of injured employees. Figure 27–2 depicts key elements of an employer-based disability management program. Employee assessment and environmental assessment are both necessary for appropriate worker-to-worksite matching whether it is during the hire phase (post-offer evaluation), concurrent with treatment, or during the post-treatment phase. Education and training of multiple stakeholders occurs throughout the health continuum from pre-injury to post-injury. Ideally, regulatory and compliance issues (e.g., OSHA, Environmental Protection Agency [EPA], Equal Employment Opportunity Commission [EEOC]) are addressed preemptively. However, the reality is that these interventions tend to be sought on a forensic basis; after the OSHA or EEOC citation is levied. Ultimately, employer-based IDM involves absence management.

Absence Management

Absence management describes lost workdays due to disability-related claims, whether they are of an occupational or non-occupational nature (Mitchell, 2000). Absence management is a vital key to serving employers' disability management needs (Geddes-Lipold, 2000). Injured or ill workers are associated with the following:

- Reduced productivity
- Increased direct medical costs
- Increased indirect medical costs
- Indemnity or wage replacement
- Decreased employee morale
- Decreased corporate competitiveness
- Increased administrative costs
- Increased legal costs

Occupational-based claims occur when an employee reports a work-related incident that is covered under WC benefits. Non-occupational claims describe those injuries or illnesses that are not directly related to one's job performance and are typically covered by automobile liability insurance, short-term or long-term disability (STD and LTD, respectively), or under group or general health (e.g., Blue Cross, HMO).

Injury and cost data support the need for innovative consultative programs. Rousmaniere and Denniston (2003) report that one of every 50 workers suffers an accident that results in at least one lost workday, whereas one of every 250 workers loses an entire month.

A survey of 476 employers conducted in 2001 indicates that an average employer spends 14.6% of payroll on absence-related benefits (Modugny, 2002). Paradoxically, although absence management is a high priority for employers, only 16% of employers provide reports on absence occurrences to supervisors. This may partly explain why poor rapport between employees and first-line supervisors accounts for a major impediment to RTW.

Figure 27–2. Key elements of an employer-based disability management program.

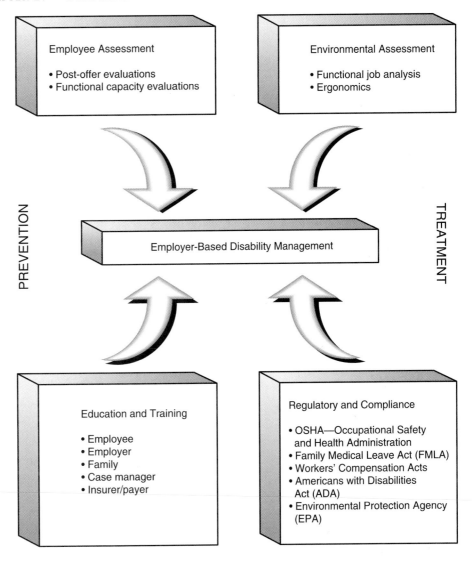

"Reasonable Accommodations"

Disability management programs strive to keep or return employees to gainful employment irrespective of whether disability results from occupational or non-occupational triggers (Hunt & Habeck, 1993). RTW is often determined by the availability of appropriate jobs in the context of the injured worker's condition. Some experts contend that transition to work (TTW) is the most important strategy an employer can implement to control workplace injury (Walker, 1998). Reasonable accommodations provide an effective means of transition to work during the pre-placement/post-offer stage or when used post-injury. Under ADA, if an employee has a disability that requires an accommodation, the employer must provide it, unless it poses an undue hardship. Although the concept of "undue hardship" continues to be the subject of legal debate, employers and their consultants may consider some guideposts (EEOC, 2004). Accommodations that rise to the level of undue hardship are generally costly

when compared with alternatives. Accommodations that are extensive or beyond the scope of an employee's or prospective employee's essential job functions can be construed as undue hardships. Accommodations that tend to be disruptive to business operations may also satisfy the undue hardship requirement under ADA, although legal rulings ultimately determine ADA compliance.

Some reasonable accommodations may require health care providers who command knowledge of function in the context of worker-worksite matching. Collaboration between physical therapists, occupational therapists, and ergonomists can be particularly effective in identifying both the human and environmental factors that come into play when attempting to match the worker to the worksite.

Esposito (1993) identified the top six reasonable accommodations under ADA:

1. Training supervisors to assist employees with disabilities
2. Modification of work procedures
3. Modification of work schedules

4. Transference of employees to vacant positions
5. Modification of worksite
6. Provision of tools and special equipment

An invaluable resource to employers and consultants is the Office of Disability Employment Policy at the U.S. Department of Labor, which sponsors the Job Accommodation Network (JAN) (http://www.jan.wvu.edu). The JAN Webpage provides a number of services including fact sheets for accommodating persons with specific disabilities, for example "Accommodating People with Cumulative Trauma Disorders" (http://www.wvu.edu/media/CTD.html) and "Ideas for Accommodating People with Chronic Pain" (http://www.wvu.edu/media/ChronicPain.html). JAN accepts ADA-related questions, provided users include the following information: (1) limitations and abilities of the individual in question; (2) specifics of the job task(s) at issue; and (3) accommodations that have been considered. JAN provides expert panels comprising mobility/motor, psychiatric/cognitive, sensory, and small business and employment.

Rehabilitation Providers' Role in Integrated Disability Management Programs

Forty-two percent of employers by 1998 offered integrated disability management programs (Watson Wyatt, 1999). This represents a significant increase in IDM programs from 26% in 1996. Employers, as they reassert control of health care expenditures, will require physical rehabilitation knowledge that can be employed through a host of integrated disability management activities (Smith & Preis, 2001). These include ergonomics, employee post-offer examinations (ADA), functional job analysis, early intervention programs, RTW program design, in-house rehabilitation management, and employee education on a number of topics including back injury prevention, cumulative trauma disorder prevention (CTDs), workstation design, and employee wellness (Dyck, 2000; Isom, 1998; Smith, 1997). Providers may have a bright future, given the growing support of their role in disability management (Smith & Preis, 2001).

Workers' Compensation: A Ripe Sector

WC costs continue to spiral upward, even for those employers with good injury and illness records (Rousmaniere & Denniston, 2003). This is due in part to the fact that managed-care strategies employed in WC have been only a modest success. A variety of psychosocial issues are present in WC that are relatively absent in other health care funding structures (Kendall, 1999).

The Bureau of Labor Statistics and U.S. Department of Labor reported 4,700,600 total non-fatal work injuries in 2002 (Bureau of Labor Statistics, 2003). Injury rates vary by industrial sector, with the manufacturing and construction sectors leading all categories. These sectors accounted for approximately 7 injuries per 100 full-time workers. These data compare with a private industry average of 5.3 injuries per 100 workers. Agriculture, forestry and fishing, wholesale and retail trade, and public transportation and public utilities all exceeded the national average. These data bode well for rehabilitation professionals who reside in parts of the country where these sectors are most prominent.

Community Rating

Because work-related injuries and illnesses are charged against an employer's WC experience or community rating, injury prevention and management programs have potential traction. Perhaps no state exemplifies the challenge of escalating WC costs more than California does. Total costs of WC in California rose from $9.5 billion in 1995 to over $25 billion by 2002 (Dembe et al, 2003). To calculate a community rating an employer's injury prevalence rate is compared to its industrial sector's overall injury experience. For instance, a trucking firm's injury occurrence rate or frequency (e.g., injuries per 200,000 hours worked) is compared to that sector's average injury frequency. If the employer's rate exceeds the industry average, the employer's premiums rise. These public domain data can be used by consultant's to target specific companies or industrial sectors.

Employer Self-Insurance or Self-Funding

Independent consultants may be particularly attractive to self-insured employers (Scott, 2002). The Society of Professional Benefit Administrators conservatively estimates that 75% of all U.S. employers use some form of self-insurance, also known as self-funding. WC is often a line of insurance that employers elect to self-insure.

Self-insured employers do not pay premiums in advance of injury occurrence. Instead, these employers pay on a claim-occurrence basis and must set aside "company reserves" for each injury or illness. Company reserves are calculated via actuarial data based on estimated medical and non-medical costs. These monies are placed into escrow accounts that cannot be accessed for employer purposes. These funds are designated for employee needs only. Since employers pay to play, disability prevention and management are critical to fiscal viability. Small companies can easily become bankrupt based on a few high-dollar, catastrophic cases. Many employers do not have resident knowledge and skill sets that rehabilitation providers often take for granted; therefore outsourcing of disability prevention solutions is a strong preference. Additionally, it is not unusual for there to be labor-management tension that prevents implementation of new initiatives (Mills, 1995).

Employees do not Assume Financial Risk Under Worker's Compensation

Injured workers do not assume financial risk under WC as they do under group or general health policies. There are no deductibles or co-payments that are commonly found in managed care. Instead, WC assures first-dollar hypothetically unlimited care, provided that medical necessity and reasonable care are established. The absence of risk erodes employers' ability to constrain medical costs, thereby providing incentive to prevent or aggressively manage disability. Litigation rates paradoxically run very high in this hypothetically no-fault system. The concepts of "medical necessity," "causality," and "maximum medical benefit" continue to plague WC claims because of the degree of litigation they attract.

Provider Panels

Unlike group health, WC does not engage the vast majority of providers in financial risk-sharing as with capitation or cases rates. However, employers do attempt to control medical costs and utilization through the selection of panel providers. Depending upon individual state laws, physical and occupational therapists may or may not be able to serve as preferred providers on WC provider panels. Employers can direct injured workers to selected panel providers. However, employers are generally restricted in terms of how long an injured worker is required to remain in treatment with a panel provider. Panel provider and care direction decisions vary under WC on a state-by-state basis.

Functional Testing

WC, unlike managed care, offers (hypothetically) unlimited first dollar medical coverage until the worker is deemed fit for return-to-work (RTW). This decision may require the assistance of therapists, particularly through functional capacity evaluations (FCEs) or functional capacity assessments (FCAs) (Vowles, 2003; Ward, 1992; Wheeler et al, 2001–2002). RTW decisions generally require a much higher standard for the cessation of health care services than the maximum medical benefit (MMB) threshold of managed care. Maximum medical benefit simply means that more health care will not improve the patient's anatomical, physiological, or psychological problem, which has stabilized. However, under WC, medical stability does not predict the ability to return to gainful employment in the performance of critical job demands, as RTW and MMI are mutually exclusive concepts. One's medical stability does not predict one's ability to RTW. This requires functional testing and assessment. Few are as qualified as physical and occupational therapists to conduct such testing. Refer to Chapter 9 for a detailed discussion of functional capacity evaluations.

Overall, the lack of benefit controls in WC makes this a very attractive market for rehabilitation consultants who can offer innovative disability prevention and management programs. Consultants do not necessarily have to hail from large corporations in order to secure consulting projects because WC involves a patchwork quilt of fifty state laws or acts. Additionally, some of the most needy employers are small to mid-size. In these companies it is not unusual for one person to serve in multiple capacities. For instance, the safety officer may also be the medical director, or the human resources person may dually function as the safety officer. When this duality exists, outsourcing is an appealing option for already overburdened staff. WC casualty insurers and employers generally prefer to collaborate with local providers who understand the intricacies of their state's compensation law or act

(Pohlman et al, 2001). Refer to Chapter 5 for a more detailed view of this unique system.

Providers can approach employers via a number of avenues in order to offer consulting services (Scully-Palmer, 2000). Employers can be approached directly, through third party casualty insurers, or by leveraging patient contacts, provided ethical standards are not breached (e.g., patient confidentiality).

Early Intervention Programs

Although treatment-based and not technically consultative services, early intervention programs serve a critical need within WC systems. Zigenfus et al (2000) illustrate the effectiveness of early intervention.

It is generally accepted within the rehabilitation community that to delay rehabilitation is to compromise rehabilitation Delays in referral to appropriate physical therapy and rehabilitation are common in WC (Rundle, 1983). Delays can be reduced when rehabilitation professionals work in collaboration with employer-customers.

On-site rehabilitation offers employers another alternative to controlling WC costs. Self-funded employers have even greater incentives to bring rehabilitation in-house. Klekamp (2003) outlines both the benefits and limitations of on-site rehabilitation, as well as its fee structure. Scruby et al (2001) describe the economic impact of on-site physical therapy.

Employers also can be directly approached if the provider needs to make a visit to the worksite to conduct a functional job analysis (FJA). The FJA can be useful as a blueprint for a RTW program. Worksite consultations are being promoted as an integral component of disability management (Grasso & Rousmaniere, 2002). During these visits, the critical job demands of the employee can be ascertained in order to craft a rehabilitation program that includes similar functional elements. The physical demands of the job can then be communicated to the attending physician or a physician who may be conducting an independent medical examination for vocational placement or fitness for duty reasons. Visits to the workplace can be conducted as a part of a discharge plan affording the provider the opportunity to sign-off on worker-to-work-site matching and reasonable accommodations. Site visits can be used for development of transitional or modified duty job banks (Fuerstein et al, 2003).

Traditionally, consultation services were considered an added expense because they could not be charged against a specific WC claim. However, insurance claim budgets are beginning to fund selective consultations such as functional job analysis, functional capacity evaluations, and ergonomic programs. Grasso and Rousmaniere (2002) contend that the return-on-investment (ROI) of worksite consultations alone justifies their use.

Case managers and casualty insurers who interface with local employers represent additional employer contact opportunities. Case managers are often retained by employers or their insurance company to facilitate a safe, cost-effective, and expeditious RTW. Case managers must balance the needs/expectations of divergent stakeholders: employees, supervisors/managers, health care providers, and claims representatives. Case managers can make referrals to therapists for consultation projects such as FJAs, reasonable accommodations, ergonomics, FCEs, and other tasks. Providers can offer an array of industrial consulting services to employers, including employee or management educational programs, ergonomics, and safety walk-through inspections.

Managed Health Versus Managed Care

Managed health involves interventions that are designed to enhance or maintain the health of targeted persons or groups, and not to simply treat the adverse consequences. Employers have traditionally been reactionary, relative to disability management. They are more apt to spend money *after* an injury or incident. However, there is a growing trend toward onsite rehabilitation and corporate wellness programs (Clifton, 1995: Daus, 1995; Ellexson, 1997; Enix & Lopez, 1998; Hebert, 1995; Joyce, 1996; Larson, 1994; Lipow, 1997; Hewitt Associates, 2001; Wynn, 1996).

Managed health differs from managed care because the emphasis is on prevention of injury and illness, not management of the beneficiary or provider. Managed health includes preventive care (e.g., vaccinations, consumer education, health screenings, disease prevention/management, and counseling). Although managed health may imply primary care involvement, primary care physicians seldom visit the workplace unless they are part of a company's medical department; therefore, therapists may be among the first to offer a visit to the workplace of an injured worker. The average physician has minimal work-injury education and virtually no training in how to handle RTW issues (Rousmaniere, 2003). A site visit can also make a positive impression on a safety officer, human resources director, first-line supervisor, or medical director when made by rehabilitation specialists.

These programs return a degree of control as well as responsibility to employers that tends to be absent when a third party insurer is involved. They also demonstrate to employees a degree of management-level commitment vital to success, both financially and morale-wise.

Physical rehabilitation providers who are qualified and are not risk-averse can seize multiple opportunities to manage health. This will require a paradigm shift from "treater" to "consultant." Table 27–4 contains a roster of employer-specific consulting opportunities that can augment one's clinical practice or treatment programs. There is great support for providers to transcend treatment. Professional rehabilitation organizations vigorously encourage providers to engage in managed health. For example, the American Physical Therapy Association's *Guide to Physical Therapist Practice* supports consumer education programs, identification of lifestyle factors, stress management, and exercise (APTA, 2001).

This document identifies consultation and education as other professional roles of the physical therapist. Pattern A of each section (musculoskeletal, neuromuscular, cardiovascular/pulmonary, and integumentary) describes primary prevention and risk reduction.

 Table 27–4 Roster of Employer-specific Consulting Opportunities

- Pre-placement employee screening
- Job matching worker-to-workstation
- Design of transitional or modified duty
- Drafting functional job analyses
- Cumulative trauma prevention training for employees and management
- Development of "reasonable accommodations" for ADA compliance
- Assistive/adaptive device identification for injured employees
- OSHA compliance
- On-site employer rehabilitation
- Service on ergonomic committees
- Ergonomic analysis and implementation of engineering and administrative controls
- Medico-legal expertise

ADA Consulting

The Americans with Disabilities Act of 1990 (ADA) can generate consulting opportunities for creative clinicians (ADA, 1990). Examples of work products permeate the clinical literature and can assist prospective consultants in getting started (Hammel & Symons, 1993; Mullins et al, 1996; Miller, 1996; Jacobs, 1992). The ADA essentially protects employees from discrimination on the basis of their real or perceived disabilities at every stage of employment, including job application, hiring stage, advancement, and from discharge for employment. Again, management commitment is one of the best predictors of program success. A 1993 National Safety Council survey demonstrated that 66% of employers used safety and health committees (Planek & Kolosh, 1994). Seventy- two percent of employer respondents indicated that management would be more dedicated to safety issues with an on-site committee. Lastly, 88% believed that employee involvement is essential. On average, committees comprised six employees for every management level member. Committee composition typically included risk managers, disability directors, health professionals, ergonomists, industrial hygienists, safety professionals, loss prevention officers, and outside consultants (Apker, 1993). These committees represent prime opportunities for therapists to position themselves as employer resources. For example, in Pennsylvania, employers who form an ergonomic committee are entitled to WC insurance premium discounts of 5% over a three-year period, provided the committee meets at least twice annually.

Therapists as Ergonomists

Piegorisch (1996) describes ergonomics as "a multidisciplinary science that interrelates information from the fields of engineering, medicine, and psychology," Ergonomics represents an extremely fertile area for therapist involvement. (Edwards, 1990; Shulenberger, 1992; Pheasant, 1991; Lutz & Hansford 1987; Kenny et al, 1995; Cosgrove, 2002). Ergonomics represents a specialty area, not an entry level competency, that can be quite cost-effective for employers. Ergonomics is the study of work and the interplay between a person, his or her environment, work tasks, and tools (Marras, 1992). Therapists who assess the injured worker's worksite can prevent reinjury and exacerbations and ensure a safe but expedient return to gainful employment. This is an appealing value proposition for employers.

Medical costs of cumulative trauma injuries average $25,000 per incident or case, often resulting in a loss of employment and also productivity for both the employee and the employer (Grasso & Rousmaniere, 2002). Costs associated with carpal tunnel range between $30,000 to $70,000 when surgery is involved (Joyce, 1988; Pinkham, 1988). Disability claims (non-working employee) routinely exceed $100,000 (National Safety Council, 1992). Consultants who understand the employer perspective can play an invaluable role that is mutually beneficial (King, 1990; Shrey & LaCerte, 1995; May, 2002; Zacharia 2002). For those therapists who may be squeamish about the engineering aspects of ergonomics, collaboration with other professionals may be the route to follow. Occupational medicine providers, ergonomists, industrial hygienists, safety professionals, and industrial engineers all possess knowledge and skill sets that when combined with those of occupational or physical therapists result in a valuable employer resource.

Table 27-5 provides an example of a collaboration between a physical therapist and certified ergonomist who is also a certified safety professional (CSP) and certified industrial hygienist (CIH). These professionals partnered in dozens of projects that focused on the amelioration of cumulative trauma. Each brought unique skill sets to consultation projects. *ERGOMED* was the operative word used to describe this collaboration. Unfortunately, their interventions were typically solicited forensically or after employers experienced a run of injuries (e.g., carpal tunnel syndrome or low back injuries). Some interventions were prompted by employers being cited by the Occupational Safety and Health Administration under the so-called "general duty clause." This clause allows OSHA to fine employers for safety violations that do not have standards of measure, as in air quality or noise abatement. "Ergonomic services" were rendered by an individual with a background in safety engineering, industrial hygiene, and ergonomics. These services included worksite analysis,

implementation of engineering controls, ergonomics training of employees, safety engineering, and industrial hygiene. "Medical/rehabilitation services" were overseen by a licensed physical therapist who provided pre-placement/post-offer employee screenings, functional job analysis, transitional or modified duty development, RTW program design and implementation, and functional capacity evaluations (FCEs). Both parties cooperatively addressed expert testimony needs, health and safety manual development, WC provider panel development, employee training, and payer education.

Ideally, consultation services like those described are best when proactively applied; however, obstacles remain to employers adopting this approach, namely, a means of funding. Again, most of these services cannot be charged against a specific insurance claim so they typically are funded through mechanisms that may be perceived as siphoning funds from production needs.

Therapists as Case Managers

What is case management? The Commission for Case Manager Certification (CCMC, 1993) defines case management as:

> *"A collaborative process that assesses, plans, implements, coordinates, monitors, and evaluates the options and services required to meet an individual's health needs, using communication and available resources to promote quality, cost-effective outcomes."*

Case managers do not directly render care but coordinate the activities of health care providers in order to expedite safe RTW. Case managers facilitate movement along the entire disability continuum through all stages of irritability (acute-subacute-chronic). Case managers, although paid by insurers or employers, represent patients/injured workers in an ombudsman fashion. Case managers can ensure that all parties are winners when injured workers achieve maximum outcome (RTW), employers receive a productive employee, care has been cost-effective (payer), and clinicians' autonomy and clinical judgment have not been compromised in the process. Physical and occupational therapists possess the requisite people skills as well as technical knowledge to serve as case managers (Lincoln et al, 2002). Therapists have a great deal of experience in dealing with the psychosocial issues that are often involved, especially in chronic conditions or catastrophic injury (Kendall, 1999). Refer to Chapter 7 for a more in-depth analysis of psychosocial issues. These factors are key determinants of success or failure, especially in WC (Shrey, 1995). Comprehensive case management services involve targeting the following three levels: primary prevention, secondary prevention, and early intervention or tertiary prevention (Martin, 1995). Rehabilitation providers offer a value proposition that can lead to reduction in both the prevalence and severity of workplace injury; decreased absenteeism or lost days; treatment cost control; minimized indemnity or lost wage replacement; and most importantly, a safe but expedient RTW.

Case management certifications can be acquired on the basis of one's individual experience and skill sets. The certified case manager or CCM designation is a widely

 Table 27-5   Example of Consulting Collaboration: The ERGO-MED Program

Ergonomic Services	Medical/Rehabilitation Services
Ergonomic work-site analysis	Pre-placement/post-offer employee screenings
Engineering controls	Functional job analyses
Ergonomics training	Transitional duty development
Safety engineering	Return-to-work programs
Industrial hygiene	Work capacity/Functional Capacity Evaluations
	Expert Testimony
	CTD prevention training
	Health and Safety Manual Development
	Insurance company training
	Employee back school

From Personnel communications between David W. Clifton, PT, Dolphin and Associates, and David Ridyard, CIH, CSP Applied Ergonomics.

acknowledged certification because it is the result of collaboration between 25 different case management associations. The Commission for Case Manager Certification (CCMC) is located in Rolling Meadows, Illinois. CCMC is solely responsible for administration of the certification examination and publication of the CCM *Certification Guide*, first published in 1993 (http://www.ccmc.org).

Resources exist for those rehabilitation providers who wish to manage but not treat injured persons. Understanding case management fundamentals is essential when dealing with persons with disabilities (Siefker, 1998; Pilling, 1992).

Professional Networking

Networking with employer representatives at conferences attended by health and safety professionals, industrial hygienists, medical directors, occupational nurses, human resource officers, employee benefits managers, and loss prevention directors is an indirect manner in which to interface with employers. These conferences provide a venue in which to learn about the concerns and unfulfilled needs of employers. Interfacement with other professionals, such as safety professional, industrial hygienists, and ergonomists, may also lead to opportunities for collaboration. Table 27-6 provides networking suggestions for rehabilitation providers.

Some professional associations have special interest groups devoted to serving the needs of employers. For instance, the American Physical Therapy Association's Orthopaedic Section has a special interest group (SIG) known as the Occupational Physical Therapist SIG. Membership is comprised of several hundred physical therapists who provide consultation services to employers of a diverse nature.

Business Coalitions and Purchasing Cooperatives

Business coalitions, or purchasing cooperatives, represent another avenue for networking with employers who may potentially need the services of a rehabilitation or disability management consultant. There are currently approximately 97 individual coalitions that are members of the National Business Coalition on Health, which is essentially a *coalition of coalitions* (Clifton, 1996). Coalitions offer a number of advantages to their employer members. Coalitions host educational programs and assist employers in managing the costs associated with disability. Coalitions and alliances pool their resources and routinely share the names of consultants among their members. These groups offer an opportunity for consultants to exponentially reach employers who are educated, to a degree, about disability prevention and management. Coalitions provide centralized purchasing options to members and routinely rate health plans and health care providers.

How to Determine What Specific Services Employers Need

Gathering data about employer needs and expectations can be expedited by reviewing survey data generated by firms who provide employee benefits, health plans, and accounting consultation services to employers. These companies include Price Waterhouse Coopers and Lybrand, Deloitte and Touche, Watson Wyatt Worldwide, Milliman and Robertson, Hewitt Associates, KPMG, and Accenture. These and other companies often conduct surveys describing employer health care purchasing and disability management trends.

Employers are generally interested in programs that manage their risk. Again, insurance premiums only finance risk and do little to manage it. Few property and casualty insurers (e.g., Liberty Mutual, Kemper/Natlsco, Wausau Insurance, Aetna/Axia) extend loss prevention or risk management programs to their insureds. Even fewer do so without additional cost incurred by the employer. One of the best means of determining which specific services are desired by employers is to secure surveys and reports published by employee benefit or actuarial firms. These firms work with employers to identify means of restraining costs while keeping the workforce healthy. For example, one survey of 65 employers offering wellness programs identified 13 service areas (Coopers & Lybrand, 1990).

Figure 27-3 depicts service areas as a percentage of those items that were ranked either first, second, or third among employer priorities.

The majority of these services fall within the skill sets of many rehabilitation providers. Exercise and fitness was reported as important by nearly 60% of respondent companies. This was followed by health assessment, ranked by more than 50% of employer respondents as important. Cholesterol screening, smoking cessation, stress management, and weight control programs rounded out the top six priorities.

Table 27-6 Networking Suggestions for Rehabilitation Providers

Subscriptions/memberships to non-clinical publications/associations

- American Industrial Hygiene Association (AIHA)
- American Society of Safety Engineers (ASSE)
- Risk Insurance Manager's Society (RIMS)
- Human Factors Society (HFS)
- Self-Insurance Institute of America (SIIA)
- National Council on Compensation Insurance (NCCI)
- Workers' Compensation Research Institute (WCRI)

Attendance of annual conferences and topical issue forums of the aforementioned groups and others. Please refer to Appendixes E, F, and H for additional listings.

Review federal and state laws/regulations

- State WC acts
- Occupational Safety and Health Administrations (OSHA)
- Americans with Disabilities Act of 1990
- National Institute of Occupational Safety and Health (NIOSH)
- National Safety Council
- U.S. department of Health and Human Services
- National Institute on Disability and Rehabilitation Research (NIDRR)

Request and review employer health care and benefit surveys conducted by firms such as those mentioned in this chapter (e.g., Watson Wyatt Worldwide, Deloitte and Touche, Price WaterhouseCoopers and Lybrand, Hewitt Associates).

Figure 27–3. Employer health care program ranking by importance. (Data from Coopers and Lybrand Consulting: Health Management: A Survey of Company-Sponsored Wellness Programs, 1990.)

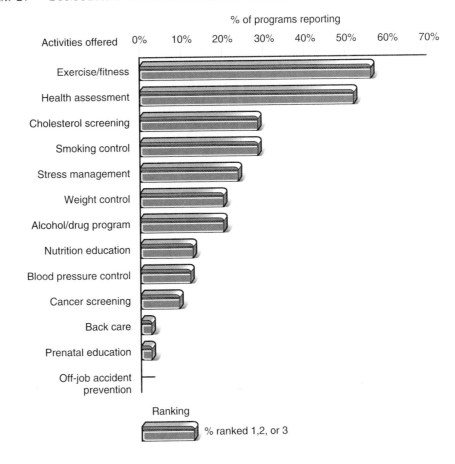

In this survey cost containment was the most frequently cited reason employers gave for service priority, followed closely by a desire to improve employee health. Employee morale and well being received third and fourth priority status, respectively. These data provide important insight for consultants in how to craft a proposal, particularly the cost-benefit section. Figure 27–4 provides a summary of these data.

A Watson Wyatt employer-based survey (1999) revealed those disability management tools most often utilized by employers. These data are summarized in Figure 27–5. This study is of particular interest because it contrasts employer responses for "occupational" versus "non-occupational" health plans. Occupational disability benefits describe WC. Non-occupational disability benefits describe sick pay, short-term disability (STD), and long-term disability (LTD).

Safety and injury prevention programs are used by 90% of employers for occupational cases, but for only 30% for non-occupational conditions. Transitional or modified RTW, case management, and independent medical examinations are used equally between occupational and non-occupational disability benefits.

A Hewitt Associates survey (2001) of 1020 companies revealed that 92% offered some form of health promotion. Employers in this survey cited three purposes for health promotion: corporate costs savings, reduced absenteeism, and increased productivity. Double-digit cost inflation was the prime motivator of health promotion programs. Seventy-one percent of employers offer

employee education/training in lifestyle choices and acute and chronic condition management. Seventy-four percent offered screenings, with 77% of these employers offering specialty programs such as disease-state management (DSM) and neonatal care. Paradoxically, although cost savings was the principal goal for employers, only 40% use financial incentives or disincentives when dealing with employees.

How Do Rehabilitation Providers Approach Employers About Consulting?

Understanding the relationship between labor and management when approaching an employer is essential to successful consulting. Mills (1995) cites an adage in labor relations that is highly relevant to consulting: "employers get the union they deserve." This statement implies that good employers get good unions, while bad employers have bad unions. Information concerning labor-management contracts (e.g., collective bargaining) must be ascertained if a consultant is to implement appropriate disability management strategies. For example, seniority rules and dispute resolution policies may dictate whether job rotation is considered as a reasonable accommodation. Responsibilities of each involved party must be delineated during a consulting project to assure accountability. Rehabilitation providers who understand a company's hierarchy, especially the functions of each distinct employer department and management level are better positioned to successfully secure and complete

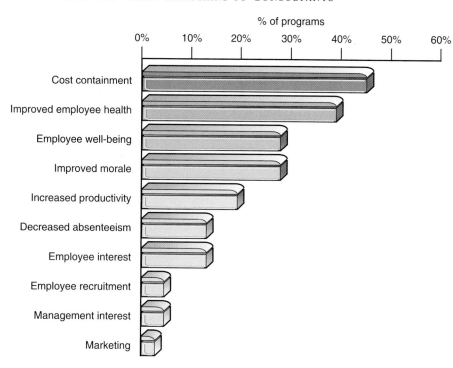

Figure 27–4. Employers' reasons for program initiation. (Data from Coopers and Lybrand Consulting: Health Management: A Survey of Company-Sponsored Wellness Programs, 1990.)

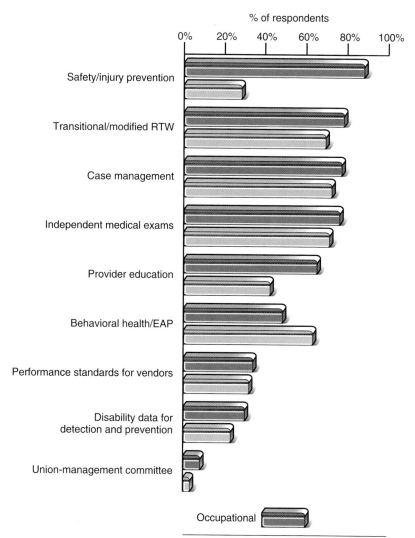

Figure 27–5. Use of disability management tools. (Reprinted with permission from Staying@Work: Increasing Shareholder Value Through Integrated Disability Management © 1999 Watson Wyatt Worldwide. For more information, visit www.watsonwyatt.com.)

consultation contracts. It is critical for prospective consultants to ascertain which elements of disability prevention and management (if any) a specific department considers a priority. Proposals to provide consultative services must be crafted in consideration of each recipient's paradigm. For instance, a chief financial officer may desire cost-based data, whereas the medical director may desire technical level or the "how to" information regarding an intervention. Again, it is critical to recognize that every employer and departmental head may possess a unique perspective. The tone of a proposal must be aligned with the perspective of its recipient. This may require some investigative work before proposal submission. Consultants should ask themselves a series of questions before submission of a proposal. These include:

- Is the proposal drafted in language its recipients will understand?
- Is the proposal being submitted at the appropriate level?
- Can I afford to allow a company representative to internally pitch my proposal? Or, should I insist on presenting it at the appropriate level?
- Is the employer a "tire kicker" who wishes to steal my ideas and methodologies or an earnest buyer? Should I demand they sign-off on a non-compete and/or non-disclosure agreement before submitting my proposal?

These and many other questions must be considered before a consultant commits capital and human resources to a project. A health and safety attitude survey is one means to determine the drivers of a company or its department heads. Table 27-7 provides a brief overview of those issues that are generally the focus of different departments.

Employer Health and Safety Attitude Survey

The key to ultimate success in employer-based consulting is to achieve alignment between the consultant's and client's goals, objectives, incentives/disincentives, and expectations. A health and safety attitude survey can accomplish this alignment.

Table 27-8 represents a sample survey instrument that may be used for a variety of consulting services. This survey instrument has utility in learning how a specific department and/or company views the importance of disability prevention and management programs. For instance, the motivation behind decision-making becomes quite clear when reviewing a completed survey. This survey will assist consultants in qualifying companies as prospective clients. It can also serve to align the goals of the company and the consultant when a suitable employer/client has been identified.

It is critical for consultants to understand that upper management (e.g., Chief Executive Officer/CEO, Chief Operating Officer/COO, Chief Financial Officer/CFO) and technical level staff (e.g., medical, health, and safety) are likely to have different priorities. Middle management can be a consultant's greatest ally, as they generally tend to covet a more balanced view of the financial and technical aspects of a proposal. Human resource directors and employee benefit specialists often straddle both the management and technical perspectives of their companies.

Table 27-7 Corporate Focus by Department

Safety Department

- Stress Environmental Protection Agency and Occupational Safety and Health Administration issues
- Not overly concerned with productivity
- Considered an expense versus profit generator
- Department head a "technician" versus a manager
- Minimal budget authority

Medical Department

- Emphasis on treating injuries and illness
- An expense item, not a profit center
- Technical level, not management, in most small-mid sized companies
- Minimal budget authority

Risk Management Department

- Stresses saving dollars through risk management, avoidance, or shifting
- Traditionally a management level position
- Relatively high budget authority
- Straddles production and safety/health
- Not technically adroit

Human Resources Department

- Emphasis on EEOC and ADA issues
- Traditionally a management level position
- Considered to be part of production team
- Relatively high degree of budget authority
- Can be at odds with medical department concerning RTW policies/procedures

Chief Financial Officer/Chief Operating Officer

- Operations focus
- Production team member
- Not technically adroit on health/safety issues
- Management level
- High budget authority

Often these persons can facilitate the acceptance of or stymie a consultant's proposal. The success of employer-sponsored health management programs hinges on a number of factors. These are depicted in Figure 27-6 as a percentage of respondents who rated the importance of different factors (Coopers & Lybrand, 1990) A full 80% of employer respondents consider "support of management" as the most predictive variable for success. "Ongoing funding" was rated highest by roughly 42%, followed closely by a "supportive culture' at 40%. Lowest importance was assigned to "program marketing" (company marketing to employees), "convenience," and "cost to employees."

TEN GENERAL PRINCIPLES OF CONSULTING

There are a number of general principles that may assist clinicians in transferring their skills, knowledge, and aptitude to consulting. First, clinicians must embrace the mindset that they are indeed consultants, not just providers who treat or providers who consult. A consultant is a person who gives professional or technical advice. Every physical rehabilitation provider, by this definition, is therefore inherently a consultant. Rehabilitation professionals simply need to learn how to identify potential customers in need of their expertise and package their services for consumption by specific target clients. This may require

Table 27–8 Sample Employer Health and Safety Attitude Survey: Department Level

Instructions: *Please have the following departmental heads complete and submit their own responses to this survey. Circle the most appropriate response(s). Please return survey results in separate envelopes to _____ @ _____ Thank you.*

Department name:

1. Which accounts for the greatest number of work-related accidents or injuries?
   a. work environment problems
   b. operator/worker behavior
   c. both
   d. other, please specify _____
2. Is health and safety at your company considered a
   a. contributor to productivity
   b. expense or cost to business
   c. both
   d. other, please specify _____
3. What is your department's per project spending limit before additional authorization is required?
   a. less than $5000 dollars
   b. $5001 to $10,000
   c. $10,001 to $20,000
   d. >$20,000
   e. other, please specify _____
4. Which best describes your department's decision-making process
   a. corporate directives
   b. departmental directives
   c. vendor or consultant input
   d. regulatory influences, e.g., OSHA, ADA
   e. other, please describe _____
5. When considering to purchase a health and safety service, do you
   a. conduct a needs analysis
   b. outright purchase
   c. consult with labor
   d. depend upon outside consultant advice
   e. other, please describe _____
6. Do you currently use criteria for consulting service purchases?
   a. yes
   b. no
   c. other, please describe _____
7. Which of the two approaches to disability best describes your department's preference?
   a. prevention-based
   b. management-based (after injury/illness)

8. Responsibility for disability prevention principally rests with
   a. the employee
   b. first-line supervisor
   c. health and safety officer _____
   d. insurance company
   e. CEO
   f. other, please describe
9. What percentage of your department's budget is spent on the following activities: _____
   a. injury/illness prevention?
   b. injury/illness management (after an occurrence)?
   c. other, please specify
10. Does your department conduct disability prevention and/or management educational and training programs for
    a. employees _____
    b. other departmental heads
    c. upper management
    d. other, please specify
11. How essential is health and safety to your company's bottom line?
    a. extremely essential
    b. moderately essential
    c. somewhat essential
    d. not essential
12. Are the majority of your company's health and safety services provided by
    a. internal staff _____
    b. external staff or out-sourced
    c. combination of a and b
    d. other, please describe
13. Do any of the following criteria apply to how your department makes its health and safety service decisions? Please check those that apply:
    ● Must be needs-driven
    ● Must have a favorable cost-benefit ratio (>20% ROI)
    ● Must be a turnkey program
    ● Must have assessment measures of success
    ● Must be customized
    ● Must be off-the-shelf and ready to go
    ● Must be first piloted
    ● Must be safe to implement
    ● Must be approved by a labor organization
    ● Must meet local, state, and federal requirements
    ● Other, please specify

Data modified from Clifton DW: If a niche doesn't exist, carve one: Tips for getting in the door. Phys Ther Today 16(2):49-51, 1993.

a paradigm shift from the medical model that emphasizes treatment to a wellness model that emphasizes health.

> **Principle No. 1:** *"All rehabilitation providers are inherently equipped with skills, knowledge and aptitudes that are of value to others."*
>
> Clifton, 1993

Rehabilitation professionals are, both by necessity and choice, great communicators. They possess in-depth knowledge in areas of vital concern to others, such as functional assessment, injury mechanisms/causality, pathophysiology, and biomechanics. Therapists are energetic and vibrant. They are skilled at assisting others in facing challenges and overcoming adversity.

> **Principle No. 2:** *Data are not information, information is not knowledge; knowledge is not wisdom unless it is tempered with experience.*

Experienced consultants understand the need to survey potential clients about their unfulfilled needs or challenges. Too often, consultants fail to do so because they embrace a "build it and they will come mentality." Experience and the wisdom that comes with it suggest that success in consulting is predicated on the following methodical steps of identifying, qualifying, selling/marketing, and servicing a client or customer. Figure 27–7 identifies stages that are necessary for successful consultation. Step 1 is to identify individual and organizational knowledge and skill sets. Step 2 involves identifying the types of businesses or organizations that may value

Figure 27–6. Factors that influence program success. (Data from Coopers and Lybrand Consulting: Health Management: A Survey of Company-Sponsored Wellness Programs, 1990.)

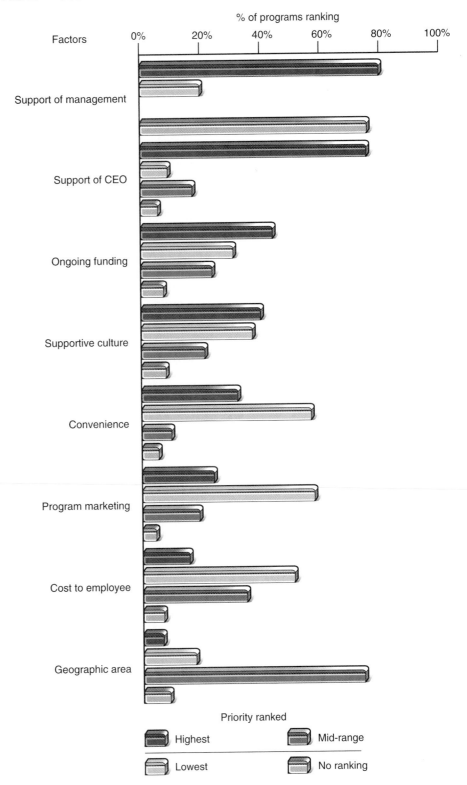

these traits. Once target clients have been identified, research specific to their disability challenges is required in order to complete a need analysis (step 3). For example, carpal tunnel syndrome is a common problem associated with a broad range of industries (Cosgrove et al, 2002; Delgrosso & Boillat, 1991; Franklin et al, 1984).

Ideally, a prospective company's data should be compared to available industry-wide data. For example,

a comparison of an employers' injury incidence and costs to similar industrial sectors (e.g., WC experience ratings, National Safety Council data, OSHA data, man-hours worked versus injury rates) may determine whether or not this company is in need of injury prevention services.

Table 27–9 provides a sample Consulting Opportunity Worksheet that assists in framing important elements of the prospecting and qualifying stages. The qualifying stage

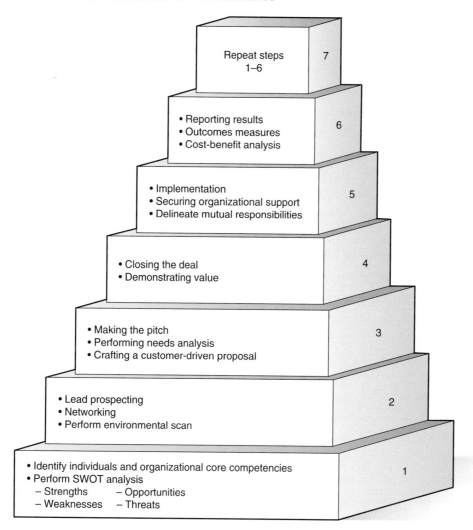

Figure 27–7. Staging model for consulting services.

represents the time spent determining of whether a particular company is a viable buyer. Some companies will be deemed non-viable for a variety of reasons, including no history of disability prevention/management spending, weak infrastructure, poor management support, low profitability, or strong labor resistance.

Next, a customized proposal is crafted, which specifies how a consultant or his or her organization will creatively address the client's challenges. Sections of a proposal should include, but not be restricted to, the following:

- Statement of the scope of the problem or challenge
- Outline of consulting steps
- Biography of key consultants
- Vignettes describing sample work products related to the proposed services
- References from satisfied clients/customers
- Project budgetary requirements and pricing information
- Consultant's responsibilities
- Clients' responsibilities
- Outcomes measures or assessment tools to be used
- Projected costs/savings expressed as cost-benefit ratios
- Relevant regulatory policies
- Follow-up steps

Measurement of success is critical to any consultation project involving work injury prevention programs. It is a common practice to compare pre-program and post-program data elements such as injury rates, costs, and productivity indicators. These data also can suggest to consultants a need to reassess their skill sets and determine whether or not additional competencies are required.

A popular dictum in consulting suggests that a majority of one's business comes from a minority of its customers. This is commonly referred to as the "80/20 rule," under which 80% of business comes from 20% of customers. However, this is true only if one delivers value in the form of reduced costs, improvements in absence management, and increased worker productivity.

> ***Principle No. 3:*** *Separate the "tire kickers" and "brain pickers" from genuine buyers of consulting services.*

Successful consultants learn to qualify the buyer of specific services through a number of mechanisms including setting priorities or establishing profiles of likely clients. For instance, if given the choice between expending

Table 27–9 Sample Consulting Opportunity Worksheet

Niche or service:

1. **Customers**
   - Who has traditionally purchased these or similar services?
   - What emerging customers are there?
   - What are the specific customer needs or problems that my service addresses?
   - What has failed to resolve the prospective customer's problems?

2. **Industry Leaders/Competitors' Analysis**
   - Who are they?
   - What do they offer that are both different and similar to our offerings?
   - How do they deliver their service? Cost? Methodology? Personnel?
   - How do they market their services?

3. **Associated Costs**
   - What are the research costs?
   - Marketing costs?
   - Start-up costs?
   - Operational costs?
   - Follow-up costs?
   - Insurance or bond costs?

4. **Risk-Benefit Ratio**
   - Total capital needs versus potential profits
   - Legal risks and liabilities versus potential profits
   - How distracting is it to our core operations?
   - What outcome measures (clinical and business) will be required?

5. **How Can the Service Be Standardized so That It Represents a Repeatable Model?**
   - Which elements can or cannot be standardized?
   - Is staff consistent in service delivery?
   - Do we need outside consultants?
   - What copyrights, trademarks or service marks (SM) are necessary?

6. **Sales/Marketing**
   - What is the message that needs to be conveyed to potential customers?
   - Which is/are the best media or vehicle for making the pitch?
   - Who will do the marketing? Clinicians? Non-clinicians? Outside consultants?

7. **Reimbursement/Financing**
   - How will we be paid for our services? Per diem? Per project? Percentage of savings or commission?
   - Are volume discounts appropriate?
   - What is the payment schedule or cycle? Down payments or advances? Timing?

8. **Access to Service**
   - How do customers access our service?
   - Do we require additional distribution sites?
   - Which elements are turnkey in nature?
   - What material is considered proprietary?

9. **Regulatory/Legislative**
   - Are there any relevant regulations or rules that could impact the project?
   - Do we have the necessary certifications or accreditations, both individually and collectively?
   - Are there any local, state, or federal filings required?

10. **Miscellaneous Concerns/Issues**
    - Will the customer provide personnel? If yes, who supervises/directs them?
    - What are the responsibilities of the customer?
    - What is the timeline for competition and are there any penalties for non-deliverables?
    - Is there any comparable industry data against which our results can be compared?

significant human and capital resources pursuing a company with a track record of disability prevention spending versus one with no history of spending, prudent consultants would select the former.

Companies with historically poor labor-management relations may not be suitable targets. Employers who are willing to open up their injury logs for analysis or afford access to employees for interviews or their facility for inspection may be appealing to consultants.

The Sample Opportunity Worksheet (Table 27–9) displays categories of data that can assist the consultant in collecting data and formulating one's thoughts prior to proposal construction. Worksheets provide a systematic method for evaluating potential consulting opportunities, thus minimizing a haphazard analysis. Responses to worksheets can form the basis for a consulting proposal itself.

Table 27–10 illustrates sample consulting sales/marketing criteria that may satisfy the needs of a consultant across a variety of service offerings. In this example, the consultant has established a reasonable profit margin (between 15% and 20%) for services. Any product/service not meeting this criterion may be excluded or not offered. Sufficient staffing, minimal legal and regulatory exposure, degree of competition, the hassle factor, consultant learning curves, timeliness of cash-flow, company size, and transferable skills/knowledge may either qualify or disqualify a consultant from offering particular services.

> ***Principle No. 4:*** *The value of a service can be a function of its price. The higher the price, the more perceived value, the lower the price, the less perceived value.*

Establishing professional fee structures can be one of, if not the, most daunting of challenges when constructing a consulting proposal. A clinician who wishes to offer consulting services to an employer must face the challenging task of pricing his or her services at a rate that is competitive and covers one's costs, while also producing a reasonable profit margin. Clinician-consultants may have a tendency to use treatment fee schedules as a means of calculating their consulting rates. This methodology may or may not reflect true and accurate value and is likely to result in an undervaluation. The following examples

Table 27–10 Sample Consulting Sales and Marketing Criteria

These criteria can be used individually or collectively to qualify buyers for a given service.

- Reasonable profit margin of at least 20%
- Minimal legal liability
- Sufficient internal staff for timely implementation
- Poor quality of competition or few competitors
- Minimal hassle factors associated with the project
- Minimal learning curve
- Readily transferable skills and knowledge
- Established working relationship with prospective customer or potential for provision of other services
- Minimal rollout time

illustrate some of the problems associated with this approach to pricing structures.

Example No. 1: A rehabilitation provider treats two patients per hour with an average visit fee billed at $50 per patient. The combined $100/hour professional fee is reduced to $60/hour when each case is reimbursed at $30 per patient. If the clinician adopts the resultant $60/hour as his or her consultation fee for non-clinical services, his or her daily or per diem (8 hr) fee equates to $480/day. This rate would be considered low for employer consulting, where a range of $1000 to $2500/day is common.

Example No. 2: A rehabilitation provider must lose one day of clinical time in order to provide expert testimony in a WC hearing. This provider, in a typical day, treats 15–20 patients. On average, the per-visit charge for this center in WC cases is $50/visit. This fee (times fifteen patients) equals $750/day, and multiplied by twenty patients/day, it equals $1000. Consultation in this case does not involve the degree of overhead (operational costs) associated with clinical care, therefore the net profit margin is higher. The therapist-consultant in this example needs to charge at east $1000 just to break even. However, one could argue that a lost clinical day can never be recovered, and therefore a higher fee is justified.

Example No. 3: A consultant has proposed to perform a plant-wide ergonomic evaluation and to make remedial suggestions of both an administrative (policies/procedures) and engineering nature (environmental changes). The project is expected to command three months, or one-quarter year's worth, of effort and time. If the therapist's annual salary equals $80,000, then conservatively the project is worth at least $20,000, which represents replacement wages and a modest profit margin. However, this would likely be too low for the type of service rendered. A three-month project fee of $100,000-plus would not be out of the ordinary. In this case, a replacement therapist must be hired to cover the clinic.

Consultants should have a consistent fee range on a per diem basis because it is their expertise, not necessarily their time, that is being purchased.

A consultant must determine whether he or she is going to compete on price or quality. It is extremely difficult to market services that satisfy these distinct goals. Generally speaking, lower price implies less service, and higher price, a higher degree of service.

Ideally, a customer's view of value is predicated on the relationship between cost and benefit. A consulting project that reduces cumulative trauma cases by 50% may be more palatable to an employer than one that only reduces incidence and cost by 10% but incurred the same costs in terms of consulting fees. Providers who enter the consulting realm should be careful not to underprice (a common tendency) or to overprice their services. When pricing their services, consultants must be mindful of a number of variables:

- Direct labor and material costs
- Potential legal liability
- Client's track record of spending
- Competitors' pricing
- Consultant's perception of his or her own value based on rarity of knowledge and skill sets
- Degree of travel associated with the project
- Time away from family
- Distraction from other core business
- Copyrighted, trademarked, licensed, or franchised materials
- Who solicited whom?
- Weekend, vacation, or holiday work
- Potential costs savings for client
- Availability of expertise
- Hidden/unforeseen costs

Beware of those employers who focus on short-term price versus long-range value (Rhomberg et al, 1995). Be equally cautious with employers who possess a reactive attitude toward work injury management. These companies tend to perceive disability prevention and management as someone else's responsibility and rarely demonstrate a top-down commitment. Their management team tends to be distant or disinterested in the technical components of a program. They also tend to delegate tasks to subordinates.

There are many companies that view health and safety initiatives as required elements only to fend off EEOC, OSHA, EPA, or other regulatory agencies and entities. These companies do not view disability prevention and management as *"the right thing to do"* for valued employees. Ultimately, each provider-consultant must use his or her own judgment in screening and selecting client companies. Risk is inherent in every business opportunity.

There are rare occasions when a consultant can enter a high-risk/high-reward agreement. Projects that pay the consultant based on outcomes such as reduced cost or increased productivity can lend themselves to this model, assuming it is legal. A percentage of savings, or commission model, requires the fullest confidence and may not be designed for the timid or inexperienced consultant, as it encumbers the greatest financial risk. Table 27–11 provides two examples of benefit-cost ratios pertaining to carpal tunnel syndrome (CTS) and low-back pain (LBP) cases.

Table 27–11 Sample Consulting Cost-Benefit Analyses

EXAMPLE NO. 1: CARPAL TUNNEL SYNDROME (CTS)

1. Indemnity/lost wage replacement under WC is calculated as follows: Employee's average weekly wage of $400 x 66% (or 2/3) wage replacement equals $264/week. This amount is non-taxable.
2. Length of disability: 36 weeks @ $264/wk = $9504 wage replacement.
3. Direct medical costs over same period:
   Diagnostic work-up = $2500
   Physician visits (generalists and specialists) = $1000
   Carpal tunnel release surgery: $5000
   Anesthesiology: $2500
   Physical and Occupational Therapy: 72 visits @ $60/visit = $4320
4. Wage replacement: 36 weeks @ $400/wk = $14,400
5. Lost productivity: Original employee produces 1000 widgets @ $12/widget or $12,000/day lost × 180 lost work days = $2,160,000 in lost productivity.
6. Replacement employee production = 800 widgets @ $12/widget = $9600/day. Total production over 180 days: $9600 × 180 = $1,728,000
   Difference between employees $2,160,000 − $1,728,000 = $432,000

Subtotal:		
$9504	wage replacement	
$2500	diagnostic fees	
$1000	physician visits	
$5000	surgical fee	
$2500	anesthesiology fee	
$4320	PT/OT fees	
$14,400	replacement wages for second employee	
$432,000	productivity loss employee #1 − employee #2	
$471,224	total losses directly attributed to one CTS case	

NOTE: These data disregard legal fees and other administrative costs.

EXAMPLE NO. 2: LOW BACK PAIN (LBP)

Problem identified: Plant population of 300 workers, of which 10 have incurred occupational LBP. The company is self-insured or self-funded and pays as they go. They do not pay insurance premiums and must reserve adequate funds (company reserves) for the treatment/management of these 10 cases.

Consultant's services: A combination of employer and employee education programs and ergonomic analysis with both engineering and administrative controls implemented.

Pre-Consultation Injury Data	Post-Consultation Injury Data
10/300 employees with lost-time LBP	1/300 employees with lost-time LBP
Aggregate indemnity (lost wages) Payments average $30,000 per employee	Aggregate indemnity payments Average $30,000 per employee
Aggregate total direct medical costs (includes rehabilitation) $400,000 or $40,000 average per injured worker	Aggregate total direct medical costs $40,000 (one LBP case)
Total direct medical and indemnity costs $700,000 for 10 cases LBP	Total direct medical and indemnity costs $70,000 for one LBP case

---

> **Principle No. 5:** *Don't wait for your ship to sail in, swim out to it.*

Whenever there is dramatic change occurring in a system, there are some who seize opportunity and others who, for whatever reason, do not. Health care has irrefutably undergone dramatic change in the past several decades. This has resulted in lost opportunities as well as the creation of new ones. Consultation services offer an immense opportunity for forward-thinking providers willing to engage in some degree of risk taking. Consultation can be the means by which a provider and/or organization can diversify to offset lost opportunities and earnings. This may require some degree of exploration and research. An environmental scan can provide invaluable direction to

the consultant and minimize a hit-and-miss approach to lead generation or sector targeting.

Use of Environmental Scans

Prospecting for consultation opportunities can be facilitated when providers are willing to explore beyond the clinical paradigm, to begin to think like and understand the perspective of potential clients. This can be accomplished in a number of ways. One means of accomplishing this is to perform a periodic environmental scan. An environmental scan identifies an issue and then systematically researches categories of information pertaining to the selected issue. Table 27–12 provides a sample of an environmental scan relative to carpal tunnel syndrome (CTS). In this case, the consultant wishes to explore the potential for consultation regarding a specific injury trend, CTS. The scan includes sections concerning the scope of the problem (the need), proposed solutions (potentially, the consultant's services), supportive data, refutative data, industrial sectors affected (do my patients come from these sectors?), and a host of other standard categories. This scan could serve as a template for other issues as well. This approach defines the magnitude of the need, the resources necessary to address the need, the competitors (or, in some cases, potential collaborators), and suggests a marketing strategy.

 Table 27–12 Sample Environmental Scan

TOPIC

Potential Consulting Opportunity for Prevention/Management of Carpal Tunnel Syndrome (CTS)

   I. Scope of the problem: American workers are reporting more cases of CTS
   II. Proposed solution: employee risk screening, ergonomics (including both engineering and administrative controls)
   III. Supportive data:
      A. Between 1981–1989 occupational repetitive motion injuries increased from 18% to 52% (Delgrosso & Boillat, 1991; Franklin et al, 1991)
      B. Surgery is palliative, not curative, and it rarely returns people to their pre-CTS status
      C. CTS disability cases can cost as much as $100,000 in direct medical costs and run into the millions for lifetime wage replacement
      D. CTS cases that involve surgery account for $30,000–$70,000 (Joyce 1988; Delgrosso & Boillat, 1991; Franklin et al, 1991)
   IV. Refutational data:
      A. Congress under President George W. Bush repealed the OSHA Ergonomic Standards, which may make employers less motivated to prevent CTS
      B. Industrial sectors affected
         1. General manufacturing
         2. Wholesale/retail trade
         3. Transportation equipment
         4. Food products, especially poultry and beef packers
         5. Apparel industry
   V. Initiatives related to CTS
      1. Steroids
      2. Functional splints
      3. Ice
      4. Rest
      5. Open or closed surgery
   VI. Public/Governmental initiatives related to CTS
      1. "Red Meat Industry Standards" for cumulative trauma disorders (CTDs)
      2. ADA and its "reasonable accommodation" clause
   VII. Cost data and market size—*to be determined based on current data*
   VIII. Competitors
      1. mobile testing companies
      2. PT centers
      3. Chiropractors
      4. Ergonomists
   IX. Available technology for remediation of the problem
      1. Sensory nerve conduction velocity (NCV) studies
      2. Ergonomic analysis of jobsites, tasks, and worksites
      3. Medical interventions
   X. Marketing targets
      1. data processing centers
      2. assembly line workers
      3. truck drivers
      4. grocery store checkers
   XI. Marketing approach
      To be determined

Other Sources of Data

Providers—if they wish to be enlightened about how other health care stakeholders view disability prevention and management—can begin by reading their literature and attending their conferences. Attendance at industrial hygiene, safety, employee benefits, risk management, and other employer conferences can lead to consulting opportunities through networking. Refer to Appendixes E, F, and H and Chapter 15 for useful references. Tap into government sources of data that may provide guidance relative to disability prevention and management. Consultants can also review state and federal regulations, laws and initiatives such as state WC acts/laws, OSHA and NIOSH publications, and National Safety Council and ADA literature.

> ***Principle No. 6:*** *Don't run with the herd because the grass gets shorter where they're going and you might get stomped on.*

It is relatively easy, non-controversial, and comfortable to run with the herd or follow what the majority does. However, the grass gets shorter if one runs with the herd, and the risk of getting stomped increases. A surplus of competitors means fewer client targets and lower fees. The alternative is to run in the opposite direction or to defy conventional wisdom. Many of today's common health care practices resulted from this approach. For example, group therapies are in direct contradiction to the traditional one-on-one patient treatment. Starting an on-site (employer site) rehabilitation clinic is an example of taking the service to the customer rather than waiting for the customer to show up (patient). Direct access in physical therapy is the opposite of awaiting a physician referral or worse yet, "prescription."

There is certainly more danger and less security when daring to explore new consulting possibilities. Performing independent consulting is not for everyone. However, risk can be minimized with the use of a number of strategies. The acronym "REHAB" can assist providers who wish to become consultants.

Research your customers and their sector
Educate your customers before you sell or market to them
Help your clients to help themselves; serve as a mentor or in a "train the trainers" capacity
Assess your efficiency and effectiveness
Benchmark results to demonstrate "value" (e.g., compare post-program injury data to industry averages)

Potential Collaborations with Other Professionals

Collaboration with well-established consultants can spread or transfer the risk associated with specific projects. The following example represents a collaboration between a physical therapy outpatient company and an ergonomic company. These entities collaborated on a number of projects that focused on the identification, prevention, and management of cumulative trauma, especially carpal tunnel syndrome (CTS) and low-back pain (LBP) (See Table 27–5).

Other natural collaborations can be explored between therapists and other experts (Frank et al., 1998). Examples include:

Project	Collaborators
Ergonomics	Certified ergonomists, certified industrial hygienists (CIH), certified safety professionals (CSP), PT, OT
Functional job analysis (FJA)	PT, OT, case manager, ergonomist
Employee screening	PT, OT, occupational medicine physician, occupational nurse
Utilization review	PT, OT, SL, case managers, utilization review organizations (UROs), bill auditing firms
Reasonable accommodations (Americans with Disabilities Act, or ADA)	PT, OT, architects, engineers, ergonomists, occupational medicine physicians and nurses
Adapative and assistive equipment	PT, OT, seating experts, rehabilitation engineers

> **Principle No. 7:** *In God we trust; all others bring data.*

Anecdotal accounts of success will not open a door or close a deal in the consulting business. Clients demand hard evidence of value and cost savings. Both the proposal and final reports should contain objective measures of accountability. It may be necessary to collect baseline data against which program performance will be gauged. This may include data related to lost workdays, medical expenditures, non-medical expenditures, reduced productivity, indemnity or wage replacement payments, litigation costs, and regulatory compliance costs.

Experienced consultants collaborate with their clients in the development of program goals, performance benchmarks, and specific responsibilities. Clients may need to open their books to consultants in order to secure baseline data against which project results can be compared. For instance, OSHA logs allow an employer to calculate its preprogram and postprogram injuries via an injury-to-man-hours-worked formula (e.g., injuries per 200,000 man-hours (an OSHA standard).

> **Principle No. 8:** *The hardest step is always the first one.*

In the movie "What About Bob," Richard Dreyfus plays a psychiatrist who attempts to help his patient (Bill Murray as "Bob") overcome intense paranoia. During therapy Dreyfus uses a technique called "baby steps" to get Murray to venture out into the world. Likewise, providers who desire consulting opportunities can do so incrementally. A good "baby step" for entering the consulting arena is to select an industry that is well represented by one's clinical patients. Next, research this sector to ascertain injury and illness patterns such as carpal tunnel syndrome in keypunch operators. An environmental scan can be constructed that serves to identify industry trends and potential threats or opportunities confronting the

consultant. Scans can be produced by exploring sources of data previously mentioned. Consultants need to identify trends versus fads. Fads tend to be brief and have little impact on an industrial sector, whereas trends tend to be at least 10 years in length and have greater impact (Naismith & Aburdene, 1990).

> **Principle No. 9:** *It is better to teach them to fish than to give them fish.*

Employers are generally more interested in turnkey projects that enable them to continue employment of disability prevention and management strategies without the need for protracted use of expensive consultants. Of course, there are always exceptions to this rule. Some companies may view self-initiated and sustained projects to be a drain of important resources that could be used in other areas, namely production. It is essential for consultants to determine before proposal submission whether or not a target company has a propensity for in-sourcing (internal) or outsourcing DM projects. A consultant cannot assume that because an employer may have a health and safety officer or ergonomist, they prefer to use them in this capacity. There are times when an employer prefers an independent, arms-length expert over its own staff. Occupational safety and health compliance initiatives such as ADA, OSHA, or the Environmental Protection Agency (EPA) are routinely outsourced in an attempt to share or transfer risk to others.

Turnkey projects can conceivably be viewed as a threat, reducing the need for consultants. On the contrary, consultants who mentor their clients tend to develop strong relationships that can lead to other areas of consultation. Once the consultant is viewed as a problem solver or resource, he or she may be called on periodically because of established credibility. The ultimate goal of consulting may be to equip clients with the necessary tools to confront their own challenges.

> **Principle No. 10:** *God gave us two ears and one mouth to use in that ratio.*

Effective consultants are reflective listeners who do not approach a client's challenge with preconceived notions about solutions. The best consultants know how to ask the right questions and where to find sources of data that will assist them in crafting customized solutions for confounding problems.

Just as in clinical practice, there are few canned solutions, and each case must be examined on its own merits. In clinical practice, the initial evaluation frames the issues and goals of treatment. There is a commensurate tool in consulting practice: the needs analysis.

The Needs Analysis

Rehabilitation providers tend to be reflective listeners who, through carefully designed questions, can elicit insightful responses from their patients or clients. This skill is readily transferable to the consultant capacity using a "needs analysis," which is the consulting equivalent to a diagnostic work-up.

Consider the following scenario. A therapist wishes to approach a local employer about offering expertise relative to industrial health, ergonomics, and ADA compliance. Marching into the company with a preconceived proposal in hand—without advance knowledge of corporate culture, operations, occupational exposures, injury records, spending patterns, corporate politics, or labor-management relations—may be an ineffective approach. It may be equally ineffective to approach the company equipped with requisite knowledge of its operations, but at the wrong corporate level. Different management levels have different biases and perspectives of problems or challenges. These have already been addressed.

A particular service and its associated marketing message must be uniquely tailored for and conveyed to the appropriate decision-making level. Therefore, a needs analysis should include the question: *"What is the most appropriate management level to query about the scope of the problem?"* A consultant can draft a meaningful proposal once the appropriate person, problem or challenge, and management level have all been determined.

A typical needs analysis should ask (and eventually answer) the six questions of journalism: Who? What? When? Where? Why? and How? Let's return to the CTS example and explore a sampler of logical questions that could be posed to corporate representatives via the needs analysis.

Who?

- Who is afflicted by CTS?
- Who is responsible for health and safety concerns?
- Who will be responsible for coordinating consultant services?

What?

- What is the extent of the CTS problem (e.g., costs, prevalence, severity)?
- What has previously been done to address this problem?
- What is your commitment to resolving this problem (human and capital resources)?
- What is your time frame for resolution?

When?

- When did this problem first reveal itself?
- When employees are hired, how are they matched to their respective jobs?
- When do you realistically believe the problem can be resolved?

Where?

- Where are the cases of CTS occurring (e.g., division, work population, work stations)?
- Where did the afflicted workers work before reporting symptoms (e.g., former jobs, tasks)?
- Where are your medical dispensary and OSHA-200 injury logs?
- Where have your injured employees received their physical rehabilitation services?

Why?

- Why do you think these CTS cases have been reported?
- Why are these specific work tasks or stations designed this way?
- Why is it important to you (and your company) to address this issue?
- Why consider an outside consultant?

How?

- How was the problem discovered?
- How do you propose to resolve it?
- How do you perceive the consultant's role?

Consultants can prepare these and other written questions and present them to the prospective client before actual submission of a proposal. This will convey to clients that preparation is pivotal to success and that *if they wish to manage it (CTS), they must first measure it.*

Responses to questions can provide revealing information about the corporate culture and assist the consultant in attempting to qualify the company as a buyer. There are contexts that necessitate walking away from a potential deal if the prospective client does not appear to be committed or possessive of the appropriate motives. Table 27–13 represents a 10-question true/false test that can be given to prospective clients as part of the qualification of buyer process. Potential clients who refuse to complete this questionnaire may, in fact, not be good clients to pursue.

SALES AND MARKETING STRATEGIES

Few clinicians are formally trained in how to design and implement a sales and marketing (SM) plan. This is especially true of hospital-based therapists with referral development. Of course, there are exceptions to this observation. Today's health care market is decidedly more competitive

---

 Table 27–13 Management Level Health and Safety

Attitude Survey

True or False

1. Executive managers do not have the time to concern themselves with health and safety issues that fall within the responsibility of the medical or safety department.
2. Executives have the principal priority of productivity or end results.
3. Safety/health professionals are considered to be technical-level rather than management-level positions.
4. Work-related accidents occur irrespective of prevention services.
5. Unsafe acts and unsafe conditions are symptoms rather than causes of problems.
6. Insurance policies cover the consequences of accidents.
7. The following quote best summarizes our corporate approach to health and safety issues: *"Work-related accidents are our problem, we don't need outside consultants' involvement."*
8. Injury/illness prevention programs are difficult to offer because of labor-management agreements.
9. There is an employee suggestion process in place concerning health and safety concerns.
10. Employees must take the primary responsibility to prevent injury or illness.

and demands that clinicians to some degree possess fundamental knowledge of sales and marketing (SM).

Covey (1990), in his book entitled *The 7 Habits of Highly Effective People,* describes effective habits as a product of the synergy between knowledge, skills, and desire; so it is with consultation. Organizations, like individuals, also have effective habits, especially when designing and implementing SM plans. These plans must package knowledge and skills in language that is understandable to the customer. Consulting customers are quite varied, and their needs represent a significant departure from the two basic customer relationships with which rehabilitation providers are familiar: patient-provider and referring doctor-rehabilitation provider. The previous discussion regarding employer departments and their unique paradigms should have utility as the consultant devises a SM plan. This plan should subscribe to the tenets described in the following quotation:

> *"Marketing is the analysis, planning, implementation, and control of carefully formulated programs designed to bring about voluntary exchanges of values with target markets for the purpose of achieving organizational objectives. It relies heavily on designing the organization's offering in terms of the target market's needs and desires, and on using effective pricing, communication, and distribution to identify, motivate and service the markets."*

> - Kotler & Clarke, 1986

Although there are legions of business texts, particularly addressing sales and marketing, these may be of little value when dealing with health care-related consultation projects.

From Prospecting to Deal Closure

Marketing of health care interventions, whether preventive or treatment oriented, requires a different approach than selling other commodities. First, health care represents a service sector, rather than a product per se. Secondly, few things in life are of a more personal nature than one's health. Lastly, health professionals who enter the consulting realm possess a dual personality as a marketer *and* consultant/resource.

There is a distinction between selling and marketing. Cooper considers marketing to be the antithesis of selling (Cooper, 1985). Selling emphasizes sales stimulants, whereas marketing identifies the customer's needs and matches the product or service to those needs. Marketing demands far more research before giving the pitch to a prospective buyer/client. Selling is product-focused or service-focused. Marketing is consumer-focused or customer-focused. Selling typically involves the pursuit of new accounts; whereas marketing prizes repeat business and long-term relationships (Clifton, 1992).

Physical rehabilitation providers are in the position of converting patient encounters into potential consulting opportunities, especially if a sound database is established. A rehabilitation center's database may enable the provider to present a pattern analysis of injuries by occupational category or job task. Employers may be unaware of injury trends and the provider may be in a position to enlighten them about emerging injury trends.

When a therapist begins to identify an emerging pattern they can approach the employer to offer educational programs. Local employers can be invited to attend breakfast or luncheon seminars relevant to their needs. For example, inviting local employers to a cumulative trauma disorders workshop offers the opportunity to interface with multiple potential clients. This could be dovetailed with a tour of a treatment center and demonstrations of specific CTD treatment techniques. Workshops should focus on education and training of employer representatives and avoid blatant infomercials. Lavishing potential clients with condition-specific information and being accessible to answer their questions is one method of developing relationships vital to consulting. Sending newsletters or e-mail transmissions about issues relevant to their employee population and industrial sector will keep providers on employers' radar screen. Sources of these data include government reports, business trade journals, topical seminars, newsletters, chambers of commerce, and the Internet.

In summary, educating the customer at every step of the process, from prospecting, the pitch, closing, implementation, and follow-up may lead to a mutually beneficial, long-term, and profitable relationship.

CONSULTING CAVEATS

> *"What we see in our roles as consultants is a great deal of emphasis on treatment efficacy, and on outcomes—but very little on injury prevention, and even still less on utilization management. People are reacting to catastrophic cases after the costs have gone through the ceiling—not trying to manage them in the first place, and insurers who many firms depend upon to fill this function have in general been slow to gather the necessary data. They're financing risk rather than managing it."*

> - Apker, 1993

Even the best-laid plans occasionally fail when offering consultative services. It is not uncommon to get through the needs analysis and sales/marketing stages, only to see an opportunity evaporate before closing the deal. This is especially common when approaching large, dynamic companies that have constantly shifting priorities. Corporate downsizing, plant layoffs, mergers, and acquisitions present risk to the consultant who has invested a great deal of time and energy.

Avoiding Common Mistakes

It has been said that one learns little from his or her successes, but the world from our failures—so it is with consulting. Consultants routinely make common mistakes, such as dwelling on processes at the expense of outcomes, especially cost and employee productivity outcomes. Ignorance of or insensitivity to labor-management negotiated agreements will easily sabotage a project. Proposals that are too technical or do not press the right client hot-buttons can be doomed to failure. Consultants who do not engage employer representatives early in the process cannot expect an automatic buy-in later on. Consultants who do not construct a "client responsibilities" listing invite full culpability should results be less than desirable. An absence of specific action steps identifying specific responsibilities, persons, and timeframes can be problematic. Egocentrism of the consultant almost certainly will destroy prospects. Egocentrism can manifest itself in situations wherein the consultant has predetermined the customer's needs and has disregarded the "customer knows best" dictum. Perhaps the ultimate flaw is offering a service that cannot be delivered because it exceeds the consulting staff's core competencies or ability to outsource it to other experts. For instance, although a therapist may have a command of CTD understanding, he or she may not be competent in selecting and/or designing equipment intended to minimize physiological stress on the wrists in the case of carpal tunnel syndrome. In this example, securing the services of a certified ergonomist or industrial engineer could prove to be a more prudent choice.

Understanding one's limitations in consulting work is equally important if not more important (from a risk management standpoint) than understanding one's capabilities. Customers tend to respect consultants more if they readily acknowledge their limitations, but work collaboratively to fulfill the client's needs.

A lack of top to bottom commitment at the client's corporate level is a common failure of consulting programs. Many managers do not involve themselves in day-to-day health and safety issues and may adopt the attitude that problems are someone else's fix. Table 27–13 provides insight into how management views disability prevention/management responsibility. Management may view injury and disability prevention programs as cost items contributing little to company productivity and, therefore, do not assign anyone direct responsibility.

SUMMARY

Physical rehabilitation providers who wish to enter the consulting world are inhibited only by their lack of creativity, risk aversion, or unwillingness to explore what others have done in this regard. This chapter has attempted to provide advice about how to transfer one's skills, knowledge, and aptitude into this exciting arena. It has supplied the reader with numerous sample forms and questionnaires toward this end. There are many providers who serve as mentors in this regard. These persons represent role models for aspiring consultants at the entry level or advanced level. A number of these persons are cited in the references. These leaders have raised the perception of the rehabilitation professions through their courage and willingness to look beyond the clinical box. Looking beyond the clinical box involves anticipating the evolving needs of potential clients and a willingness to assume some risk through consulting.

R EFERENCES

Americans with Disabilities Act of 1990 (ADA), Public Law 101-336, 42 U.S.C. 12101, 1990.

American Physical Therapy Association: Guide to physical therapist practice, second edition, part one: A description of patient/client management, part two: Preferred practice patterns. Phys Ther J 81(1):768, 2001.

Apker C: Covering the spectrum. Risk and Benefits J Fall:10-13, 32, 1993.

Bryan JM, Geroy GD, Isernhagen SI: Nonclinical competencies: A survey of occupational health physical therapists. J Orthop Sports PT 19(5):305-311, 1994.

Bryan JM, Geroy GD, Isernhagen SI: Nonclinical competencies for physical therapists consulting with business and industry. J Ortho Sports PT 18(6):673-681, 1993.

Bureau of Labor Statistics, U.S. Department of Labor. OSH Summary Estimates Chart Package. Washington DC, Government Printing Office, December 18, 2003.

Chandler J, O'Brien P, Weinstein L: The role of occupational therapy in transition from school to work for adolescents with disabilities. WORK 6(1):55-59, 1996.

Clifton DW: Marketing and reimbursement of work therapy services. Orthop Phys Ther Clin 1(1):133-147, 1992.

Clifton DW: If a niche doesn't exist, carve one! Phys Ther Today 16(2):49-51, 1993.

Clifton DW: Diversifying for success in the '90s. Rehabil Manage 8(3):52-53, 55, 57, 59-60, 1995.

Clifton DW: Payer-provider alliances. Rehabil Manage 9(5):100-102, 1996.

Commission on Health & Safety and Workers' Compensation. Fact Sheet: Workers' Compensation Medical Care in California: Costs, Aug. 2003, 455 Golden Gate Avenue, 10th Floor, San Francisco, (telephone): (415) 703-4220, No.1:1-4, 2003.

Cooper PD: Health Care Marketing: Issues and Trends. Rockville, MD, Aspen 1985.

Coopers and Lybrand Consulting: Health Management: A Survey of Company-Sponsored Wellness Programs, 1990, www.pwcglobal.com, accessed July 13, 2004.

Cosgrove JL, Chase PM, Mast NJ: Carpal tunnel syndrome in railroad workers. Am J Phys Med Rehabil 81(2):101-107, 2002.

Covey SR: The 7 Habits of Highly Effective People. New York, Simon and Schuster, 1990.

Coy JA, Davenport M: Age changes in the older worker: Implications for injury prevention. WORK (2):38-46,1991.

Darphin LE: Work hardening and work conditioning perspectives. In Isernhagen SJ (ed): The Comprehensive Guide to Work Injury Management. Gaithersburg, Md, Aspen, 1995, p 443-462.

Daus C: On-site rehab. Rehabil Manage 8(3):25-26, 28-29, 1995.

Delgrosso I, Boillat MA: Carpal tunnel syndrome: role of occupation. Int Arch Occup Environ Health (Germany) 63(4):267-270, 1991.

Dembe AE, Sum J, Baker C: Workers' Compensation Medical Care in California: Costs, Fact Sheet, Number 2, August 2003, California Healthcare Foundation and Commission on Health & Safety and Workers' Compensation, www.chcf.org and www.dir.ca/gov/chswc, accessed July 14, 2004.

Dyck DE: Disability management: Theory, strategy, and industry practice. Toronto, Butterworths, 2000.

Edwards CH: Applied ergonomics. WORK 1(1):27-38, 1990.

Equal Employment Opportunity Commission (EEOC): Enforcement guidance on reasonable accommodation: An undue hardship under the Americans with Disabilities Act, http://www.eeoc.gov/policy/docs/accommodations.html, accessed February 3, 2004.

Ellexson MT: Worksite rehabilitation programs: The future for industrial rehabilitation? Work Programs Special Interest Section Quarterly. Am Occup Ther Assoc 11(2):1-3, 1997.

Enix DH, Lopez SD: How early is early? On-site early return-to-work programs cut losses and cots. Rehabil Manage 11(2):28,33-35, 1998.

Esposito MD: Implementing the ADA: A guide to the new employment regulations and how to comply, Englewood Cliffs, NJ, Maxwell MacMillen, 1991.

Fernberg PM: Integrated disability management works, but who's looking? Occup Hazards 61(2):25-26, 1999.

Fitzpatrick MA, King PM: Disability management pays off. Am Society Safety Engineers J (ASSE) January:39-41, 2001.

Frank J, Sinclair S, Hogg-Johnson S: Preventing disability from work-related low back pain: New evidence gives new hope-if we can just get all the players onside. Can Med Assoc J 158(12):1625-1631, 1998.

Franklin GM, Haug J, Heyer N et al.: Occupational carpal tunnel syndrome in Washington state, 1984–1988. Am J Pub Health 81(6):741-746, 1991.

Fuerstein M, Shaw WS, Lincoln AL et al.: Clinical and workplace factors associated with a return to modified duty in work-related upper extremity disorders. Pain J 102(1–2):51-61, 2003.

Geddes Lipold A: Managing the guy who isn't there. Business & Health Nov/Dec:25-30, 2000.

Gilpin SL: Disability management: It takes a PRO to solve the puzzle. Business & Health 18(2):37-39, 2000.

Grasso M, Rousmaniere P: An emerging strategy for high cost claims: Worksite consultations-which can reveal barriers to return to work and remedies that would otherwise be overlooked-are underused in the assessment of cumulative trauma injuries—Workers' comp. Risk & Insurance November 2002, http://www.fidnarticles.com/cf_0/MOBJK/14_13/94666510/print.jhtml, accessed February 11, 2004.

Hablutzel N, McMahon BT: The Americans with Disabilities Act: Access and Accommodations: Guidelines for Human Resources, Rehabilitation and Legal Professionals. Orlando, FL, PMD Press, 1992.

Hammel J, Symons J: Evaluating reasonable accommodations in the workplace: A team approach. WORK 3(4):12-20, 1993.

Hebert LA: OSHA ergonomics guidelines and the PT consultant. PT Magazine 3(7):54-61, 1995.

Hewitt Associates: Employers continue offering programs to promote health and productivity, http://www.hewitt.com, press releases dated July 24 2001, accessed August, 27, 2001.

Hewitt Associates: Health promotion/managed health provided by major U.S. employers in 2000, http://www.hewitt.com, accessed August, 27, 2001.

Hochanadel CD, Conrad DE: Evolution of an on-site industrial physical therapy program. J Occup Med 35(10):1011-1016, 1993.

Hunt HA, Habeck RV: The Michigan Disability Prevention Study, Kalamazoo, MI, W.E. Upjohn Institute for Employment Research, May 1993.

Isom RN: Disability management: Building the program. J Rehabil Adm 22(2):137-139, 1998.

Jacobs K: Integrating the Americans with Disabilities Act of 1990 into client intervention. Am J Occup Ther 46(5):445-449, 1992.

Jacobs K: Ergonomics for Therapists, 2nd ed. Boston: Butterworth-Heinemann, 1999.

Job Accommodation Network (JAN), http://www.jan.wvu.edu, accessed February 23, 2004.

Johnson W et al: Why is the treatment of work-related injuries so costly? New evidence from California. Inquiry 33:3-65, 1996.

Joyce M: Ergonomics offer solutions to numerous health complaints. Occup Health & Safety 57(4):58-66, 1988.

Joyce S: Reshaping corporate wellness. Case Rev 2(3):26-28, 30, 1996.

Kendall NA: Psychosocial approaches to the prevention of chronic pain: The low back paradigm. Balliere's Best Practice Res Clin. Rheum 113(3):545-554, 1999.

Kenny D, Powell NJ, Reynolds-Lynch KR: Trends in industrial rehabilitation: Ergonomics and cumulative trauma disorders. WORK 5(2):133-141, 1995.

King JW: An integration of medicine and industry. J Hand Ther 3:45-49, 1990.

Klekamp JK. In the workplace: On-site physical therapy a win-win option Occupational Health Tracker J 6(3): 2003, http//:www.systoc.com/Tracker/Autumn03/PT, accessed August 28, 2004.

Kornblau BL, Ellexson M: Hiring employees under the disabilities act. Risk Manage 38(11):38-50, 1991.

Kotler P, Clarke RN: Creating the responsive organization. Healthcare Forum 29(3):26-32, 1986.

Larson BA: On-site work rehabilitation: The employer insurer, and provider connection. Work Programs Special Interest Section Quarterly AOTA 8(4):1-2, 1994.

Lincoln AE, Fuerstein M, Shaw WS et al: Impact of case manager training on worksite accommodations in workers' compensation claimants with upper extremity disorders. J Occup Environ Med 44(3):237-245, 2002.

Lipow VA: Aging workers: Disability management strategies. Rehabil Manage 10(1):32, 34, 36, 1997.

Lunda KA: Americans with Disabilities Act consulting: The role of physical therapy and ergonomics, ergonomics part II. Orthopaedic Phys Ther Clin North Am 5(3):353-373, 1996.

Lutz G, Hansford R: Cumulative trauma disorder controls: The ergonomic program at Ethicon Inc. J Hand Surg 12A:863-866, 1987.

Marras WS: Toward an understanding of dynamic variables in ergonomics, occupational medicine. State Art Rev 7(4):55-66,1992.

Martin KJ: Workers' compensation case management strategy. Am Assoc Occup Health Nurses (AAOHN) 43(5):245-250, 1995.

May DC: Results of an OSGHA ergonomic intervention program in New Hampshire. Appl Occup Environ Hyg 17(11):768-773, 2002.

McGinty SM, Cicero MC, Cicero JM et al.: Reason as given by California physical therapists for not belonging to the American Physical Therapy Association. Phys Ther 81(6):1224-1232, 2001.

Mills D. Building joint labor-management initiatives for worksite disability management. In Shrey DE, Lacerte M (eds). Principles and Practices of Disability Management in Industry. Winter Park, FL, GR Press, 1995, pp 225-247.

Modugny A: No time off for employers seeking to control absence costs. New York, Marsh and McLennan Companies, 2002, http://www.mercerhr.com, accessed August 2004.

Miller M: The ADA offers unique opportunities for physical and occupational therapists. WORK 6(1):47-52, 1996.

Mills DL: Building joint labor-management initiatives for worksite disability management. In Shrey DE, Lacerte M (eds): Principles and Practices of Disability Management in Industry. Winter Park, FL, GR Press, 225-247, 1995.

Mitchell RW: Absence management can save big bucks. National Underwriter 104:50, 113, 2000.

Mullins JA, Rumrill PD, Roessler RT: The role of the rehabilitation placement professional in the ADA era. WORK 6(1):3-10, 1996.

Naismith J, Aburdene P: Megatrends 2000: Ten new directions for the 1990s. New York, Avon Books, 1990, p 416.

National Safety Council: Accident Facts, Washington, DC, Bureau of Labor Statistics, 1992.

Office of Inspector General (OIG). "Operation Restore Trust," Fact Sheet 1997.05.20, Operation Restore Trust Accomplishments. Washington, DC, OIG Press Office, www.hhs.gov/news/press/1997/pres/970520d.html, accessed July 16, 2004.

Pheasant S: Ergonomics, Work and Health. Gaithersburg, MD, Aspen, 1991.

Pilling D. Approaches to case management for people with disabilities. London: J. Kingsley; Rehabilitation Resource Centre, City University, 1992.

Pinkham J: CTS impacts thousands and costs are skyrocketing. Occup Saf & Health 57(8):6-7, 1988.

Planek TW, Kolosh K: Survey shows support for safety-and-health committees. Saf Health J January:76-78, 1994.

Pohlman J, Poosawtsee C, Gerndt K et al: Improving work programs delivery of information and service to workers' compensation carriers, WORK 16(2):91-100, 2001.

Reis E: In sickness and in wellness. PT Magazine 11(9):44-48, 51, 2003.

Rhomberg S, Wolf L, Evanoff B: An integrated program for the prevention and management of musculoskeletal work injuries. WORK 5(2):105-122, 1995.

Rothman J, Levine RE: Prevention Practice: Strategies for Physical and Occupational Therapy. Philadelphia, WB Saunders, 1992.

Rousmaniere P, Denniston P: Getting workers comp costs under control: Workers' comp insurance costs may accelerate as employers with good records continue to opt for self-insurance. Risk and Insurance, March 3, 2003, http://www.findarticles.com/o/mOBJK/3-14/98416383/print.jhtnl, accessed February 11, 2004.

Rundle RL: Move fast if you want to rehabilitate workers. Business Insurance May:10-12, 1983.

Scott LR: Post-offer screening. Am Assoc Occup Health Nurses J (AAOHN) 50(12):559-563, 2002.

Scott MB: Insurers support services focus on enabling return to work from disability. Employee Benefit Plan Rev 54(9):16-22, 2000.

Scruby DJ, Denham S, Larkin GN: Economic impact of on-site physical therapy. J Occup Environ Med 43:670-671, 2001.

Scully-Palmer C: Outcome study: An industrial rehabilitation program. WORK 15(1):21-23, 2000.

Shrey DE, LaCerte M: Principles and Practices of Disability Management in Industry. Winter Park, FL, GR Press, 1995.

Shulenberger CC: Ergonomics in the workplace: Evaluating and modifying jobs. Occup Med: State Art Rev 7(1):105-112, 1992.

Siefker JM. Fundamentals of Case Management: Guidelines for Practicing Case Managers. St. Louis, Mosby, 1998.

Smith D: Implementing disability management: A review of basic concepts and essential components. Employee Assistance Q 12(4):37-50, 1997.

Smith PJ, Preis I: A systematic approach to provider-based disability management. Hawaii Med J 60(12):318-320, 2001.

Society of Professional Benefit Administrators. What % of Employer Health Plans Use Self-Funding? Chevy Chase, MD, Society of Professional Benefit Administrators, undated.

Threlkeld AJ, Jensen GM, Royeen CB: The clinical doctorate: A framework or analysis in physical therapist education. Phys Ther 79(6):567-578, 1999.

U.S. Office of Disability Employment Policy. Making Management Decisions about Accommodations. Washington DC, U.S. Department of Labor, Office of Disability Employment Policy, 2002.

Vowles KE, Gross RT: Work-related beliefs about injury and physical capability for work in individuals with chronic pain. Pain J 101(3): 291-298, 2003.

Walker JM: Understanding disability. Risk Manage J 45(11):14-22, 1998.

Watson Wyatt Worldwide Consulting: Staying @ Work: Increasing Shareholder Value Through Integrated Disability Management, Third Annual Survey Report 1998/1999. Washington, DC, Washington Business Group on Health, 1999, p 12 .

Ward SR: Impairment rating. Clin Manage 12(5):38-45, 1992.

Wheeler PM, Kearney JR, Hanson CA: The U.S. study of work in capacity and reintegration. Soc Secur Bull 64(1):32-44, 2001–2002.

Wiersma RN: Ergonomics analysis of work stressors, ergonomics: Part I. Orthop Phys Ther Clin North Am 5(2):207-230, 1996.

Winters JM: Rehabilitation engineering training for the future: Influences of trends in academics, technology and health reform. Assistive Technol 7(2):95-110, 1995.

Wynn KE: Setting corporate trends with on-site PT. PT Magazine 4(7):66-71, 1996.

Zacharia D, Robertson J, MacDermaid J: Work-related cumulative trauma disorders of the upper extremity: Navigating the epidemiologic literature. Am J Ind Med 423(3):258-269, 2002.

Zigenfus GC, Yin J, Giang GM et al. Effectiveness of early physical therapy in the treatment of acute low back musculoskeletal disorders. J Occup Environ Med 42:35-39, 2000.

RECOMMENDED READINGS

Isernhagen SJ (ed): Industrial physical therapy. Orthop Phys Ther Clin North Am 1(1):1-189, 1992.

Piegorisch KM (guest ed): Ergonomics: Part I. Orthop Phys Ther Clin North Am 5(2):ix, 1996.

Piegorsch KM: Ergonomics: Part II, Orthop Phys Ther Clin North Am 5(3):ix-x (Foreward), 1996.

Shrey DE, LaCerte M: Principles and Practices of Disability Management in Industry. Winter Park, FL, GR Press, 1995.

Stoddard S, Jans L, Ripple JM, Knaus L (eds): National Institute on Disability and Rehabilitation Research, Chartbook on Work and Disability in the United States, Washington, DC, U.S. Department of Education, 1998, p 60.

Government Sources of Disability Data/Information

Agency/Organization	Website
Administration on Aging (AOA) Administration on Developmental Disabilities	www.aoa.gov
Agency for Health Care Quality & Research (formerly Agency for Health Care Policy & Research or AHCPR)	www.ahrq.gov
Bureau of the Census	www.census.gov
Bureau of Health Professions	www.bhpr.hrsa.gov
Bureau of Labor Statistics (BLS)	www.bls.gov
Centers for Disease Control (CDC)	www.cdc.gov
Centers for Medicare & Medicaid (CMM) Services (formerly Health Care Financing Administration or HCFA)	www.cms.hhs.gov
Congressional Budget Office (CBO)	www.cbo.gov
Congressional Quarterly Researcher (CQR)	www.cq.com
Department of Health & Human Services (DHHS)	www.ddhs.gov
Department of Labor (DOL), Bureau of Labor Statistics	www.dol.gov
Department of Veteran Affairs (VA)	www.va.gov
Department of Defense (DOD)	www.dod.gov
Equal Employment Opportunity Commission (EEOC)	www.eeoc.gov
Food & Drug Administration (FDA)	www.fda.gov
Government Accounting Office (GAO)	www.gao.gov
Government Printing Office (GPO)	www.gpo.gov
Health Care Financing Administration (now Centers for Medicare & Medicaid CMM)	www.hcfa.gov www.cms.hhs.gov
Institute of Medicine (IOM)	www.iom.gov
Interagency Committee on Disability Research (ICDR)	www.icdr.gov
Library of Congress	www.loc.gov
National Center for Education Statistics (NCES)	www.ed.gov
National Center for the Dissemination of y Disabilit Research (NCDDR)	www.ncddr.gov
National Center for Health Statistics (NCHS)	www.nchs.gov

Agency/Organization	Website
National Center for Medical Rehabilitation Research (NCMRR)	www.nichd.nih.gov
National Council on Disability (NCD)	www.ncd.gov
National Information Center for Children & Youth with Disabilities (NICHCY)	www.nichcy.org
National Institute on Aging	www.nia.nih.gov
National Council on Disability (now known as Disability Rights Commission)	www.ncd.gov
National Health Center	www.health.gov
National Institute on Disability & Rehabilitation Research (NIDRR)	www.ccddr.org
National Institutes of Health	www.nih.gov
National Institute of Occupational Safety & Health (NIOSH)	www.niosh.gov
National Library of Medicine	www.nlm.gov
National Rehabilitation Information Center	www.ncddr.org/icdr
National Science Foundation (NSF) (NIDRR funded)	www.nsf.gov
National Technical Information Service Technology Administration, U.S. Department Of Commerce	www.fedworld.gov
Office of Special Education & Rehabilitation Services (OSERS)	www.ed.gov/offices/ OCERS/NIDRR
Office of Disability, Aging & Long-term Care (DALTCP)	www.aspe.hhs.gov/ daltcp
Office on Disability & Health (division of CDC)	www.cdc.gov
Office of Disease Prevention & Health Promotion	www.dhhs.gov
Occupational Safety & Health Administration (OSHA) Social Security Administration (SSA)	www.osha.gov www.ssa.gov
Rehabilitation Services Administration (RSA)	www.ed.gov
Social Security Administration (SSA)	www.ssa.gov
U.S. Administration on Aging (division of DHHS)	www.dhhs.gov
U.S. Bureau of the Census	www.census.gov
U.S. Department of Commerce	www.commerce.gov

State Insurance Commissioners

Alabama
Department of Insurance
201 Monroe St., Ste 1700
Montgomery, AL 36104
Tel: (334) 269-3550

Alaska
Department of Commerce
Division of Insurance
PO Box 110805
Juneau, AK 99811
Tel: (907) 465-2515

Arizona
Department of Insurance
2910 N. 44th St.
Suite 210
Phoenix, AZ 85018
Tel: (602) 912-8400

Arkansas
Department of Insurance
1200 W. 3rd St.
Little Rock, AR 72204
Tel: (501) 686-2600

California
Insurance Commissioner
300 Capitol Mall
Suite 1500
Sacramento, CA 72204
Tel: (916) 492-3500

Colorado
Division of Insurance
1560 Broadway
Suite 850
Denver, CO 80202

Connecticut
Insurance Commissioner
Dept. of Insurance
State Office Building
P.O. Box 816
Hartford, CT 06142
Tel: (860) 297-3802

Delaware
Insurance Commissioner
841 Silver Lake Blvd.
Dover, DE 19901
Tel: (302) 739-4251

District of Columbia
Insurance Superintendent
Insurance & Securities
810 First St., N.E.
Washington, D.C. 20013
Tel: (202) 727-8000

Florida
Insurance Commissioner
Department of Insurance
State Capitol
Plaza Level Eleven
Tallahassee, FL 32399
Tel: (850) 922-3101

Georgia
Insurance Commissioner
Floyd Building
704 West Tower
2 Martin Luther King Dr.
Atlanta, GA 30334
Tel: (404) 656-2056

Hawaii
Insurance Division
Consumer Affairs
250 S. King St.
5th Floor
Honolulu, HI 96811
Tel: (808) 586-2790

Idaho
Department of Insurance
700 W. State St.
3rd Floor
Boise, ID 83720
Tel: (208) 334-4250

Illinois
Department of Insurance
320 W. Washington St.
4th Floor
Springfield, IL 62767
Tel: (217) 782-4515

Indiana
Commissioner of Insurance
311 W. Washington
Indianapolis, IN 46204
Tel: (317) 232-2385

Iowa
Division of Insurance
Lucas Off. Bldg
Des Moines, IA 50319
Tel: (515) 281-4025

Kansas
Department of Insurance
420 S. W. 9th St.
Topeka, KS 66612
Tel: (800) 432-2484

Kentucky
Department of Insurance
215 W. Main St.
P.O. Box 517
Frankfurt, KY 40601
Tel: (502) 564-6027

Louisiana
Commissioner of Insurance
950 N. 5th St.
Baton Rouge, LA 70802

Maine
Superintendent of
  Insurance
State House Station 34
Augusta, ME 04333

Maryland
Insurance Commissioner
525 St. Paul Place
Baltimore, MD 21202

Massachusetts
Division of Insurance
470 Atlantic Ave.
2nd Floor North
Boston, MA 02210
Tel: (617) 521-7794

Michigan
Insurance Bureau
611 W. Ottawa St.
Lansing, MI 48933
Tel: (517) 373-9273

Minnesota
Department of Commerce
133 E. 7th St.
St. Paul, MN 55101
Tel: (612) 296-6848

Mississippi
Commissioner of Insurance
1804 Walter Sillers
Jackson, MS 39201
Tel: (601) 359-3569

Missouri
Department of Insurance
301 W. High St.
Jefferson City,
  MO 65102
Tel: (800) 726-7390

Montana
Insurance Commissioner
126 N. Sanders
Helena, MT 59601
Tel: (406) 444-2040

Nebraska
Department of Insurance
Terminal Building
Suite 400
941 O Street
Lincoln, NE 68508
Tel: (402) 471-2201

Nevada
Insurance Division
Nye Building—Capitol
1665 Hot Springs Road
Carson City, NV 89710
Tel: (702) 687-7650

New Hampshire
Insurance Department
56 Old Suncock Road
Concord, NH 03301
Tel: (603) 271-2261

New Jersey
Commissioner of Insurance
20 W. State St.
CN 325
Trenton, NJ 08625
Tel: (609) 292-5363

New Mexico
Superintendent of
   Insurance
P.O. Box Drawer 1269
Santa Fe, NM 87504
Tel: (505) 827-4601

New York
Insurance Department
25 Beaver St.
New York, NY 10004
Tel: (212) 480-2289

North Carolina
Department of Insurance
P.O. Box 26387
Raleigh, NC 27611
Tel: (919) 733-7349

North Dakota
Insurance Department
Capitol Bldg.
Bismarck, ND 58505
Tel: (701) 328-2440

Ohio
Department of Insurance
2100 Stella Court
Columbus, OH 43215
Tel: (614) 644-2658

Oklahoma
State Insurance Department
3814 N. Santa Fe
Oklahoma City, OK 73118
Tel: (405) 521-2686

Oregon
Insurance Department
350 Winter St.
Room 200
Salem, OR 97310
Tel: (503) 378-4100

Pennsylvania
Insurance Department
1326 Strawberry Square
13th Floor
Harrisburg, PA 17120
Tel: (717) 787-0442

Rhode Island
Department of Business
Regulation Ins. Sect.
233 Richmond St.
Providence, RI 02903
Tel: (401) 277-2223

South Carolina
Department of Insurance
1612 Marion St.
Columbia, SC 29201
Tel: (803) 737-6160

South Dakota
Department of Insurance
118 W. Capitol Ave.
Pierre, SD 57501
Tel: (605) 773-3563

Tennessee
Department of Commerce
   & Insurance
500 James Robertson
Parkway
Nashville, TN 37243
Tel: (615) 741-3563

Texas
Department of Insurance
333 Gaudalupe
Austin, TX 78701
Tel: (512) 463-6464

Utah
Insurance Commissioner
3110 State Off. Bldg.
Salt Lake City, UT 84114
Tel: (801) 538-3800

Vermont
Department of Banking &
   Insurance
89 Main St., Drawer 20
Montpelier, VT 05620
Tel: (802) 828-3301

Virginia
State Corporation
   Commissioner
Insurance Bureau
1300 E. Main St.
Richmond, VA 23209
Tel: (804) 371-9694

Washington
Office of Insurance
   Commissioner
P.O. Box 40255
Olympia, WA 98504
Tel: (360) 753-7301

West Virginia
Insurance Commissioner
Box 50540
Charleston, WV 25305
Tel: (304) 558-3354

Wisconsin
Office of Commissioner of
   Insurance
121 E. Wilson St.
Madison, WI 53702
Tel: (608) 267-1233

Wyoming
Insurance Department
Box 50540
Herschler Bldg.
122 W. 25th St.
3rd East
Cheyenne, WY 82002
Tel: (307) 777-7401

Foundations and Research Institutes

FOUNDATIONS THAT SUPPORT THE STUDY OF HEALTH CARE

The following foundations are involved in a variety of health care and disability related initiatives. This list intentionally excludes condition-specific or constituency-specific foundations because these are too numerous and narrow in focus.

These foundations have supported research and demonstration projects on a variety of clinical care, health policy, financing, managed care, Medicare, and delivery issues. Their Websites are great and, in most cases, research results are available.

Name/Address	Website
The Commonwealth Fund 1 E. 75th St. New York, NY 100021 Fax: (212) 606-3875	www.cmwf.org
Families U.S.A. Foundation 1334 G St., N.W. Washington, D.C. 20005	www.familiesusa.org
Foundation for Physical Therapy 1111 N. Fairfax St. Alexandria, VA 22314 Tel: (800) 875-1375 Fax: (703) 706-8519	www.foundation@apta.org
The John Hartford Foundation 55 E. 59th St. New York, NY 10022-1178 Tel: (212) 832-7788 Fax: (212) 593-4913	www.jhartfound.org
Henry J. Kaiser Family Foundation 2400 Sand Hill Road Menlo Park, CA 94025 Fax: (650) 854-8037	www.ikff.org
W. K. Kellogg Foundation 1 Michigan Ave. East Battle Creek, MI 49017-4058 Tel: (616) 968-1611	www.wkkf.org

Name/Address	Website

Milbank Memorial Fund
646 Madison Ave.
New York, NY 10022
"Evaluating the Quality of
  Health Care: What Research
  Offers Decision Makers"
"Patients as Effective Collaborators
  in Managing Chronic Conditions"
"Better Information, Better Outcomes?"
	www.milbank.org

The Pew Charitable Trusts 1 Commerce Square 2005 Market St., Suite 1700 Philadelphia, PA 19103-7077 Fax: (215) 575-4939	www.pewtrusts.com
Robert Wood Johnson Foundation Route 1 and College Ave. East P.O. Box 2316 Princeton, NJ 08543-2316 Tel: (609) 452-8701	www.rwjf.org
The American Occupational Therapy Foundation 4720 Montgomery Lane, P.O. Box 31220 Bethesda, MD 20824-1220 Tel: (301) 652-2682 Fax: (301) 656-3620 Web site/e-mail: aotf@aotf.org	www.aotf.org

HEALTH POLICY RESEARCH INSTITUTES

Name/Address	Website
American Enterprise Institute For Public Policy Research 1150 17th St., N.W. Washington, D.C. 20036 Tel: (202) 862-5800 Fax: (202) 862-7172	http://www.aei.org
The Brookings Institute 1775 Massachusetts Ave., N.W. Washington, D.C. 20036 Tel: (202) 797-6000 Fax: (202) 747-6004	http://www.brook.edu

Name/Address	Website
Citizens Council on Health Care 1954 University Ave. West, Suite 8 St. Paul, MN 55104 Tel: (651) 646-8935 Fax: (651) 646-0100	www.cchc-mn.org
Coalition for Healthier Cities and Communities	www.healthycommunities.org
Economic and Social Research Institute 1015 18th St., N.W. Suite 210 Washington, D.C. 20036-3203 Tel: (202) 833-8877 Fax: (202) 833-8932	http://www.ndpolicy.com

Name/Address	Website
Institute for Health Policy Solutions 1441 I St., N.W. Washington, DC 20005 Tel: (202) 789-1491 Fax: (202) 789-1879	http://www.ihps.org

The Levy Institute of Bard College
Blythewood
P.O. Box 5000
Annandale-on-the-Hudson,
  NY 12504-5000
"Physician Incentives in Managed
  Care Organizations"
"Regulating HMOs"
	http://www.levy.org

Accreditation and Certification Bodies

PAYER FOCUS

Agency/Organization	Website
Consumer Assessments of Health Plans Study (CAHPS)	www.qahcpr.gov
National Council on Quality Assurance (NCQA)	www.ncqa.org
American Accreditation Healthcare Commission (formerly known as Utilization Review & Accreditation [URAC])	www.urac.org

PROVIDER FOCUS

Agency/Organization	Website
Accreditation Association for Ambulatory Healthcare (AAAHC) Wilmette, IL Info@aaahc.org	www.aaahc.org
Commission on the Accreditation of Rehabilitation Facilities (CARF)	www.carf.org
Joint Commission for the Accreditation of Healthcare Organizations (JCAHO)	www.jcaho.org
The Medical Quality Commission (TMQC)	www.tmqc.org
The National Practitioners Data Bank, Healthcare Integrity and Protection Data Bank	www.npdb-hipdb.com

Associations/Organizations

AGING-RELATED ASSOCIATIONS/ORGANIZATIONS

The following groups may be useful to rehabilitation providers who specialize in long-term care, disease state management, and chronic illness/injury management.

Name/Address	Website
American Association of Homes and Services for the Aging 901 E St., N.W. Washington, D.C. 20004-2011 Tel: (202) 783-2242	www.aahsa.org
American Society of Aging 833 Market St. San Francisco, CA 94103	www.asaging.org
Gray Panthers 1424 16th St., N.W., Suite 602 Washington, D.C. 20036	www.graypanthers.org
National Council on the Aging 409 3rd St., S.W., Suite 200 Washington, D.C., 20024 Tel: (202) 479-6653	www.ncoa.org
National Association of Area Agencies On Aging, Suite 100 1112 16th St., N.W. Washington, D.C., 20024	www.n4a.org
National Senior Citizens Law Center (NSCLC) 1101 14th St., N.W., Suite 400 Washington, D.C. 20005 Tel: (202) 289-6976	www.nsclc.org
The National Institute on Consumer-Directed Long-Term Services c/o National Council on the Aging Washington, D.C., 20024 Tel: (202) 479-6653	www.ncoa.org

HEALTH CARE INFORMATION MANAGEMENT ORGANIZATIONS

The following organizations may serve as vital links for data concerning information management, including electronic mail, billing, and reimbursement; practice guidelines; and regulatory, legislative, compliance, patient confidentiality, HIPAA, financial management, and outcomes measures.

Name/Address	Website
American Health Information Management Association 233 N. Michigan Ave., Suite 2150 Chicago, IL 60601 Tel: (312) 233-1100	e mail: info@ahima.org
American Association of Health Care Administrative Management 1200 19th St., N.W., Suite 300 Washington, D.C. 20036 Tel: (202) 857-1179	e-mail: aaham@dc.sba.com
American Medical Informatics Association 4915 St. Elmo St., Suite 401 Bethesda, MD 20814 Tel: (301) 657-1292	e-mail: mail@.amia.org
American Telemedicine Association 1010 Vermont Avenue, N.W., Suite 301 Washington, D.C. 20005 Tel: (202) 628-4700	e-mail: atmeda@atmeda.org
Association of Electronic Healthcare Transactions 3513 N. McKinley St., N.W. Washington, D.C. 20015	e-mail: afehct@aol.com
Association for Repetitive Motion Syndromes (formerly CTS/RSI Association) P.O. Box 471973 Aurora, CO 80047	health.gov/NHIC
Association of Telemedicine Service Providers 7276 S.W. Beaverton-Hillsdale Highway Portland, OR 97225 Tel: (503) 222-2406	e- mail: info@atsp.org
College of Healthcare Information Management Executives 3300 Washington Ave., Suite 225 Ann Arbor, MI 48104 Tel: (734) 665-000	e-mail: staff@chime-office.org

Name/Address	Website
Healthcare Financial Management Association 2 Westbrook Corporate Center, Suite 700 Westchester, IL 60154 Tel: (708) 531-9600	www.hfma.org
Health Care EDI Coalition 1405 N. Pierce St., Suite 100 Little Rock, AR 72207 Tel: (501) 661-9408	e-mail: hedic@hedic.org

HOME HEALTH CARE ASSOCIATIONS

American Association for Homecare, www.aahomecare.org. Tel: (703) 836-6263.

American Federation of Homecare Providers, www.amerifed. net. Tel: (301) 588-1454.

National Association for Home Care, www.nahc.org. Tel: (202) 547-7424.

Visiting Nurses Association of America, see each state's VNA Website. Tel: (202) 737-3707.

INSURANCE/PAYOR ASSOCIATIONS

The following organizations offer conferences, seminars, white papers, and journal publications on selected topics that may be of interest to rehabilitation providers. Some of these groups also offer associate memberships.

Name/Address	Website
Alliance of American Insurers 3025 Highland Parkway, Suite 800 Downers Grove, IL 60515 Tel: (630) 724-2100	www.allianceai.org
American Association of Health Plans (AAHP), merger of Group Health Association of America (GHAA) and Managed Care and Review Assn (AMCRA) 1129 20th St., N.W. Washington, D.C. 20036 Tel: (877) 291-AAHP	www.aahp.org
American Association of Preferred Provider Associations 2300 Clarendon Blvd., Suite 611 Arlington, VA 22201-3367 Tel: (703) 351-5638	www.aappo.org
American Risk and Insurance Association (ARIA) 716 Providence Road Malvern, PA 19355 Tel: (610).640-1997	
Health Insurance Association of America (HIAA) 555 13th St., N.W. Washington, DC 20004 Tel: (202) 824-1600	www.ana.org
Insurance Institute of America 720 Providence Road P.O. Box 3016 Malvern, PA Tel: (610) 644-2100	www.aicpcu.org

Name/Address	Website
Insurance Rehabilitation Study Group (IRSG)	None
International Association of Accident Boards & Commissions (IAABC)	www.iaabc.com
National Association of Independent Insurance Adjusters (NAIIA) 300 W. Washington St. Chicago, IL 60606	www.naiia.com
National Association of Insurance Commissioners (NAIC) 2301 McGee, Suite 800 Kansas City, MO 64108-2604 Tel: (816) 842-3600	www.naiac.org
National Council on Compensation Insurance (NCCI) 750 Park of Commerce Drive Boca Raton, FL 33487 Tel: (561) 997-1000	www.ncci.com
Pam Pohly's Net Guide "Health Professional Associations, Academies and Organizations"	www.pohly.com/assoc2
Risk & Insurance Management Society (RIMS) 655 R Third Ave. New York, NY 10017-5367 Tel: (212) 286-9292	www.rims.org
Self Insurance Institute of America (SIAA) 12241 Newport Ave., Suite 100 Santa Ana, CA 92705 Tel: (714) 508-4920	www.siia.org
Workers Compensation Research Institute (WCRI) 955 Massachusetts Ave. Cambridge, MA 02139	www.wcrinet.org

PROVIDER PROFESSIONAL ASSOCIATIONS

Name/Address	Website
American Academy of Disability Evaluating Physicians	www.aadep.org
American Academy of Orthopedic Surgeons	www.aaos.org
American Academy of Physical Medicine & Rehabilitation One IBM Plaza Suite 2500 Chicago, IL 60611-3604 Tel: (312) 464-9700	www.aapmr.org
American Board of Chiropractic Consultants	www.accc-chiro.org
American Board of Independent Medical Examiners	www.abime.org
American College of Occupational & Environmental Medicine	www.acoem.org

Name/Address	Website
American Health Care Association 1201 L Street, N.W. Washington, D.C. 20005 Tel: (202) 842-4444	www.ahca.org
Association of Rehabilitation Facilities (formerly National Association of Rehabilitation Facilities (NARF)) P.O. Box 17675 Washington, D.C. 2004 1-0675 Tel: (703) 648-9300	www.naranet.org
American Health Quality Association 1140 Connecticut Ave., N.W. Washington, D.C. 2003 Tel: (202) 331-5790	www.ahqua.org
American Hospital Association (AHA) 325 Seventh St., N.W. Washington, D.C. 20004 Tel: (202) 638-1100	www.aha.org
American Medical Association (AMA) 515 North State St. Chicago, IL, 60610 Tel: (800) AMA-3211	www.ama-assn.org
American Medical Rehabilitation Provider Association 1606 20th St., N.W. 3rd Floor Washington, D.C. 20009 Tel: (202) 265-4404	www.amrpa.org
American Occupational Therapy Association (AOTA) 4720 Montgomery Lane P.O. Box 31220 Bethesda, MD 20824-1220 Tel: (301) 652-2682	www.aota.org
American Pain Society 4700 West Lake Ave. Glenview, IL 60025 Tel: (847) 375-4715	www.ampainsoc.org
American Physical Therapy Association (APTA) 1111 North Fairfax St. Alexandria, VA 22314-1488 Tel: (800) 999-APTA(2782)	www.apta.org
American Public Health Association(APHA) 800 I Street, N.W. Washington, D.C. 20001-3710 Tel: (202) 777-APHA (2742) Fax: (202) 777-2532	www.apha.org
American Rehabilitation Counseling Association (ARCA) 5999 Stevenson Ave. Alexandria, VA 22304 Tel: (800) 545-2223	www.counseling.org
Association of Rehabilitation Nurses (ARN) 4700 West Lake Ave. Glenview, IL 60025-7530 Tel: (800) 229-7530	www.rehabnurse.org

Name/Address	Website
American Subacute Care Association 1440 Kennedy Causeway, Suite 412 North Bay Village, FL 22141 Tel: (305) 864-0396 Fax: (305) 868-0905 e-mail: ascamail@aol.com	www.asca.org
Healthcare Billing & Management Association (HBMA) 1540 S. Coast Highway, Suite 203 Laguna Beach, CA Tel: (877) 640-HBMA	www.hbma.com

International Association of Rehabilitation
   Professionals (IARP), formerly National
   Association Rehabilitation Professionals
in the Private Sector (NARPPS)
783 Rio Delmar Blvd., Suite 61
Aptos, CA 95003
Tel: (800) 240-9059
	www.rehabpro.org

National Association of Disability Evaluating Professionals	www.nadep.com
National Association for Healthcare Quality (NAHQ) 4700 West Lake Ave. Glenview, IL 60025 Tel: (800) 966-9392 "Journal for Healthcare Quality"	www.nahq.org
National Association of Managed Care Physicians (NAMCP) 4435 Waterfront Dr., Suite 101 P.O. Box 4765 Glen Allen, VA 23058 Tel: (804) 527-1905	www.namcp.com
National Council on Rehabilitation Education (NCRE) 2011 Eye St., N.W., Suite 300 Washington, D.C., 20052 Tel: (202) 973-1550	www.rehabeducators. com
National Rehabilitation Counseling Association (NRCA) 8807 Sudley Road, Suite 102 Manassas, VA 2210-4719 Tel: (703) 361-2077	www.nrca-net.org

National Rehabilitation Association
   Of Job Placement and Development
   (NRAJPD)
633 South Washington St.
Alexandria, VA 22314
Tel: (703) 836-0850
	www.nationalrehab.org

National Rehabilitation Association (NRA) 6335 Washington St. Alexandria, VA 22314 Tel: (703) 836-0850	www.nationalrehab.org
National Subacute Care Association (NSCA) 655 15th St., N.W. Suite 210 Washington, D.C. 20005	www.nsca.net
Vocational Evaluation and Work Adjustment Association (VEWAA) 202 E. Cheyenne Mountain Blvd. Suite N Colorado Springs, CO 80906 Tel: (719) 527-1801	www.vewaa.org

APPENDIX F

Coalitions and Consulting Companies

BUSINESS COALITIONS AND ALLIANCES

Employer health care alliances, business coalitions, and purchasing groups represent potential customers for rehabilitation providers who offer prevention/wellness, treatment, provider network, and post-treatment consultation services that focus on disability management.

Name/Address	Website
Buyers' Health Care Action Group 3639 Elmo Road Minnetonka, MN 55305 Tel: (612) 854-7066	www.bhcag.com
Colorado Health Care Purchasing Alliance 3033 E. First Ave., Suite 810 Denver, CO 80206 Tel: (303) 333-6767	www.coloradohealthonline.com
Employer Health Care Innovation Project 1350 I. St., N.W., Suite 870 Washington, D.C. 20005 Tel: (202) 638-0551	www.capalliance.com
National Business Coalition on Health 18th St. N.W., Suite 450 Washington, D.C. 20036 Tel: (202) 775-9300 ● Represents more than 100 business coalitions ● More than 34 million employees & family covered	www.nbch.org
National Coalition on Health Care 1200 6th St., N.W., Suite 750 Washington, D.C. 20005 Tel: (202) 638-7151	www.nchc.org
Pacific Business Group on Health 33 New Montgomery St., Suite 1450 San Francisco, CA 94105 Tel: (415) 281-8660	www.pbgh.org
Washington Business Group on Health (WBGH) 50 F St., N.W., Suite 600 Washington, D.C. 20001 Tel (202) 628-9320	www.wbgh.org

Note: This represents a partial listing of business coalitions in the U.S. For a comprehensive directory, refer to Faulkner & Gray Health Care Pub., NY: NY.

PROFESSIONAL SERVICES CONSULTING COMPANIES

The following companies routinely survey employer health care costs, needs, and programs. A number of them publish annual employer health care trend and cost surveys, (e.g., Wyatt Watson Worldwide, KPMG Peat Marwick) that are especially useful to provider organizations for strategic planning and marketing purposes. Samples are listed below selected company names.

Name/Address	Website
Arthur Andersen	www.arthureandersen.com
Deloitte & Touche	www.deloitte.com
Ernst & Young	www.ey.com
KPMG Peat Marwick	www.kpmg.consulting.com
McKinsey Company	www.mckinsey.com
Milliman & Robertson "Research Report: Provider Reimbursement" "A Comparative Analysis of Claims-based Methods of Health Risk Assessment" "Provider Incentives in the Optimally Managed Delivery System"	www.milliman.com
Price Waterhouse Coopers Lybrand "Health Cost Tactics: A Blueprint for the Future" "Health Management: A Survey of Company-Sponsored Wellness Programs"	www.pwcglobal.com
Towers Perrin "The Changing Face of Healthcare: Balancing Employer and Employee Needs" "Towers Perrin 2003 Health Care Cost Survey"	www.towers.com
US Mercer/Foster Higgins "National Survey of Employer Sponsored Health Plans" "State-of-the-Art in Long-Term Care Insurance"	www.mercerhr.com
Watson Wyatt Worldwide "Employer Health Costs Worse than Budgeted in 2002"	www.watsonwyatt.com

Managed Care Models and Structures

Accountable health plan	An organization that combines health insurance services with actual delivery of care
Exclusive provider organization (EP)	A model similar to a PPO in which enrollees use network providers for specialty services
Group model HMO	An HMO that contracts with an independent group practice for the delivery of services
Health insurance purchasing cooperative (HIPC)	A not-for-profit organization that has a selection of accountable health plans (AHPs) it offers to its enrollees
Hybrid HMO	Any combination of the aforementioned models
IPA HMO mode	An HMO that contracts predominantly with independent providers, but not to the exclusion of provider associations and multi-specialty group practices
Independent	An association of providers typically of similar profession, discipline, provider, or specialty that align in order to gain critical mass, association (IPA) market distribution, contract negotiation leverage, and intensified marketing efforts
Point of service (POS)	An indemnity managed care structure that allows beneficiaries to use a preferred panel of providers, but also allows out-of-network provider selection, however, at greater financial risk (e.g., co-pays, higher deductibles). Provider reimbursement is typically fee-for-service (FFS). This model is also known as an open-ended HMO.
Preferred provider organization (PPO)	A benefits structure that uses a collection of providers who have agreed to financial arrangements (e.g., fee-for-service) to offer services to health plan members, PPOs are the dominant model under workers' compensation
Network model HMO	An HMO that predominantly contracts with two or more independent provider groups and solo practitioners when geographic coverage or specialized services are required
Staff model HMO	An HMO that employs providers to deliver services

Useful Links and Additional Information

INTERNET: HEALTH CARE LINKS

Name/Address	Website
Achoo Internet Health Care	http://www.achoo.com
American Cancer Society	http://www.cancer.org
American College of Healthcare Executives	http://www.ache.org
America's Health Network	http://www.ahn.com
American Heart Association	http://www.americanheart.org
American Lung Association	http://www.lungusa.org
American Medical Association	http://www.ama-assn.org
American Medical Informatics Association	http://www.amia.org
APTA (American Physical Therapy Association)	http:///www.apta.org
"Hooked on Evidence" Caresoft Inc.	http://www.caresoft.com
Doctors' Guide	http://www.docguide.com
EINet Galaxy, Medicine	http://galaxy.einet.net
Food and Nutrition Information Center	http://www.nalusda.gov/fric/
Hardin Meta Directory of Health Resources	http://www.arcade.uiowa.edu
Health AtoZ	http://www.healthatoz.com
Healthcare Information & Management Systems Society (HIMSS)	http://www.himss.org
Healthcare Information Systems Directory	http://www.health-infosys-dir.com
Healthcare Open Systems & Trails	http://www.hostnet.org
Healthfinder (Department Of Health and Human Services)	http://www.healthfinder.gov
Health Information Resources	http://www.nnlm.nlm.nih.gov
Health Sciences Professional	http://www.lib.uwaterloo.ca
Healthtouch: Online for Better Health	http://www.healthtouch.com/
Hospital Web	http://www.neuro-www.mgh.harvard.edu
Intelihealth-John Hopkins Health Information	http://www.intelihealth.com
Mayo Health Oasis	http://www.mayohealth.org
MD Consult LLC.	http://www.mdconsult.com
Medical Matrix	http://www.medmatrix.org
MedicineNet	http://medicinenet.com/
MedLine Plus-National Library of Medicine	http://medlineplus.nlm.nih.gov/
Medical Network Inc.	http://www.medconnect.com
Medscape	http://www.medscape.com
Medweb: Telemedicine Merck's Health Infopark	http://merck.com/disease/
New England Journal of Medicine	http://nejm.org
Onhealth	http://www.onhealth.com/onhealth

Name/Address	Website
The Virtual Hospital	http://www.vh.radiology.uiowa.edu
The Visible Human Project	http://www.nlm.nih.gov/research/visible/visible_human.html
Virtual Medical center	http://www.mediconsult.com
Well-Connected Patient Education Reports	http://www.healthgate.com
WWW Virtual Library: Medicine	http://www.ohsu.edu/clinweb
NOAH.New York Access To Health	http://www.noah.cuny.edu

Disclaimer: The authenticity and accuracy of data contained on these sites have not been established. Readers should exercise caution when accessing sites and using data and refer to Chapter 15 for advice about how to screen Websites.

ADDITIONAL SOURCES OF DATA AND INFORMATION

Name/Address	Website
American Bar Association (ABA) 740 15th St., N.W. Washington, D.C. 20005-1022	www.abanet.org/disability
Americans with Disabilities Act ADA home page	www.usdoj.gov
● ADA Document Center	www.janweb.icdi.wvu.edu
● ADA Information Center	www.access.gpo.gov
American Medical Information, Inc. 5711 S. 86th Circle P.O. Box 27347 Omaha, NE 68127-0347 Tel: (402) 596-7570 Fax: (402) 331-8177	www.salesleadsUSA.com
The Bureau of National Affairs (BNA) 1231 25th St., N.W. Washington, D.C. 20037 Tel: (202) 452-4200 "State Health Care Regulatory Developments"	www.bna.com
Center for Consumer Healthcare Information P.O. Box 16067 Irvine, CA 92713 Tel: (714) 752-2335 Fax: (714) 752-8433	
Dictionary of Occupational Titles	www.wave.net/upg/immigration/dot_index
Disability Evaluation Study Disabled Sports U.S.A. 451 Hungerford Dr., Suite 100 Rockville, MD 20850 Tel: (301) 217-9840	www.ssa.gov/statistics/des

Name/Address	Website
ErgoWeb evaluation exchange	www.ergoweb.com
Job Accommodation Network	www.Janweb.icdi.wvu.edu
Harvard Conference on American Health Care	www.hsph.harvard.edu
Harvard School of Public Health	
12 State St.	
Boston, MA 02109	
Hospital Blue Book	
2100 Powers Ferry Rd.	
Atlanta, GA 30339-9909	
Tel: (404) 955-5656	
Fax: (404) 952-0669	
Managed Care Information Center (MCIC)	www.themcic.com
1913 Atlantic Ave., Suite F4	
Manasquan, NJ 08736	
Tel: (732) 292-1100	
Musculoskeletal Disorders (MSDS) and Workplace Factors	www.cdc.gov/niosh/ergosci1.html
National Health Information, LLC	www.nhionline.net
P.O. Box 15429	
Atlanta, GA 30333	
Tel: (800) 597-6300	
Fax: (404) 607-0095	
National Managed Care Congress	www.nmhcc.org
Tel: (888) 882-2500	
National Rehabilitation Information Center (NARIC)	www.naric.com
1010 Wayne Ave., Suite 800	
Silver Spring, MD 20910	
Tel: (800) 346-2742	
Fax: (301) 562-2401	
World Health Organization	www.who.int

CASE MANAGEMENT/DISABILITY MANAGEMENT CERTIFICATIONS

- Certified case manager (CCM)
- Certified disability evaluator (CDE)
- Certified disability management specialist (previously certified insurance rehabilitation specialist or [CIRS])
- Certified registered rehabilitation nurse (CRRN)
- Certified rehabilitation counselor (CRC)
- Certified vocational counselor (CVE)
- Licensed professional counselor (LPC)
- National certified counselor (NCC)

LEGAL AND REGULATORY DATA SEARCHES

Name/Address	Website
American Bar Association (ABA) Commission on Mental & Physical Disability Law	www.abanet.org/disability/home.html
American Law Source On-Line	www.lawsource.com
American Law Sources	www.lawsource.com
Code of Federal Regulations	www.access.gpo.gov
EmedicoLegal	www.emedicolegal.com
Law.com	www.law.com

Name/Address	Website
Legal Information Institute	www.law.cornell.edu
Lexis, Mead Data Central	
9393 Springboro Pike	
Dayton, OH 45401	
Westlaw, West Publishing Co.	
50 W. Kellogg Blvd.	
St. Paul, MN 55164	
Heinonline	www.heinonline.org
State Health Watch	www.statehealthwatch.com
Bureau of National Affairs	www.bna.com
Workers Compensation Law Materials	www.law.cornlell.edu

ASSISTIVE AND ADAPTIVE TECHNOLOGY RESOURCES

ABLEDATA　　　　**www.ABLEDATA.com**

Database with information on more than 29,000 assistive technology products, including descriptions, pricing, and vendor/company data pertaining to each product.

The Alliance for Technology Access (ATA)　　　**www.ataccess.org**

A network of community-based resource centers, developers, and vendors. Serves as a resource center for persons with disabilities through a consumer-directed model.

disAbility　　　　**www.disability.gov**

A government-based Website managed by the Presidential Task Force on Employment of Adults with Disabilities. Provides an employers section for the purpose of recruiting and hiring of persons with disabilities. This Webpage is linked to other well-known employment Websites (e.g., Brassring.com, Monster.com).
Provides information about low-cost accommodations that facilitate gainful employment.

JAN (Job Accommodation Network)　　**www.jan.wvu.edu**

JAN has teams of consultants available to assist employers and individuals with job accommodations. These teams include experts in the following areas: motor/mobility, psychiatric/cognitive, sensory, and small business and self-employment.

RESNA (Rehabilitation Engineering & Assistive Technology Society of North America)　　　**www.resna.org**

RESNA is an interdisciplinary association chartered for the advancement of rehabilitation and assistive technology. RESNA is located in Arlington, Va.

WebAble　　　　**www.webable.com**

Website for disability-related Internet resources and information. Maintains a library of books, white papers, plans, standards and guidelines, and journals focusing on accessibility and assistive and adaptive technology for persons with disabilities.

APPENDIX I

Fact Sheets

The following Fact Sheets are included as reference material that may prove invaluable resources for rehabilitation professionals. The organizations, entities, and initiatives that are covered represent some of the most potent agents of change in today's disability prevention and management sector. This listing is not all-inclusive, but does represent a broad sampling of activities.

JOINT COMMISSION ON ACCREDITATION OF HEALTH CARE ORGANIZATIONS

Who/What?   JCAHO originally was created by the American College of Physicians to accredit hospitals (JCAH). As health care delivery systems evolved, it became clear that accreditation had to expand beyond hospitals—hence, JCAHO. JCAHO's self-policing policy traditionally focused on prose and structure, and only in the past decade has it emphasized outcomes as well. **JCAHO's mission:** *To continuously improve the safety and quality of care provided to the public through the provision of health care accreditation and related services that support performance improvement in health care organizations.*

When?   JCAHO has required quality assurance programs since 1983. In 1987 the Joint Commission announced "The Agenda for Change," which outlined a series of major steps designed to modernize the accreditation process through the ORYX initiative.

How?   JCAHO has codified its standards in an accreditation manual for hospitals and health care organizations. JCAHO's approach now stresses the importance of outcomes and the integration of clinical *and* financial data sets. JCAHO develops clinical quality indicators through expert panels and beta site testing. JCAHO supports the use of electronic data exchange for comparison purposes. The ORYX (2002) permitted rigorous comparison of actual results of care across institutions. JCAHO accredits more than 16,000 health care organizations throughout the United States.

Where?   http://www.jcaho.org

THE FOUNDATION FOR ACCOUNTABILITY (FACCT)

Who or what?   FACCT is a not-for-profit organization dedicated to helping Americans make better health care decisions. It is a collaboration of consumers and purchasers representing 80 million persons. It is organized as a forum in which parties work toward a quality-focused health care system.

When?   FACCT was formed in 1995 and established offices in 1996.

How?   FACCT publishes an accountability resource series, *Prototype Guidebook for Performance Measurement*, and consumer satisfaction sets. It also conducts seminars/symposiums on quality-related topics.

Where?   Offices in Portland, OR; Website: http://www.facct.org/htm.

Vision?   **Consumers**
1. Appreciate the value of quality in health care.
2. Make decisions based on clear, reliable quality data.
3. Provide direction to the health care system about important consumer needs and expectations.
4. Balance personal and societal needs in health care decision making.

Purchasers
1. Hold the health care system accountable for quality and value.
2. Provide data and support for quality-based decisions.
3. Provide real choices for employees and beneficiaries.
4. Create health-focused partnerships with beneficiaries, providers, and the community at large.

Providers and plans
1. Understand what consumers want.
2. Monitor and improve performance in the areas that matter most to consumers.
3. Mobilize consumers as partners in their health care.
4. Compete on quality as well as price.

Data from: http://www.facct.org/about/vision.html, accessed July 15, 2000.

NATIONAL COMMITTEE FOR QUALITY ASSURANCE (NCQA)

Who or What? NCQA is a non-profit external accreditation organization for managed care organizations (MCOs). NCQA's accreditation is voluntary and its "Quality Compass 1999" database contains data on more than 50 quality measures, 250 organizations, and 410 HMOs and POS plans covering nearly 70 million people.

When? NCQA's accreditation program was launched in 1991.

How? NCQA assessment areas include the following:

- Quality improvement
- Member responsibilities and rights
- Utilization management
- Preventive services
- Medical record keeping

NCQA's Committee on Performance Measurement developed the Health Plan Employer Data and Information Set, or HEDIS 3.0. NCQA also released the report *State of Managed Care Quality*, which used comparative data from 329 MCOs and 37 million individuals.

Employers routinely use NCQA data in their MCO selection/retention process, and NCQA encourages MCOs to use it in their marketing and recruitment as well.

Mission/vision? *To provide information that enables purchasers and consumers of managed health care to distinguish among plans based on quality, thereby allowing them to make more informed health care purchasing decisions.*

Where? NCQA, 2000 L St. N.W., Washington, DC; Website: http://www.ncqa.org/htm.

HEALTH PLAN EMPLOYER DATA AND INFORMATION SET (HEDIS)

Who or What? HEDIS is a set of 50 performance measures used to evaluate and compare health plans. HEDIS was developed and refined by NCQA. HEDIS was developed through the input of more than 1700 organizations, including health plans, public and private purchasers, and consumer groups. HEDIS is currently considered the "gold standard" for health plan performance measures. As such, it enjoys widespread use and support.

When? NCQA released HEDIS 2.0 in 1993, and it released HEDIS 3.0 along with Medicaid HEDIS in 1996.

How? HEDIS measures address performance in the following eight key areas:

1. Effectiveness of care
2. Access and availability of care
3. Satisfaction with care
4. Health plan financial stability
5. Use of services
6. Cost of care
7. Informed health care choices
8. Health plan descriptive data

The latest version of HEDIS addresses women's health issues and chronic care.

HEDIS produces "patient-centered report cards" and covers cost control, value purchasing, accountability, and standard reporting mechanisms.

Mission/vision? Same as NCQA's.

Where? NCQA , 2000 L St. N.W., Washington, DC; Website: http://www.ncqa.org/pages/hedis/htm.

COMMISSION ON ACCREDITATION OF REHABILITATION FACILITIES (CARF)

Who or What? CARF is a private not-for-profit organization dedicated to fostering improvement in the following two key areas:

1. Organizational management
2. Service delivery

CARF accredits a variety of entities including:

- Adult daycare services
- Assisted living
- Behavioral health
- Employment and community services
- Medical rehabilitation

When? CARF was formed in 1966 through the merger of two national organizations: the Association of Rehabilitation Centers (ARC) and the National Association of Sheltered Workshops and Homebound Programs (NASWWHP).

In 1970, the Council of State Administrators of Vocational rehabilitation adopted a resolution urging state agencies to require CARF accreditation. This proved to be the seminal point in CARF's brief history. By 1973 CARF had published program evaluation standards, *Standards Manual for Rehabilitation Facilities*.

How? CARF develops standards in collaboration with providers, consumers, and purchasers through a peer review process. Standards are reviewed/revised annually. CARF publishes a number of documents including *How to Choose a Provider Guide, Accreditation Sourcebook, The Persons Served: Ethical Perspectives on CARF's Accreditation Standards & Guidelines*.

Vision/mission? *To improve the quality of care provided to the public through an accreditation process that promotes continuous improvement in organization performance. To serve as the preeminent standards and accrediting body promoting and advocating for the delivery of quality rehabilitation services.*

Where? CARF, 4891 E. Grant Rd., Tucson, AZ 85712; Website: http://www.carf.org/htm.

UTILIZATION REVIEW & ACCREDITATION COMMISSION (URAC)

Who or What? URAC, also known as the American Healthcare Commission, is a non-profit charitable organization. URAC's membership comprises diverse constituents, including employers, consumers, regulators, health care providers, and workers' compensation and managed care industries. URAC offers at least 10 different voluntary accreditations, to include:

- Case management organization standards
- Credential verification organization (CVO) standards
- Health call center standards
- Health network standards
- Health utilization management standards
- Health provider credentialing standards
- Workers' compensation network standards
- Workers' compensation utilization managment standards
- External review standards

When? URAC was created in 1990 and has issued more than 1600 accreditation certificates to more than 300 organizations.

How? URAC uses a "modular approach to accreditation in recognition of the diversity of healthcare delivery networks and organizations that exist today. Accreditation generally involves the following three-step process: submission of required documentation, an onsite visit by URAC staff, and final application review conducted by an executive committee and accreditation committee.

Where? URAC, 1275 K St. N.W., Washington, D.C.; Tel: (202) 216-9010; Website: http://www.urac.org

NATIONAL COUNCIL ON COMPENSATION INSURANCE (NCCI)

Who? NCCI is a nationally recognized workers' compensation insurance information services company.

When? NCCI was established in 1922.

How? NCCI offers insurers a single point of data collection, analysis, and management that supports the delivery of advisory/rating services, production of experience modifications, and evaluation of proposed legislative initiatives. NCCI boasts the nation's largest workers' compensation database, which contains hundreds of millions of data records used by actuaries, analysts, researchers, technicians, policy makers, and others. NCCI publishes the *Basic Manual for Workers' Compensation and Employers Liability Insurance*. This text contains the rules and procedures that insurers use when writing workers' compensation insurance. NCCI reports data to the International Association of Industrial Accident Boards and Commissions (IAIABC).

Where? National Council on Compensation Insurance (NCCI), 750 Park of Commerce Drive, Boca Raton, FL 33487, Tel: (561) 997-1000; Website: http://www.ncci.com

WORKERS' COMPENSATION RESEARCH INSTITUTE (WCRI)

Who? The Workers' Compensation Research Institute (WCRI) is a nationally recognized independent not-for-profit research organization that studies workers' compensation issues. WCRI provides unbiased data regarding how workers' compensation (WC) systems perform and compare to each other. WCRI analyzes cost drivers and legislative changes and discusses alternative solutions to vexing problems. WCRI constituents include WC administrators, industry groups, provider organizations, and policy makers.

When? WCRI was organized in 1983.

How? WCRI disseminates information through a number of publications available to both members and non-members. A full range of reports (more than 110) are listed in an online alphabetized directory. These include: *WCRI Research Report, WCRI Video Briefs,* and *WCRI Research Briefs.*
WCRI Research Briefs are published 10 to 12 times a year.

Where? Workers' Compensation Research Institute, 955 Massachusetts Ave., Cambridge, MA, 02139; Tel: (617) 661-WCRI; Website: http://www.wcri.org

NATIONAL CLEARINGHOUSE OF REHABILITATION TRAINING MATERIALS (NCRTM)

Who? NCRTM is funded by a grant from the Rehabilitation Services Administration (RSA).

What? NCRTM locates, collects, and distributes a variety of training materials, reference materials, and research services. The *NCRTM Quarterly* is a free publication available to assist users in staying abreast of current rehabilitation training materials. Free reference and research services are available for use by rehabilitation professionals, educators, researchers, and providers.

Where? Tel: (800) 223-5219 or (405) 624-76650; Website: http://www.ncrtm@okstate.edu

NATIONAL INSTITUTE FOR SAFETY & HEALTH (NIOSH)

Who? NIOSH is the federal agency responsible for conducting research and providing recommendations for the prevention of work-related disease and injury. NIOSH is a component of the Centers for Disease Control & Prevention (CDC). NIOSH comprises a diverse collection of disciplines including industrial hygienists, nurses, physicians, engineers, biostatisticians, and others.

What? NIOSH investigates potentially hazardous working conditions when requested by employees or employers. Recommendations and training are offered following onsite investigations. A National Occupational Research Agenda (NORA) is a tool that provides a framework to NIOSH and the occupational safety and health community at large. Approximately 500 organizations and individuals external to NIOSH provided input into the development of NORA. A consensus of top priorities resulted.

How? NIOSH's mission is *delivering on the nation's promise: safety and health at work for all people through research and prevention.*

- Specific NIOSH responsibilities include the following:
- Enumerate hazards present in the workplace
- Identify the causes of work-related diseases and injuries
- Evaluate the hazards of new technologies and work practices
- Create ways to control hazards
- Train safety and health professionals
- Recommend occupational safety and health standards

When? NIOSH was established by the Occupational Safety & Health Act of 1970, which is the same act that led to OSHA or the Occupational Safety & Health Administration. These two agencies are distinct, but they share priorities working in collaboration.

Where? NIOSH is headquartered in Washington, D.C., with regional offices in Atlanta, Ga., Cincinnati, Ohio., Morgantown, W. Va., Bruceton, Penn., and Spokane, Wash.; Website: http://www.cdc.gov/niosh

OCCUPATIONAL SAFETY & HEALTH ADMINISTRATION (OSHA)

Who? OSHA is a federal agency housed within the U.S. Department of Labor (DOL). OSHA has responsibility for more than 100 million American workers' job site health and safety.

What? The mission of OSHA is to save lives, prevent injuries, and protect the health of workers through a combination of rules/regulations, investigations, citations, research, training, and education. Virtually every American worker falls under OSHA's jurisdiction, which extends throughout 200 offices nationwide. OSHA cites employers with poor safety and health records, but also offers them technical assistance. The prevention of cumulative trauma disorders has been a priority of OSHA's during the past decade or so. An attempt to promulgate national ergonomic standards failed; however, many employers have been cited under the "General Duty Clause" of OSHA. This clause is used whenever there is no specific rule or regulation as in air quality.

Where? OSHA is headquartered in Washington, D.C., with 200 offices nationwide; Website: http://www.osha.gov

OCCUPATIONAL INFORMATION NETWORK—O*NET

Who? O*NET is a comprehensive database of worker attributes and job characteristics. O*NET replaces the Dictionary of Occupational Titles. The database contains information about knowledge, skills, abilities (KSAs), interests, general work activities (GWAs) and work context for thousands of jobs. The O*NET project is sponsored by the U.S. Department of Labor's Employment and Training Administration.

How? O*NET uses a common language that transcends all job classifications across the economy. O*NET objectives include the following:

- Create occupational clusters based on KSA information
- Develop job descriptions
- Facilitate employee training
- Identify criteria to guide vocational selection and placement decisions
- Create skills-match profiles
- Target recruitment efforts to maximize person-job-organizational fit
- Improve vocational and career counseling efforts
- O*NET uses a "content model" comprising the following six major domains: worker characteristics, worker requirements, experience requirements, occupational requirements, occupational characteristics, and occupation-specific information.

Where? http://www.onetcenter.org

NATIONAL LIBRARY OF MEDICINE (NLM)

Who?
The NLM contains a vast array of data useful to rehabilitation professionals. Perhaps best known to health care providers are NLM's MEDLINE and Index Medicus databases. Index Medicus indexes articles in more than 2800 journals in medicine and related areas. MEDLINE is this index's online equivalent with more than 3700 journals represented.

How?
LOCATOR*plus* is NLM's online catalog that can be accessed via the Internet at http://www.locatorplus.gov. LOCATOR*plus* is one component of NJM's integrated library system. This database is continuously updated and contains catalog records for books, audiovisuals, journals, computer files, and other materials found in the Library's collection.

LOCATOR*plus* allows searching by keyword, title, journal title, author, MeSH (medical subject headings), call numbers, and a combination of other search menus.

Where?
Reference & Customer Services, National Library of Medicine (NLM), 8600 Rockville Pike, Bethesda, MD, Tel: (888)FINDNLM; Website: http://www.nlm.nih.gov/pubs

AGENCY FOR HEALTHCARE RESEARCH & QUALITY (AHRQ)

Who?
AHRQ (formerly known as Agency for Healthcare Policy & Research, or AHCPR) falls within the U.S. Department of Health & Human Services (USDHHS, or HHS). This is the federal agency charged with enhancing the quality of health care through evidence-based medicine, outcomes and effectiveness studies, technology assessment, preventive services, and clinical practice guidelines. AHRQ houses the National Guideline Clearinghouse (www.guideline.gov). The National Quality Measures Clearinghouse is an online database of health care quality measures. AHRQ is responsible for a number of health care surveys, including the Medical Expenditure Panel Survey (MEPOS) and the Healthcare Cost & Utilization Project (HCUP).

How?
AHRC, through the National Quality Measures Clearinghouse, defines a quality measure according to the Institute of Medicine's definition: *the degree to which health care services for individuals and populations increase the likelihood of desired health outcomes and are consistent with current professional knowledge* (Lohr 1990).

AHRC's quality measures are used for quality improvement within an institution (internal quality improvement), or across systems of care and institutions (external quality improvement). AHRC's National Guideline Clearinghouse's mission is *to provide physicians, nurses, and other health professionals, health care providers, health plans, integrated delivery systems, purchasers and others an accessible mechanism for obtaining objective, detailed information on clinical practice guidelines and to further their dissemination, implementation, and use.*

NGC provides an annotated bibliographic database from which users can search and retrieve citations for publications and resources concerning guideline development, methodology, structure, evaluation, and implementation. Users can browse by condition or diagnosis and treatment or intervention. Structured abstracts (summaries) about the guidelines and their development as well as links to full-text documents are available through NGC.

Where?
Agency for Healthcare Research and Quality (AHRQ), 540 Gaither Road, Rockville, MD 20850, Tele: (301) 427-1364; Website: http://www.ahcpr.gov

Reference: Lohr KN (ed): Medicare: A Strategy for Quality Assurance/Committee to Design a Strategy for Quality Review and Assurance in Medicare, Division of Health Care Services, Institute of Medicine, volume 1, Report of a study. Washington, DC, National Academy Press, May 1990, p 468.

Glossary and Abbreviations

INSURANCE TERMS

Adverse selection
The opposite of favorable selection or a situation in which an insured person or insured pool consume more benefits than are projected by insurance company actuaries

All-payer system
A uniform or set price that all purchasers of health care services by regulation must pay

Allocated loss expense
Carrier expenses that can be directly tied to a particular claim

Business coalitions/ alliances
Groups of employers that are aligned in order to achieve the necessary critical mass and resources to purchase disability prevention and management products and services

Capitation
A fixed payment mechanism that defines a specific period of time, and a fixed per capita payment level (e.g., per-person-per–month, or PMPM)

Captive insurance company
An insurance company owned and operated by the corporation(s) to which it provides insurance coverage

Claim lag
The time that elapses between an incurred injury or claim and its submission to the insurer for payment

Closed claim
A claim in which all benefits have been honored or paid; it may or may not still involve disability

Case management
Either an internal (within the provider organization) or external process (insurer, health plan, utilization review organization, or case management firm) whereby health care delivery efficiency and effectiveness are fostered by resource allocation

Co-insurance or cost sharing
The portion of health care cost that the patient or beneficiary is expected to pay (e.g., 20% co-pay); co-pays can vary when in-network versus out-of-network providers are selected

Company reserves
A specific pool of money that must be set aside by self-funded or self-insured employers for projected costs associated with an injury/ illness; typically includes direct medical and indemnity costs

Community rating
A method used to determine insurance premium levels and spreading risk among an established group of insured individuals

Controverted claim
A claim in which there is conflict over the compensability on work-relatedness and involves a dispute over disability and compensability

Cost shifting
The act of shifting costs from one insurance plan to another in order for providers to maximize their reimbursement or for beneficiaries to reduce cost sharing

Diagnostic related groups (DRGs)
A system of classifying treatments by diagnosis and other variables (e.g., age, sex, complications, co-morbidities) in relation to the relative costs or resource use

Distal causal factors
Those factors or circumstances that did not directly set in motion an accident; distal causes usually do not occur in the same time frame as the accident itself

Employer contribution
The employer's financial obligation toward premium costs

Evidence of insurability
Statement of proof that a beneficiary's condition is a covered item

Exclusions
Exclusions are those items not covered under an insurance or health plan; exclusions may include provider types, treatment settings, specific interventions, or diagnoses and conditions

Experience rating
A method used by actuaries to determine the premium amount for a particular insured group based on their use of resources and loss history

Indemnity
An insurance program that covers expenses for insured persons, typically, medical and lost wages

Integrated benefits
The combined administration of insurance or employee benefits programs designed to control costs while assuring quality clinical outcomes, for example workers' compensation and group health or group health (general health) and disability insurance

Length of stay (LOS)
A measurement of resource use typically expressed as days or units of treatment

Loss ratio
The ratio between premium collected and payouts/losses

Maximum benefit
The maximum amount, in dollars or time, during which an individual's claim is covered (e.g., $10,000 personal injury protection limit, or PIP)

Participating provider
A provider who is contracted with a health plan or insurer to provide medical services in exchange for specific payment schedules

Permanent partial disability (PPD)
A condition that results in permanent disability, but partial recovery is expected, enabling return-to-gainful employment in some capacity

Permanent partial scheduled
A permanent partial injury with a specific period of time that a claimant can collect benefits under compensation law

Permanent partial non-scheduled
A permanent partial injury not designated under a payment schedule, benefit period may be limited or lifetime depending upon compensation law

Physician or Provider contingency (PCR) or withhold	The "at-risk" portion of an insurance reserve claim that is deducted or withheld by the health plan before payment is made to the provider based upon their utilization rates as compared to a database
Point of service plan, or POS	A hybrid of a prepaid and indemnity plan wherein patients may select in-network or out-of-network providers subject to co-payment differentials
Preexisting conditions	An illness or injury that pre-dates the period of insurance coverage
Prepaid health plans (PHP)	Health plans that offer specific benefits in exchange for set premium payments
Prospective payment system (PPS)	A Medicare system of diagnosis related groups or DRGs in which hospitals receive payments driven by resource usage
Proximate cause	The cause(s) that directly set in motion an uninterrupted chain of events leading to an accident
Reinsurance	Reinsurance is coverage of losses above the stipulated primary coverage amount. Reinsurance companies typically underwrite this excess or "stop loss" amount, reinsurance is bought from a reinsurer by another insurance company, provider organization, or a self-funded employer
Resource-base relative scale (RBRVS)	A classification system that reimburses providers depending on the education, training, and skill associated with specific treatment interventions
Risk management	The process of identifying and controlling elements of a business enterprise in order to prevent or minimize the effects of accidental losses or injuries
Self-funding or self-insurance	A health plan in which employers do not pay insurance premiums to an insurer, but instead, pay as losses are incurred, typically company reserves are required to be set aside to cover projected costs on a case by case basis
Single payer system	A one-payer system such as Medicare or a state-based or monopolistic workers' compensation system
Small group pools	A system that allows small businesses to join a larger group in order to share risk and negotiate better insurance premiums
Subrogation	The right of an insurance company to recover partial or full financial losses from a third party through other coverages
Temporary partial disability (TPD)	A condition that results in partial loss of earning capacity, but from which a full recovery is expected
Third party administrator (TPA)	An entity that administers insurance claims on behalf of another entity (e.g., self-funded or insured employer)
Third party payer	A private or public entity that insures or pays for health expenses incurred by an insured group, the patient is the first party, the employer or organization is the second party, and the payer the third party under these arrangements
Total vocational rehabilitation costs	Sum of the evaluation expense, job placement, indemnity benefits, and educational expenses
Vocational rehabilitation evaluation expenses	All expenses that are incurred during the testing and evaluation of a claimant's knowledge, aptitude, and ability when attempting to determine employment suitability
Vocational rehabilitation educational expenses	All costs associated with vocational training, including: tuition, books, living expenses, and travel
Vocational rehabilitation incurred expenses	Temporary disability indemnity payments that are incurred during a beneficiary's participation in a vocational training/education program

COMMONLY USED ACRONYMS AND ABBREVIATIONS

AAAHC	Accreditation Association for Ambulatory Health Centers
AAHC	American Accreditation Healthcare Commission
AAHP	American Association of Health Plans
AARP	American Association of Retired Persons
ADA	Americans with Disabilities Act of 1990
AEP	Associate Ergonomics Professional
AFDC	Aide to Families with Dependent Children
AGS	American Geriatrics Society
AH	alternative health
AHA	American Hospital Association
AHCA	American Health Care Association
AHCPR	Agency for Health Care Policy & Research
AHFP	Associate Human Factor Professional
AHP	accountable health plan
AHRQ	Agency for Healthcare Research & Quality
ALC	assisted living center
AMA	American Medical Association
AMRPA	American Medical Rehabilitation Providers Association
ANSI	American National Standards Institute
AOA	Agency on Aging
AOTA	American Occupational Therapy Association
APGs	ambulatory payment groups
APHA	American Public Health Association
APTA	American Physical Therapy Association
ARM	Associate in Risk Management
ARN	Association of Rehabilitation Nurses
ASCA	American Subacute Care Association
ASHRM	American Society for Healthcare Risk Management
AWP	any willing provider laws
BBA	Balanced Budget Act of 1997
BNA	Bureau of National Affairs
CAM	Complementary and alternative medicine
CAP	Computer Accommodation Program
CARF	Commission for the Accreditation of Rehabilitation Facilities
CBO	Congressional Budget Office
CCD	Consortium for Citizens with Disabilities
CCM	Certified Case Manager
CCMC	Commission for Case Management Certification
CD	consumer directed (also [CDC], consumer-directed care)
CDC	Centers for Disease Control
CDE	Certified Disability Evaluator
CDMS	Certified Disability Management Specialist
CDS	clinical decision support
CEA	Certified Ergonomics Associate
CHAMPUS	Civilian Health & Medicaid Program of the Uniformed Services
CHFP	Certified Human Factors Professional

CHIP	Childrens Health Insurance Program
CIQ	Community Integrated Questionnaire
CITA	Center for Information Technology Accommodation
CLCP	Certified Life Care Planner
CM	case management
CMN	Certificate of Medical Necessity
CMS	Centers for Medicare & Medicaid
COBRA	Consolidated Omnibus Budget Reconciliation Act of 1995
CON	Certificate of Need
CORF	comprehensive outpatient rehabilitation facility
COTA	Certified Occupational Therapist Assistant
CPI	clinical practice improvement
CPR	computerized patient record
CPS	Current Population Survey
CQ	Congressional Quarterly
CQI	continuous quality improvement
CRA	comprehensive rehabilitation agency
CRC	Certified Rehabilitation Counselor
CREATE	Committee on Resources for Electronic Accessible Technology to End- Users
CRRN	Certified Registered Rehabilitation Nurse
CRS	Current Rehabilitation Survey
CTDs	cumulative trauma disorders
CVE	Certified Vocational Evaluator
DHHS	Department of Health & Human Services
DHS	designated health service
DM	disability management
DME	durable medical equipment
DOL	Department of Labor
DRG	Diagnostic Related Group
DSM	disease state management
DSS	decision support system
EAP	employee assistance program
EBC	evidence-based care
EBM	evidence-based medicine
EBP	evidence-based practice
EDI	electronic data interchange
EEOC	Equal Employment Opportunity Commission
EHR	electronic health records
EMR	electronic medical records
EPSDT	early and periodic screening, diagnosis, and treatment
ERISA	Employment Retirement Insurance & Security Act Transfer
FACCT	Foundation for Accountability
FCA	functional capacity assessment
FCE	functional capacity evaluation
FDA	Food & Drug Administration
FFS	fee-for-service reimbursement
FI	fiscal intermediary (Medicare)
FIMs	functional inventory measures
FJA	functional job analysis
FJD	functional job description
FLCTT	Federal Laboratory for Technology
FMLA	The Family Medical Leave Act of 1993
FRGs	functionally related groups
FSM	functional status measure
GAO	Government Accounting Office
GSA	Government Services Administration
HCFA	Health Care Financing Administration

HCPPs	health care prepayment plans (managed Medicare)
HEDIS	health plan employer data information sets
HFMA	Health Financial Management Association
HHA	home health agency
HHC	home health care
HI	health insurance (Part-A Medicare hospital insurance)
HIAA	Health Insurance Association of America
HIPAA	Health Insurance Portability and Accountability Act of 1996
HRQL	Health-Related Quality of Life Measures
IAABC	International Association of Accident Boards & Commissions
IADLs	instrumental activities of daily living
IARP	International Association for Rehabilitation Professionals
ICD	International Classification of Diseases
ICDR	Interagency Committee on Disability Research
ICDS	International Center for the Disabled Survey
ICFs	intermediate care facilities
ICIDH	International Classification of Impairment, Disability & Handicaps
IDM	integrated disability management
IDN	integrated delivery network
IDS	integrated delivery system
IN	Internet
IOM	Institute of Medicine
IP	inpatient
IPA	independent practitioner association
ISNs	integrated service networks
ISP	Internet service providers
IT	information technology
IVR	interactive voice response
JAN	Job Accommodation Network
JCAHO	Joint Commission for the Accreditation of Healthcare Organizations
LIM	lifestyle inventory measures
LLC	limited liability corporation
LOS	length of stay
LTC	long-term care
LTD	long-term disability
MCBS	Medicare Current Beneficiary Survey
MCO	managed care organization
MDS	minimum data sets
MDS	musculoskeletal disorders
MEDPAC	Medicare Payment Advisory Commission
MEDPAR	Medicare Provider analysis and review
MFFS	managed fee-for-service
MIS	managed information systems
MMI	maximum medical improvement
MPFS	Medicare Physician Fee Schedule
MPI	master patient index
MSA	medical savings accounts
MSO	managed services organization
NAHC	National Association of Home Care
NAIC	National Association of Insurance Commissioners
NAMCS	National Ambulatory Medical Care Survey
NARA	National Association for Rehabilitation Agencies
NARIC	National Rehabilitation Information Center

NASL	National Association for the Support of Long-Term Care
NBCH	National Business Coalition on Health
NCCI	National Council on Compensation Insurance
NCDDR	National Center for the Dissemination of Disability Research
NCES	National Center for Education Statistics
NCHES	National Center for Health Education Statistics
NCHS	National Center for Health Statistics
NCMRR	National Center for Medical Rehabilitation Research
NCQA	National Committee for Quality Assurance
NHIS	National Health Interview Survey
NIA	National Institute on Aging
NIDRR	National Institute on Disability & Rehabilitation Research
NIH	National Institutes of Health
NIOSH	National Institute of Occupational Safety & Health
NLM	National Library of Medicine
NLTCS	National Long-term Care Survey
NPDB	National Practitioners Data Bank
NRIC	National Rehabilitation Information Center
NSCA	National Subacute Care Association
NSF	National Science Foundation
OASIS	Outcome Assessments Information Set
OBQI	outcomes-based quality improvement
OIG	Office of Inspector General
OM	outcomes measures
OP	outpatient
ORES	Office of Research, Evaluation & Statistics
ORT	Operation Restore Trust (Medicare)
OSERS	Office of Special Education & Rehabilitation Services
OSHA	Occupational Safety & Health Administration
PACE	program of all-inclusive care for the elderly
PBR	performance-based reimbursement
PCC	patient-centered care
PCEPD	President's Commission on Employment of People with Disabilities
PCN	primary care network
PCP	primary care physician
PECS	patient evaluation and conference system
PEO	professional employment organization
PFC	patient-focused care
PHO	physician-hospital organization
PHP	pre-paid health plan
PIP	personal injury protection
PMPM	per member per month (capitation)
POC	provider of care or plan of care
POS	point-of-service HMO
PPD	permanent partial disability
PPO	preferred provider organization
PPR	pre-payment review
P&Ps	policies and procedures
PPRC	Physician Payment Review Commission (Medicare)
PRO	peer review organization
PSN	provider sponsored network
PSO	provider-sponsored organizations
PSRO	Professional Standards Review Organization
PTA	Physical Therapist Assistant
PTD	permanent total disability
PTIP	physical therapist in independent practice
PVA	Paralyzed Veterans of America
QA	quality assurance
QAUR	quality assurance and utilization review
QHP	qualified (federally) health plans
QOL	quality of life measures
RAI	resident assessment instrument
RAPS	resident assessment protocols
RM	risk management
ROI	return-on-investment
RSA	Rehabilitation Services Administration
RSI	repetitive strain injuries
RTW	return-to-work
RUGS	resource utilization groups
SF-36	Short Form-36 (John Ware)
SIPP	Survey of Income & Program Participation
SIU	special investigation unit
SLMB	specified low-income Medicare beneficiary
SNF	skilled nursing facility
SSA	Social Security Administration
SSDI	Social Security Disability Insurance
SSI	Social Security Insurance
STD	short-term disability
TEFRA	Tax Equity & Fiscal Responsibility Act
TMQC	The Medical Quality Consortium
TPA	third party administrator
TPD	temporary partial disability
TQM	total quality management
TTD	temporary total disability
UCRs	usual-customary-reasonable fees
UDS	Uniform Data Sets
UDSMR	Uniform Data Sets for Medical Rehabilitation
UM	utilization management
UPN	universal product number
UR	utilization review
URAC	Utilization Review Accreditation Commission
VA	Department of Veterans Affairs
VR	vocational rehabilitation
WBGH	Washington Business Group on Health
WC	workers' compensation
WCA	work capacity assessment
WCE	work capacity evaluation
WHO	World Health Organization
WRMSDS	work-related musculoskeletal disorders

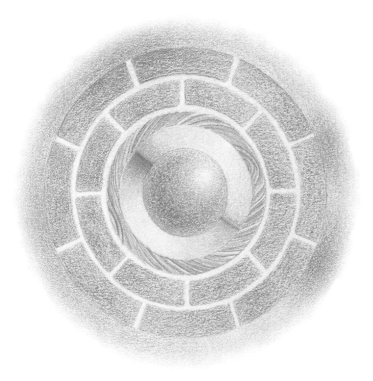

Index

V

W